Chris → 292-5061
Jeremy →

INDUSTRIAL HYGIENE ENGINEERING

INDUSTRIAL HYGIENE ENGINEERING

Recognition, Measurement, Evaluation and Control

Second Edition

Edited by

John T. Talty, P.E.

National Institute for Occupational Safety and Health
Cincinnati, Ohio

Reprint Edition

NOYES DATA CORPORATION
Park Ridge, New Jersey, U.S.A.

Copyright © 1988 by Noyes Data Corporation
Library of Congress Catalog Card Number 88-17863
ISBN: 0-8155-1175-2
Printed in the United States

Published in the United States of America by
Noyes Data Corporation
Mill Road, Park Ridge, New Jersey 07656

10 9 8

Library of Congress Cataloging-in-Publication Data

Industrial hygiene engineering : recognition, measurement, evaluation,
    and control / edited by John T. Talty. -- 2nd ed.
            p. cm.
    Includes bibliographies and index.
    ISBN 0-8155-1175-2 :
    1. Industrial buildings--Environmental engineering. 2. Sanitary
engineering. 3. Industrial hygiene. I. Talty, John T.
TH6057.I53I53   1988
628.5'1--dc19   88-17863
                        CIP

Foreword

This book provides an advanced level of study of industrial hygiene engineering situations. Emphasis is on the *control* of exposure to occupational health hazards. Primary attention is given to industrial ventilation, noise and vibration control, heat stress, and industrial illumination. Other engineering topics covered include industrial water quality, solid waste control, handling and storage of hazardous materials, personal protective equipment, and costs of industrial hygiene control.

The creation of this text came out of an attempt to design a course to teach the fundamentals of industrial hygiene engineering as related to the design of controls for exposure to health hazards in the workplace. During the design of the course, it was necessary to research the field of industrial hygiene. As this research was being conducted, it became evident that no single source provided sufficient coverage of the subject. In fact, control received very little attention in many of the existing texts on industrial hygiene. For the most part, existing texts emphasized recognition, measurement and evaluation of occupational health hazards. Though this is an important concern of the industrial hygiene engineer, the sparse coverage of *control* topics indicated a need for an additional text.

The first objective of this text then, is to provide a single reference source on the subject of industrial hygiene engineering *and* control. The *control* of occupational health hazard exposures requires a broad knowledge of a number of subject areas. To provide a text that includes the necessary theoretical foundation as well as the practical application of the theory is a significant undertaking. It is hoped this objective has been reached and that this text will be a valuable and needed addition to the literature of industrial hygiene.

A second objective was to provide the reader with a systematic approach to problem solving in the field of industrial hygiene. Throughout the text, the systems approach to problem solving is emphasized.

The text has been divided into eight sections, each of which covers a particular subject area. This structure allows for reference to a single topic area without the need to consult other sections of the book.

It should be noted that recommended and mandatory codes and standards change over time. Therefore, when faced with practical problems, the industrial hygiene engineer must consult the latest references to obtain up-to-date requirements of concern.

The information in the book is from *Advanced Industrial Hygiene Engineering,* edited by John T. Talty of the National Institute for Occupational Safety and Health (NIOSH), for NIOSH, June 1986, and is an update of the first edition of *Advanced Industrial Hygiene Engineering* prepared by Bruce B. Byers, Ronald J. Hritz and James C. McClintock for NIOSH.

The table of contents is organized in such a way as to serve as a subject index and provides easy access to the information contained in the book.

Advanced composition and production methods developed by Noyes Data Corporation are employed to bring this durably bound book to you in a minimum of time. Special techniques are used to close the gap between "manuscript" and "completed book." In order to keep the price of the book to a reasonable level, it has been partially reproduced by photo-offset directly from the original report and the cost saving passed on to the reader. Due to this method of publishing, certain portions of the book may be less legible than desired.

ACKNOWLEDGMENTS

This text was developed under the sponsorship of the National Institute for Occupational Safety and Health (NIOSH), Division of Training and Manpower Development, Cincinnati, Ohio. Serving as Project Officer was Robert B. Weidner.

Authors of the first edition of the text were Bruce B. Byers, Ronald J. Hritz, and James C. McClintock. Also assisting as consultants to the development of the material were Ralph J. Vernon and Richard B. Konzen of the Department of Industrial Engineering, Texas A&M University. Art work for the first edition was prepared by Carole D. Byers; manuscript preparation was the responsibility of Elaine S. Holmes.

Based on NIOSH technical review of the first edition, the document was revised and edited. This was done under the editorial direction of John T. Talty. Technical assistance was provided by William F. Martin, Glenda M. White and John M. Yacher. Layout and proofreading assistance for the second edition was provided by Pauline J. Elliott. Wapora, Inc. provided contractual assistance in word processing and graphics.

NOTICE

Contents and Subject Index

SECTION 1
INTRODUCTION TO INDUSTRIAL HYGIENE ENGINEERING AND CONTROL

1. RECOGNITION OF HEALTH HAZARDS. 2
   Introduction. 2
   An Easy Way to Recognize Hazards 3
   The Classification of Hazards. 5
   Methods That Can be Used to Recognize Hazards 7
      Accident or Injury Reports. 7
      Physical Examinations 7
      Employee Nofifications 7
      Required Inspections 7
      Literature and Discussions with Other Professionals. 8
      Walk-Through Inspections. 8
      Sampling and Spot Inspections. 8
      Preliminary Hazard Analysis 8
      Review of Process Flows. 8
      Fault-Tree Analysis 9
      Critical Incident Technique. 9
      Failure Mode and Effect. 9
      Job Safety Analysis. 9
   Summary. 9

2. METHODS FOR MEASURING AND EVALUATING HEALTH HAZARDS 11
   A Suggested Analysis Study Outline 12
      Recognition of Hazards 12
         Walk-Through Survey. 12
         Preliminary Hazard Recognition. 12
      Hazard Assessment Study Design 15
         Preliminary Hazard Assessment 15
         Hazard Assessment Study 17
   Summary. 22
   Case Study. 22
      Introduction. 22
      General Description. 22

3. HUMAN SYSTEMS. 36
   Introduction. 36
   The Study of Human Systems 37
   The Basic Unit of Life—The Cell. 39
   The Structure of the Body—The Skeleton. 41
   The Moving Force—The Muscles. 44
   The Control System—The Nervous System 46
   Fuel Processing—The Digestive System. 47
   The Distribution System—The Circulatory System 48
   The Combustion Fuel Supply System—The Respiratory System 50
   The Filtering System—The Renal System 51
   The Defense Systems—Skin and Sense Organs 51
   Other Systems—Reproductive and Chemical Control 52
   Summary. 53

4. INDUSTRIAL TOXICOLOGY. 54
   Introduction. 54
   Toxicology. 55
   Exposure Routes of Toxic Materials and Protective Mechanisms That Exist 57
   The Physiological Classification of Toxic Materials in Air 59
      Irritants. 59
      Asphyxiants. 59
      Anesthetics 59
      Hepatotoxic Agents. 59
      Nephrotoxic Agents. 59
      Neurotoxic Agents. 59
      Blood Damaging Agents 59
      Lung Damaging Agents. 60
   The Physical Classification of Toxic Materials. 60
   Summary. 61

5. PHYSICAL HAZARDS 62
   Introduction. 62
   Physical Hazards—Noise 63
   Physical Hazards—Vibration. 64
   Physical Hazards—Ionizing and Nonionizing Radiation 64
   Physical Hazards—Thermal 65
   Physical Hazards—Mechanical. 66
   Physical Hazards—Pressure. 67
   Physical Hazards—Illumination. 67
   Physical Hazards—Traumatic 68
   Other Hazards—Biological 68
   Other Hazards—Psychological. 69
   Summary. 69

6. GENERAL METHODS OF CONTROL AVAILABLE TO THE INDUSTRIAL
   HYGIENE ENGINEER 70
   Introduction. 70
   General Methods of Control—Substitution 71
   General Methods of Control—Isolation of Source. 72
   General Methods of Control—Ventilation. 73
   General Methods of Control—Administrative. 74
   General Methods of Control—Personal Protective Equipment. 75
   Determining the Control Method to Use 76

Summary. 77

7. LEGAL ASPECTS OF OCCUPATIONAL SAFETY AND HEALTH 79
  Introduction. 79
  OSHA—Prescribed Duties 80
  Inspections. 80
  Citations 81
  Recordkeeping: Posting of Periodic Reports 81
  Penalties 81
  Contest of Citations and Penalties. 82
  Variances. 82

8. REFERENCES. 84

SECTION 2
INDUSTRIAL VENTILATION

1. CHARACTERISTICS OF AIR. 88
  Pressure. 88
  Heat Intensity—Temperature. 89
  Heat Quantity. 91
  Perfect Gas Law 93
  Application of the Gas Laws 94
  The Effect of Moisture in Air. 97
  Relative Humidity. 100
  Summary. 102

2. PROPERTIES OF AIRBORNE CONTAMINANTS 103
  Properties of Gases and Vapors 103
    Toxic Properties of Gases or Vapors 104
    Combustibility 105
    Motion of Gases and Vapor 107
  Properties of Particulate Matter 108
    Dust 108
    Fumes. 109
    Smoke. 109
    Mists. 110
    Particulate Size. 110
    Toxicity of Particulate Matter 111
    The Motion of Particulate Matter 111
    Dust That Is Projected 113
    Brownian Motion 113
  Causes of Initial Dispersion of Particulates in the Air 113
    Thermal Convection. 114
  Summary. 114

3. PRINCIPLES OF AIR MOVEMENT. 115
  General Concepts of Ventilation. 115
  Components of a Ventilation System 116
  Pressure in a Ventilation System. 117
  Measurement of Pressures in a Ventilation System 120
    Manometer. 120
    Inclined Manometer. 121
    The Impact Tube. 121

The Pitot Tube 122
Flow in a Ventilation System 122
How Air Flows in a Ventilation System 123
The Effect of Friction on Air Flow 124
The Effect of Changes in Duct Diameter 129
The Effect of Changes in Direction of Airflow 130
Summary 134

4. DILUTION VENTILATION 135
Principles of Dilution Ventilation 135
Components of a Dilution Ventilation System 137
Contamination Generation 138
Purging of a Concentration Buildup 139
Maintaining a Steady State Concentration 140
Determination of the Safety Factor (K) 144
Substitution of Materials 144
Dilution Ventilation for Mixtures 145
Dilution Ventilation for Fire and Explosion Control 146
Thermal Ventilation for Dilution 148
General Rules for Application of Dilution Ventilation 149
Problems Related to the Use of Dilution Ventilation 150
Summary 150

5. LOCAL EXHAUST VENTILATION 152
Components of a Local Exhaust System 152
Blow Versus Exhaust 153
Rate of Flow in a Hood 155
The Application and Advantage of Local Exhaust Ventilation 155
General Categories of Local Exhaust Ventilation Hoods 156
Enclosing Hoods—Total Enclosures 156
Enclosing Hoods—Booths and Tunnels 157
Rate of Flow for Enclosing Hoods 158
Exterior Hoods 158
Summary 161

6. MAKE-UP AIR 162
General Principles of Make-Up Air 162
Volume Requirements 162
Location 163
Conditioning of the Air 163
Signs of Inadequate Make-Up Air 163
Components of a Make-Up Air System 164
Methods of Tempering the Air 164
Steam Coil 165
Direct-Fired Heaters 166
Indirect-Fired Heaters 166
Recirculated Air 167
Heat Recovery 167
Determining the Amount and Cost of Tempering the Required Make-Up Air 169

7. DESIGN OF EXHAUST HOODS 171
Determination of Capture or Control Velocity 172
Capture Velocity for an Exterior Hood 172
Limitations of Theoretical Model 175

Experimental Determination of Contours. 176
Efficiency of Exhaust Hoods. 177
   Coefficient of Entry—C_e. 179
   Hood Entry Loss—h_e. 180
   Hood Design Relationships 181
Hood Design. 183
Hood Design Procedure 185
Summary. 187

8. PRINCIPLES OF AIR CLEANING. 188
   The Reasons for Cleaning Air. 188
      Remove Hazardous Contaminants. 188
      Remove Nuisance Contaminants. 188
      Protect Air-Moving Equipment. 188
      Recover Valuable Materials. 189
      Enable Recirculation 189
      Meet Environmental Requirements. 189
   Factors Affecting Air Cleaning. 190
      The Type of Contaminant. 190
      The Volume of Air Handled 190
      The Degree of Collection Required. 190
      The Toxicity of the Contaminant. 191
      Radioactivity of the Contaminant. 191
      Temperature and Humidity. 191
      The Presence of Corrosive Contaminant Material. 191
      The Presence of Abrasive Particulates 191
      Disposal of the Collected Contaminant 191
      Flammability of the Carrier Gas or the Contaminant 191
      Chemical Reactions. 192
      Pressure Losses. 192
      The Integrity of the Air Cleaner. 192
      Variations in Contaminant Loading. 192
      The Cycle for Cleaning. 192
      The Cost of Cleaning the Air 192
      The Efficiency of the Air Cleaner. 193
   Characteristics of the Contaminant. 193
   General Methods of Air Cleaning 194
      Gravitational Force 194
      Centrifugal Force 194
      Inertial Impaction 195
      Direct Interception 196
      Diffusion. 196
      Electrostatic Precipitation. 196
      Adsorption. 197
      Absorption. 197
      Incineration. 197
      Catalytic Combustion. 197
   Summary. 197

9. AIR-CLEANING DEVICES. 198
   Air Cleaners for Particulate Contaminants—Mechanical Separators 198
      Gravity Settling Chamber 198
      Cyclone Cleaners. 200
      Impingement or Impaction Devices. 201

Dynamic Collectors. 202
Air Cleaners for Particulate Contaminants—Filters. 203
Deep-Bed or Mat Filters 203
Fabric Filters—Bag Houses. 203
High-Efficiency Panel Filters 204
Air Cleaning for Particulate Contaminants—Wet Collectors 205
Chamber Scrubbers—Spray Towers. 206
Cyclonic Scrubbers (Wet Cyclones). 206
Self-Induced Spray Scrubbers 206
Wet Impingement Scrubbers 207
Venturi Scrubber. 207
Mechanical Scrubbers. 208
Air Cleaning for Particulates—Electrostatic Precipitators. 208
Air Cleaning for Gases—Absorption. 209
Recirculating Adsorbing Systems 210
One-Pass Nonregenerative Systems 210
One-Pass Regenerative Systems 210
Air Cleaning for Gases—Absorption. 210
Air Cleaning for Gases—Incinerators 211
Air Cleaning for Gases—Catalytic Combustion (Oxidation) 212
Summary. 212

10. AIR-MOVING DEVICES 215
Terminology Relating to Fan Operation. 215
Fan Laws. 220
Fan Curves. 221
Correcting for Nonstandard Conditions 223
Categories of Fans. 225
Types of Axial Fans. 226
The Propeller Fan 226
Tube-Axial Fans 226
Vane-Axial Fan. 226
Types of Centrifugal Fans. 226
Selecting and Installing a Fan. 227
Type of Fan to Use 227
The Type of Drive Mechanism. 228
The Direction of Rotation of the Fan 228
Duct Connections 228
Fan Installation. 229
Other Factors to be Considered in Installation 229
Changing the Rate of Flow of the Fan. 229
Injectors 229
Summary. 230

11. DESIGN OF DUCTS 231
Components of a Duct System. 231
Straight Duct 231
Expansions and Contractions. 235
Elbows 236
Branch Connections. 238
Other Components of a Duct System 239
Dampers 239
Equalizer. 239
Switch. 239

Slip Joints 240
Cleanouts. 240
Weather Cap or Stackhead. 240
Supports 240
Transitions. 241
Summary. 242

12. PRINCIPLES OF SYSTEM DESIGN. 242
The Effect of Branches in a Ventilation System. 246
Sizing the Duct. 248
Determining the SP_f. 249
The Calculation Worksheet 254
Some Final Comments on the Principles of System Design 258
Velocity Pressure Method of Calculation 262
Summary. 262

13. VENTILATION SYSTEM DESIGN 264
Introduction. 264
A Design Procedure for Ventilation Systems. 264
Types of Ventilation System Design 267
Balanced-System Design. 267
Blast-Gate Design 267
Plenum Design 267
Advantages and Disadvantages of the Three Methods of Design 268
Other Design Considerations 270
Transport Velocity 270
Fire and Explosion Hazards. 270
Make-Up Air. 271
Maintenance. 271
Noise 271
Summary. 272

14. RECIRCULATION OF EXHAUST AIR 273
Problems Relating to Recirculation. 273
Obtaining Clean Air to Be Recirculated 274
Necessity to Monitor Incoming Recirculated Air. 275
Contaminants Not to Be Recirculated 275
An Approach to Recirculation. 275
Some General Considerations in Designing a Recirculation System 276
Other Alternatives to Conserve Energy Usage 278
Summary. 280

15. CORRECTING FOR NONSTANDARD CONDITIONS 281
Standard Versus Nonstandard Conditions. 281
Need for Correction. 281
Summary. 288

16. THERMAL VENTILATION EFFECTS 289
General Principles of Air Motion About a Hot Process 289
Draft Pressure. 289
Velocity of Air in a Heated Column 289
Formula for Rate of Flow of Hot-Air Column. 290
Convectional Heat Loss Formula 291
Control of Contaminants from Processes—The Low Canopy Hood 292

Control of Contaminants from Hot Processes—High Canopy Hood 296
Enclosures for Hot Processes 297
Natural Ventilation in Buildings 298
Summary 299

17. TESTING PROCEDURES IN THE PLANT 300
Reasons for Ventilation System Tests 300
Types of Ventilation System Tests 301
The Location and Purpose of Ventilation System Tests. 302
Testing Local Exhaust Systems 302
Determining the Static Pressure of the System 302
Determining Velocity Pressure—The Pitot Tube. 304
Determining Velocity Pressure—Other Instruments 308
Testing Dilution or Make-Up Air Systems. 310
Other Methods Available for Testing Ventilation Systems 312
Determining Where Problems Exist. 313
Summary 314

18. ENVIRONMENTAL AIR POLLUTION. 315
Beyond the Plant. 315
The Effects of Air Pollution 315
Determining the Extent of Air Pollution—Measuring the Ambient Air 316
Determining the Extent of Pollution—Measuring at the Source. 318
Control of Environmental Air Pollution. 320
Cleaners for Particulate Matter. 320
Cleaners for Gases and Vapors 320
Weather Considerations for Pollution Control 320
Summary 321

19. REFERENCES 323

SECTION 3
THERMAL STRESS

1. HEAT EXCHANGE AND ITS EFFECTS ON MAN 326
Heat Exchange 326
Methods of Heat Exchange 328
Sources of Heat. 330
Physiological Responses to Extreme Temperatures. 330
Stress and Strain. 331
Indicators of Thermal Strain 331
Factors in Heat Stress. 334
Age. 334
Acclimatization. 334
Other Effects of Heat Stress 335
Summary 335

2. THERMAL MEASUREMENT 336
Introduction. 336
Measurement of Air Temperature. 336
Measurement of Radiant Heat 338
Measurement of Air Velocity. 339
Measurement of Humidity. 340
The Psychrometric Chart 342

Equipment for Measuring Humidity 342
Summary. 344

3. THERMAL STRESS INDICES. 345
Introduction. 345
Effective Temperature 346
Heat-Stress Index 349
The Predicted Four-Hour Sweat Rate 354
The Wet-Bulb Globe Temperature Index 354
The ACGIH Guide for Assessing Heat Stress. 356
The Wind-Chill Index. 358
Summary. 358

4. METHODS FOR CONTROLLING THERMAL EXPOSURES 360
Introduction. 360
General Administrative Methods for Reducing Heat Stress. 360
Decreasing the Work Required. 360
Modifying the Worker's Exposure to Heat Stress 361
Screening of Workers. 361
Education and Training of Workers. 362
Acclimatization of Workers. 362
Other Administrative Controls. 362
Modifying the Thermal Environment for Radiant Heat. 363
Lower the Radiant Heat Level 363
Shielding for Control of Radiant Heat. 364
Personal Protective Equipment. 364
Modifying the Thermal Environment for Convective Heat. 365
General Dilution Ventilation 365
Removing Heat from the Air 366
Protection from Climatic Conditions. 366
Modifying the Environment for Moisture. 366
Modifying the Environment for Cold. 367
Personal Protective Clothing 367
Summary. 368

5. REFERENCES 369

SECTION 4
SOUND

1. PHYSICS OF SOUND 372
Introduction. 372
What is Sound?. 372
An Example of Sound 372
Sound Wave. 373
Velocity of Sound. 375
Frequency of Sound 375
Wavelength. 376
Summary. 377
Sound Pressure 378
Sound Power 380
Sound Intensity 382
Relationship Between Sound Power and Sound Pressure. 386
Summary. 387

2. PHYSICS OF SOUND 390
   Introduction. 390
   Complex Sound 390
   Frequency Bands. 393
   Decibels. 395
   Adding and Subtracting Decibels 401
   The Relationship Between Sound-Power Level and Sound-Pressure Level. 402
   Correction for Atmospheric Conditions. 404
   Correction for the Directivity of a Sound Source. 405
   Summary. 408

3. PHYSICS OF SOUND 410
   Introduction. 410
   Sound in a Room 410
   Absorption. 413
   Room Constant. 415
   Room Constant and Sound Pressure 416
   Critical Distance 419
   Sound in an Adjoining Room. 425
   Transmission Loss of Combined Materials 427
   Secondary Room. 430
   Summary. 433

4. THE EAR AND THE EFFECTS OF SOUND 438
   Introduction. 438
   The Threshold of Hearing 438
   Hearing Loss and Age. 440
   Other Causes of Hearing Loss. 440
   Other Effects of Noise 441
   Sound (Noise) Level, dBA. 448
   Extra-Auditory Effects. 452
   Damage-Risk Criteria 452
   Summary. 453

5. VIBRATION 455
   Introduction. 455
   Definition of Vibration. 455
   Periodic Vibration. 455
   When to Use What. 458
   Resonance 459
   Vibration Measurement 459
   The Effects of Vibration. 461
      Raynaud's Syndrome. 462
   Control of Vibration 462
   Summary. 469

6. NOISE CONTROL 470
   Introduction. 470
   Does Noise Control Pay?. 470
   Basics of Noise Control. 471
   Plant Planning. 471
   A Simple Example of a New Plant Noise Prediction 471
   New Plant Planning and Substitution of Equipment—Some General Rules 472
   Controlling Noise in an Existing Facility 473

Controlling Noise at the Source 473
Mufflers. 477
Controlling Noise Along Its Path 478
Enclosures. 479
Additional Notes About Total Enclosures 482
Enclosures Inside a Noisy Work Area. 483
Partial Enclosures 486
Shields and Barriers. 486
Controlling Noise Along Its Path Using Room Absorption. 488
Noise Control at the Receiver 490

7. **REFERENCES**. 492

SECTION 5
INDUSTRIAL ILLUMINATION

1. **LIGHT** 494
Introduction. 494
What Is Light? 494
Electromagnetic Spectrum 502
The Quantum Theory. 503
The Emission Spectra. 505
Incandescence. 505
Fluorescence and Fluorescent Lamps 506
Comparing Different Light Sources. 507

2. **LIGHT AND SEEING/DESIGN OF A LIGHTING SYSTEM** 509
Behavior of Light 509
The Human Eye 512
Variables in the Seeing Process. 514
Terminology Used in the Science of Light 516
Luminous Flux (F) 516
Luminous Intensity 518
Illumination. 519
Luminance. 519
Reflectance 520
The Measurement of Light 520
Foot-Candle Measurements. 522
Light Survey Procedures. 523
Evaluation of Results. . . . .

3. **LIGHTING DESIGN** 524
Introduction. 524
Quantity of Light 524
Quality of Light 526
Glare. 526
Luminaire Classification 531
Indirect Lighting. 531
Semi-Indirect Lighting. 531
General Diffuse or Indirect Lighting and Direct-Indirect Lighting. 531
Semi-Direct Lighting 532
Supplementary Lighting. 532
Lighting Systems or Illumination Methods 533
General Lighting. 533

    Localized General Lighting 534
    Supplementary Lighting. 534
  Other Factors to Consider When Designing a Lighting System 534
  Lumen Method of Lighting Design 536
    Introduction. 536
    The Formula 537
    Coefficient of Utilization 538
    The Light Loss Factor 554
    Summary of Steps Involved in Computing Lumen Method 559

4. **REFERENCES**. 561

SECTION 6
RADIATION

1. **PRINCIPLES OF NONIONIZING RADIATION** 564
  Introduction. 564
  Radiation—Overview 564
    Units of Measure. 565
  Nonionizing Radiation—General. 567
  Nonionizing Radiation—Specific Regions. 568
    Ultraviolet Region. 568
    Exposure Criteria 573
  Visible Light. 575
  Infrared Radiation. 575
    Threshold Limit Values 577
  Radio Frequencies. 578
  Microwaves 582
    Biological Effects 585
    Threshold Limit Values 585
  Lasers 587
    Biological Effects 591
    Threshold Limit Values 591
  Summary. 597

2. **CONTROL OF NONIONIZING RADIATION** 598
  Ultraviolet Radiation. 598
    Personnel Protection 602
    Shielding. 602
  Lasers. 608
    Medical Surveillance. 614
  Microwaves 615
    Hazard Control. 618
  Summary. 620

3. **PRINCIPLES OF IONIZING RADIATION** 621
  Atomic Structure 621
  Radioactivity 621
    Alpha Particles 623
    Beta Particles 624
    Gamma Radiation. 626
    X-Radiation. 629
    Neutrons. 630
  Units of Measure. 631

Units of Energy. 631
Units of Activity. 631
Exposure. 631
Absorbed Dose. 633
Dose Equivalent 635
Fluence. 635
Flux Density 635
Biological Effects of Ionizing Radiation. 635
Industrial Uses of Ionizing Radiation. 636
Radiation Gauges 637
Radiography and Fluoroscopy. 639
X-Ray Diffraction and Fluorescent Analysis. 639
Electron-Beam Equipment 640
Activation Analysis 641
Radioactive Tracers. 641
Aerosol Fire Detectors. 642
Luminescent Dials. 642
Large Radiation Sources. 643
Agricultural Uses. 643
Medical Uses. 645
Hazards. 645
Maximum Permissible Dose. 647
Summary. 648

4. INSTRUMENTATION. 648
Introduction. 649
Instrumentation 649
Ionization Chamber Instruments 650
Proportional Counter Instruments 651
Geiger-Mueller (G-M) Counter 653
Scintillation Detector. 654
Photographic Devices. 656
Solid-State and Activation Devices 657
Personnel Monitoring Devices 657
Film Badges 658
Pocket Dosimeter 658
Pocket Chamber 658
Choice and Use of Instruments. 659

5. CONTROL OF IONIZING RADIATION 659
Identification of Radiation Safety Problems. 660
Authorization for Radionuclide Use 662
Protection from Radiation Hazard 662
Time. 663
Distance 664
Shielding. 665
Gamma Radiation Shielding 676
X-Radiation Shielding 682
Survey and Monitoring Procedures for Radiation Hazards 684
Personnel Monitoring. 685
Facilities 687
Posting the Area 688
Trays and Handling Tools 688
Storage and Disposal of Radionuclides. 688

Personnel. 692
Radiation Accidents. 695
Emergency Instructions in the Event of Release of Radioactivity and
  Contamination of Personnel 695
  Objectives of Remedial Action. 695
  Procedures for Dealing with Minor Spills and Contamination. 696
  Personnel Decontamination. 696
  Reporting Radiation Accidents 697
Responsibilities of the Industrial Hygiene Engineer 697
Summary. 698

6. REFERENCES. 699

SECTION 7
ERGONOMICS

1. INTRODUCTION TO ERGONOMICS. 702
What Is Ergonomics? 702
The Man/Machine System 705
The Systems Approach. 706
  Function and Task Analysis. 707
  Procedure for Conducting a Functional and Task Analysis. 710
Summary. 711

2. THE WORKER AS THE PHYSICAL COMPONENT 712
Introduction. 712
The Average Man. 712
Using Anthropometrical Data 714
  Structural Anthropometry 714
  Functional Anthropometry. 715
Biomechanics. 719
  Classification of Body Movements 721
Factors Affecting the Performance of Physical Tasks 725
  Range of Movement. 726
  Strength 726
  Endurance. 727
  Speed 728
  Accuracy. 728
Summary. 729

3. THE WORKER AS THE CONTROLLING COMPONENT. 730
Introduction. 730
The Worker As a Sensor—Visual. 731
  Visual Discrimination. 731
The Worker As a Sensor—Auditory. 733
The Worker As a Sensor—Tactual. 734
Displays. 734
Qualitative Visual Displays 737
  Status Indicators. 737
  Auditory Range Displays 738
  Tactual Display. 738
Choosing the Type of Stimulus 739
Grouping of Visual Displays 740
Summary. 740

4. DESIGN OF THE JOB. 741
   The Worker's Function in the Workplace 741
      The Job Functions. 741
   A General Procedure for Determining Where Controls for Hazard Exposures
   Are Required. 742
   The Data Gathering Function 743
   Processing Information. 745
   Controlling the System. 746
      The Recommended Direction of Control Movements 748
   General Control Design Principles. 748
   Physical Requirements—Material Handling 750
   Summary. 751

5. DESIGN OF THE WORKPLACE 752
   General Work Station Design Principles 752
   Design for Visibility and Hearing 753
   Design for Worker Operations 754
      Provision for Equipment in the Workplace 755
      Standard Design 756
      Provide Adequate Storage. 756
   Workplace Space Considerations. 756
   The Design of the Plant Equipment Layout 758
      Use of Color Coding in the Plant 759
   Traffic Spaces. 759
      Aisles and Corridors. 759
      Exits and Entrances. 760
   Ladders, Stairs, and Ramps 762
   Summary. 763

6. REFERENCES 765

SECTION 8
OTHER TOPICS

1. CONTROL OF INDUSTRIAL WATER QUALITY 768
   Introduction. 768
   Water Treatment. 770
      Sedimentation 770
      Control of pH. 771
      Coagulation and Flocculation 771
      Filtration. 772
      Bacterial Digestion. 773
      Control of Disease-Causing Organisms 773
      Aeration 774
      Removal of Waste Sludge 774
      Other Water Treatment. 774
   Thermal Pollution. 775
   Cross Connection of Water Sources. 776
   Control of Hazardous Materials in Water Treatment. 777
   Summary. 779

2. CONTROL OF SOLID WASTE 780
   Introduction. 780
   The Objectives of a Solid Waste Disposal Program 780

The Sources of Industrial Waste 781
   Raw Material Extraction. 781
   Process Industries 782
   Manufacturing and Assembly. 782
   Packaging. 783
   Consumer Use. 783
The Solid Waste Disposal Methods 783
   Sanitary Landfill. 783
   Incineration. 784
   Recycling. 785
   Grinding-Compaction. 785
Meeting the Objectives of a Solid Waste Disposal Program 786
Summary. 788

3. PURCHASE, HANDLING, AND STORAGE OF HAZARDOUS MATERIALS 789
   Introduction. 789
   Areas for Control of Hazardous Materials. 790
   The Purchase of Hazardous Materials. 791
   Information Required for Potentially Hazardous Materials 793
   A Suggested Data Base for Hazardous Materials. 794
      Computerization of Data Base. 796
   Handling of Hazardous Materials 797
      Some Basic Rules for Handling of Hazardous Materials. 798
   Storage of Hazardous Materials 799
   Summary. 799

4. PERSONAL PROTECTIVE EQUIPMENT 800
   Introduction. 800
   Personal Protective Equipment As a Control. 801
   Protection from Respirable Hazards 801
      The Air-Purifying Respirator 802
      Cartridge Type Respirators 804
      Mechanical Filter Type Respirator 805
      Air-Supplied Respirators. 805
      The Self-Contained Breathing Unit 807
   Precautions That Should Be Taken When Using Respirators. 808
   Other Personal Protective Equipment 809
   Summary. 810

5. COSTS OF INDUSTRIAL HYGIENE CONTROL 812
   Introduction. 812
   Economic Cost of Not Providing Controls 813
      Workers' Compensation 813
      Disability Insurance. 814
      Legal Costs. 814
      Replacing Lost Employees 815
      Medical Insurance 815
      Availability of Labor Pool. 815
      Production Losses. 815
      Public Relations 815
      Social Costs 815
   The Assessment of Risk 815
   The Economic Cost of Providing Industrial Hygiene Controls. 816
      Equipment Costs. 817

Effects on Production 817
Costs of Control Operation 817
Cost of Training 817
Equipment Life. 817
Other Related Costs. 817
Selecting a Control Method 818
Identify the Exposure 818
Choosing Alternatives. 818
Predicting Results 819
Evaluation of Alternatives. 819
Summary 820

6. BASIC ECONOMIC ANALYSIS 821
Introduction 821
The N-Year Payback 822
Economic Analysis Using the Present Worth Approach 824
Effects of Taxes on Economic Analysis 828
Summary 830

7. REFERENCES 831

Section 1

Introduction to Industrial Hygiene Engineering and Control

1. Recognition of Health Hazards

<u>Introduction</u>

The workplace is a potentially hazardous environment. This fact has been recognized for a long time. With the increased interest in protection of the environment, both internal and external to the plant, the number of alleged threats to man's health and safety, both as a worker and as a resident of an industrial neighborhood, have multiplied. Hardly a day goes by when one does not open a newspaper and find some new threat to human health and safety that originates within the industrial complex. And with the introduction of new technology occurring as quickly as it does, one should not expect that this situation will improve. Who knows what new chemical will be introduced tomorrow that has long-range, serious, chronic effects upon those who come in contact with it, either as workers or consumers. The governmental order concerning "red dye" is an example of a material that was widely used that has been recognized as a potential health hazard.

For every claim concerning the existence of a hazard, there also exist those individuals who are willing to stake their reputations that such a hazard does not exist. As an example, consider the turmoil created by the ban of cyclamates and the existence of some experimental results that would seem to indicate that this ban may have been hastily made and ill conceived. Similar situations exist in the area of the use of nuclear power as an alternative to oil and coal, and the limitations on the use of DDT as a pesticide. One can quickly see that the issues are not always clear cut and the problems are not necessarily well defined. It is in this tumultuous climate that the industrial hygiene engineer must operate. Perhaps no better reason exists than that presented above for the need for an industrial hygiene engineer to remain objective and systematic in the recognition, evaluation and control of occupational hazards. The true professional must operate as much as possible in the realm of facts. There is no room for emotionalism when considering problems with the potential impact of those in areas such as occupational safety and health.

The occupational aspects of the total field of environmental health may be considered industrial hygiene, which has been defined by the American Industrial Hygiene Association as "the science and art devoted to the recognition, evaluation, and control of those environmental factors and stresses, arising in or from the workplace, which may cause sickness, impaired health and well-being, or significant discomfort and inefficiency among workers along with citizens of the community."

Some of the classical communicable diseases have been shown to have a specific agent which gives rise to a specific disease. This is very seldom

2

the case with occupationally-caused diseases as the etiology is often quite complex. Many times the situation is such that there are multiple chemical and physical caused factors. Although an infectious agent may have a pathognomonic (disease-specifying) characteristic, there may be no apparent unique relationship to the stressing agent when chronic exposures to chemical or physical factors are involved.

There is usually a short and fairly definite period of time between invasion of the host and the development of the disease with diseases that are caused by living microorganisms. In contrast to such short incubation periods, occupational diseases, in most instances, usually require long periods to develop the observable effects as a result of exposures to physical and chemical agents. These are exceptions, however.

The objective of industrial hygiene has been primarily to reduce the incidence and mortality of occupational disease. It is now being called upon to improve the effective quality as well as the length of life. Inasmuch as occupational diseases arise from multiple factors having a complex etiology, evaluation is often difficult and, as a consequence, environmental control measures evolve slowly.

Many biological agents are important in the field of occupational health. However, in the overall picture, they are not of as major concern in the area of industrial hygiene as are the various chemical and physical agents. The qualities of these contaminants which are of importance in assessing the effect of the harmful agents to the industrial hygiene engineer are: concentration, level, type of matter and energy, and the length of time that a potentially harmful agent has in which to act on susceptible tissues (of prime importance).

Although this text is directed specifically to industrial hygiene engineering and control, it is necessary to discuss at least briefly the area of recognition and evaluation. It has often been said that recognizing and defining the problem is more than one-half of the job. Obviously, it is very difficult to establish controls for a problem when, in fact, the problem is not recognized and its extent is not known. The first three chapters of this text will emphasize the recognition and evaluation of potential hazards within the industrial environment. Of major concern will be the structuring of procedures for recognizing and evaluating industrial hazards. Little emphasis will be placed on specific equipment that is used. This information can be found elsewhere. The major objective of this material is to provide a logical and systematic method which will enable the user to evaluate objectively the problems as they are recognized. With this as a basis, the industrial hygiene engineer can begin to develop methods for control. This is not to say that the industrial hygiene engineer through the use of such an orderly method can solve all the problems concerning the existence or nonexistence of a particular health hazard. However, by using such a logical approach and by remaining objective, the industrial hygiene engineer may be able to act as a stabilizing influence.

An Easy Way to Recognize Hazards

There is no easy way to recognize hazards. We are constantly looking for an easy way out, but in this case we will look in vain. Many methods have been developed that purport to identify hazards. Each of these methods has its advantages and works, but none is easy to implement. Many of the methods that have been developed will be further discussed later in this chapter.

If there is only one general method that is best used to recognize potential hazards in the work environment, it is that of the experience of the observer. If you can remember the first time you walked into an industrial plant operation and looked around, you probably remember the feeling of awe that you experienced. And if you were to be responsible for understanding the operation, you probably felt frustrated with the seemingly impossible scope of the task. If you can reconstruct your feeling when walking into the same industrial plant six months or so later, you can remember that the feeling of helplessness was no longer present. When you looked at the operation, you saw things that you never saw before. The man operating the punch press is not keeping up with the rest of the production. There is a strange noise emanating from one of the grinders that seems to indicate that some major repair will be required. Now it's easy to recognize problems. Your powers of observation are sharpened through a better understanding of what is going on and what is supposed to go on. Thus, experience has become an easy way to recognize potential problems.

However, experience is not the only answer. One can have two kinds of work experience. One can work on a job and have the same experience over and over again; or one can work and have a series of new experiences, each one adding to the knowledge and skill of the individual. It is obvious that the latter is the more desirable type of experience to gain. But, in approaching a new problem, one does not always have the benefit of experience to rely on. Certainly many of the problems that were faced in the past have application to the new problem that is currently being faced; however, this has its limitations. You must investigate the problem in some logical manner and attempt to gather data and form conclusions as a result of your investigation.

The above is especially true in the area of health and safety hazards. When the industrial hygiene engineer is walking through a plant and observing the work being performed, the hazards are readily apparent. Depending on his or her experience, certain hazards will be evident. However, many of the problems will be hidden from view. For example, potential health hazards that might exist as a result of the use of a certain chemical compound in the process may not be evident unless the observer has an intimate knowledge of the process and the various chemical reactions that occur. These hazards cannot be noted just by watching the process. The industrial hygiene engineer must review the chemical process flow sheets and use experience as well as the experience of others to determine if a potential hazard is present. Once it is determined that a potential hazard exists, the industrial hygiene engineer must then ascertain the extent of the hazard. When making this determination, the industrial hygiene engineer must also consider what other hazards may be present and if too much time is being spent on a particular potential hazard. Other hazards that may be present may go undetected and uncontrolled. Good judgment is then necessary to determine what potential hazards should be investigated in what order and which of the potential hazards present a real hazard that must be controlled within the workplace.

In summary, the industrial hygiene engineer does not have an easy job to recognize potential hazards in the industrial environment. If there is one thing that more than any other will enable the industrial hygiene engineer to do a good job in recognizing potential hazards, it is experience. However, this experience is not all that is required. The industrial hygiene engineer must remain objective and organized in the approach to assure that experience does not lead to unwarranted conclusions concerning a new problem that is faced.

The Classification of Hazards

Hazards encountered in the work environment may be classified using any one of a number of systems. No one classification system is better than another. In addition, within the varying classification systems, the level of specificity may be different. Classification of hazards can provide a framework that can be of assistance to the industrial hygiene engineer in recognizing potential hazards in the workplace. It can also provide a basis for evaluation of the extent of the seriousness of the hazard present.

Perhaps one of the more obvious types of classifications of hazards is the type of hazard involved; i.e., either a health hazard or a safety hazard. Quite often this classification rule is used to define the difference in duties between the industrial hygienist and the safety professional within a given organization. However, the system is imperfect. It is not always easy to classify a hazard as being a health hazard or a safety hazard. For example, consider an area where a 95 dBA noise level is present. Is this a health hazard or is it a hazard to the worker's safety? Certainly, it is probable that long-term damage to the worker's hearing will be realized at this noise level, and thus it can be considered a health hazard. But it is also a fact that because of the high noise level it will be difficult to communicate; and because of this difficulty, the workers may become psychologically distressed, thus becoming subjected to potential traumatic injury. If the problem is looked at in this manner, the noise becomes a hazard to the worker's safety. As is evident, it is not always easy to define clearly the difference between the two classifications. Many of the problems that exist in defining the duties of an industrial hygienist or safety professional are encountered because of the overlap that is encountered when trying to distinguish between a health hazard and a safety hazard. The field of industrial hygiene deals mainly with health hazards.

Another classification system that can be helpful when attempting to determine the priority of solution for a given hazard is considering the hazard by its level of effect to the human system.

Three possible categories within such a classification system are as follows:

A.   Low--annoyance and possible harmful effect.

B.   Medium--dangerous to the health of humans.

C.   High--cause death or severe injury to health.

It is obvious that those hazard exposures falling within the High category should be solved as quickly as possible, whereas those falling within the Low category will receive a lower priority. This classification system also helps to identify those areas where immediate interim steps such as personal protective equipment should be used to protect the worker until a more permanent solution can be developed.

Another method somewhat similar to that presented above is to consider the potential hazard in terms of its type of effect on the human system. Some hazards are acute, causing an immediate reaction of the human system to an exposure to the hazard. Other hazards are chronic and result in a long-term human system response to exposure. This distinction between types of effect can be helpful when attempting to identify hazards of an acute nature. It is also useful because hazards with chronic effects are not necessarily easily recognized by observing the workers. More sophisticated recognition and evaluation techniques are required to determine if a hazard is present.

A fourth useful method of classifying hazards is by type of exposure. If a hazard can be classified within a particular type of exposure, this classification may be helpful in identifying general methods of control that can be used. The various types of exposure classifications are as follows:

A.   Airborne contaminants--relating to contaminants that are airborne such as respirable dust, vapors, and gases.

B.   Physical--hazards that are of a physical nature (not including air quality hazards) including such things as noise, ionizing radiation, nonionizing radiation, and thermal hazards.

C.   Surface contacting materials--non-respirable toxic materials, generally in liquid or solid form, that affect the human system through physical contact.

D.   Flammable materials--materials that are flammable or explosive.

E.   Material handling--hazards that result because of physical stress created on the human system in moving materials from one place to another.

F.   Mechanical and electrical--hazards involving mechanical and electrical equipment that can cause traumatic injury to the worker.

G.   Facilities--hazards relating to the general facilities of the plant such as waste disposal, housekeeping, adequate safe water supply, and traffic flow inside and outside the plant.

In general, the first three categories of hazards are primarily the concern of the industrial hygienist, while the last three categories are primarily the concern of the safety professional. The flammable material category may fall under the special function of the fire protection engineer, or it may be included in the duties of the safety professional.

All of these classification systems can be useful in helping the industrial hygienist to identify and categorize the hazard that is encountered, thus providing for a more logical approach to solving the problems that exist. In addition, these classifications can assist in providing a mechanism whereby the priority of solution can be set. Also, the categorization can help to define the general types of control procedures that might be applicable.

Methods That Can Be Used To Recognize Hazards

There are a number of different methods that can be used to recognize hazards. The following will briefly discuss some of these methods. No one method is best to assure that all hazards will be recognized. Probably the best recognition system will include at some point all the methods that will be discussed.

1. Accident or injury reports--In terms of recognizing hazards that cause traumatic injury, a study of accident or injury reports can be useful. Group statistics from such reports can indicate areas of the plant and processes that are involved in large numbers of accidents or injuries. In addition, a detailed analysis of the accident or injury report can help to point out methods being used by the workers that increase the risk of an accident. It is true that writing a detailed accident report is somewhat akin to "closing the barn door after the horse has been stolen." However, in many cases it is only after the accumulation of such data that it is possible to identify hazards that are not necessarily obvious to the observer.

2. Physical examinations--Pre-employment examinations along with periodic physical examinations can help to identify chronic conditions that may be a result of contact with a hazard in the work environment. For example, if a number of workers demonstrate a hearing threshold shift in the 4000 to 6000 Hz frequency range when a comparison is made between pre-employment and periodic audiometric tests, noise exposure should be considered as a potential cause. It is then necessary to determine if any common factors exist between the workers exhibiting the threshold shift; i.e., work in the same location, work on the same shift, etc. Again, as in the preceding method, this is an after-the-fact method of recognizing a problem. Certainly it would be better to identify the noise problem in advance. However, any hearing threshold shifts identified indicate a problem that might otherwise go unnoticed.

3. Employee notifications--In some cases, the employee will recognize a health or safety hazard before it is recognized by any other plant personnel. Given the right management atmosphere, the employee will bring this problem to the attention of those responsible for rectifying the problem. Such employee contributions can be stimulated by stopping to talk to individual workers concerning health and safety during normal plant rounds.

4. Required inspections--Certain pieces of equipment are on a schedule of required inspections. These required inspections can indicate problems before they become a hazard to the health or safety of the worker. For example, boilers must be inspected on a periodic basis

by a state inspector. If the results of these inspections are provided to the occupational health and safety personnel, they can provide information that may be useful in eliminating potential hazards.

5.   <u>Literature and discussions with other professionals</u>--It is the responsibility of the professional to keep abreast of changes that are occurring within the occupational safety and health field. This can be done by reviewing periodicals relating to the subject as well as by attending meetings and training sessions where individual problems may be discussed with other professionals. It is also valuable to maintain contact with professionals working in other organizations so that, when a problem does come up, additional input and experience can be obtained. Quite often the problem that you face today has been faced previously by someone else in the field. The difficulty is in finding out who has encountered this problem and what was done to solve it.

6.   <u>Walk-through inspections</u>--This method for recognizing hazards is well established in the field. However, as previously discussed, this method requires significant experience to be an effective tool for recognizing potential hazards. One must be aware of the various types of hazards that can be encountered if they are to be recognized when one is walking through the plant. In addition, not all potential hazards are recognizable during a walk-through inspection. The walk-through inspection is not a "cure all" for recognizing hazards.

7.   <u>Sampling and spot inspections</u>--Though quite often limited to air-quality studies, this method can be used to recognize many types of hazards. The problem is one of defining a statistical method that assures adequate sampling and proper selection of the inspection locations. Using such a method can result in significant savings of time.

8.   <u>Preliminary hazard analysis</u>--A preliminary hazard analysis should be conducted prior to any extensive study of a potential hazard. The preliminary hazard analysis attempts to organize logically the currently known facts to determine the variables to be included in the study and the methods to be used to determine if a hazard exists. This approach is valuable in the investigation of new or modified operations to determine if potential hazards are being introduced into the system.

9.   <u>Review of process flows</u>--Quite often the only way to identify certain chemical and air-quality hazards is to review the process flows to determine where reactions are occurring and what intermediate and final products are being produced. This same approach can be used to identify hazards related to mechanical and electrical equipment where the review is for potential human contact with moving equipment, ergonomic stress, and thermal exposure.

10. <u>Fault-tree analysis</u>--Using fault-tree analysis, a probabilistic model of the system events is constructed. With the application of fault-tree analysis, it is possible to determine the likelihood that a given event will occur and that a given series of events will cause this event to occur. Though typically considered to be a technique used for safety analysis, this approach also provides a powerful tool that the industrial hygiene engineer can use to recognize potential health hazards. The procedures used in this approach have been well documented in the literature, and the reader is encouraged to become familiar with the use of fault-tree analysis.

11. <u>Critical incident technique</u>--Using the critical incident technique, a number of workers from a given location or plant are interviewed to determine unsafe practices or errors that have occurred while they have been on the job. These critical incidents are categorized, and the result is a systematic list of areas where potential hazards may exist that should be controlled.

12. <u>Failure mode and effect</u>--A technique wherein failure of a given component or element within a system is assumed to occur, and the effect of this failure on components or elements in the system is determined. This technique helps to point out the possibility of a minor failure resulting in a major catastrophe.

13. <u>Job safety analysis</u>--Using this technique, each individual job is broken down into tasks that must be performed and elements that are required to perform these tasks. Each task and element is reviewed to determine if a potential hazard exposure to the worker may exist. Where potential hazard exposures do exist, action is taken to modify either the procedures used, the equipment involved, or the protection afforded the worker to eliminate the exposure.

There are other hazard recognition methods that may be used in the work environment. New methods are being identified on a regular basis. The key that allows the industrial hygiene engineer to recognize potential hazards effectively is the use of a number of techniques rather than relying on only one or two. An unsafe ladder is easily recognized during a walk-through inspection, while an exposure to a toxic chemical may not be obvious. The hazards are there; the problem is to find them before the worker becomes seriously ill or injured.

Summary

Although the emphasis in this text is the engineering control of the working environment, it is important not to forget the recognition of potential health hazards. If the hazard has been identified properly and if the cause and effect relationship has been well described, it is possible to exercise engineering control to eliminate the hazard. If a good job has not been done in recognizing the potential hazards, it becomes more difficult, if not impossible, to control the environment. Obviously, if one is to control the work environment, one must be aware of the potential problems that exist and the mechanisms by which these problems can be of danger to the worker.

Quite often the individual responsible for solving a problem tends to jump to a conclusion without adequate data to support that conclusion. This danger is faced by all occupational safety and health personnel. If the groundwork is not done and the hazard recognized for what it is, it is very easy to jump to a conclusion that is only a partial solution to the problem. The importance of a logical, systematic approach toward recognizing and defining the potential hazard exposures that exist within the occupational environment cannot be underestimated. If this job is done properly, the job of control becomes much simpler.

2. Methods for Measuring and Evaluating Health Hazards

Assume for a moment that you have been called to a local plant to act as an occupational safety and health consultant. The plant manager tells you that he has only recently become aware of the OSHA law and feels that his plant may be in violation of that law in some areas. He would like you to study the plant for potential health hazard exposures, identify those exposures that exist, and make recommendations concerning controls that can be effected to remove these health hazard exposures. In this situation, what would you do? How would you proceed to identify the problems? Obviously you cannot go helter-skelter throughout the plant looking here and there in hopes that you will identify a health hazard exposure. As a consultant, your daily rate is high enough that you must provide the plant manager with a maximum return for his dollar invested. Therefore, it is imperative that you organize your approach in such a manner that the results obtained will be the best possible.

Although the same general considerations should exist if you were hired as a full-time employee on the staff of the plant, it may not be the case. The individual who works as an employee of an organization may not be asked to justify his salary and the results obtained for that salary as is the case with the consultant. Consequently, the employee may be caught up in the act of being a member of the "fire brigade," putting out "little fires" as they occur rather than attempting to organize and plan the work in such a manner as to show major accomplishments. It is suggested that whether one is a consultant or an employee of a plant, one should attempt to obtain the maximum result for each dollar expanded.

In the field of occupational safety and health, it is desirable that, rather than reacting to problems, the professional plan and organize his work to seek out problems before they become emergencies that need immediate solutions. This is not always going to work; but as a general rule, most emergencies could be prevented with proper planning.

The purpose of this discussion is to present an organized method for recognizing and evaluating health hazards within the occupational environment. The method that is presented is a suggested organization method and is not the only way this can be done. However, the basic principles employed here should be present in any occupational safety and health study. As a matter of fact, the general principles presented here are applicable to other professions as well. Only the specific details would be changed.

A Suggested Analysis Study Outline

Your overall objective as an industrial hygiene engineer is to recognize potential hazard exposures, determine if they are in fact really exposures, and develop methods for controlling those hazard exposures that do exist. This seems simple enough. However, consider the case study presented at the end of this chapter. In the case study, you are to assume the position of a consultant responsible for occupational health and safety within the facility. On further consideration, the job is not so simple as it seemed at first glance. Many potential hazards exist. Many real hazards may be present. Alternate methods for control are available to be considered. Where do you start and what do you do to attempt to bring some order to the situation? In the following pages, a suggested method for accomplishing your job in a reasonable amount of time and with a reasonable amount of effort is presented.

Recognition of Hazards

Walk-Through Survey. Perhaps the first thing you might do on completing initial discussions with the plant manager is to conduct a walk-through survey of the plant. It is of value to carry a portable tape recorder with you to make notes on things that you see during this survey. The purpose of such a survey is not to identify all hazard exposures that may exist or to identify solutions that might be used to control hazards that you may feel exist but rather to gain a general feel for the operation. Your first objective is to become familiar with the overall plant, its products, its people, its general layout, and the work environment as a whole. Notes concerning these can be made for later reference. Remember, this is only an initial walk-through survey; it may be necessary to go back and look at things in more detail later.

Preliminary Hazard Recognition. After becoming familiar with the overall operation of the facility, you should make a more detailed study of the plant to identify potential hazard exposures. To do this, you will need your notes from the initial walk-through survey, layouts of the individual plant areas and the plant as a whole, process flows, process descriptions, job descriptions, and procedures in use. Now organize your thoughts in terms of a given plant area: for example, metal fabricating, vapor degreasing, paint shop, etc. Each of these areas must be studied in detail using the layouts, process flows, and other information that pertains to it.

Beginning with one of the areas chosen, consider the types of exposures that may exist: for example, airborne contaminants, physical hazards, surface-contacting materials, flammable materials, etc. By considering the types of exposures that a worker in the area might face, you will be less likely to miss potential hazards. In each of these types of exposures, consider where a possible potential hazard exposure to the worker may exist within the plant area. This can be done by reviewing your notes, the process, job descriptions, and procedures that are available. The emphasis is on identifying all potential hazard exposures, not just those that appear to exist. In this way it is possible to include exposures that may be present but easily overlooked.

In reviewing the operation for the various types of exposures, tools such as fault-tree analysis, job-safety analysis, and failure mode and effect are of value. These methods were discussed in the previous chapter. Through the use of these tools, it is possible to describe where potential problems mayexist that are not necessarily obvious. The industrial hygiene engineer should become familiar with the use of these and similar tools to improve the results obtained from a preliminary hazard analysis.

The preliminary hazard worksheet (Figure 1.2.1) presents a method for listing the results of your initial survey. For each type of exposure, a description of the potential hazard is given. This description should contain an explanation of what the potential hazard is, the probable source of the hazard, and the possible cause. The description must of necessity be brief; however, it should be concise enough to pinpoint the problem being considered.

The next important item to consider is the number of employees potentially affected by the hazard. This information will help to identify those hazards that require the most immediate action. Obviously all hazards should be controlled, but this may not be feasible given the time required to accomplish the control. The important thing is to solve first things first and go from there in an organized manner.

It is important to note the methods that are currently being used to control the hazard exposure. Just because controls exist, one cannot assume that the exposure is being controlled. Quite often malfunction of a control system can create a hazard exposure more serious than that which would exist in the absence of any control. If a control exists, it should be carefully evaluated to assure that it is working properly.

The next item to consider for a given hazard exposure is its level of effect on the human system. For purposes of this discussion, this level of effect has been broken down into three categories: a low level, where the hazard is of annoyance to the workers and has possible harmful effects; a medium effect, including those hazards that are dangerous to the health of humans; and a high effect, including those hazards that cause death or severe injury to the worker's health. This classification system is only suggested. Other classification systems can be developed that may be more useful. The major use of such a classification is to provide criteria upon which the decision concerning the priority of action can be made.

One further determination is useful before deciding the priority of study for each of the hazard exposures identified. It is desirable that the professional make some judgment concerning the probability that the hazard does, in fact, exist. In many cases, it is possible to determine that there is little likelihood that the exposure is not being controlled even though the potential hazard is a very serious one. For example, the absence of layers of dust in an area that would be expected to have a high concentration of airborne particles certainly indicates that the controls being used are relatively effective. Other factors such as experience and the presence or absence of worker complaints can help the professional to determine whether there is a high likelihood that a problem exists.

Figure 1.2.1

PRELIMINARY HAZARD RECOGNITION WORKSHEET

Area _____

Date _____

Investigator _____

TYPE OF EXPOSURE	DESCRIPTION OF POTENTIAL HAZARD	EMPLOYEES POTENTIALLY AFFECTED	PRESENT CONTROLS	LEVEL OF EFFECT LOW MED HIGH	PROBABILITY OF HAZARD EXISTING LOW MED HIGH	PRIORITY

Finally, after all potential hazard exposures in each given area have been identified and described, it is desirable to determine those exposures that should be studied and in what order they should be studied. To determine the order in which problems will be studied, a subjective priority should be placed on each hazard as it relates to the other potential hazards. This priority is determined by considering both the level of effect and the probability of existence for each exposure. Those hazard exposures with a high level of effect and a high probability of existence should be studied first, while those potential hazard exposures with a low level of effect and a low probability of existence can be considered only after the more likely and dangerous exposures have been controlled.

Upon completion of preliminary hazard recognition, the industrial hygiene engineer has a list of hazard exposures that can serve as a basis for planning and organizing his work for a long time in the future. Such a method can also provide a justification for neglect of a particular problem at a given time while others may feel that this problem should be under study. Without such a system, it is likely that the industrial hygiene engineer will be forced to react to every request for study that comes up, since there is no way to compare this hazard to other potential hazards that also require study.

Hazard Assessment Study Design

Preliminary Hazard Assessment. The first step in a hazard assessment study design is to make a preliminary determination concerning the possible extent of the hazard. If such a determination was made during the preliminary hazard recognition stage, it will not require repetition at this point. If such a determination was not made, it should be, since quite often a complete study of potential hazard exposure requires a significant expenditure of time and money. If preliminary results indicate that the problem is not significant, then this expenditure of time and money can be avoided.

Various alternatives exist to accomplish a preliminary hazard assessment, depending on the type of exposure being assessed. For example, if an air quality problem is being studied, colorimetric indicators can be used to obtain initial results. If the function of a ventilation system is in question, smoke tubes might be used to gain a quick estimate concerning the capture velocity of the system. Sound level readings might be made at key spots within an area to determine if a noise problem appears to be significant, or the industrial hygiene engineer might assess the difficulty in conversation within an area to gain a quick estimate concerning the level of noise that is present. These and similar techniques can provide an initial screening of the problem to determine whether further study is required, thus saving valuable time and money.

Hazard Assessment Study. If the results of the preliminary hazard assessment seem to indicate the need for further study, then a complete hazard assessment study must be conducted. The specific methods to be used will depend on the problem being faced. There are, however, certain general characteristics of a hazard study design that should be considered by the industrial hygiene engineer.

The first consideration is: Has the hazard exposure been defined completely? Do you know what type of hazard exposure may exist? Where is the likely source of the exposure? In what form will the hazard be found? This information should be available from the preliminary hazard recognition, but it is worthwhile to reconsider the problem definition at this point to be sure that the study will obtain the information necessary to determine whether or not the hazard exposure is present.

A second major consideration is choosing between alternative methods for obtaining desired results. Quite often the tendency is to design a study without considering possible alternative designs that might be used. Some time should be taken to assure that alternative designs do not exist that will provide better results or are easier to implement.

Related to the above consideration is the selection of equipment to be used to determine the hazard level. There are various types of measuring instruments available that can be used in a hazard assessment study. Each of these types of equipment has advantages and disadvantages and is best suited for certain types of assessment studies. The description of the hazard and the results to be obtained must be considered in choosing the appropriate equipment to use. Again alternatives should be considered to assure that the best equipment is used. One restraint on this choice of alternatives is the equipment that is available within the plant. Although gas chromatography may be the best method for analyzing a given air sample, this equipment may not be available for use either within the plant itself or in the local area. Thus, it may be necessary to choose an alternate method to obtain the results.

The definition of the problem will help define the kind of equipment that is required. For example, in an air quality study, the sampling train that is to be used may be set up to provide instantaneous samples or integrated samples, depending on the desired results. This decision must be considered, given the definition of the problem.

A clear definition of the target limit that the study results should not exceed is required. Such a definition in terms of the units to be considered will assist in defining the equipment and sampling methods to be used. Is the desired result in terms of peak levels, or is it in terms of a time-weighted average concentration of the hazard? What is the upper limit to be considered as safe? This may be the published threshold limit value, or it may be some other figure, depending on the existence of a threshold limit value or other requirements. This should be clearly defined at the outset of the study so that the decision criteria for further action are known.

When designing the study, consider the possibility of installing continuous monitoring equipment if the hazard is extremely dangerous to the worker and could get out of control quickly. Such a continuous monitoring system can be used to determine the levels present during the study and can remain in effect to assure that the limit is not exceeded in the future.

Another important consideration in designing a hazard assessment study is the location at which the sampling is to take place. Again this depends on a definition of the problem that may be faced. Where are the workers within the potential hazard area? Are they stationary, or do they move from area to area? The use of dosimeters can provide useful information concerning workers who move about. A stationary sampling point is certainly adequate when the worker does not move about the work area. It is also important to consider the method of entry of the sample into the human system. If the pollutant is likely to enter the human system as a result of respiration, the sampling point should be at the breathing zone level, either on the individual worker or stationary at this level within the area.

With the exception of a continuous sampling device, the time at which samples are taken is important. Hazard exposures may vary according to the time of day, and this variation should be considered when setting up the sampling plan. Quite often a buildup over a particular shift will occur, or the buildup may occur in relation to processing cycles. If this type of situation is expected, it is desirable to obtain multiple samples during the various expected cycles to determine if such a buildup is occurring. Another point to consider in terms of time is that, although the operation may be shut down during a third shift, there may be requirements for maintenance workers to operate in the area at this time. The exposure of maintenance workers should also be considered, and samples may be required during this third shift.

The next step in designing a hazard assessment study is to develop a step-by-step procedure that identifies what is to be done to assess the hazard exposure. This step-by-step procedure should include any evaluation steps and define any calculations that are necessary. This is done to assure that the study design plan is well thought out before entering into the study itself. If the study has not been well designed, it is possible that a number of false starts will occur, each requiring unnecessary expenditure of time and money; or that the results obtained will not be adequate to make the decision. Then the study will have to be repeated using different procedures. The procedure being used may be of a branching nature so that, given a certain occurrence, certain calculations or procedural steps must be performed; while given another occurrence, other steps or calculations will be performed. It is also possible that interim procedural steps may indicate that the study is no longer necessary. This type of branching can save time and money in accomplishing the study.

One important consideration in a hazard assessment study is the documentation of the study and its results. This documentation can provide information that will be useful in the future should other studies be required. The documentation can also justify the study and the results obtained. If a question arises concerning the results, it will be easy to identify exactly what was done and how the results were obtained. A sample for documenting the study design is given in Figure 1.2.2. A study outline is shown in Figure 1.2.3.

Summary

The preceding discussion has been presented to outline a procedural method that can be used to recognize and evaluate hazard exposures that may be present within the work environment. The objective of this discussion was to provide a logical method of approach that can be used for any hazard exposure. Obviously, certain types of exposures require that specific methods be used to assess their level. Regardless of these specific methods, it is necessary to approach the problem in a systematic manner.

It is not within the scope of this text to review the various types of measurement and evaluation techniques that are available and that can be used for a given hazard exposure. To do so would require much more space than is available. This subject matter has been covered well in other documents. Within the later chapters of this text, certain specific measurement equipment will be considered for the particular type of exposure being discussed. For example, in the area of ventilation, the various devices that can be used to measure and evaluate the effects of a ventilation system will be discussed in some detail.

Figure 1.2.2

Hazard assessment design.

Area _____   Type of Exposure _____

Date _____

Potential Hazard Description_____

_____

_____

Number of Employees Potentially Exposed _____

Desired Level To Be Maintained (TLV) _____

Results Obtained from Study _____

Action Recommended _____

_____

PRELIMINARY HAZARD ASSESSMENT

Equipment _____

Procedure _____

_____

Result/Recommendation _____

_____

_____

_____

_____

_____

_____

Figure 1.2.2 (Continued)

Equipment _____

_____

Location of Sampling Points _____

_____

Time Schedule for Sampling _____

_____

Procedure _____

_____

_____

_____

_____

_____

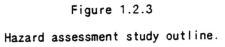

Figure 1.2.3

Hazard assessment study outline.

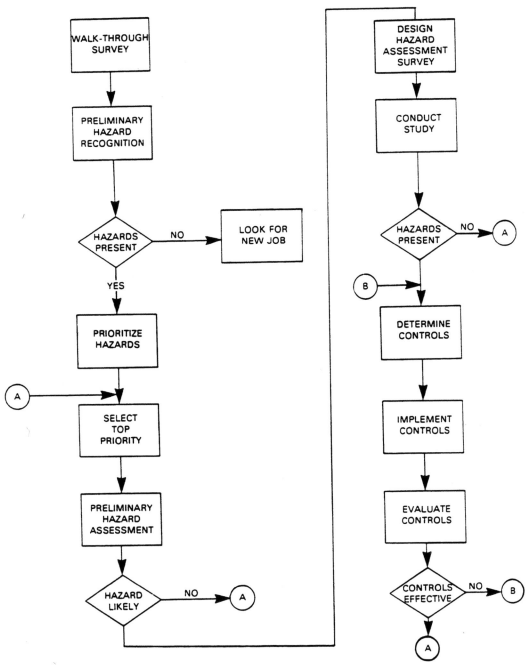

CASE STUDY

Introduction

The following pages describe a case concerning an industrial firm, Acme Metal Fabricating, Inc. (AMF). This case may be used for study throughout the text. The case attempts to describe a realistic industrial plant that faces many occupational health and safety problems. The reader may chose to return to this case study and analyze it in an attempt to make his learning experiences more realistic.

General Description

Acme Metal Fabricating, Inc. (AMF) is a small metal fabricating firm operating on the west side of Centertown, Ohio (population 16,500). AMF employs 94 people including office and design engineering staff. The plant is a large, single-story building with dimensions of 270 ft. by 120 ft. and open ceiling heights of 16 ft. in the production and storage areas. Office ceilings are 10 ft. AMF fabricates large and small metal parts used by other manufacturers in the local area.

The Plant Manager, Jim Brown, has recently become aware of the possible existence of conditions that are hazardous to the health and safety of the workers. Having no one who is responsible for the health and safety of the workers, he has contacted your firm, Health and Safety, Inc., for the purposes of determining if hazards are present and, if so, recommending controls to alleviate the hazards. You and some other members of the firm's staff have been chosen to act as consultants to AMF. Mr. Brown has provided the following descriptive information concerning the operation of AMF to your group.

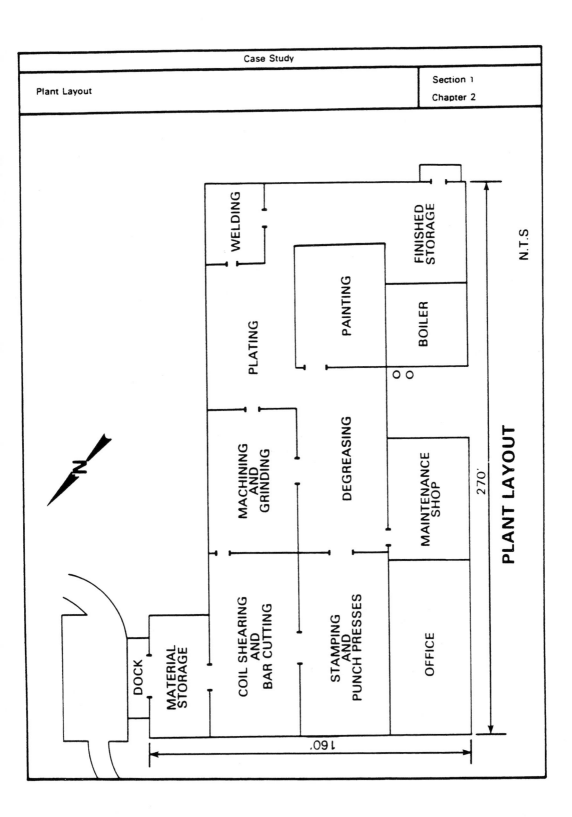

Case Study

Plant Layout

Section 1

Chapter 2

PLANT LAYOUT

Case Study	
Material Storage	Section 1 Chapter 2

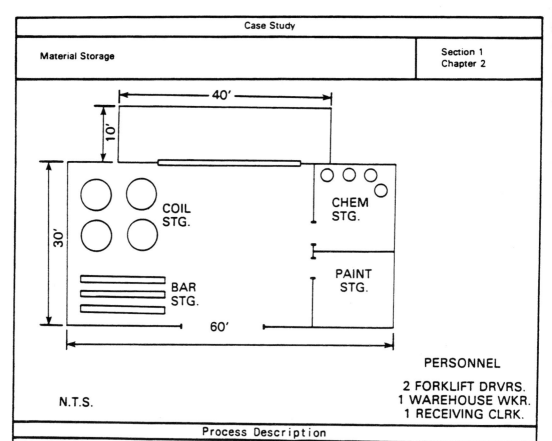

N.T.S.

PERSONNEL

2 FORKLIFT DRVRS.
1 WAREHOUSE WKR.
1 RECEIVING CLRK.

Process Description

Steel Coils
1. Steel coil is delivered by truck.
2. Forklift truck (LPG) moves coils from truck to storage. Coils weigh from 8,000# to 15,000# each depending on steel gauge.
3. Coils are stored on end.

Bar Stock
1. Bar stock is delivered by truck.
2. Forklift (LPG) moves bar stock to storage racks. Bars may vary in size from 1" x 2" x 6' to 6" x 8" x 6'.

Chemicals and Welding Materials
1. Chemicals delivered by truck in 55-gal drums. Acetylene, carbon dioxide, LPG, and oxygen are delivered in cylinders.
2. Forklift truck moves chemicals and cylinders to storage room door.

3. Drums and cylinders are moved manually using a hand cart which is pushed to storage area and tilted to slide drum or cylinder off into storage.
4. Drums are stored on end. Cylinders are stored horizontally on the floor.
5. Forklift trucks are charged with LPG in the area outside the chemical storage room.

Paint
1. Paint is delivered by truck on a pallet in 5-gal cans.
2. Forklift truck moves the pallet to storage room door.
3. Cans are manually carried to a 3-level rack and placed in labeled positions.

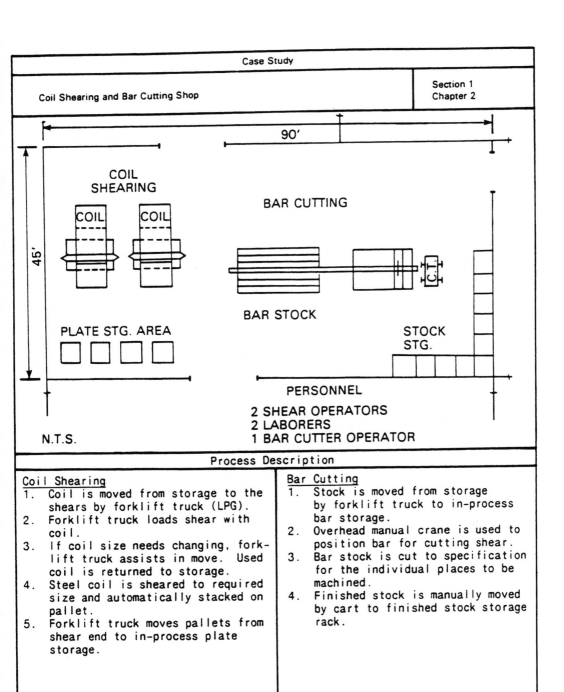

Case Study	
Coil Shearing and Bar Cutting Shop	Section 1 Chapter 2

90'

45'

COIL
SHEARING

COIL   COIL

BAR CUTTING

BAR STOCK

PLATE STG. AREA

STOCK
STG.

C.T.

PERSONNEL

2 SHEAR OPERATORS
2 LABORERS
1 BAR CUTTER OPERATOR

N.T.S.

Process Description

Coil Shearing
1. Coil is moved from storage to the shears by forklift truck (LPG).
2. Forklift truck loads shear with coil.
3. If coil size needs changing, forklift truck assists in move. Used coil is returned to storage.
4. Steel coil is sheared to required size and automatically stacked on pallet.
5. Forklift truck moves pallets from shear end to in-process plate storage.

Bar Cutting
1. Stock is moved from storage by forklift truck to in-process bar storage.
2. Overhead manual crane is used to position bar for cutting shear.
3. Bar stock is cut to specification for the individual places to be machined.
4. Finished stock is manually moved by cart to finished stock storage rack.

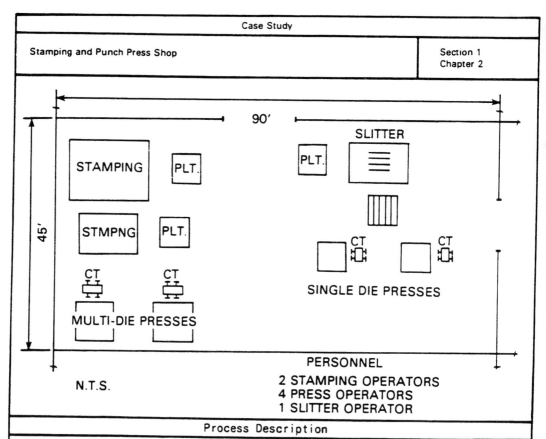

Case Study	
Stamping and Punch Press Shop	Section 1 Chapter 2

Process Description

Stamping
1. Plate is delivered by forklift truck to stamping machine.
2. Single plate is automatically fed by vacuum to stamping area.
3. Operator activates stamping mechanism approximately once every 1-2 minutes.
4. Stamped part is placed in truck wagon by operator who manually removes the part from the stamping machine.
5. Operator changes dies and press punch to meet specifications.

Slitting
1. Plate is moved from storage to slitting operation by forklift truck.
2. Plate is slit to specified size by manually moving plate through slitters.

3. Finished slit plate is manually stacked for punching.

Punch Presses
1. Two single die punch presses are used for punching split plate. Two multi-die presses are used for plate punching.
2. Plate is moved to multi-die presses by forklift truck. Slit plate is manually loaded in single die presses.
3. All presses operate automatically with operator feeding stock and removing finished product from stacker.
4. Finished products are stored in tote boxes in small cart that can be pulled manually or by forklift.
5. Operator changes punches and dies to meet specifications.

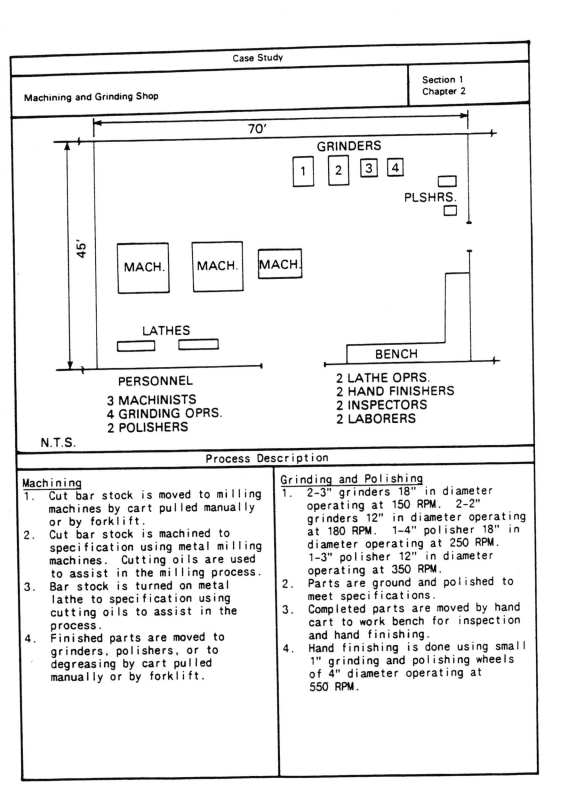

Process Description

Machining

1. Cut bar stock is moved to milling machines by cart pulled manually or by forklift.
2. Cut bar stock is machined to specification using metal milling machines. Cutting oils are used to assist in the milling process.
3. Bar stock is turned on metal lathe to specification using cutting oils to assist in the process.
4. Finished parts are moved to grinders, polishers, or to degreasing by cart pulled manually or by forklift.

Grinding and Polishing

1. 2-3" grinders 18" in diameter operating at 150 RPM. 2-2" grinders 12" in diameter operating at 180 RPM. 1-4" polisher 18" in diameter operating at 250 RPM. 1-3" polisher 12" in diameter operating at 350 RPM.
2. Parts are ground and polished to meet specifications.
3. Completed parts are moved by hand cart to work bench for inspection and hand finishing.
4. Hand finishing is done using small 1" grinding and polishing wheels of 4" diameter operating at 550 RPM.

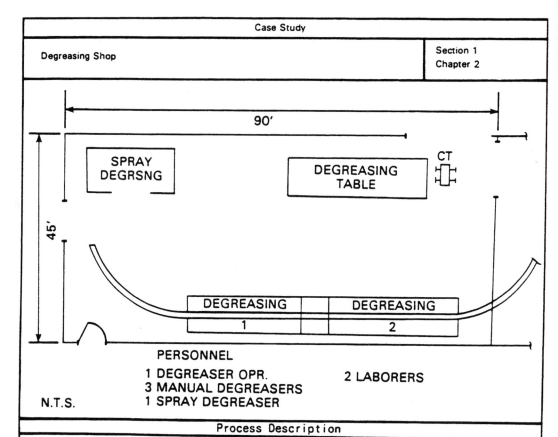

Case Study	
Degreasing Shop	Section 1 Chapter 2

PERSONNEL

1 DEGREASER OPR.   2 LABORERS
3 MANUAL DEGREASERS
1 SPRAY DEGREASER

N.T.S.

Process Description

Large Parts

1. Large parts moved by forklift truck pulling cart to vapor degreaser.
2. Degreaser workers remove parts from wagon and attach to overhead conveyor.
3. Degreaser operator operates controls to move part into degreaser. Operator is responsible for timing part in degreaser.
4. Degreaser consists of 2-tank process. Part immersed in first tank; vapor bathed in second tank.
5. Tanks are steam heated to 190°. Solvent used is trichloroethylene with stabilizers added. Thermostat controls vapor line.
6. Tanks are cleaned and charged every 48 hours of operation.
7. Each tank is 23' long, 5' wide, and 10' high. Solvent is 4' deep.

Small Parts

1. Small parts are delivered from either machining/grinding or the punch press operation by cart to degreasing tables and booth.
2. At degreasing table small parts are attached to hand operated conveyor chain and dipped into small tank of trichloroethylene at room temperature, removed, brushed with paint brush to loosen oil and grease, and allowed to dry while hanging on chain conveyor.
3. Other small parts are attached to chain in a small spray booth. Operator sprays parts to remove oil and grease and moves to drying position to air dry. Small hand spray is used to apply solvent.
4. Dried parts put in cart for painting, electroplating, or welding as required.

Case Study	
Electroplating Shop	Section 1 Chapter 2

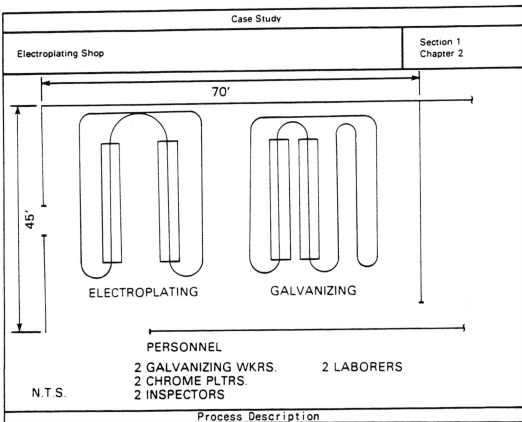

70'

45'

ELECTROPLATING   GALVANIZING

PERSONNEL

2 GALVANIZING WKRS.   2 LABORERS
2 CHROME PLTRS.
N.T.S.   2 INSPECTORS

Process Description

Chrome Plating

1. Parts are delivered by hand cart to the overhead conveyor.
2. Parts are attached to overhead conveyor, which is a manually operated motor-driven system, to move parts through the plating process.
3. A pre-plating acid cleaning process is accomplished by dipping the parts into a solution of sulfuric acid.
4. The chrome plating dip tank is filled with chromic acid with additives to reduce misting.
5. Chrome plated parts are inspected while on the conveyor.
6. Parts are removed from the conveyor to hand carts.

Galvanizing

1. Parts are delivered by hand cart to the overhead conveyor.
2. Parts are attached to the overhead conveyor, which is a manually operated motor-driven system, to move parts through the plating process.
3. A pre-plating acid cleaning process is accomplished by dipping the parts into a solution of sulfuric acid.
4. Galvanizing is accomplished by dipping parts into the molten zinc tank.
5. Galvanized parts are inspected on the conveyor.
6. Parts are removed from the conveyor to hand carts.

Case Study	
Paint Shop	Section 1 Chapter 2

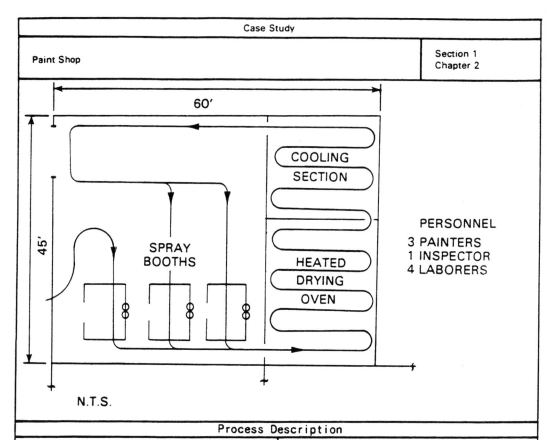

N.T.S.

Process Description	

1. Small parts are delivered by hand cart and attached to one of two parallel overhead conveyors. Large parts that are to be painted are delivered to the spray booth conveyor. Parts not painted are removed from conveyor in paint shop and carried by hand cart to electroplating, welding, or storage as required.
2. Painter sprays parts using hand-held spray gun.
3. Paint used is leaded zinc oxide base paint.
4. Parts moved from spray booth to a pickup conveyor.
5. Parts are moved continuously through drying oven operating at 300°F.

6. Final stage of drying is at cool temperature, 60°-70°F.
7. Parts are removed from conveyor and placed on cart equipped with racks to be moved to storage by forklift truck.

Case Study	
Welding Shop	Section 1 Chapter 2

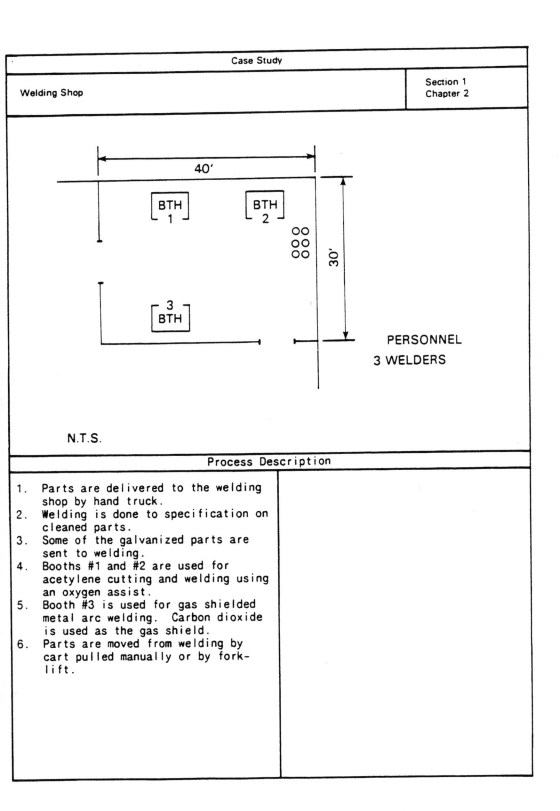

N.T.S.

Process Description

1. Parts are delivered to the welding shop by hand truck.
2. Welding is done to specification on cleaned parts.
3. Some of the galvanized parts are sent to welding.
4. Booths #1 and #2 are used for acetylene cutting and welding using an oxygen assist.
5. Booth #3 is used for gas shielded metal arc welding. Carbon dioxide is used as the gas shield.
6. Parts are moved from welding by cart pulled manually or by fork-lift.

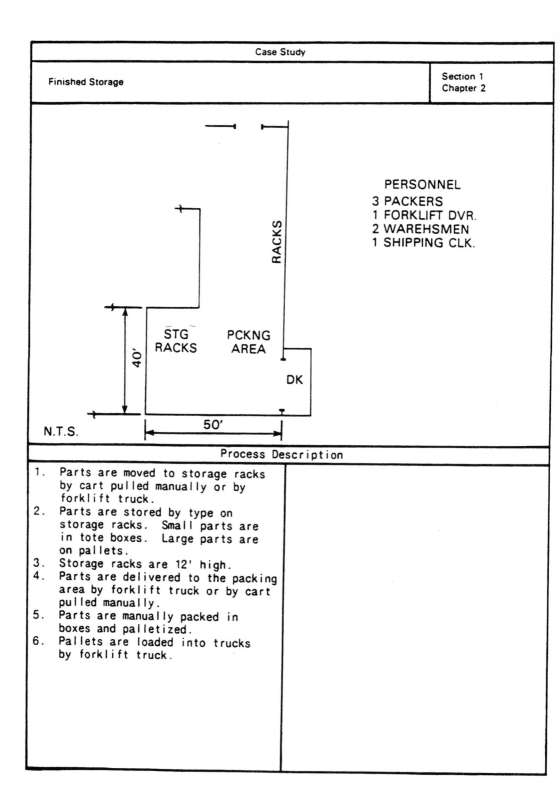

Case Study	
Finished Storage	Section 1 Chapter 2

RACKS

PERSONNEL
3 PACKERS
1 FORKLIFT DVR.
2 WAREHSMEN
1 SHIPPING CLK.

40'

STG RACKS   PCKNG AREA

DK

N.T.S.   50'

Process Description

1. Parts are moved to storage racks by cart pulled manually or by forklift truck.
2. Parts are stored by type on storage racks. Small parts are in tote boxes. Large parts are on pallets.
3. Storage racks are 12' high.
4. Parts are delivered to the packing area by forklift truck or by cart pulled manually.
5. Parts are manually packed in boxes and palletized.
6. Pallets are loaded into trucks by forklift truck.

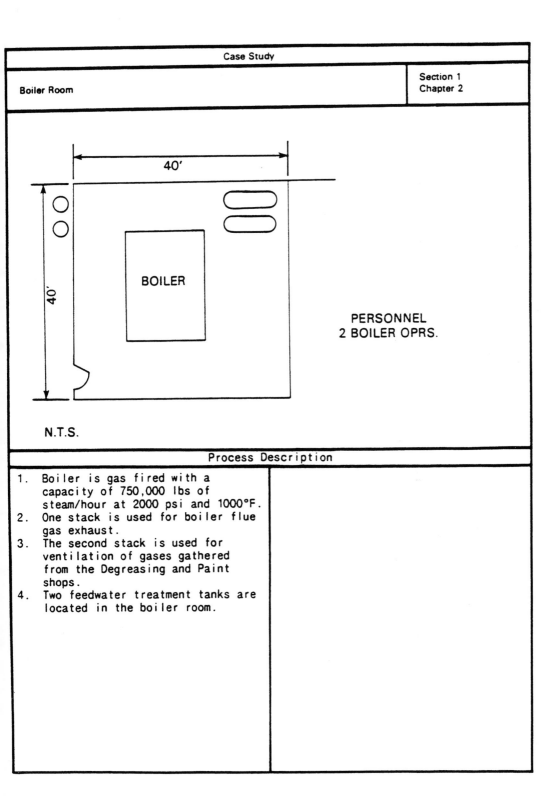

Case Study	
Boiler Room	Section 1 Chapter 2

40'

40'

BOILER

PERSONNEL
2 BOILER OPRS.

N.T.S.

Process Description

1. Boiler is gas fired with a capacity of 750,000 lbs of steam/hour at 2000 psi and 1000°F.
2. One stack is used for boiler flue gas exhaust.
3. The second stack is used for ventilation of gases gathered from the Degreasing and Paint shops.
4. Two feedwater treatment tanks are located in the boiler room.

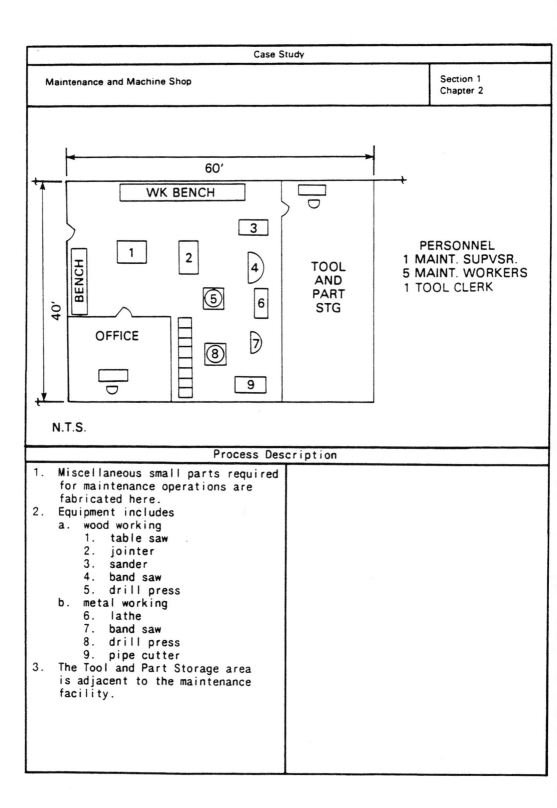

Case Study	
Maintenance and Machine Shop	Section 1 Chapter 2

PERSONNEL
1 MAINT. SUPVSR.
5 MAINT. WORKERS
1 TOOL CLERK

N.T.S.

Process Description

1. Miscellaneous small parts required for maintenance operations are fabricated here.
2. Equipment includes
    a. wood working
        1. table saw
        2. jointer
        3. sander
        4. band saw
        5. drill press
    b. metal working
        6. lathe
        7. band saw
        8. drill press
        9. pipe cutter
3. The Tool and Part Storage area is adjacent to the maintenance facility.

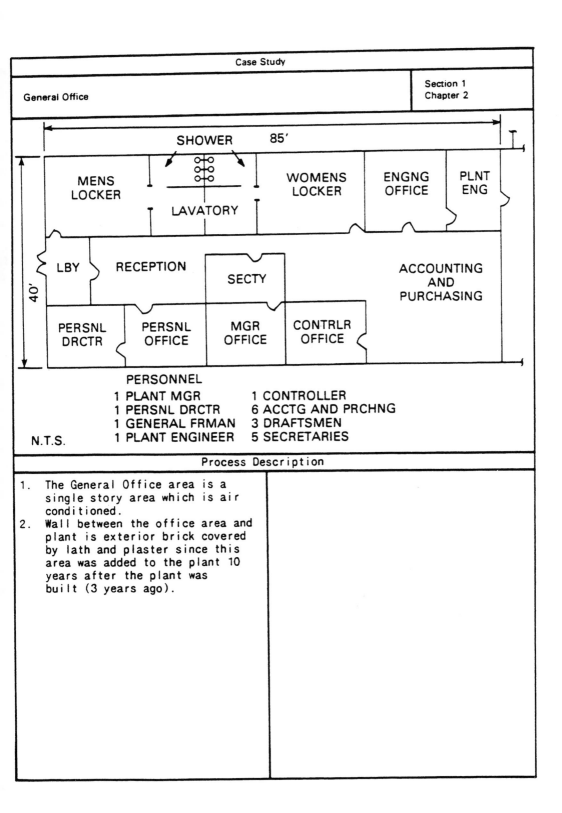

Case Study

General Office	Section 1 Chapter 2

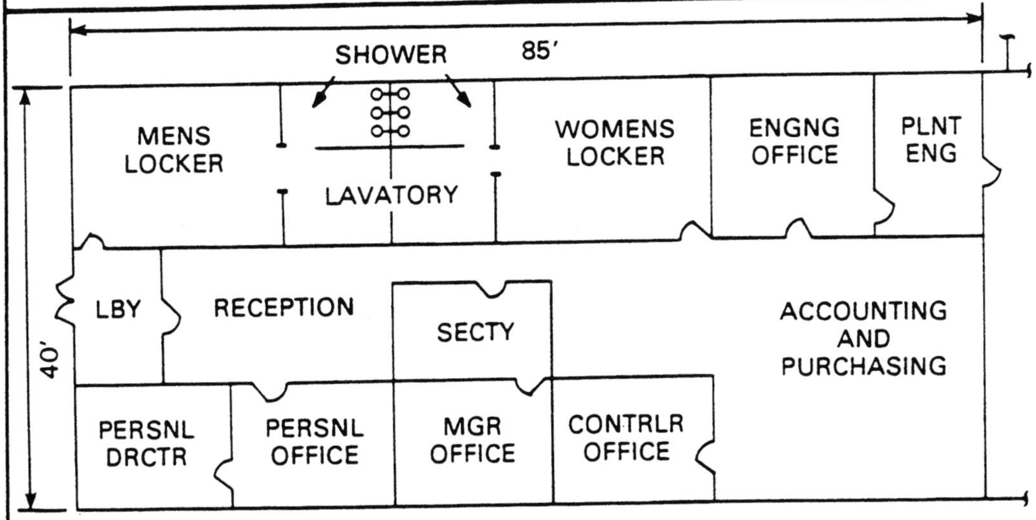
85′
40′
SHOWER
MENS LOCKER
LAVATORY
WOMENS LOCKER
ENGNG OFFICE
PLNT ENG
LBY
RECEPTION
SECTY
ACCOUNTING AND PURCHASING
PERSNL DRCTR
PERSNL OFFICE
MGR OFFICE
CONTRLR OFFICE

PERSONNEL

1 PLANT MGR	1 CONTROLLER
1 PERSNL DRCTR	6 ACCTG AND PRCHNG
1 GENERAL FRMAN	3 DRAFTSMEN
1 PLANT ENGINEER	5 SECRETARIES

N.T.S.

Process Description

1. The General Office area is a single story area which is air conditioned.
2. Wall between the office area and plant is exterior brick covered by lath and plaster since this area was added to the plant 10 years after the plant was built (3 years ago).

3. Human Systems

Introduction

It is important that the industrial hygiene engineer have a basic understanding of the structure and functioning of the human system. With such an understanding, the industrial hygiene engineer can communicate with other individuals on the health team concerning the probable cause and effect of potential hazard exposures within the industrial environment. Results obtained from the physical examination of workers can provide useful information to the industrial hygiene engineer concerning potential hazards to which the worker may have been exposed. The malfunctioning of the human system may indicate the potential effect of an outside influence, such as the occupational environment.

The occupational environment can affect the performance of the human system in a number of ways. First in the effect to the human system is the physical health of the worker. Many hazard exposures will result in a change in the physical functioning of body systems for those individuals exposed. These changes can be identified by certain symptoms that the worker exhibits. The occupational environment may also affect the emotional health of the worker. This effect is not always as evident as a change in physical health. It is also very difficult to document changes in emotional health and to relate these changes to occupational exposures. The most obvious effect on the human system, and the one in which a cause-and-effect relationship is easiest to identify, is the traumatic injury to the worker. If a worker puts his hand in a band saw and loses three fingers, it is obvious that the effect, the loss of three fingers, was caused by an occupationally related incident. However, it is not always easy to determine the factors that caused the worker to put his hand in the band saw in the first place.

To assess the extent of a hazard, it is necessary to determine the effect of the hazard on the human system. Generally, this effect results in a change in the normal function of a particular system within the human body. Such changes may or may not indicate the existence of a problem. Also, the changes may or may not be occupationally related. However, it is important that problems identified during normal physical examination of workers be investigated to determine if there is a cause-effect relationship between the problem and the occupational environment.

From the above it can be implied that determination of the existence of a problem in the functioning of the human system is the responsibility of the physician. The industrial hygiene engineer should not jump to conclusions concerning symptoms observed in the worker without first referring the worker

1.3.2

to a qualified physician to determine if these symptoms do indicate a
malfunction of the worker's body system. Having determined that a malfunction
exists, the industrial hygiene engineer should consult literature prepared by
various health researchers concerning the probable cause-and-effect
relationship to determine whether the worker's problem can be related to the
occupational work environment. Once a probable cause-effect relationship has
been established, it is the responsibility of the industrial hygiene engineer
to determine if an occupational exposure present within the work environment
caused the identified health problem.

In this crucial position, the industrial hygiene engineer must be able to
interpret the results obtained by the physician and the health researcher and
apply these results to determine if the potential cause is present. When
interpreting these results, it is important that the industrial hygiene
engineer have a basic understanding of the functioning of the human system and
the terminology used to describe the system.

The Study of Human Systems

There are four major classifications of study related to the human
system. The first classification is the study of the anatomy. This study
involves the form of living systems. The study of <u>anatomy</u> is concerned with
the identification of the various components of the body. It is also
concerned with the structure and location of these components within the
body. Figure 1.3.1 presents some common prefixes and suffixes used in medical
terminology related to the human system. Figure 1.3.2 presents some common
anatomical terms. Knowledge of these terms will help the industrial hygiene
engineer to interpret the common medical terminology that may be encountered.

The second major classification related to the study of the human system
is physiology. <u>Physiology</u> involves the study of the function of living
systems. In simple terms, physiology is involved with the study of what the
system does. It is involved with why the system does what it does and how the
system performs its functions. It is important that an understanding of
anatomy be obtained to relate the system function with its location,
structure, and the terminology used to describe its components.

The study of biochemistry is the third major classification of the study
of human systems. <u>Biochemistry</u> is related to the chemistry of living systems.
The human body, as well as that of other living organisms, is a chemical
system. The body manufactures chemicals and uses these chemicals to perform
its various functions. Chemical changes within the body often are indicative
of a problem within the human system.

The fourth major category of human system study is <u>biophysics</u>. This
discipline is related to the study of physical methods used within human
systems. The human system is composed of bones, joints, and muscles. The
biophysicist is interested in the workings of these components to accomplish
the requirements that are placed upon the body.

Figure 1.3.1

Terminology--the human system.

Common Prefixes

a- (or an-)	absence of	hypo-	below, deficient
ambi-	both	hystero-	uterus
angio-	tube or blood vessel	in-, intra-	in, inside
ante-	before	leuko-	white
anti-	before	macro-	large
anthro-	joint	mal-	disordered, bad
bi-	two	mamma-	breast
brady-	slow	meno-	monthly, menstrual
cardio-	heart	micro-	small
cephalo-	head	myo-	muscle
cerebro-	brain	nephro-	kidney
chole-	biled	neuro-	nerve
circum-	around	oto-	ear
contra-	against	para-	side
cyt-	sac	pneumo-	air, lung
derma-	skin	poly-	many
dys-	disordered, painful, difficult	post-	after
		pre-	before
		pseudo-	false
en-	in	pulmo-	lung
entero-	intestine	pyelo-	kidney
erythro-	red	pyo-	pus
gastro-	stomach	retro-	behind
glyco-	sugar	rhino-	nose
hem-, hema-, hemato-	blood	semi-	half
		sub-	under
hemi-	half	super-, supra-	above, greater
hepa-, hepato-	liver	tachy-	fast
hydro-	water	trans-	across
hyper-	above, excess		

Common Suffixes

-algia	pain	-oma	tumor
-asthenia	weakness	-ostomy	opening
-cyte	cell	-paresis	weakness
-ectomy	surgical removal	-pathy	disease
-emia	blood	-phobia	fear
-esthesia	feeling	-pnea	breathing
-genic	causing	-scopy	see
-graphy	visualization	-uria	urine
-itis	inflammation		

Figure 1.3.2

Anatomical terms.

Relating to Location

anterior (ventral)	toward the front of the body
posterior (dorsal)	toward the back of the body
superior	upper
inferior	lower
superficial	near the surface
deep	remote from the surface
internal	inside
external	outside
proximal	part nearest (with reference to the heart)
distal	part furthest (with reference to the heart)
medial	toward the center of the body
lateral	away from the center of the body; to the side

Relating to Direction

craniad (cephalad)	toward the head
caudad	toward the feet

Relating to Position and Movement

supine	lying horizontal on the back, face upward
prone	lying horizontal, face down
abduction	a movement away from the body
adduction	a movement toward the body
flexion	the act of bending, or the condition of being bent
extension	the movement that brings the parts of a limb toward a straight condition

---

The Basic Unit of Life--The Cell

As the atom is the building block of all substances, so the cell is the building block of all living organisms. All tissue in the human body is made up of individual cells, each of which acts as a site for conversion of nutrients into energy and waste materials. The principal functions of cells are essentially the same regardless of where the cells are located in the human body. These functions are:

A.   Exchange of materials with the immediate environment. The exchange between the environment and the cell occurs by diffusion through the cell membranes.

B.   The production of energy from nutrients (metabolism). Carbohydrates, fats, and protein are broken down, yielding energy, heat, and a variety of chemical waste products. This breakdown of carbohydrates, fats, and protein is accomplished through the use of oxygen supplied by the blood. The resultant metabolism yields waste products, including carbon dioxide, lactic acid, ketones, and urea.

C.   The synthesis of proteins. Within the cell, proteins are built from the various chemicals that are present. These proteins are the building blocks of the body.

D.   Reproduction. Reproduction occurs through the division of cells, with some cells reproducing more readily than others. This is evident where regenerative tissue, such as skin, is compared to less regenerative tissue, such as the heart muscle.

Figure 1.3.3

The cell.

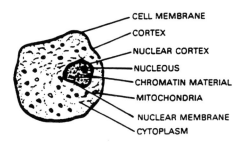

All cells, regardless of their location and purpose as a part of the body tissue in which they are present, perform the above functions in the same manner. Specialization of cells occurs when groups are formed together to accomplish different functions of the human body. The general term used for the specialization of these cell groups is tissue. The four main types of tissues in the human body are:

A.   Epithelial tissue--the covering of the outer surface of the body and its organs.

B.   Connective tissue--the supporting and connecting tissue of the body, including tendons, ligaments, cartilage, and bones.

C.   Muscle tissue--the tissue that functions to move the body and its organs.

D.   Nervous tissue--the tissue that acts to send messages to and from the various organs and muscles of the body.

The cell is composed of many types of molecules. The most important of these is water which comprises approximately eighty percent of the total weight of the cell. Water is the basis for practically all processes that occur within the cell and thus within the human body. The major constituents of the cell structure are the organic molecules (compounds of carbon) that occur in a large number within the cell. These organic molecules include proteins, lipids (fats), carbohydrates, and the two important nucleic acids, deoxyribonucleic acid (DNA) and ribonucleic acid (RNA). The DNA is the blueprint of genetic information in the cell nucleus, and the RNA transmits this information in forms that can be used by the cell to reproduce itself and its products in the same form. The third class of chemical cell components is inorganic electrolytes such as phosphorus, potassium, sulphur, chlorine, iron and other trace elements.

The basic process which transforms food to energy is as follows. Proteins are broken down into simple amino acids in the digestive system. Carbohydrates and fats are similarly broken down within the digestive system. These chemicals are then absorbed into the blood stream and transported to the various cells of the body. When the nutrients reach the cell, they penetrate the cell membrane through the process of diffusion. Within the cell proper, a process called metabolism occurs. In metabolism, a chemical reaction within the cell fragments large molecules into smaller ones and synthesizes large molecules of a different structure from the raw materials that have been fragmented. During this action, energy is released.

While the cells and tissues within the body are performing their functions, the body remains in system balance, or homeostasis. The rate of metabolism within the body must constantly change in reaction to external stimuli from the environment in which the body is living. The changes that occur within the body to allow the metabolic rate to change must balance each other to assure that the system does not get out of control It is because of homeostasis that, for example, an individual shivers when placed in a cold environment. Shivering is the body's attempt to generate heat through muscle activity to compensate for the lower environmental temperature. Another example of the maintenance of system balance occurs when the human is exposed to an extremely hot environment. The body attempts to maintain a temperature equilibrium by evaporating perspiration and dilating surface blood vessels to allow more blood to pass near the surface of the skin and become cooled. The system balance is very delicate. Although the balance can be maintained within a wide range of certain environmental stimuli, once an imbalance occurs, the result can quickly become a significant danger to the individual.

The Structure of the Body--The Skeleton

The structure upon which the human body is built is the skeleton. The skeleton is composed of 206 bones. It provides the basis for the shape of the body as well as protection within its cavities for vital organs, such as the brain, heart, and liver.

The <u>axial skeleton</u> is made up of the bones of the skull, vertebrae, and thorax. The skull contains 29 bones, many of which are fused and appear as one bone structure. The spinal column is made up of 26 bones called <u>vertebrae</u>. The vertebrae serve as the support that enables the body to remain erect. The vertebrae also have a hollow cavity through which the spinal cord passes. Attached to the vertebrae are the 12 pairs of ribs that meet in the center at the breastbone (sternum).

Figure 1.3.4

The skeleton.

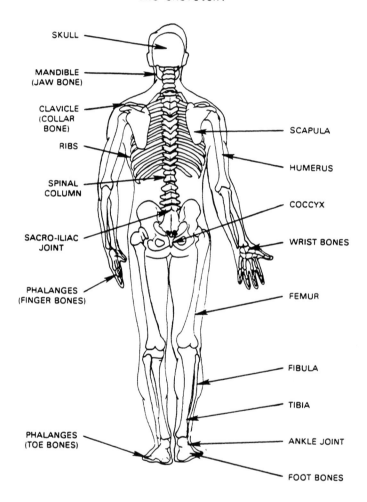

The appendicular skeleton consists of the bones of the upper extremities and the lower extremities. The upper extremities include four bones within the pectoral girdle and 60 bones in the arms and hands. The lower extremities consist of two bones within the pelvic girdle and 60 bones within the legs and feet. The bones of the appendicular skeleton provide the structure for the most mobile parts of the body--the arms and legs.

Where bones come together, a joint or articulation is formed. Such articulations occur at the knee and elbow. The joints permit various types of movement. The degree of movement between joints can be very slight--as that which occurs between bones in the skull, or very large--as that which occurs at the thumb. Articulations are classified as follows:

A. Gliding--as in the joints between vertebrae.
B. Hinge--as at the elbow.
C. Ball and socket--occurs in the hip and shoulder joints.
D. Pivot--allows for rotation of the forearm.
E. Ellipsoidal--allows for movements at the wrist.
F. Saddle--allows for the unique movement of the thumb.

There are many types of motions that occur at the joints. A standard nomenclature has been developed for these motions. The following presents the various movements that have been described:

A. Flexion-extension. Flexion is the movement of a joint in which the angle between the bones is decreased, such as bending the arm at the elbow. Extension is the opposite of flexion where the movement increases the angle between the bones, such as straightening the arm.

B. Abduction-adduction. Abduction is the movement of a part away from the center plane of the body or a part of the body, such as lifting the arm outward away from the body. Adduction is the opposite of abduction: a movement toward the center plane of the body or of a part of the body.

C. Supination-pronation. Supination is the turning of the hand so that the palm faces upward, while pronation is the turning of the hand so that the palm faces downward.

D. Rotation. Rotation is a movement in which a part turns on its longitudinal axis, such as turning the head or turning an arm or leg outward or inward.

E. Circumduction. Circumduction involves rotary movements which circumscribe an arc, such as swinging the arm in a circle.

F. Inversion-eversion. Inversion is the movement of the ankle joint in which the sole of the foot is turned inward. Eversion is the movement of the ankle in which the sole of the foot is turned outward.

G. Elevation-depression. Elevation is a movement in which a part is raised, while depression is a movement in which a part is lowered.

For example, the movement of the jaw up and down illustrates elevation-depression.

H.   Protraction-retraction. Protraction is the movement of a part forward, while retraction is the backward movement of a part. An example is jutting the jaw forward or pulling it backward.

I.   Hyperextension. Hyperextension includes movements of the wrist and other joints in which a part is extended beyond the straight line formed by normal extension. An example is a ballet dancer standing on his or her toes.

In addition to the bones of the skeleton, the body is comprised of connective tissue that holds the skeleton together. Three types of connective tissue are present within the body. Tendons, which are cords of strong, elastic fibrous tissue, attach the muscles to the bones. Ligaments, which are bands of tough, flexible connective tissue, join the bones at the articulations. Ligaments tend to inhibit movement beyond a certain point at the joints. Thus, when a joint moves beyond its normal pattern, ligaments may become torn. The third type of connective tissue, cartilage, is a relatively hard, smooth-surface tissue. Cartilage serves as a compression cushion that minimizes jolts and bumps to the skeletal system and protects the bones from breaking or chipping.

Figure 1.3.5

Connective tissue.

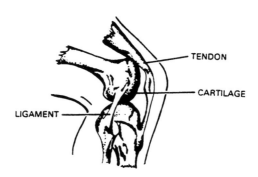

The bones of the skeleton have one other function beyond that of providing a structure for the human system. In the center of the bone is a cavity that contains red bone marrow. This bone marrow is important in the production, maintenance, and disposal of blood cells in the adult. Thus, the bone is a living group of cells just like any other part of the human body.

The Moving Force--The Muscles

The muscles are made up of many separate fibers that are able to contract and relax. There are many hundreds of muscles within the human body. If a muscle is viewed under a microscope, it will appear either as a group of fibers or as an essentially smooth tissue. Those muscles that appear as a group of fibrous tissues are called <u>striated muscles</u>. The skeletal muscles are striated muscles. The smooth-appearing muscles are called <u>smooth muscles</u>. The muscles moving the internal organs within the body are smooth muscles.

There are three major classifications of muscles. The first classification is the <u>voluntary muscle</u>: for example, the biceps, triceps, flexors, and extensors. The muscles are called voluntary because they are set in motion by the conscious direction of the human. A second group of muscles involves the <u>involuntary muscles</u>: for example, the diaphragm, esophageal, and stomach muscles. These muscles act independently of conscious will and thus are called involuntary. The third muscle classification is <u>cardiac muscle</u>. This is the heart muscle. The heart muscle acts as an involuntary muscle, but is generally classified separately from the other involuntary muscles because of its structure: striated muscle joined together in a continuous manner.

Voluntary muscles perform two major functions. The first of these is the maintenance of posture. The voluntary muscles tend to hold the body in the position in which it rests. Certain muscle contraction is required to maintain a given position, which is why a person can get tired while being seated or standing in one position. The second major function of the voluntary muscles is the movement of the human body. By relaxing and contracting, the muscles cause the articulations to move, thus propelling the body or part of the body in the desired direction.

The involuntary muscles provide propulsion of substances through the body passages, as in the case of the movement of blood through the circulatory system and the movement of food from the mouth to the stomach through the esophagus. These muscles also provide for the expulsion of stored substances, such as the action of the intestinal muscles. Other involuntary muscles involve the regulation of opening and sizes of tubes, thus providing for the change in pupil size and the expansion and contraction of blood vessels.

The muscles, whether voluntary or involuntary, receive a stimulus from the brain through the nerves to the muscle. This stimulus causes the muscle to either contract or relax. In order to accomplish this contraction or relaxation, glucose is converted to energy (metabolism). Oxygen is required to burn the glucose in this conversion process. The conversion process results in movement of the muscle that allows work to be performed while much of the energy created is dissipated as heat.

When a muscle performs its function for a long period of time, it is subject to muscle <u>fatigue</u>. Fatigue occurs because of either a lack of nutrients or a lack of oxygen being supplied to the muscle. Thus, the individual operating at a less than adequate nutritional level will feel fatigue much more quickly than an individual who has maintained the proper diet. Lack of oxygen can, in the short run, be compensated for by the body's buildup of an <u>oxygen debt</u>. For this reason, the human, after performing strenuous work, often becomes winded and must breathe hard for a period of time to repay the oxygen debt.

The Control System--The Nervous System

The human body is constantly bombarded by stimuli from the environment. The nervous system acts as the control mechanism that interprets the stimuli received and translates this interpretation into the appropriate action required by the body.

Anatomically, the nervous system can be broken down into two components--the <u>central nervous system</u> and the <u>peripheral nervous system</u>. Functionally, the nervous system can be broken down into the <u>automatic nervous system</u> and the <u>voluntary nervous system</u>.

The central nervous system is composed of the <u>brain</u> and <u>spinal cord</u>. The brain acts as the computer that directs all actions of the human body. The brain has several functions:

A. <u>As a regulatory center</u>. In response to impulses that are received about the state of the body's system and the external environment, the brain sends out messages to enable the system to make the appropriate adjustments.

Figure 1.3.6

The brain.

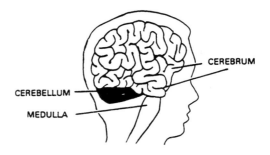

B. <u>As the seat of sensations</u>. It is the brain that makes us aware of ourselves and our surroundings.

C. <u>As the center of sensations</u>. The individual's perception of the environment received from the various sensory organs is interpreted by the brain. It is the brain that decides that an individual prefers the taste of a medium-rare sirloin steak to that of a hot dog.

D. <u>As a source of voluntary acts</u>. The brain sends signals to the various muscles of the body, causing them to relax or contract depending on the wishes of the individual. These voluntary acts can become programmed, as in typing, so that they appear to be automatic.

E. <u>As a seat of emotions</u>. The brain is the source of emotions, such as happiness, sadness, fear, and all other feelings that affect human behavior.

F. <u>As a seat of higher mental processes</u>. The brain acts as the basis for all thought, reasoning, judgment, memory, and learning. It is through learning that the voluntary act of typing becomes similar to reflex action.

The spinal cord serves as a conducting pathway from the brain to the various parts of the body. It is also a reflex center where actions, such as the well-known knee-jerk reflex, originate.

The <u>peripheral nervous system</u> connects the central nervous system with the distant parts of the body. It acts as a telegraph wire transmitting messages to and from the central nervous system. The <u>sensory nerves</u> or <u>afferent nerves</u> carry impulses from receptors located in all parts of the body to the brain. The <u>motor nerves</u> or <u>efferent nerves</u> carry impulses from the central nervous system to the muscles or other organs that must react to stimuli.

The <u>autonomic nervous system</u>, which is part of the peripheral nervous system, is important in regulating the automatic or involuntary functions of the body. The autonomic nervous system can be divided into two separate systems--the <u>parasympathetic nervous system</u>, which controls the body functions such as heart rate and respiration, and the <u>sympathetic nervous system</u>, which controls the body's response to stress and danger. The parasympathetic nervous system regulates the body functions, while the sympathetic nervous system regulates the body balance or homeostasis.

The <u>voluntary nervous system</u> is the system that carries messages from the brain to the voluntary muscles. Conscious control over the voluntary muscles of the body is maintained by messages transmitted over the voluntary nervous system.

The nervous system works on a combined electrical-chemical process. Although this process is not completely understood, it appears that an electrical impulse is transmitted along the nerve fibers while chemicals help control the rate of the impulses at the junctions of the nerves (synapses).

Fuel Processing--The Digestive System

The digestive system acts both chemically and mechanically to transform food into a form that the cells can use. The digestive system is made up of the <u>mouth</u>, including the <u>salivary glands</u>, <u>esophagus</u>, <u>stomach</u>, <u>intestines</u>, <u>liver</u>, <u>gall bladder</u>, and <u>pancreas</u>.

Digestion begins in the mouth. Food is mechanically broken down into small pieces, and the salivary glands release an enzyme that begins the chemical breakdown of starches. Whether our mothers know it or not, they were assisting the digestive process when they told us to chew our food well.

After leaving the mouth, the food travels through the pharynx or throat into the esophagus. The esophagus is the muscular tube that extends from the pharynx to the stomach. Liquids travel through the esophagus by gravity, while solid foods are propelled by muscular contractions of the esophagus.

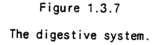

Figure 1.3.7

The digestive system.

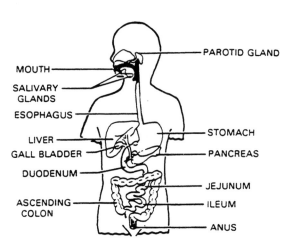

In the stomach, digestion of protein is initiated. The food is mixed with gastric juices containing acid and digestive enzymes, and the stomach walls move to churn the food and mix it with the gastric juices.

After a sufficient time, the food enters the upper part of the small intestine, the duodenum, where the partially digested food is subjected to enzymes secreted into the duodenum by the pancreas. Bile, which is produced in the liver and stored by the gall bladder, also enters the duodenum to aid in the digestion of fats.

The liver, in addition to forming bile, also functions in the metabolism of carbohydrates, the formation of red blood cells and clotting agents, and the detoxification of potentially harmful substances. The detoxification function of the liver is the reason it becomes important in the study of long-term exposures to potentially hazardous chemicals. Quite often these exposures cause pathological changes to occur in the liver, such as an increase in size or a modification of function.

After leaving the upper portion of the small intestine, the foods move through the remainder of the small intestine where the digested proteins, fats, and carbohydrates are absorbed through the intestinal walls into the blood and lymph. The remainder of the waste products pass into the large intestine or colon where water is extracted to produce a semi-solid waste form. This waste is then passed out of the body.

The Distribution System--The Circulatory System

The circulatory system is involved in transporting the body fluids from one region of the body to the other. It is made up of two separate and distinct systems: the blood vascular system and the lymphatic system.

Figure 1.3.8

The circulatory system.

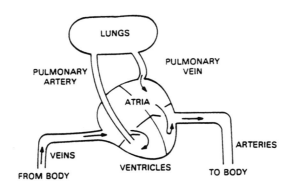

The blood vascular system consists of the heart and associated blood vessels. The heart is a hollow muscular organ that lies between the lungs in the center of the chest directly behind the sternum. The heart is divided into four chambers: two atria and two ventricles. Blood collected from the veins returning from the various portions of the body enters the right atrium. The blood then passes to the right ventricle from which it is pumped through the pulmonary arteries into the lungs. In the lungs, the blood is oxygenated and passes through the pulmonary vein to the heart where it enters the left atrium. From the left atrium, the blood enters the left ventricle where it is pumped through the aorta to be distributed throughout the system.

The circulatory system is composed of veins and arteries. The pulmonary artery previously mentioned carries blood from the heart to the lungs. The pulmonary vein returns the blood to the heart to be distributed through the aorta, arterioles, and capillaries to the body tissues. The venules, veins, and venae cavae return the blood to the heart to begin the cycle once again.

Blood itself is made up of red blood cells, white blood cells, platelets, and plasma. The red blood cells contain hemoglobin that plays the key role in transporting oxygen to the peripheral tissues. The white blood cells are responsible for the body's defense against microorganisms. Platelets are the component of the blood that cause clotting. The remaining liquid of the blood is called plasma.

The second major component of the circulatory system is the lymphatic system. The lymphatic system is made up of capillaries, vessels, and ducts. It also includes special function tissues, such as the lymph nodes, the spleen, the tonsils, and the thymus. The lymphatic system differs from the circulatory system in that it is a one-way system carrying fluids from the peripheral tissues back to the blood vascular system.

Fluid that has filtered out of the blood capillaries into the peripheral tissues must be returned to the blood stream to maintain the plasma volume of the system. This fluid (lymph) is returned to the blood stream by the lymphatic system. Certain special function tissues add lymphocytes and other antibodies to the lymph that, upon entering the blood stream, will be used to fight various infections.

The Combustion Fuel Supply System--The Respiratory System

All living cells require a constant supply of oxygen to carry out the metabolic processes necessary for life. The metabolic process generates waste in the form of carbon dioxide that must be removed from the system. The respiratory system is responsible for providing the oxygen supply and eliminating carbon dioxide waste.

Air enters the respiratory system through the nose and mouth. Near the middle of the nasal cavity, a series of bones (turbinates) is present. The turbinates are covered by a mucous membrane surface and serve to condition the incoming air by adding heat and moisture and trapping bacteria and dust. The turbinates are also coated with cilia or hair-like filaments that wave back and forth to help the mucous membrane to clean the incoming air. The nasal cavity has several small openings that lead to eight sinuses. The sinuses function to equalize the air pressure in the nasal cavity.

The conditioned air that has entered through the nasal cavity passes into the pharynx and into the trachea (windpipe). The opening to the trachea is blocked by the epiglottis during swallowing to prevent food from entering the respiratory system. The trachea divides into the right and left bronchi that further divide and subdivide many times before entering the bronchiole that end in tiny air sacs called alveoli. Each alveolus has a thin membrane wall surrounded by a network of blood capillaries.

Oxygen is supplied to the body tissue by the air that is inspired and passed through the respiratory system to the alveoli. The oxygen within the alveoli diffuses across the membranes and attaches to the hemoglobin in the blood. The blood carries hemoglobin to the various cells of the body where it is used to burn glucose for energy. The waste product of this metabolism, carbon dioxide, is released and carried in the blood stream back to the lungs. Carbon dioxide is transported by attaching to the hemoglobin in the same manner as oxygen and also by entering into a solution with the blood itself. The carbon dioxide is released to the environment from the lungs during expiration.

The primary moving force of the lungs is the diaphragm, a large group of muscle fibers and tendons separating the thorax from the abdomen. When the muscles of the diaphragm contract, the chest cavity is increased; and a partial vacuum is created within the chest that causes air to flow into the trachea, bronchi, and alveoli. Expiration occurs when the diaphragm muscles relax, thus squeezing the lungs and forcing the air out. This respiration normally occurs at a rate of approximately twelve to eighteen respirations per minute, depending on the activity of the individual. The carbon dioxide level within the blood triggers the respiration rate. As a high carbon dioxide level is sensed, the respiration rate increases.

The Filtering System--The Renal System

The renal system or urinary system controls the production and elimination of waste fluids from the body. The system consists of the kidney, bladder, and excretory passages. The kidney acts as a filter for removal of toxic and waste substances from the blood stream. It also is important to the maintenance of the salt and water balance and acid-base balance within the human system.

The bladder serves as a storage area for waste liquids. From the bladder the waste material passes out of the body.

The Defense Systems--Skin and Sense Organs

As is evident from the above, the human system is a complicated group of subsystems that function in unison to permit life. This system must remain in a delicate balance called homeostasis in order to survive. Many dangers in the outside environment can act to modify this system balance, in some cases to the point where the system goes out of control, and life ceases to exist.To protect the body from these outside influences, nature has provided a series of defensive mechanisms that act in various ways to insure that life goes on. The major components of this defensive system are the skin, with its various layers, and the sense organs, including the eyes, tongue, ears, and nose. Other organs of the body such as the liver and the kidney also provide protection to the body as a part of their normal function. The detoxification action of the liver and kidney has been previously discussed. The maintenance of the delicate system balance by the autonomic nervous system and the involuntary muscles as a defense against such hazards as heat or cold has also been discussed. In this section, the sense organs and the skin as defensive mechanisms will be discussed.

The eye, which enables man to see, is the first of these defensive systems. To make vision possible, the structures of the eye convert light rays to nerve impulses that are then transmitted directly to the brain. Since the distance between the eye and the brain is so short, the reaction time between sight and action is quick. The eye itself is protected by a system of lachrymal glands and ducts that secrete tears and convey them to the surface of the eye to remove foreign matter before damage to the lens mechanism occurs. The dilation and constriction of the pupil, controlled by the autonomic nervous system and the involuntary muscles of the eye, allow for sight in areas where limited or excessive light is present.

The ears provide a second defense for the body. Although the eyes cannot see what is going on behind a person, the ears can hear noises that are generated from any direction. Everyone is aware of what happens to an individual when a loud sound occurs immediately behind him. The ear is the first receptor of the initial signal that a potential danger exists. Upon hearing such a sound, the individual turns so that the eyes might determine if a danger does exist. In addition to providing for hearing, the ear also has the function of maintaining the body's physical balance. This is accomplished within the semicircular canals in the inner ear. Further discussion on the anatomy and physiology of the ear will be presented in a later chapter.

The sense of smell, which originates in the <u>olfactory mucosa</u> of the nose, is another defensive mechanism. The sense of smell protects the individual from hazards such as fire or the presence of noxious gases.

The <u>taste</u> buds present on the tongue act as a defensive mechanism and provide the pleasure that accompanies eating a piece of chocolate cake. Certain unpleasant tastes, such as that received from spoiled food, help the individual to protect the digestive system from the invasion of unwanted materials.

The skin is one of the more complex defensive systems in the body. In addition to providing the outer covering that holds the tissues together, it protects against the loss of fluid and heat. The skin acts as the principal barrier between man and the hazards that exist within the environment. Through nerve receptors in the skin, communication between man and the environment is maintained. The skin is made up of the <u>epidermis</u> or outer surface, the <u>dermis</u> or inner surface, <u>hair</u> and <u>hair follicles</u>, <u>sebaceous glands</u> for secretion of oil, <u>sweat glands</u> for secretion of sweat, <u>nerve receptors</u>, <u>fat</u>, <u>small muscles</u>, and <u>blood vessels</u>. Through the skin man is able to experience sensations of pain, touch, heat or absence of heat, traction or pinching, and tickling. The reflex action that occurs when someone touches a hot surface is an example of one of the ways the skin acts as a protection to the body. The sebaceous glands secrete oil that acts as a protective layer to the skin and prohibits the entry of potentially hazardous substances into the body.

In today's modern world we tend to overlook the fact that the sense organs provide primary protection to the human body. However, if one can put himself in place of prehistoric man, the protection provided by these sense organs becomes much clearer. The primary purpose of sight in prehistoric man was not to watch television or read the newspaper but to survey his environment and determine if any dangers were lurking therein. In the same manner, the primary purpose of hearing was not to listen to a politician's speech or to enjoy a symphony orchestra but rather to listen for sounds that indicated the presence of danger. Though these sense organs have found other uses today, they are still important in the defense of the human system.

Other Systems--Reproductive and Chemical Control

For completeness, it is important that two other major systems of the body, the <u>reproductive system</u> and the <u>endocrine system</u>, be mentioned. The reproductive system obviously allows man to continue in existence through the reproduction of the human species. The endocrine system provides the chemical control for the human system.

The endocrine system and the reproductive system are linked together, since many of the organs that are important for reproduction are also important in providing for the chemical balance of the human system. The endocrine system is a very complicated system, the operation of which is not totally understood. We do know that this system of glands exerts a profound influence on man, his activities, and the metabolic processes within the human body. Some of the functions that the endocrine system performs are:

A.   Regulation of growth, development, and sexual maturation of the young.
B.   Regulation of water excretion and retention.
C.   Regulation of electrolyte salt balance.
D.   Regulation of lactation for the new mother.
E.   Regulation of sexual development, activity, and reproduction.
F.   Regulation of body composition and ability to adapt and resist stress.

The major glands of the endocrine system are the pituitary gland, which acts to regulate growth, water balance, and electrolyte salt balance in the blood; the thyroid, which controls metabolic processes and the rate of metabolic processes; the adrenals, which assist the body in coping with stress; and the gonads, or ovaries and testes, which are essential in the development of secondary sex characteristics.

Summary

The industrial hygiene engineer is required to communicate with medical personnel concerning health problems of workers that may be related to an occupational exposure. During such communications, it is necessary for the industrial hygienist to be familiar with the terminology related to the human system as well as to have a basic understanding of the functions performed by the various systems within the human body. With this information, the industrial hygiene engineer has a basis for determining the relationship between the conditions exhibited by the worker and the potential exposure to a particular occupational hazard.

4. Industrial Toxicology

Introduction

As was pointed out in the last chapter, the human system exists in a delicate balance. As the human body functions within the environment, it is constantly being assaulted with many foreign substances and physical phenomena. This is especially the case when the human is working within the industrial environment where many foreign substances and physical phenomena exist in highly concentrated forms because of the work that is being performed. Some of these substances and phenomena present a potential danger to the human system; many are harmless; and a large category of substances and phenomena exist for which the results are not yet in.

Some of the major defense mechanisms that protect the human system were discussed in the previous chapter. These defensive mechanisms are useful when the concentration of potentially hazardous materials is relatively low. However, in the industrial environment where high concentrations of such materials may exist, the defense mechanisms of the human system often fail to provide adequate protection for the body. Thus, a hazard exposure exists for the worker.

The industrial hygiene engineer should consider certain major factors when attempting to determine the hazardous effect of a material of phenomenon. The first of these considerations is the type of substance or phenomenon. Some materials are inherently more dangerous than others. Many substances in the industrial environment are materials for which either no potential hazard has been proved or no hazard exists. A previous discussion pointed out that for those materials and phenomena judged to be hazardous, there exist varying levels of effect on the human system. For example, though carbon tetrachloride and asbestos are both toxic materials, one would not likely consider carbon tetrachloride in the same classification as asbestos in terms of toxicity.

The next major consideration in determining the hazardous effect of a material or phenomenon is the route of entry of the hazardous material into the human system. The route by which the hazardous material enters the human body can have a relationship to the reaction of the body to the material. Certainly those materials that enter the body through the respiratory system are generally more difficult to handle and present a significantly greater potential danger to the worker than those materials that are hazardous when touched by the worker's unprotected skin.

The amount of exposure or concentration of the material or phenomenon is also important. Too much of anything can be hazardous. For example, although water is not hazardous in normal amounts, it is certainly likely that physical harm will occur to an individual who is submerged in water without breathing apparatus for over six minutes. A general rule in terms of the amount of exposure is that the more toxic the material or phenomenon, the less exposure the human system can tolerate.

Quite often the duration of the exposure is also important. Again using the water problem, submersion for thirty seconds is not likely to cause a problem, while submersion from four to six minutes can result in drowning. Quite often the duration of exposure that can be tolerated by the human system is not known. Presently much controversy surrounds the hazard potential of a short exposure to asbestos or vinyl chloride in the air.

With deference to the Declaration of Independence, not all men (and women) are created equal, particularly in terms of their ability to withstand exposure to hazardous materials. Individuals often respond differently as a result of their age, sex, and general overall health. As an individual ages, his or her ability to withstand long exposures to high temperatures lessens. The same result can be expected for individuals who are in poor physical condition.

Another reason that individual responses might not be the same for a given hazard is that each individual may have other interfaces with the environment which affect that person's response to a particular substance or phenomenon. In the example of heat tolerance, it may be that a particular individual, through other circumstances or jobs, has become acclimatized and thus has a higher tolerance for the hot environment. On the other hand, there may exist synergistic effects, as in the relationship between alcohol and certain barbituates, which has been well publicized as the apparent cause of death for a number of Hollywood celebrities. Again returning to the effects of thermal stress, the worker who was on a "binge" the night before is more likely to be adversely affected by exposure to heat than if the evening had been spent with the family.

Toxicology

The study of industrial toxicology involves the study of chemical agents that are found in the industrial environment and that are thought to cause potentially harmful effects on the function of the human system. Many substances have been known to be toxic for hundreds of years: for example, lead and mercury. Other substances have only recently been identified as toxic: for example, asbestos, coke gases, and vinyl chloride. Many substances have been identified as potentially toxic, although no cause-and-effect relationship has yet been determined. And with the rate of entry of new chemicals into the industrial environment, it is likely that harmful effects exist for many chemicals that have not been studied at all.

How does one determine whether a substance is toxic or not? Obviously it is not desirable for this determination to wait until proved harmful effects to the human system have been exhibited by a number of individuals who have been exposed to the substance. As a result, the determination of toxicity is dependent upon animal studies. In these studies, certain animals--quite often rabbits, rats, or primates--are exposed to the substances under study, and the dose-response relationship is determined. In more preliminary studies, the response to be identified is cessation of life in the test animal. Other studies may be conducted for the pathological changes in the major organs, such as the liver and kidney, of such animals. Two terms are used by toxicologists to identify the dose-response results obtained from a study. The first of these is the dose which will produce death in fifty percent of the dose animals. This value is abbreviated in the following manner: LD_{50}. The value is the best estimate that can be made based upon the results of the study, and it is obtained statistically. The second major term is used to designate the concentration in air that may be expected to kill fifty percent of the animals exposed for a specified length of time. This statistical estimate is abbreviated as LC_{50}.

The results of toxicological studies are presented using the same general format and providing the same types of data. The data that are important in a toxicological study are as follows:

A.   Compound--the material that is under study and was used in the test.

B.   Animal used--a description of the animal that was used in the study.

C.   Route of administration--how the material under study was administered to the animal. This may have involved inhalation in an exposure chamber, administration of an oral dose, or an intraperitoneal injection (normally abbreviated ip).

D.   Transport medium--the material in which the test material was mixed for administration.

E. LD_{50} or LC_{50}--the dose rate that was administered that yielded the fifty percent mortality.

F.   Time period elapsed--the time period that elapsed after the mortality count was made to establish the LD_{50} or the LC_{50}.

G.   Confidence limits--since the dose-response is statistically determined, it is necessary that confidence limits be placed on the dose administered.

The results of such studies provide a basis for determining the relative toxicity of a given material when compared to other materials. The following table, which is reproduced from a table presented in The Industrial Environment: Its Evaluation and Control, NIOSH, 1973 (page 63), presents an overview of the relative toxicity classes as found in toxicological study reports. The nomenclature has been developed to prevent confusion concerning the use of terms such as toxic, nontoxic, and mildly toxic. The table presented assumes the subject of study to be rats. The dose-response for a different subject can differ from that presented in the table.

Table 1.4.1

Toxicity classes for LC_{50}/LD_{50} studies.

Toxicity Rating	Descriptive Term	LD_{50}-Wt/kg Single Oral Dose Rats	4 hr. Inhalation LC_{50}--PPM Rats
1	Extremely toxic	1 mg or less	< 10
2	Highly toxic	1-50 mg	10-100
3	Moderately toxic	50-500 mg	100-1,000
4	Slightly toxic	0.5-5 g	1,000-10,000
5	Practically nontoxic	5-15 g	10,000-100,000
6	Relatively harmless	15 g or more	> 100,000

Exposure Routes of Toxic Materials and Protective Mechanisms That Exist

One route by which exposure to hazardous materials may occur is the oral route. Hazardous materials may enter the body as a result of handling materials prior to eating or smoking. It is possible that hazardous materials may be ingested in large amounts accidentally; however, this is of minor concern in considering the working environment. As parents are aware, this route becomes very important when considering the exposure of small and inquisitive children to hazardous materials.

In general, absorption in the system through the oral route is low. The major danger is the corrosive action to the gastrointestinal tract. The low absorption of materials ingested through the oral route is a result of the protection offered by the poor permeability of the gastrointestinal lining to many hazardous substances.

The major area of concern for the industrial hygiene engineer is with those materials that may enter the body through the respiratory tract. Much of the industrial hygiene engineer's work involves determining the concentration of hazardous pollutants that exist in the air of the work environment. This emphasis of concern is justified both in terms of the hazardous effect of respirable toxic substances on the human system and the ubiquitous nature of toxic substances that become suspended in the air.

The dose rate for respirable toxic substances is difficult to determine. The respiration rate and depth between individuals varies. This is particularly the case when, in a given work place, some individuals remain sedentary, and others are required to do more physical labor, thus increasing the respiration rate and depth. In addition, the concentration of pollutants in the air may vary at different locations of the work environment. Concentrations can also build up and reach peaks based upon production cycles that occur in the work environment. The variance in concentration as a result of location and time make the measurement of the pollutant difficult. This subject was discussed in Chapter 2.

Certain protective mechanisms in the respiratory system provide a first line of defense against toxic materials that may be inspired. Soluble gases are absorbed in the moist mucous membrane of the upper respiratory tract, thus limiting their effect to that of an irritant in this area of the respiratory system. Particulate matter is filtered out of the respiratory system at various stages. The nasal structure and turbulent air flow that results cause the settling of large particles that are then captured by the mucous membrane of the nose. The cilia, small hair-like filaments in the nose and upper respiratory tract, help the mucus filter particulate matter from incoming air. The large number of branches that occur in the bronchi also act to filter out large particulate matter. Usually, only the smallest particles will reach the alveoli of the lung. These particles are of a diameter of less than 10 micrometers. Once these particles have reached the lowest level of the lungs, phagocytic cells (macrophages) entrap the particles to slow their potential harmful action in the body. Some particles are filtered out of the system through the lymph that circulates in the lymphatic system.

The most common route of exposure that exists in the industrial environment is the action of toxic substances on the skin. Substances coming in contact with the skin may react with the skin, causing a dermatitis in the worker, or the material may be absorbed through the skin into the human system. Though dermatitis is unsightly, it is not nearly so severe as the harmful effects that can occur through respiration of toxic material. Only very toxic materials that are systemic in nature are likely to cause harm by absorption through the skin.

The skin has certain protective mechanisms that inhibit exposure to toxic material through this route. The first mechanism is the multiple layers of skin that provide a less permeable surface. Perspiration from the sweat glands will dilute toxic substances that come in contact with the skin. The lipid film left on the skin surface as a result of the action of the sebaceous glands also provides a protective layer that must be penetrated. A breakdown of any of these protective mechanisms will cause a more serious hazard exposure to exist. Thus, if the oily film is removed by cutting oils, or if a break in the skin occurs through a wound, the danger to the worker of exposure through the cutaneous route is much higher.

Another route of entry for toxic materials into the body route is through the eyes. In a toxic environment, the eyes are subjected to splashing of toxic material. In addition, mists, vapors, or gases will also act upon the eyes. The first protective mechanism available to prevent harm to the eyes is the eyelids, which can be closed to prevent damage to the eyes. The second line of defense is the lachrymal action of the tear ducts, which act to dilute or wash away any harmful substances. In general, any damaging effects from ocular exposure to a hazardous material are limited to the area of the eye.

The Physiological Classification of Toxic Materials in Air

Toxic materials in the air produce many physiological responses in the human system. The following discussion presents a system for classifying toxic materials in terms of the physiological response obtained. This system, though generally accepted, is somewhat arbitrary, since the type of physiological response depends on the dose concentration of the toxic material. The system is based on The Industrial Environment: Its Evaluation and Control, NIOSH, 1973 (pp. 70-73).

1. Irritants. An irritant can cause inflammation of the mucous membrane of the respiratory tract. Toxic materials can be either primary irritants, where inflammation is the major physiological reaction (for example, acids), or the toxic materials may be secondary irritants. Secondary irritants, along with causing inflammation of the respiratory tract, also result in more serious toxic action to the human system. Examples of secondary irritants include hydrogen sulfide and many of the aromatic hydrocarbons.

2. Asphyxiants. Asphyxiants deprive the cells of the body of their oxygen supply. Simple asphyxiants are inert elements that, in sufficient quantity, exclude oxygen from the body. Examples of simple asphyxiants include nitrogen, carbon dioxide, and helium. Chemical asphyxiants act in the body to limit the use or availability of an adequate oxygen supply. Examples of chemical asphxyiants are carbon monoxide and cyanides. The action of carbon monoxide in attaching to the hemoglobin of the body, thus disabling the transport of oxygen, is well known.

3. Anesthetics. Anesthetics act to depress the central nervous system. The most common example of an anesthetic is alcohol. Other anesthetics include acetylene hydrocarbons, ethyl ether, paraffin hydrocarbons, and aliphatic ketones.

4. Hepatotoxic Agents. Hepatotoxic agents damage the normal functioning of the liver. Examples of hepatotoxic agents are carbon tetrachloride, tetrachloroethane, nitrosamines, and certain compounds of plant origin.

5. Nephrotoxic Agents. Nephrotoxic agents damage the functioning of the kidney. Examples of nephrotoxic agents include some halogenated hydrocarbons and uranium.

6. Neurotoxic Agents. Neurotoxic agents damage the nervous system. Examples of neurotoxic agents include organo-metallic compounds such as methyl mercury and tetraethyl lead and carbon disulfide.

7. Blood Damaging Agents. Blood damaging agents break down the red blood cells or chemically affect the hemoglobin in the blood. Examples of blood damaging agents include benzene, arsine, and aniline.

8.   <u>Lung Damaging Agents</u>. Lung damaging agents produce their effect on
the pulmonary tissue. This effect goes beyond the irritant action
that certain acids and other materials produce. Examples of lung
damaging agents are silica, asbestos, coal dust, and organic dusts.

The Physical Classification of Toxic Materials

There are four major categories for the physical classification of toxic
materials. These classifications are gases and vapors, particulate matter,
liquids, and solids. The latter two, liquids and solids, though a concern of
the industrial hygiene engineer, do not pose nearly the problem that is posed
by gases and vapors and particulate matter.

A <u>gas</u> is defined as a material that exists in natural form as a gas at
25°C and 760 mm Hg. Gases are normally compressible, formless fluids which
occupy the space of an enclosure and which can be changed to the liquid or
solid state only by the effect of increased pressure or decreased temperature
or both. On the other hand, a <u>vapor</u> is the gaseous stage of a material that
is a liquid or solid in its natural state at 25°C and 760 mm Hg, and which can
be changed to these states either by increasing the pressure or decreasing the
temperature alone.

The next physical classification of toxic materials is <u>particulate</u>
<u>matter</u>. Particulate matter is generally in the form of an <u>aerosol</u>: i.e., a
dispersion of solid or liquid particles in a gas. There are five major types
of aerosols that can exist. These are as follows:

A.   Smoke--aerosol mixture that results from incomplete combustion of
carbonaceous material such as coal, tar, oil, tobacco, etc.

B.   Fog--high concentrations of very fine droplets that are more
frequently airborne.

C.   Mist--a dispersion of liquid droplets generated by condensation from
the gaseous to the liquid state or by breaking up a liquid into a
dispersion such as by splashing, foaming, and atomizing, many of
which are individually visible.

D.   Fume--solid particles created by condensation from a gaseous state,
generally as a result of volatilization of molten metal or by
chemical reaction such as oxidation.

E.   Dust--particles that result from a mechanical action on a solid
(handling, crushing, grinding, and detonation of organic and
inorganic materials such as rock, metal, coal, wood, etc.)

The physical classification of toxic materials is important both in the
methods that are used to evaluate the level of contaminants in the atmosphere
and in the control methods that are available to remove the contaminants.
Controlling gases and vapors is a different problem from attempting to remove
particulate matter from the air.

Summary

Determining the toxicity of a substance is not simple. Many substances exist for which no determination of toxicity has been made. For those materials for which toxic determinations have been made, the determination in the great majority of cases has been as a result of animal studies in which the LD_{50} or LC_{50} has been determined. Even in these cases, the toxic effect on humans is not necessarily clearly identified. Many factors such as individual differences, duration of exposure, other interfaces with the environment, and the route of entry are important in determining the toxic effect of a particular material.

Toxic substances may enter the human through a number of routes. Entry may be oral, through the respiratory tract, through the skin, or through the eyes. The major concern of most industrial hygiene work is the entry of toxic materials through the respiratory tract. Thus, materials in the form of gases, vapors, and aerosols are the targets of most industrial hygiene engineering studies. However, in certain cases other routes of entry are important; and the toxicity of liquids and solids must be considered.

Once in the body, toxic materials act in different ways to harm the system. Among the various actions of toxic materials are irritant action, asphyxiant action, and anesthetic action. In many cases it is through the resulting action and the symptoms exhibited by the worker that the particular substance involved can be identified.

5. Physical Hazards

Introduction

The hazards that the worker encounters in the work environment can be classified into three major groupings. The first grouping includes the toxic hazards that are a result of a chemical action on the human system. These toxic hazards were covered in the last chapter. The second major classification involves physical hazards. Physical hazards are a result of a physical force that is exerted on the human body by some action within the work environment. A third classification of hazards, which we shall call other hazards, includes psychological and biological stresses placed on the human system.

In this chapter, we will discuss briefly the various types of physical hazards and other hazards that the worker encounters. The effect of physical hazards on the worker may be twofold. Certain physical hazards may damage the health of the worker. Also, the worker may receive traumatic injury as a result of exposure to a physical hazard. Those physical hazards that produce the possibility of traumatic injury are generally considered to be within the realm of responsibility of the safety professional. However, the traumatic injury may be secondary to a toxic hazard or a physical hazard that exists in the work environment. For example, exposure to many of the aliphatic halogenated hydrocarbons can disorient a worker, thus making the worker subject to potential traumatic injury. This situation may occur even though the exposure level of the toxic substance is insufficient to cause a chronic or acute toxic reaction in the worker.

In the following paragraphs, the various types of physical and other hazards will be discussed. For each hazard, its characteristics and effect on the human system will be covered. Where protection mechanisms of the human system are brought into action, those protective mechanisms will also be presented. Each of the following hazards will be covered:

Physical Hazards

A. Noise
B. Vibration
C. Ionizing and nonionizing radiation
D. Thermal
E. Mechanical
F. Pressure
G. Illumination
H. Traumatic

Other Hazards

    A.   Biological
    B.   Psychological

Physical Hazards--Noise

When one first enters an industrial plant, the first impression received is usually that of the presence or absence of high levels of noise. Certain operations are noisy by nature.

The level of noise in an industrial operation can constitute a physical hazard to the exposed workers. The extent of hazard depends not only on the overall noise level, but also on the time period for which the worker is exposed, the frequency of the noise to which the worker is exposed, and the type of noise: i.e., whether it is continuous or intermittent. All these factors must be considered when determining if a noise hazard exists. A more thorough discussion of the determination of the existence of a noise hazard exposure will be presented in the section related to noise.

The existence of a noise exposure can have various effects on the worker. First, the worker who is exposed to a high-level noise for a short period of time can exhibit a temporary hearing threshold shift. This hearing threshold shift is a loss in hearing that can be recovered within a short time after removal of the noise source. In general, most of this recovery occurs within one to two hours of exposure, with complete recovery occurring in approximately 14 to 16 hours. If the worker is continually exposed to the same excessive noise for a long period of time, the temporary hearing threshold shift can become permanent. This permanent hearing loss cannot be recovered by the worker.

Another effect of excessive noise levels is its resultant interference with communication between workers. This interference with communication can be an annoyance to the worker and may result in a lowering of the efficiency of the operation. There also exists the possibility of traumatic injury because of this loss of communication.

Certain temporary physiological changes can occur in the human body when it is exposed to excessive noise levels. For example, the heart rate and blood pressure tend to increase. At present there are no data to indicate that these temporary physiological changes result in any chronic damage to the worker's system.

The temporary hearing loss exhibited when exposed to excessive noise is in itself a protective mechanism. It can serve as a warning to the worker who is temporarily exposed that unless something is done a more permanent hearing loss may be incurred. In addition, when more permanent hearing loss begins to occur, it can be diagnosed in the 3000-6000 Hz frequency range, with most affected persons showing a loss or "dip" at 4000 Hz. If high-level exposures are continued, the loss of hearing will further increase around 4000 Hz and spread to lower frequencies. Periodic audiometric tests can identify threshold shifts in the 3000-6000 Hz frequency range, thus providing for corrective action prior to any hearing loss that might affect the worker's ability to understand voice communication.

Physical Hazards--Vibration

Vibration is often closely associated with noise. One of the reasons for this close association is the fact that generally if a vibration is present, a noise is also present. However, the noise that is present may not be at a level that can cause damage to the worker's hearing, while the vibration may be serious enough to merit concern.

Vibration results in the mechanical shaking of the body or parts of the body. These two types of vibration are called whole-body vibration and segmental vibration. Vibration originates from a mechanical motion generally occurring at some machine or series of machines. This mechanical vibration can be transmitted directly to the body or body part, or it may be transmitted through solid objects to a worker located at some distance away from the actual vibration.

The effect of vibration on the human body is not totally understood. Research has only begun to indicate where problems might exist. Initial research indicates that whole-body vibration increases the physiological activity of the heart and respiration. The results have also shown that there is an inhibition of tendon reflexes as a result of vibration. There seems to be reduced ability on the part of the worker to perform complex tasks, and indications of potential damage to other systems of the body also exist.

More research has been done in the area of segmental vibration, such as that received when using a pneumatic hammer. One recognized indication of the effect of segmental vibration is impaired circulation to the appendage that has been named Raynaud's Syndrome. Such segmental vibration can also result in the loss of the sense of touch in the affected area. There have also been indications of decalcification of the bones in the hand as a result of vibration transmitted to that part of the body. In addition, muscle atrophy has been identified as a result of segmental vibration.

As with noise, the human body can withstand short-term vibration even though this vibration might be extreme. In addition, the dangers of vibration are related to certain frequencies that are resonant with various parts of the body. Vibration outside these frequencies is not nearly so dangerous as vibration that results in resonance.

Physical Hazards--Ionizing and Nonionizing Radiation

Ionizing and nonionizing radiation are becoming increasingly prevalent in the industrial work environment. Ionizing radiation results from electromagnetic radiation with energy sufficient to cause the loss of an electron from the matter with which it interacts. Nonionizing radiation is caused by rays from the electromagnetic spectrum having energy which is insufficient to cause the loss of an electron. Ionizing radiation includes X-, gamma, alpha, beta, and neutron rays. Nonionizing radiation is caused by ultraviolet, infrared, laser, and microwave rays from the electromagnetic spectrum.

The effects of nonionizing radiation on the human are not well documented. However, some major effects that have been identified include damage to the eye and its ability to function, damage to the reproductive system, and burns of the skin. Ionizing radiation can produce skin burns as well as deep tissue burns for certain types of ionizing radiation. Ionizing radiation can also produce chronic effects on the human system. For example, ionizing radiation has certain carcinogenic and gene-damaging properties that can affect the long-term health of the exposed individual and potentially his or her progeny. Ionizing radiation can occur as both an external and an internal exposure in the human. External exposure can occur as a result of unprotected proximity to gamma rays or X-rays. Internal exposure results from inspired radioactive material that can cause tissue damage in the lungs and transmit damage throughout the human system by way of the blood stream.

The body has very little protection against radiation. The skin acts as a protective mechanism for small doses of both ionizing and nonionizing radiation. The normal phagocytic action that occurs in the lungs for respirable dust is not nearly so effective a protective mechanism for inspired radioactive materials as it is for other respirable dusts.

Physical Hazards--Thermal

Workers may be exposed to thermal hazards involving extreme heat, extreme cold, or rapid changes in temperature. Most exposures involve workers in high temperature areas. However, those exposures related to cold and rapid change in temperature can also exist.

There are various effects of high temperature on the worker as well as a number of factors that affect the individual's response to exposure to high temperatures. Among the important factors are the age of the individual, the surface-area-to-weight ratio of the individual, and the acclimatization that the individual has attained. The ability to withstand high temperatures while performing work lowers in older workers. As an individual becomes more obese, his ability to withstand temperatures is also lowered. Individuals working in a hot area will be more effective when they have had a chance to become acclimatized to the heat. Another factor that affects the human's response to heat is the amount of physical activity performed while subjected to the hot environment. As the physical activity increases, the time that a given temperature can be tolerated without adverse effect decreases.

Certain physiological changes in the body result from exposure to extreme heat. The first of these is the loss of salt that occurs because of perspiration. In addition to this loss of salt, a loss of body water and dehydration occur. The sweat glands can exhibit fatigue after prolonged exposure to high temperature. Also, because of the dilation of blood vessels near the surface of the skin, a pooling of blood in the extremities can occur.

The physiological changes in the body can result in various heat illnesses. These illnesses are as follows:

A. Heat cramps--painful spasms of the muscles as a result of hard work during exposure to high temperature.

B. Heat exhaustion--the worker experiences fatigue, nausea, and headache. The worker may lose consciousness from heat exhaustion.

C. Heat stroke--generally results in mental confusion or loss of consciousness and can result in convulsions and coma if left untreated. Shock can result because blood pools in the blood vessels of the extremities.

D. Skin rash--a body rash resulting from the inflammatory reaction of the skin to perspiration and the plugging of the sweat glands.

Exposures to extreme cold can result in frostbite occurring in exposed areas of the body. In addition, long-term exposure to cold temperatures can lower the core temperature of the body, thus presenting a more acute danger to human life.

The human body can regulate its internal body temperature within narrow limits by perspiration and dilation and constriction of the blood vessels. The variation in blood vessel size occurs to cause blood to flow to the surface for cooling in the case of high temperature and to restrict flow in the case of low temperature. In addition, after exposure to high temperatures, the worker can become acclimatized, thus allowing the body to withstand hard work at high temperatures with less chance of adverse effects. The muscle movement or shivering that occurs in cold temperature is a reaction of the body to attempt to generate heat within the body tissue.

Physical Hazards--Mechanical

Mechanical hazards can occur when stress is placed on the musculoskeletal system beyond the limits that the system can endure. This stress can be the result of a blow, a constant pulling, or a pushing on the body structure. Mechanical stress can also be caused as a result of fatigue in the muscles that results in the worker performing tasks in an improper manner, thus causing undue stress to be placed on the body structure.

Mechanical hazards can result in traumatic injury. For example, the most likely effect of a blow to the body is a traumatic injury. Another example is the worker who is required to lift heavy objects repeatedly, thus becoming fatigued. As the worker becomes fatigued, the probability increases that he will drop one of the objects or cause damage to another part of his body by improper lifting.

Chronic disabilities can result from mechanical hazards. Workers who are required to maintain a particular position for prolonged periods of time can develop chronic ailments of the vertebrae or joints that are affected by the required position.

Fatigue is a protective mechanism the body employs to prevent mechanical damage from occurring. If the worker can heed the fatigue signals and rest, the likelihood of injury occurring is lessened. Body muscles, when allowed to rest, have great recuperative powers. To take advantage of these recuperative powers, however, it is necessary that the worker be given sufficient rest time for the muscles to regenerate.

Physical Hazards--Pressure

The exposure of workers to abnormal pressures is generally limited to a few occupational areas. Two of the most obvious of these are the individuals who work as sand hogs constructing tunnels under bodies of water, and individuals working in diving apparatus. In both of the above cases, the workers are exposed to higher-than-atmospheric pressures. It is possible that workers can be exposed to lower-than-atmospheric pressure. This may become more prevalent in the future as space travel expands.

At high pressures, workers may experience an acute syndrome called "oxygen poisoning." Nitrogen poisoning, which has a narcotic effect on the body, can also occur at high pressures. The most commonly known effect of high pressure is the necessity to decompress the workers from the high pressure to normal atmospheric pressure. If decompression is not handled properly, the worker develops decompression sickness, otherwise known as "the bends." High pressures can act on the fluids and tissue of the body to compress these fluids and tissue into the cavities of the body, such as the sinuses.

Low pressure can result in an oxygen deficiency to the body; also, the expansion of gases into the cavities of the body is noticed under low pressure. Such expansion of gases can cause severe pain. In addition, the worker entering a low-pressure area is, in effect, being decompressed and is thus subjected to the same decompression sickness that occurs during decompression from high pressures.

The body attempts to adjust for low pressures by increasing the number of red blood cells in the blood at higher altitudes, thus allowing for increased oxygen transported to the tissues. At low pressure, respiration will increase, thus bringing more oxygen to the respiratory system. In addition, individuals can become acclimatized to low pressures, especially in the case of low pressure at high altitudes.

Physical Hazards--Illumination

Inadequate illumination is a hazard to the worker and can cause a number of detrimental effects. Eyestrain can develop if the worker is required to perform close and exacting work with inadequate illumination. In addition to eyestrain, inadequate illumination can also cause errors and reduced efficiency. Attempts to compensate for these errors and reduced efficiency can increase the chance for traumatic injuries. In poorly illuminated areas, the potential for accidents is high.

The body's basic protective mechanism to adjust for low illumination is dilation of the pupils. This mechanism does not react quickly; an individual subjected to a glare or a quick change in the amount of illumination will not react immediately. These changes in illumination and the presence of glare, therefore, result in the individual being subjected to a period of time during which vision is inadequate. During this period, the probability of traumatic injury increases greatly.

Physical Hazards--Traumatic

The number of potential causes of traumatic injury to the worker are legion. Some of these, such as changes in illumination and fatigue, have been mentioned. Four general causes of traumatic injury can be stated. In some cases, these causes may be secondary to a primary cause. The first of these is the potential for fire and explosion. The primary result of a fire or an explosion is injury to the individuals in close proximity. The second potential cause of traumatic injury is through mechanical means. This can . occur when an individual interfaces with a piece of machinery such as a radial saw or punch press. A third major cause of physical injury involves the interface of the individual with electrical systems. Finally, the worker may be injured as a result of a structural failure, such as when a ladder breaks or the worker falls on a slippery floor.

The obvious effects of traumatic injury are the physical damage that the body incurs as well as the possibility of death. Organizationally, the effects of traumatic injury are felt in terms of property damage and the cost of lost-time injuries on the part of the workers.

As opposed to the health hazards that are faced, the individual worker has adequate protection to avoid many of the potential traumatic injuries that are encountered. This protection exists in the proper use of the senses of the body. The worker must learn to identify through sight, sound, smell, touch, and taste those factors in the work environment that can result in an unsafe situation. However, the amount of concentration required on the part of the worker to do this consistently makes these protective mechanisms only partially useful.

Other Hazards--Biological

Biological hazards consist of exposure to bacteria, viruses, and parasites. This exposure can be a direct result of the work being performed or the result of unhealthy conditions in the work environment. The obvious example of exposure as a result of the work being performed is the worker in the hospital whose job requires contact with various communicable diseases. Exposure in the work environment can result from unsanitary conditions in rest rooms, eating areas, and locker rooms. The obvious result of biological exposures is the illness of the worker and the transmission of the disease to other associated workers.

The body has an internal mechanism that creates white blood cells to fight infections. In addition, the individual can be protected from many diseases by immunization, which produces antibodies that protect against possible future infection of a particular disease. Since immunization is disease specific, it is not a cure-all protective device.

Other Hazards--Psychological

Consideration has only recently been given to psychological job stress. Workers may be affected psychologically by pressures that are inherent within the job or pressures that exist outside the job. Endogenous pressures include such things as unrealistic production schedules, demanding management, and unclear directions concerning the work to be performed. Exogenous factors include the worker's peer group relationship, the general atmosphere in which the work is accomplished, and the person's satisfaction with his home life.

Research is only beginning in this area of job stress. No conclusions have been reached, although many hypotheses have been put forth. There currently is a feeling that psychological stress can result in physiological changes in the body. Behavior changes are also hypothesized. It is felt that some workers develop somatic complaints and become ill as a result of psychological stresses. There does appear to be some correlation between individuals under psychological stress and the accident rate encountered by individuals in similar jobs.

Man adjusts and makes decisions. As a result of this fact, individuals will tend to modify their behavior patterns when faced with psychological stress. This modification of behavior patterns can result in a lower stress on the worker involved. In addition, workers faced with undue psychological stress will tend to self-select out of the job, thus removing themselves from the hazard. This, however, does not prohibit other workers from entering into the same job and facing the same psychological stress.

Summary

It is evident from the previous discussion that a given worker can face many potential physical hazards while performing his work. In any given situation, not all of these hazards are important. In fact, certain groups of jobs encounter only a few of the hazards that have been mentioned. It is the job of the industrial hygienist or safety professional to identify the hazards that the worker faces on a given job and to take action to control the worker's exposure to these hazards.

Although certain protective mechanisms do help the human system adapt to its surroundings, these protective systems operate only within a small range. It should be remembered that a hazard exists when the stress placed on the human system cannot be compensated for by the internal mechanisms of the system without resulting in strain. In such a situation, it is the responsibility of the industrial hygienist or safety professional to remove the stress or to cause it to be lowered to such a level that the compensating mechanism within the human system will provide protection without strain on the workers.

6. General Methods of Control Available to the Industrial Hygiene Engineer

Introduction

In the previous chapters, the role of the industrial hygiene engineer in recognizing and evaluating the industrial environment has been discussed. This chapter will deal with the general methods of control available to the industrial hygiene engineer when he is faced with the necessity to control a hazard exposure.

The job of the industrial hygiene engineer involves four major functions. These functions are:

A. <u>Recognition</u> of potential hazards in the work environment.

B. <u>Measurement</u> of the work environment to determine the extent of the hazard present and the subsequent evaluation of the measurements obtained to determine if a hazard exists.

C. <u>Identification and recommendation of controls</u> that can be implemented to remove or reduce the hazard exposure of the worker.

D. <u>Anticipation of potential hazards</u>, so these problem hazards can be avoided in the planning stage, if possible.

There are certain principles that relate to the methods that can be used to control hazards. The first principle is that <u>all hazards can be controlled</u> in some manner and to some degree. This is not to say that all hazards are equally easy to control. Some hazard exposures by their very nature present difficult problems to the industrial hygiene engineer. However, through perseverance, exposure to the hazard can be limited. Application of the Golden Rule, "Do unto others as you would have them do unto you," is useful when faced with the temptation to overlook a hazard exposure because of the difficulty required to solve it. As an industrial hygiene engineer, you might put yourself in the worker's shoes: would you be willing to work in the same environment? When you answer this question, you will agree that all hazards can be controlled.

The second general principle relating to the control of hazards is that <u>there are usually many alternate methods of control</u> that are available. As an industrial hygiene engineer, it is your responsibility to identify the alternate methods of control available and to select the most appropriate method. You must resist the temptation to jump to the first solution that is identified.

The third principle is that <u>some methods of control are better than others</u> in a given situation. This principle is almost a corollary to the second principle. In any given situation, there are usually not only many alternate solutions available, but also probably a best solution. The choice is not always easy since there are many factors to consider: the cost of implementation; worker acceptance; enforceability; effect on other operations within the production system; and the continuing operating cost that will be incurred by implementation of the chosen alternative.

The fourth principle of control is that <u>some situations will require more than one control method to obtain optimum results</u>. This is easy to overlook when faced with a problem. Just as there is a tendency to jump to the first solution that is identified, so there is a tendency to use only the single solution chosen as a method of control. Though the chosen solution may improve the situation, it is possible that implementing other alternatives will give greater control of the hazard exposure.

General Methods of Control--Substitution

The first general method of control available to the industrial hygiene engineer is substitution. Substitution can take three forms:

A.   Substitution of materials

B.   Substitution of process

C.   Substitution of equipment

Any one or combination of these forms of substitution may provide a method of control for a given hazard. Referring to the preceding discussion, don't forget that you can substitute using all three forms if necessary to obtain optimum results.

When considering substitution as a method of control, the first question which must be asked is: "Is there a less toxic or flammable material that can do the job?" Given the abundance of materials currently available in the industrial world, substitute material may do the job as well or better than the hazardous material being used. Or it may be necessary to give up some production efficiency to obtain the required control of the hazard exposure to the worker.

Common examples of material substitution include the use of trichloroethylene for carbon tetrachloride and aliphatic chlorinated hydrocarbons for benzene. In each of these cases, the material substituted is less toxic than the original material. In the case of solvents, a further substitution of alkali-and-water detergent solutions may yield equal results with an even greater margin of safety for the worker. Thus, given a particular situation, the material being used might be replaced by another material which involves no hazard exposure.

The second question that might be asked is: "Can the process be changed, thus removing the hazard exposure?" Or worded differently, "Is there a better way to do the job?" It may be possible to change the overall process or some procedures within the process to eliminate the worker's exposure to hazardous materials or operations. One general principle is usually applicable: a continuous operation is generally less hazardous than an intermittent operation.

For example, when spray-painting a part, consider the possibility of changing to an alternative process such as dipping the part in a paint bath or flow coating it. Either of those processes presents less potential contamination by toxic materials in the air. Another example would be the substitution of automated material handling devices for manual or mechanical methods. This substitution has the additional benefit of eliminating costly manual labor. The substitution of closed system continuous processing for batch processing is an example of the general principle stated above. Where containers of toxic materials must be opened and dumped into a system, consider pumping or conveying the toxic materials from the storage area to the process rather than requiring that they be transported and dumped. Another example is the use of wet methods to reduce dust generation in mining and quarrying operations.

The final type of substitution is substitution of equipment. Is there a better type of equipment to do the job? Can engineering changes be made on the existing equipment to make the equipment less hazardous?

Examples of such substitution include the use of machine guarding on existing mechanical equipment and the substitution of automated equipment for manual methods. Adding the catalytic converter to the automobile to reduce the emission of pollutants is an example of making changes to existing equipment that reduce the hazard potential. The next logical step is to develop an automobile that operates on a nonpolluting fuel: for example, an electric or steam automobile. This approach has led to the use of LPG and electric-powered lift trucks in place of gasoline-powered trucks.

General Methods of Control--Isolation of Source

Another method available for controlling hazard exposures is removing the source of the hazard exposure from the worker's environment. This isolation can be accomplished in a number of ways. First, the source of the hazard exposure can be separated from the work area by placing it in another location where the workers are unlikely to come in contact with it. A second method is to enclose or shield the source with physical barriers. Thus, although the source remains in the work area, it is separated from the workers and the work environment. A third method that was briefly mentioned in relation to substitution of equipment and process is to automate the process so that it operates within a closed system. A fourth method of isolation that controls potential exposure from toxic or flammable materials stored in the production area is the removal and storage of these materials in a separate location.

There are many examples of isolation that have been used in industry. Tank farms that are used for storing toxic or flammable materials in areas apart from the work environment are a type of isolation. The automated processes that are used in chemical processing and petroleum refining are also examples. Heat barriers and soundproof enclosures have also been used in industry. Another common type of isolation is the removal of the worker to a control room that is separate from the processing area.

General Methods of Control--Ventilation

Ventilation is a useful method for controlling the air quality and the thermal exposures that the worker encounters. Ventilation can be used to remove air pollutants from the breathing zone of the workers. It can also be used to condition the air for worker comfort. In addition, ventilation systems can be designed to supply air to assure the proper operation of any local exhaust system in use.

There is no single type of ventilation system that solves all problems. Ventilation systems come in different sizes and shapes, depending on the requirements of the process and the hazard exposure that is to be controlled. The various categories of ventilation that can be used are:

A. Comfort ventilation. Comfort ventilation moves and conditions the air to assure the comfort of the workers. It is useful in controlling the amount of heat or cold to which the worker is exposed. Also controlled by comfort ventilation are the humidity level and any unpleasant odors that might be present in the work environment.

B. Local exhaust ventilation. Local exhaust ventilation is used to remove contaminants that are generated at a local source. Air is drawn from a source at a rate capable of removing any air contaminants generated at that source before they can be dispersed into the work environment.

C. Local supply ventilation. Local supply ventilation involves supplying air to a specific point or operation where it is required. Local supply ventilation can be used to provide spot cooling for workers in hot areas, or it can be used as one component of a local push-pull ventilation system.

D. Make-up air. Make-up air is air supplied to the work environment to make up for air that is being exhausted through a local system. Without adequate make-up air, local exhaust systems will not operate effectively.

E. Dilution ventilation. Dilution ventilation supplies or exhausts air from a large area in order to control a pollutant in the total area by diluting the pollutant. In general, dilution ventilation is not applicable to highly toxic hazards and proves to be expensive in order to obtain the desired results.

F. Natural ventilation. Natural ventilation systems use the characteristics of air movement created by thermal differences to attain pollution control without mechanical assistance.

The air-conditioning system within an office building, computer room, or factory is an example of comfort ventilation. Such a system provides for the comfort of the worker by adding or removing heat and moisture from the work environment. Exhaust hoods installed over laboratory benches are examples of local exhaust systems. The push-pull ventilation system used over an open tank to capture pollutants before they enter the work environment is an example of a local supply and local exhaust system. The ventilation system that is installed in a traffic tunnel to eliminate carbon monoxide buildup is an example of a dilution ventilation system. Exhausting polluting materials away from a plant through stacks is an example of both natural ventilation and dilution ventilation.

General Methods of Control--Administrative

General administrative controls are those controls available to the organization that do not directly remove the source of hazard exposure from the workplace. These controls are usually effective when used with one of the other control methods previously outlined. Examples of general administrative controls available include worker training, monitoring the work area or the worker, scheduling workers into the area, good housekeeping, and preventive maintenance scheduling to assure proper functioning of the existing controls.

The training of workers has a valuable, though sometimes overemphasized, part in control of hazard exposures. Through training, workers can be taught to identify potential hazards and report these hazards before an incident occurs. Training can be used to provide workers with methods and procedures that are useful in avoiding hazards and to develop error avoidance behaviors in workers.

Another type of administrative control is monitoring the work area or worker. Continuous monitoring equipment can be placed in the work area. This equipment can sound a warning should the potential hazard exceed limits that can become harmful to the workers. Personnel samplers or dosimeters can also be used to monitor the exposure of the worker when he is required to move in and out of the areas where potential hazards exist.

After-the-fact biological monitoring of workers can be of value in determining if a worker has been exposed to a hazard. This biological monitoring can involve pre- and post-employment medical exams to provide data upon which a comparison can be made. Periodic medical examinations should be scheduled for all workers who must work in potentially hazardous areas of the plant. However, the results of such monitoring occur after exposure and may be too late for the worker involved unless the biological monitoring has the sensitivity to identify symptoms before the worker's body is damaged. Therefore, other control techniques should be implemented.

The rotation of worker schedules can control the exposure of any individual worker. Workers can be rotated in and out of hazardous areas during a shift. Workers can be rescheduled to different areas of the plant after a period of time to control possible cumulative effects of the potential hazard. Workers required to perform extremely physical tasks or to work in hot or cold areas can be given rest periods during which their systems can recover from the exposure. In using this technique caution is required to insure that it does not result in the spreading of serious risk to workers as compared to the institution of permanent corrective action.

Good housekeeping procedures can go a long way to helping control hazards. This includes, but is not limited to, cleanliness of the workplace, waste disposal, healthful drinking water, adequate washing and eating facilities, and control of insects and rodents.

The use of preventive maintenance schedules is a valuable administrative control to eliminate potential hazard exposures. Maintenance on a regularly scheduled basis for potentially hazardous operations is a must. If the worker is to be protected, the system must operate as it was designed to operate. Normal wear can often cause problems to develop that will expose the worker to a hazard that could have been avoided had the equipment been maintained properly. This is also true for any control or monitoring equipment in the workplace. Filters become clogged, fans do not always work as they were designed to work, and monitoring equipment can malfunction.

Other administrative controls that are available include such things as reports and statistics gathered from previous work-related injuries and illnesses and a recognition program that emphasizes regular inspections to identify potential hazard exposures before they become a problem. The existence of adequate emergency aid and emergency procedures can also be used, not as a control of a hazard but as a method to minimize the extent of individual injury and the number of people exposed when an emergency occurs.

General Methods of Control--Personal Protective Equipment

Personal protective equipment should be used only as a last resort and as a temporary measure until more permanent controls can be installed. In somecases there is no immediate alternative but to use personal protective equipment. However, the industrial hygiene engineer should continue to look for other solutions where personal protective equipment is currently being used.

Each type of protective equipment and clothing used should be tested to assure it will do the job for which it was designed. It is also important to be sure the protective equipment and clothing are adequate to provide protection from the hazard. The use of goggles will protect the eyes from damage but will not provide protection for the face. Perhaps a face shield is more appropriate for the potential hazard exposure.

Protective equipment should be designed to provide minimum interference with the job being done. If this is not considered, the worker is likely to discard the protective equipment very quickly and risk being exposed to the hazard. For example, large gloves may interfere with the requirement to perform small psychomotor manipulation of parts. These gloves may be replaced by latex form-fitting gloves that allow the required movements but provide the same protection to the hands.

Personal protective equipment can be categorized as follows:

A.   Skin protection--including gloves, suits, and aprons.

B.   Eye protection--including safety glasses, goggles, face shields, and hoods.

C.   Ear protection--including plugs and ear muffs.

D.   Respiratory protection--including air-purifying respirators, air-supplied respirators, and self-contained breathing units.

E.   Other protection--including safety shoes, diving suits, and environmental control suits.

Determining the Control Method to Use

The first step necessary to determine the appropriate control method(s) to use for a particular hazard is to be sure that the hazard has been identified correctly. You must know what is being controlled to control it effectively. You should be aware of the entry routes that the hazard may take to the human body. The use of the procedures suggested in Chapter 2 should provide the information that is necessary to establish effective control of the hazard.

After the hazard has been identified and described, it is desirable to identify alternate methods for controlling the hazard. The first method selected as a potential control may not necessarily be the best. Alternate methods should be identified. The problem may be such as to require that a combination of controls be implemented to obtain optimum results. Identification of alternate methods can help to point out the possible application of multiple control methods.

After all the potential alternatives have been identified, it is necessary to determine which alternative(s) provide the best solution to the problem. Which alternative is most effective in controlling the worker's exposure to the hazard? What is the cost of implementing the various alternatives, and which is the most cost effective? What are the ongoing and operational costs in terms of maintenance and other requirements? These questions must be asked to determine which of the alternatives is the most appropriate for implementation.

The best alternative should be selected for implementation. Some of the criteria for selection were mentioned above. Quite often the best alternative involves a trade-off between factors.

The next step is to implement the control(s) that have been selected. This implementation should include a series of tests of the system to assure that, upon operation, the controls will provide the protection for which they were designed.

After the system has been implemented and is operating, periodic follow-up is desirable. Inoperable control mechanisms give a false sense of security while exposing the worker to a hazard level even higher than that to which he was exposed prior to the implementation of controls. Changes in procedures and processes can make the controls ineffective. Tests on the system are necessary to assure that the controls are doing the job for which they were designed. A proper preventive maintenance schedule should be instituted. Any rules and procedures that govern the workers should be reviewed for compliance, and enforcement must be uniform to assure that the rules and procedures will be followed.

Anticipation of potential hazards is another way of saying that an integral part of the control procedure is to be involved in the planning stages. Proper design of equipment during plant construction is very important in reducing industrial health problems. Provisions must be made for the safe handling of hazardous materials. The health professional should make sure that he is included in the plan-checking procedures. Then he can discover health and safety hazards and correct conditions that would result in hazardous exposures or unsafe practices. Otherwise such conditions may be built into the facility and its equipment.

Many companies have implemented a system requiring that drawings or specifications be approved by the health professional before use. Hazards involved in making products should be minimized insofar as possible. Instructions and warnings developed for employee use should be reviewed for safe manufacturing procedures. The health professional should also make sure that company policies and applicable standards are followed in purchase specifications for new materials and equipment and for modification of existing equipment.

The engineering department, with the help of the health professional, should check with the purchasing department to determine the necessary safety and health measures to be built on or into a machine before it is purchased. The health professional must have as complete a grasp as possible of the occupational disease and accident losses to the company in terms of specific machines, materials and processes. If he is to recommend the expenditure of large sums of money for protection of health to be used throughout the plant, he should have evidence that the investment is justified.

Summary

The industrial hygiene engineer has many methods available for control of hazards in the industrial environment. Using one or more of these methods, it is possible for the industrial hygiene engineer to control to some degree all hazards to which the worker is exposed. The problem becomes one of selecting the control or controls that best provide for the protection of the worker.

The general control methods available to the industrial hygiene engineer include substitution of materials, process, or equipment; isolation of source; ventilation; administrative controls; and personal protective equipment. In many cases, the situation may merit the use of more than one method to provide optimum results in controlling the hazards.

To maximize the potential for success in selecting and implementing the appropriate control method(s), it is desirable that the industrial hygiene engineer use a structured problem-solving approach. Such an approach has been outlined in the chapter.

7. Legal Aspects of Occupational Safety and Health

<u>Introduction</u>

The Occupational Safety and Health Act was signed into law December 29, 1970. Its purposes were to assure safe and healthful working conditions for the nation's working men and women and to preserve human resources. The Act delegated certain major responsibilities and authorities to the Department of Labor:

1. To promulgate, modify, and improve mandatory occupational safety and health standards.

2. To enter plants.

3. To prescribe regulations for maintaining accurate records.

4. To develop and maintain statistics on occupational safety and health.

5. To establish and supervise programs for the education and training of employee and employer personnel.

6. To make grants to states.

Certain other responsibilities and authorities were delegated to the Department of Health, Education, and Welfare (HEW); authority has since been delegated to the Department of Health and Human Services (HHS):

1. To conduct, directly or by grants or contracts, research, experiments, or demonstrations relevant to occupational safety and health.

2. To develop criteria for dealing with toxic materials and harmful physical agents.

3. To make toxicity determinations on request by employer or employee groups.

4. To publish an annual listing of all known toxic substances.

5. To conduct directly, or by grants and contracts, educational programs aimed at providing an adequate supply of qualified personnel.

6. To establish a National Institute for Occupational Safety and Health.

Congress also established several committees to fulfill the provisions of the act: the 12-member National Advisory Committee on Occupational Safety and Health; the Occupational Safety and Health Review Commission to adjudicate disputes; and the National Commission of State Workmen's Compensation Laws to study and evaluate such laws.

The Occupational Safety and Health Act applies directly to all employers except Federal installations and states or political subdivisions of the states. It covers every workplace except those for which other Federal agencies and specified state agencies (such as the Atomic Energy Commission) exercise statutory authority to prescribe and enforce standards and regulations affecting occupational safety and health.

OSHA--Prescribed Duties

The General Duty Clause states that every employer is obligated "...to furnish to each of his employees employment and a place of employment which are free from recognized hazards that are causing or likely to cause death or serious physical harm to his employee."

There are two types of standards defined by the General Duty Clause. The first type, General Standards, is applicable to all employees and is contained in Title 29, Code of Federal Regulations, Part 1910. The second type, Particular Standards, (such as the Safety and Health Regulations for Construction) which is applicable to specific industries and is contained in Title 29, Code of Federal Regulations, Part 1518.

Inspections

The Act contains a general prohibition against giving advance notice of inspection, except in limited circumstances:

1.   In cases of apparent imminent danger to enable the employer to abate the danger as quickly as possible.

2.   In circumstances where the inspection can most effectively be conducted after regular business hours or where special preparations are necessary for an inspection.

3.   Where necessary to assure the presence of representatives of the employer and employees or the appropriate personnel needed to aid in the inspection.

4.   In other circumstances where the Area Director determines that giving advance notice would enhance the probability of an effective and thorough inspection.

Inspectors are authorized to enter without delay at reasonable times where work is performed by employees of an employer; and to conduct investigations during regular working hours at other reasonable times within reasonable limits and in a reasonable manner.

The Act also authorizes an inspector to examine pertinent conditions, including structures, machines, apparatuses, devices, equipment, and materials; and to question privately any employer, owner, operator, agent or employee.

Citations

The OSHA Area Director issues citations when appropriate. OSHA Form 2A--Citation for Serious Violation is issued when investigation reveals a serious violation; OSHA Form 2B--Citation is issued when investigation reveals a "de minimis" violation.

OSHA Form 3--Notification of Proposed Penalty is issued to accompany each Citation for Serious Violation. If the citation being issued is for a violation found after the second investigation and indicates a failure to correct a previous violation, the Area Director issues OSHA Form 3A--Notification of Failure to Correct Violation and of Proposed Additional Penalty to accompany the Citation.

Recordkeeping: Posting of Periodic Reports

OSHA defines recordable occupational injuries and illnesses as occupational illnesses and injuries which result in fatalities, or nonfatal cases which result in loss of work days, transfer to another job, or termination of employment; and illnesses and injuries which require medical treatment other than first aid or involve the loss of consciousness or restriction in motion.

Any recordable injury or illness must be entered in OSHA Form 100--Log of Occupational Injuries and Illnesses as soon as practical, but no later than six days after the responsible party has received word that such an injury or illness has occurred. (An equivalent form that contains all details provided in OSHA Form 100 may be used.) OSHA Form 101--Supplemental Record of Occupational Illnesses and Injuries may be used when Form 100 has been filed.

Form 102--Annual Summary must be completed for the previous year no later than January 31. It must be certified by the employer to be true and correct, and it must be posted at each of the employer's establishments for 30 consecutive days, beginning no later than February 1.

Penalties

The Act provides criminal sentences, criminal fines, and civil penalties to be assessed against an employer for violation of either the General Duty Clause or of specific standards. The types of violations defined by the Act are:

    --willful violations causing death of an employee;
    --willful or repeated violations;
    --serious violations;
    --nonserious or other violations;

-- "de minimis" violations;
-- daily penalties for failure to abate;
-- failure to post notice of employee rights under Act;
-- failure to post citations;
-- failure to report employment deaths;
-- failure to maintain records;
-- penalty for giving false information; and
-- penalties for killing, assaulting, or hampering the work of
   enforcement personnel.

Contest of Citations and Penalties

An employer who receives a citation and proposed penalties has the right to contest either the citation or the proposed penalties, or both, to the Occupational Safety and Health Review Commission. The contest must be filed within 15 working days from receipt of the citation and proposed penalty.

Within seven days of receipt of the notice of contest, the Area Director must file with the Commission the notice of contest, or modification of abatement, and all citations and notifications of failure to correct violations.

Within 20 days of receipt of the notice of contest, the Secretary of Labor files with the Commission a complaint against the employer. The employer will receive a copy of the complaint, as will the representative(s) of the employees who have elected-party status. The employer must file an answer within 15 days after receipt of the complaint.

After the Commission has received the employer's notice of contest from the Area Director, the Commission appoints a judge to conduct the hearing. The appointed judge will control all proceedings, discovery, depositions, and production of documents in the case.

After the hearing, the employer or other party against whom the Commission has filed an adverse order has the right to have the Commission's order reviewed by the Court of Appeals. The appellate review is limited to only those questions of law or objections raised before the Commission.

Variances

The Act provides that any affected employer may be granted a temporary variance from a standard, a permanent variance from a standard, or a variance, tolerance, or exemption for any or all provisions of the Act.

To obtain a temporary variance, the employer must establish that:

-- he is unable to comply with a standard by its effective date because
   of the unavailability of professional or technical personnel or of
   materials and equipment needed to come into compliance with the
   standard, or because necessary construction or alteration of
   facilities cannot be completed by the effective date;

-- he is taking all available steps to safeguard his employees against the hazards covered by the standard;

-- he has an effective program for coming into compliance with the standard as quickly as possible.

The application requirements for a temporary variance are detailed in 29 CFR Section 1905.10(b)(1972).

To obtain a permanent variance, an employer must establish, by a preponderance of evidence, that the conditions, practices, means, methods, operations and processes he uses or proposes to use will provide employment and a place of employment for his employees which are as safe and healthful as those which would prevail if he complied with the standard. Application requirements for a permanent variance are detailed in 29 CFR Section 1905.11(b)(1972).

Any employer must request a variance, tolerance, or exemption from the Act if it is necessary to avoid serious impairment of the national defense. Application requirements for this type of variance are detailed in 20 CFR Section 1905.12(b)(1972).

When an employer files an application with the Assistant Secretary for a temporary variance, permanent variance, or a variance, tolerance or exemption from the Act, the request will be referred to a hearing examiner. The hearing examiner will preside over the hearing and conduct and control all proceedings.

The hearing examiner will make his decision based upon the evidence presented at the hearing. The decision will become final 20 days after it has been rendered unless exceptions are filed.

If any exceptions are filed, the Assistant Secretary will review the hearing record and transcript and then rule on the exceptions and the rule or order of the hearing examiner. Only the decision of the Assistant Secretary may be appealed and reviewed by the Court of Appeals.

8. References

American Conference of Governmental Industrial Hygienists. <u>Air Sampling Instruments for Evaluation of Atmospheric Contaminants</u>, 4th ed. Cincinnati: American Conference of Governmental Industrial Hygienists, 1972.

American Conference of Governmental Industrial Hygienists. <u>Threshold Limit Values for Chemical Substances and Physical Agents in the Workroom Environment with Intended Changes for 1974</u>. Cincinnati: American Conference of Governmental Industrial Hygienists, 1974.

American Conference of Governmental Industrial Hygienists. Committee on Recommended Analytical Measurements. <u>Manual of Analytical Methods</u>. Cincinnati: American Conference of Governmental Industrial Hygienists, 1958.

American Medical Association. <u>The Wonderful Human Machine</u>. Chicago: American Medical Association, 1967.

American Public Health Association. <u>Intersociety Committee Methods of Sampling and Analysis</u>. Washington: American Public Health Association, 1972.

Elkins, H. B. <u>The Chemistry of Industrial Toxicology</u>, 2d ed. New York: John Wiley and Sons, Inc., 1959.

Giever, Paul M., ed. <u>Air Pollution Manual Part 1-Evaluation</u>, 2d ed. Akron: American Industrial Hygiene Association, 1972.

Green, H. L. and W. R. Lane. <u>Particulate Clouds: Dusts, Smoke, and Mists</u>. London: E. and F. N. Spon, Ltd., 1964.

Guyton, Arthur C., M. D. <u>Function of the Human Body</u>, 3d ed. Philadelphia: W. B. Saunders Company, 1969.

Jacobs, M. B. <u>The Analytical Toxicology of Industrial Inorganic Poisons</u>. New York: Interscience Publishers, Inc. 1967.

Kusnetz, Howard L. "Evaluation of Chemical Detector Tubes." Paper presented at Chemical Section, National Safety Congress, October 7, 1965. Chicago.

Magill, P. L., F. R. Holden, C. Ackley, F. G. Sawyer, eds. <u>Air Pollution Handbook</u>. New York: McGraw-Hill Book Co., 1956.

Olishifski, Julian B. and Frank E. McElroy, eds. <u>Fundamentals of Industrial Hygiene</u>. Chicago: National Safety Council, 1971.

Patty, Frank A. <u>Industrial Hygiene and Toxicology</u>, 2d ed. 2 vols. New York: Interscience Publishers, Inc., 1958.

Steen, Edwin B., Ph.D. and Ashley Montague, Ph.D. Anatomy and Physiology, 2 vols. New York: Barnes and Noble Books, 1959.

U. S. Department of Health and Human Services, Public Health Service, National Institute for Occupational Safety and Health. The Industrial Environment: Its Evaluation and Control. Washington: U. S. Government Printing Office, 1973.

Willard, H. H., L. L. Merrit, and J. A. Dean. Instrumental Methods of Analysis. New York: D. Van Nostrand Co., Inc., 1965.

Section 2

Industrial Ventilation

1. Characteristics of Air

In order to provide a background for the design of industrial ventilation systems, it is desirable to review the characteristics of air and the properties of airborne contaminants. The purpose of this and the following chapter is to undertake such a review. It is expected that the reader will find that some of the material included in these chapters has been encountered previously, while other material may be totally new. However, it is important that this material be covered to assure that all will be at the same level when beginning the discussion concerning the design of industrial ventilation systems.

The air that blankets the earth is a mixture of gases with approximately the following concentration:

–Nitrogen	78.088%
–Oxygen	20.949%
–Argon	0.930%
–Carbon dioxide	0.030%
–Neon	0.0018%
–Helium	0.0005%
–Methane and krypton	0.0001%

Air also contains traces of hydrogen and other elements. The proportion of the above mixture varies slightly in different locations. However, these differences in concentration are not significant.

As a gas, air can be compressed: that is, the molecules can be moved closer together. If no force compresses the air, it will expand indefinitely to fill the space available. The compressibility of air is conveniently ignored when considering air moving in a ventilation system. This subject will be covered in much more detail during the discussions concerning the design of ventilation systems.

As with any other gas, there is no cohesive force that attracts the molecules of air to one another. These molecules are in constant movement. During this movement, the molecules collide with one another and with the walls of their container. The molecular collisions occur without any loss of kinetic energy; thus, the molecules remain in continuous motion.

Pressure

The molecular movement and the tendency of air to expand indefinitely cause a force to be exerted on a given unit of any containing object. Thus, if more air is pumped into a container, there are more molecules colliding with the same unit area of the sides of the container. This results in a higher pressure inside the container.

The air that surrounds the earth exerts a pressure on a given unit area of the earth's surface as a result of the earth's gravitational attraction for the air. Without the pull of gravity, air would disperse into space, and life could not exist on earth. Since gravitational attraction varies inversely with distance from the center of the earth, air becomes thinner and weighs less at higher altitudes. In fact, 99 percent of the atmosphere is found below 20 miles above the surface of the earth. The heat of the sun causes higher molecular motion in the air. This higher molecular motion results in thinner air or less atmospheric pressure. Differences in atmospheric pressure cause the earth's weather patterns.

Standard atmospheric pressure is generally measured using a mercury barometer. If the temperature is assumed to be constant at a specified reference value, the standard atmospheric pressure at sea level is 29.92 inches of mercury or 760 millimeters of mercury. Mercury is much heavier than water; thus, if a water barometer were used, it would yield as standard atmospheric pressure 33.96 feet of water at sea level. Another convenient method of expressing standard atmospheric pressure is 14.7 pounds per square inch or 1.03 kg/cm^2. These values will become important when working with industrial ventilation systems.

As has been discussed previously, the volume occupied by a given amount of gas varies with the temperature and pressure of the gas. This fact yields several important standard values that are useful when working with air. The first of these is the specific weight. The specific weight is the weight in pounds of one cubic foot of a gas at a given temperature and pressure. The reciprocal of the specific weight is the specific volume; that is, the volume one pound of a gas will occupy at a given temperature and pressure. The specific weight of air is .075 pounds per cubic foot at 70 degrees Fahrenheit and 29.92 inches Hg or 1.20 kg/m^3 at 21.1°C and 760 mm Hg. The specific volume at the same temperature and pressure is 13.35 ft^3 per pound or 832.9 cm^3/g. One other important constant is obtained from these relationships: the specific gravity. Specific gravity is the ratio of the density of a gas to the density of air at standard conditions. The specific gravity of air equals 1.

Heat Intensity--Temperature

Temperature is a measure of the average kinetic energy of the molecules that move about in a substance. A given temperature value states this molecular energy in relation to a standard. The relationship of temperature to molecular motion can be demonstrated by bending a paper clip or wire coat hanger back and forth in order to break it. As the material is bent, the molecules become more active. This activity can be sensed by touching the metal near the point at which it is being bent and noticing that the metal has become hot. The higher molecular motion results in heat.

Temperature is measured on a thermometer that is divided into one of three different scales which are used to measure temperature. The first of these is the Fahrenheit scale where water freezes at 32 degrees Fahrenheit and boils at 212 degrees Fahrenheit. The second is the Celsius scale where water freezes at 0 degrees Celsius and boils at 100 degrees Celsius. The third is the absolute scale. The absolute scale starts at 0 degrees absolute, where no molecular movement exists, and extends upward indefinitely.

Often during industrial ventilation work, it is necessary to convert from one scale to the other in order to compare standards. To convert from Celsius to Fahrenheit, one only has to remember that the Celsius scale is divided into an interval of 100 degrees from freezing to boiling, while the equivalent interval for the Fahrenheit scale is 180 degrees. The result is a ratio of 5:9. This ratio, along with the fact that water freezes at 0 degrees Celsius, which is equivalent to 32 degrees Fahrenheit, yields the following equation:

(2.1.1) Celsius degrees   = 5/9(°F − 32)°
(2.1.2) Fahrenheit degrees = 9/5 °C + 32°

The equivalent Celsius value for 0 degrees absolute is −273°C.

The absolute scale can be divided into degree intervals equivalent to either Celsius or Fahrenheit intervals. Since the pressure of a gas increases or decreases by 1/273 of its pressure at 0°C for each degree the temperature is raised or lowered, there is a direct relationship between the Celsius and absolute scales. Thus, 1 Celsius degree is equal to 1 Kelvin degree, where Kelvin degrees denote the use of the absolute scale. Such a direct relationship does not exist between Kelvin and Fahrenheit degrees; thus a separate scale, the Rankine scale, has been developed to express Fahrenheit degrees in terms of absolute temperature. The following relationships can then be developed:

(2.1.3) Rankine degrees = (460 + °F)°
(2.1.4) Kelvin degrees = (273 + °C)°

Just as there is a standard atmospheric pressure at which most measurements are to be compared, there is a standard temperature value. Unhappily, scientists and engineers have not been able to agree on the standard temperature that should be used. This lack of agreement will cause some consternation when working in the field of industrial hygiene. However, it is a fact to live with. The varying standards are as follows:

Chemistry--0°C and 760 mm Hg

Industrial Hygiene--25°C and 760 mm Hg

Ventilation--70°F and 29.92 in Hg

You will note that all standards at least agree on the atmospheric pressure, so that compensation must be made for differences in temperature only. The industrial hygiene engineer must take care in interpreting tables to determine which of the above standards is being used in the table. In

Figure 2.1.1

Temperature scales.

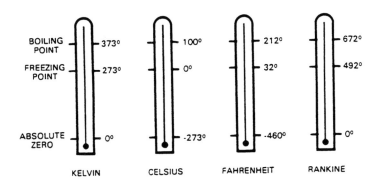

	KELVIN	CELSIUS	FAHRENHEIT	RANKINE
BOILING POINT	373°	100°	212°	672°
FREEZING POINT	273°	0°	32°	492°
ABSOLUTE ZERO	0°	-273°	-460°	0°

general, the difference between the industrial hygiene standard and the ventilation standard does not create a significant error in any calculations (25°C = 77°F). However, the difference between the industrial hygiene standard and the chemistry standard is significant and can introduce large errors if correction is not made for the difference.

Heat Quantity

All materials possess thermal energy. Thermal energy is the measure of a material's total potential energy. Materials differ in the amount of total potential energy or thermal energy available per unit mass. Thus, 1 gram of wood has a higher potential energy than 1 gram of sand. Temperature is the measure of the average kinetic energy of the molecules in a material. As a material is heated, the molecules become more active, and part of the total potential energy is converted to kinetic energy. The average kinetic energy that each molecule possesses is the measure of the total temperature of the body.

Heat is the quantity of internal energy that is transferred from one material or one body to another. Heat transfer occurs as a result of a difference in temperature of the two materials or bodies and, as such, is independent of the quantity of material involved in the transfer. Heat always flows from the hotter material to the colder material unless external work is performed.

The difference between thermal energy, heat, and temperature can be illustrated by placing a small container of water and a large container of water on a stove and heating them at the same rate for the same period of time. If temperature measurements are made, the small container will yield a higher temperature than the large container. However, if the contents of the two containers are mixed, the resulting temperature of the mixture will be closer to that of the large container than to that of the small container. If the containers were of equal size, and one contained water while the other contained a solid block of iron, it would be found that the solid block of iron yielded a higher temperature than that of the water for the same thermal energy supplied. In both cases, the same amount of energy was supplied to each container, but a temperature difference was obtained. The energy that was supplied relates to the quantity of heat available.

Figure 2.1.2

Thermal energy vs. temperature.

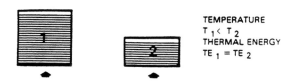

CONSTANT THERMAL ENERGY SUPPLY

The difference in temperature noted between the iron and water illustrates a relationship called specific heat. As is evident in this example, not all materials have the same ability to absorb the thermal energy transmitted to them. The heat capacity of a material is the amount of heat that is required to raise the temperature of the material 1°. The specific heat of a substance is the ratio of heat required to raise a unit weight of a substance one degree Fahrenheit or one degree Celsius to the heat required to raise the same unit weight of water through one degree Fahrenheit or one degree Celsius. If the temperature is being measured in degrees Fahrenheit, then the specific heat or quantity of heat is measured in British Thermal Units (BTU). If the temperature is being measured in degrees Celsius, the quantity of heat is measured in calories. One BTU is the heat required to raise one pound of water through one degree Fahrenheit. One calorie is the heat required to raise one gram of water through one degree Celsius at approximately 16.5°C–17.5°C. In all cases, the specific heat value assumes a constant atmospheric pressure of 760 mm Hg or 29.92 in Hg.

The following examples illustrate the calculation of BTU's and calories.

What quantity of heat is required to raise 100 pounds of water from 68°F to 77°F where the specific heat of water is equal to 1?

100 pounds x (77°F – 68°F) x 1 BTU/lb-°F = 900 BTU

What quantity of heat is required to raise 100 pounds of air from 68°F to 77°F where the specific heat of air is equal to 0.241?

100 pounds x (77°F - 68°F) x .241 BTU/lb-°F = 217 BTU

If the above problems were translated into metric equivalents (100 pounds = 45,360 grams), the following would be obtained:

For water
45,360 grams x (25°C - 20°C) x 1 calorie/g-°C = 226,800 calories

For air
45,360 grams x (25°C - 20°C) x .241 calorie/g-°C = 54,658.8 calories

Perfect Gas Law

All gases, including air, obey certain laws that exhibit the temperature, volume, and pressure relationships discussed earlier. The first of these laws illustrates the pressure-volume relationship that exist.

Boyle's Law--For a perfect gas at a constant temperature, the volume will vary inversely with the pressure.

$$(2.1.5) \quad P_1 V_1 = P_2 V_2$$

In other words, if a given amount of air were made to occupy one-half the space, then the pressure exerted on a unit area would be twice that in the original volume.

A second important law relates the volume with the temperature. This law is stated as:

Charles' Law--For a perfect gas at a constant pressure, the volume will vary directly with the absolute temperature.

$$(2.1.6) \quad \frac{V_1}{V_2} = \frac{T_1}{T_2}$$

This law relates the molecular action of the gas to the amount of heat that is added to the gas. As heat is added, the molecules become more active, thus the volume expands.

The Perfect Gas law combines these two laws into a useful expression:

$$(2.1.7) \quad PV = WRT$$

where
P = absolute pressure in pounds/ft^2 or Newtons/m^2
V = the total volume of gas in ft^3 or m^3
W = the total mass of the gas in pounds or kilograms; determined by the product of the molecular weight x the number of moles
R = the gas constant in ft/mole-°R or Nm/kg mole-°K
T = the absolute temperature in °R or °K

The gas constant is calculated by using the fact that this constant, when multiplied by the molecular weight of a gas, will always equal 1545.4. Thus the gas constant for air can be calculated by determining the molecular weight of air to be as follows:

Calculation of the Gas Constant for Air

Element	Part.Volume	Mol.Wt.(MW)	Part.Vol. x MW
Nitrogen	.781	38	21.866
Oxygen	.210	32	6.720
Argon	.009	39.9	.355
	1.000	MW (Air)	28.941

$$R = 1545.4/28.941$$
$$R = 53.4 \ ft/°R$$

If metric units are used, the universal gas constant is 8314 Joules/kg mol-K° and then R becomes 8341/28.94 = 287.27 Nm/kg-°K. In general, the English system is used throughout this text since the basic charts, dimensions for ducts, etc., use this system.

When a mixture of gases is present, then Dalton's Law is important. Dalton's Law states that the total pressure of a mixture of gases is equal to the sum of the partial pressures of the component gases. Dalton's Law points out that a mixture of gases will occupy the same volume at the same time.

Application of the Gas Laws

The following examples are presented to indicate how the above laws can be used to predict the volume, pressure, temperature, and weight relationships of a given amount of gas as compared to standard.

Example 1--If 1 cubic foot of air at 70°F is heated 10°F, what volume of air will be present? Assume standard atmospheric pressure.

Solution

Using Charles' Law (2.1.6)

$$\frac{T_1}{T_2} = \frac{V_1}{V_2}$$

$$\frac{460° + 70°}{460° + 80°} = \frac{1}{V_2}$$

$$V_2 = 1.019 \ ft^3$$

Example 2--A tire is inflated to 28 pounds per square inch gauge at a temperature of 70°F. At what pressure will the tire be after operation resulting in an internal air temperature of 110°F in the tire? Assume the barometer reads 30 in Hg and that the volume remains constant.

Solution

Atmospheric Pressure = 14.7 pounds/in^2

$$\frac{29.92 \text{ in Hg}}{30 \text{ in Hg}} = \frac{14.7 \text{ pounds/in}^2}{P_2}$$

Using Charles' Law (2.1.6)

$$\frac{P_1}{P_2} = \frac{T_1}{T_2}$$

$$\frac{28 + 14.74}{P_2 + 14.74} = \frac{460° + 70°}{460° + 110°}$$

$$P_2 = 31.22 \text{ pounds/in}^2 \text{ or psi}$$

In example 2, note that the pressure used in the calculations is the total pressure; i.e., the gauge pressure plus the atmospheric pressure.

Example 3--The barometer reads 30.23 in Hg and the temperature is 70°F in the classroom. What is the weight of air that is contained in the room?

Solution

Using the Perfect Gas Law (2.1.7)
PV = WRT

To determine the pressure in pounds/square feet, use standard values at 29.92 in Hg and P = 2116.3 lb/ft^2

$$\frac{29.92}{2116.3} = \frac{30.2}{P_2}$$

$$P_2 = 2136.1 \text{ lb/ft}^2$$

Substituting this pressure in the Perfect Gas Law
2136.1 V = W x 53.4 x (460° + 70°)
2136.1 V = 28302 W
W = .0755 V pounds/ft^3
Where V is the volume of the room in ft^3.

Example 4--To solve the above problem using metric units.

Solution

A reading of 30.23 in Hg = 767.84 mm Hg
Pressure is measured in N/m^2
2116.3 lb/ft^2 = 10,333.9 kg/m^2

$$10,333.9 \text{ kg/m}^2 \times 9.8 \text{ m/sec}^2 = 101,272.22 \text{ N/m}^2$$

Temperature equivalent

$$°C = 5/9(°F - 32)$$
$$C = 21.1°$$

then

$$\frac{760 \text{ mm Hg}}{767.87 \text{ mm Hg}} = \frac{101,272.22 \text{ N/m}^2}{P_2} \text{ ; } P_2 = 102,334.23 \text{ N/m}^2$$

Using the Perfect Gas law (2.1.7)

$$102,334.23 \text{ N/m}^2 \times V \text{ m}^3 = W \text{ kg} \times 287.27 \text{ Nm/Kg-°K} \times (273 + 21.1)°K$$

$$W = 1.215 \text{ V kg/m}^3$$

Where V is the volume of the room in m^3.

Example 5--Air is heated to a temperature of 600°F. What is its
density? What is the ratio of this density to that of
standard air (density factor)? What is the ratio of the
volume of air at 600°F to that of standard air? For the
above, assume a standard barometric pressure of 29.92 in Hg.

Solution

Density at 600°F
$$PV = WRT$$
$$V = 1 \text{ ft}^3$$
$$2116.3 \times 1 = W \times 53.4 \times (460 + 600)$$
$$W/V = .0374 \text{ pounds/ft}^3$$
Density at 70°F
$$2116.3 \times 1 = W \times 53.4 \times (460 + 70)$$
$$W/V = .0748 \text{ pounds/ft}^3$$
$$\text{or } W/V = 0.0012 \text{ g/cm}^3 = 1.2 \text{ kg/m}^3$$

Density Factor

$$\frac{.0374}{.0748} = .50$$

To determine the volume at 600°F

$$\frac{V_1}{V_2} = \frac{\rho_1}{\rho_2}$$

$$\frac{1}{V_2} = \frac{.0374}{.0748}$$

$$V_2 = 2.0$$

$$\text{or } V_2 = \frac{1}{\text{Density Factor}} \times V_1$$

Example 6--5000 ft^3 of air at 600°F is equivalent to how many cubic feet of air at standard temperature? Assume standard barometric pressure.

Solution

From the results obtained in example 5,

$$\text{or } V_2 = \frac{1}{\text{Density Factor}} \times V_1$$

The density factor was .50 in example 5.

$$V_2 = \frac{1.0}{0.50} \times V_1$$

$$V_1 = 2500 \text{ ft}^3$$

The Effect of Moisture in Air

The standard conditions that were previously stated assume no moisture content in the air. However, this is not a normal situation. Air usually has some moisture content. In many cases this moisture content is low enough that the error introduced by not including the measurement in calculations is not significant. However, there are situations where the amount of moisture in the air is significant and must be considered while designing ventilation systems. The general rule of thumb is that if the air temperature is under 100°F, no correction for humidity is necessary; and if the temperature exceeds 100°F, and the moisture content is greater than .02 pounds of water per pound of dry air, a correction factor must be used.

The standard barometric pressure for the atmosphere at sea level is 29.92 in Hg. If the air contains water vapor, this water vapor will exert an additional pressure. The barometric reading obtained is the total pressure of both the air and the water vapor. From Dalton's Law, it can be shown that the partial pressure exerted by water vapor can be deducted from the total pressure to obtain the actual air pressure. This is shown as follows:

$$(2.1.8) \quad P_{total} = P_{air} + P_{vapor}$$

$$P_a = P_t - P_v$$

Water vapor, like air, obeys the gas laws. For example, as the temperature increases, the volume of water vapor in air will also increase (Charles' Law). As the volume of an air-water vapor mixture decreases, the pressure of the mixture will increase (Boyle's Law). For an air-water vapor mixture, application of Dalton's Law indicates that the water vapor and air will occupy the same volume at the same time. Any volume differences from standard air exist because of the partial pressures exerted by the water vapor and air in the mixture rather than the fact that water vapor displaces air. Barometric readings indicate the sum of the partial pressures of air and any water vapor content in the air.

Let us now look at how the presence of water vapor can affect the results of calculations. Using the Perfect Gas Law and using the subscript (a) to denote air and the subscript (v) to denote water vapor, we have the following:

(2.1.9) $P_aV_a = W_aR_aT_a$

(2.1.10) $P_vV_v = W_vR_vT_v$

$$\text{where } R_v = \frac{1545.4}{\text{mole weight } H_2O} = \frac{1545.4}{18.02}$$

$$R_v = 85.76$$

then

(2.1.11a) $P_vV_v = 85.76 \, W_vT_v$

and from previous calculations

(2.1.11b) $P_aV_a = 53.4 \, W_aT_a$

By Dalton's Law, the air and water will occupy the same space.
Volume of vapor = volume of air
$$V_v = V_a$$

Solving (2.1.11a) and (2.1.11b) for V_v and V_a and substituting gives

$$\frac{85.76 \, W_vT_v}{P_v} = \frac{53.4 \, W_aT_a}{P_a}$$

but $T_a = T_v$ so that

$$\frac{85.76 \, W_v}{P_v} = \frac{53.4 \, W_a}{P_a}$$

Assuming 1 pound of dry air

$$\frac{85.76 \, W_v}{P_v} = \frac{53.4}{P_a}$$

$$W_v = \frac{53.4 \, P_v}{84.76 \, P_a}$$

But, $P_a = P_{tot} - P_v$ and P_{tot} at standard = 2116.3 pounds/ft^2 so that the following is obtained:

(2.1.12) $W_v = \dfrac{.623P_v}{2116.3 - P_v}$

and

(2.1.13) $P_v = \dfrac{2116.3\ W_v}{623 + W_v}$

From the preceding, either the weight or the vapor pressure of a given saturation of air can be found if the other is known at a given temperature and pressure.

Example 1--What is the vapor pressure exerted in saturated air at standard conditions?

Solution

Using the relationship developed in (2.1.13) for 70°F and 29.92 in Hg:

(2.1.13) $P_v = \dfrac{2116.3\ W_v}{.623 + W_v}$

From the Psychrometric Chart (Industrial Ventilation Manual, pp. 13-21) at 70°F and 29.92 in Hg
$W_v = .0157$ pounds water/pound dry air
Substituting

$P_v = \dfrac{2116.3 \times .0157}{.623 + .0157}$

$P_v = 52.02$ pounds/sq. ft.

Converting this value to inches Hg, the ratio is used:

$\dfrac{52.02}{2116.3} = \dfrac{P_v}{29.92}$

$P_v = .74$ in Hg

Example 2--What volume will 1 pound of dry air occupy given the partial pressure relationships calculated above?

Solution

Using Dalton's Law
$P_a = P_t - P_v$ (2.1.8)

Substituting
P_v = 52.02 pounds/ft^2 from above problem
P_a = 2116.3 pounds/ft^2 - 52.02 pounds/ft^2
P_a = 2064.3 pounds/ft^2

One pound of dry air then occupies:
$P_a V_a = W_a R_a T_a$

$$V = \frac{1 \times 53.4 \times (460° + 70°)}{2064.3}$$

V = 13.7 ft^3

Example 3--What volume will one pound of the saturated air occupy?

Solution

The total weight of the mixture can be expressed as:
$W_t = W_a + W_v$
W_t = 1.00 + .0157
W_t = 1.0157 pounds

Thus, if 1.0157 pounds of the mixture occupies 13.7 ft^3 (the same area as 1 pound of dry air), then

$$V/pound = \frac{13.7 \ ft^3}{1.0157 \ pounds} = 13.49 \ ft^3/pound$$

Relative Humidity

Air does not always exist in a saturated condition in the industrial environment. Most often the moisture content is less than the saturation level. This lower moisture content can be expressed using the term, "relative humidity." Relative humidity is defined as the ratio of the partial pressure of water vapor present at a given temperature to the partial pressure of water-saturated air at the same temperature. This is stated as follows:

$$(2.1.15) \quad \text{Relative humidity(\%)} = \frac{P_v \ (\text{water vapor})}{P_v \ (\text{saturated air})} \times 100\%$$

Example 1--At a relative humidity of 50%, what is the partial pressure of water vapor in the preceding example?

Solution

Using formula (2.1.15)

$$RH = \frac{P_{vu}}{P_{vs}}$$

$$.50 = \frac{P_{vu}}{.74 \text{ inches Hg}}$$

$P_v \text{unsaturated} = .37$ inches Hg or 26.2 pounds/ft^2

Example 2--What volume will one pound of the 50% saturated air occupy?

Solution

From the above example, the partial pressure of the water vapor is 26.2. The partial pressure of dry air is

$P_a = P_t - P_v$ (2.1.8)
$P_a = 2116.3 - 26.2$
$P_a = 2090.1$ pounds/ft^2

The volume occupied by one pound of dry air that exerts this pressure is calculated as follows:

$P_a V_a = W_a R_a T_a$ (2.1.9)

$$V = \frac{53.34 \times 530}{2090.1}$$

$V = 13.53$ ft^3

The volume occupied by one pound of water vapor and air mixture is found in the following way:

The total weight of 13.53 ft^3 of the mixture is
$W_t = W_a + W_v$ (2.1.14)
$W_t = 1.00 + (.50 \times .0157)$
$W_t = 1.00785$

The volume occupied by one pound of the mixture is

$$V = \frac{13.53 \text{ ft}^3}{1.00785}$$

$V = 13.42$ ft^3

Summary

In this chapter, the characteristics of air have been described. The basic formulas for determining the relationship between volume, pressure, temperature, and water vapor content have been described. The following table summarizes the formulas that have been discussed:

REFERENCE	RELATIONSHIP	FORMULA
2.1.1	Converting Fahrenheit degrees to Celsius degrees	$°C = 5/9(°F - 32)$
2.1.2	Converting Celsius degrees to Fahrenheit degrees	$°F = 9/5°C + 32$
2.1.3	Converting Fahrenheit degrees to Rankine degrees	$°R = 460 + °F$
2.1.4	Converting Celsius degrees to Kelvin degrees	$°K = 273 + °C$
2.1.5	Boyle's Law (pressure-volume)	$P_1V_1 = P_2V_2$
2.1.6	Charles Law (temperature-volume)	$\dfrac{V_1}{V_2} = \dfrac{T_1}{T_2}$
2.1.7	Perfect Gas Law	$PV = WRT$
2.1.8	Dalton's Law (partial pressures of components of air-water mixture)	$\delta P_m = \delta P_1 + \delta P_2 + ... \delta P_n$ $P_{total} = P_{air} + P_{vapor}$
2.1.12	Weight of water vapor in a given air-water mixture	$W_v = \dfrac{.623P_v}{2116.3 - P_v}$
2.1.13	Partial pressure of the water vapor in a given air-water mixture	$P_v = \dfrac{2116.3W_v}{623 + W_v}$
2.1.14	Total weight of air-water mixture	$W_t = W_a + W_v$
2.1.15	Relative Humidity	$RH\% = \dfrac{P_v(unsaturated)}{P_v(saturated)} \times 100\%$

2. Properties of Airborne Contaminants

In the preceding chapter, the characteristics of air were discussed. In this chapter, the discussion will center around the behavior of contaminants that are airborne. Airborne contaminants are those materials that are part of the air mixture but that are foreign to the normal state of the mixture. The contaminants in air may be harmful, irritating, or a nuisance to man. These contaminants may be the result of natural occurrences or the result of man's activity.

The natural contaminants found in the air are legion. For example, ozone, which is formed photochemically or by electrical discharge during storms, can be found in the atmosphere. Hydrogen fluoride, hydrogen chloride, and hydrogen sulfide, resulting from volcanic disturbances, can also be found in the atmosphere. Salt particles from sea water condensation, dust becoming airborne as a result of wind disturbances, bacteria spores, and pollen are also examples of natural contaminants that can be found in the air.

In addition to these natural contaminants, the industrial revolution has brought about the addition of a number of man-made contaminants to the atmosphere. These contaminants include gases (a material which assumes a gaseous state at 25°C and 760 mm Hg), vapors (a material which assumes a liquid state at 25°C and 760 mm Hg), and particulate matter including dusts, fumes, mists, etc., which are dispersed as solid particles in the air (aerosol). It is these man-made contaminants that are of interest to the air pollution engineer and the industrial hygiene engineer, and that will be discussed in this chapter.

Properties of Gases and Vapors

Gases and vapors, like air, obey the laws discussed in the previous chapter (Boyle's Law, Charles' Law, the Perfect Gas Law, Dalton's Law). It is important to realize the significance of Dalton's law as it applies to a mixture of gases and vapors in air. In general, Dalton's Law predicts that a complete mixing action will occur in which a gas or vapor will occupy the same space as the air. A gas that is allowed to escape into the air will tend to diffuse equally throughout the entire area occupied by the air.

One of the properties of a gas or vapor is its density. Density is the mass of a unit volume of a substance expressed as pounds per cubic foot or grams per cubic centimeter. In the preceding chapter, it was pointed out that the density of air is .075 pounds per cubic foot. If one takes the density of air as the base and forms a ratio with the density of any other gas, the specific gravity of that gas is obtained. A similar property, which is closely related to density, is <u>viscosity</u>. Viscosity describes the tendency of a fluid or gas to resist flow. Gases and vapors generally have very low viscosity and flow easily.

<u>Toxic Properties of Gases or Vapors</u>. Gases and vapors that contaminate the air may be harmless, or they may exhibit toxic properties. If a gas or vapor is known to be toxic, this fact is generally indicated by placing a threshold limit value (TLV) in terms of parts per million of the amount of the gas or vapor that can be present in the air without causing harm to individuals exposed to that contaminant.

It is useful to review the determination of parts per million of a toxic substance present in the air. When the industrial hygiene engineer takes samples of the workroom air, the temperature and pressure are also noted. The measurements are then analyzed to determine the number of milligrams per liter of the substance that are found in the samples. These milligrams per liter can be converted to parts per million by the following formula:

(2.2.1)
$$ppm = \frac{1000 \times 24.45}{molecular\ weight} \times concentration\ (mg/l)$$

The above formula is based on the fact that 1 gram mole of a perfect gas at 25°C and 760 mm Hg occupies a volume of 24.45 liters. In order to illustrate the above formula and how that formula can be corrected for varying temperature, the following example problems are presented.

<u>Example Problems--Toxicity</u>

> <u>Example 1</u>--Suppose analysis of samples of workplace air yielded a concentration of .0074 mg/1 of HCl. Is this a toxic concentration? Assume industrial hygiene standard conditions exist.

> <u>Solution</u>

>> Molecular weight of HCl = 36.47
> then

>> $$ppm = \frac{24.45 \times 10^3}{36.47} \times 0.0074\ mg/1$$

>> ppm = 670.4 x .0074

>> ppm = 4.96

> The TLV for HCl is 5 ppm, and the TLV is not exceeded in the above situation.

> <u>Example 2</u>--Assume that the above results were obtained at a temperature of 90°F. Is the TLV exceeded?

Solution

$$ppm = \frac{24.45 \times 10^3}{36.47} \times .0074 \times \frac{460 + 90}{460 + 70}$$

ppm = 5.15

In this case, the TLV of 5 ppm is exceeded. From this example, it is easy to see the effect of temperature on the results obtained in the sample measurements. If correction were not made for the higher temperature, the results would be understated.

Combustibility. Some gases and vapors are combustible. In general the concentration that is required to support combustion is much greater than the TLV level for toxic combustible gases. For this reason, the combustible limits are normally expressed as a percent of the volume of air rather than in parts per million. In terms of combustibility, the values of concern are the flash point, lower explosive limit, and upper explosive limit.

The flash point is the lowest temperature at which a liquid gives off enough vapor to form an ignitable mixture. By this definition, gases do not have a flash point, since they exist as a mixture in the air regardless of temperature. It should be noted that combustion does not occur spontaneously by this definition. An ignition source must be present in order for combustion to occur.

The lower explosive limit (LEL) indicates the minimum concentration of a vapor or gas in the air that will burn if an ignition source is present. The upper explosive limit (UEL) indicates the maximum concentration of the vapor or gas in the air that will burn if an ignition source is available. Concentrations of combustible gases or vapors that exist between these two limits are those that present a potential fire hazard.

Example Problems--Combustibility

Example 1--Hydrogen cyanide is found to be present in the workroom air at a concentration level of 0.015 mg/1. Does this concentration represent a fire hazard?

Solution

Using the previous formula to determine the concentration in parts per million:

$$ppm = \frac{24.45 \times 10^3}{27.03} \times .015 \text{ mg/l}$$

ppm = 904.55 x .015
ppm = 13.57
Percent concentration = .001357

Since the LEL for hydrogen cyanide is 5.6%, the above concentration does not represent a potential fire hazard.

Example 2--A concentration of how many mg/liter of hydrogen cyanide will be necessary to yield a potential fire hazard?

Solution

$$ppm = \frac{24.45 \times 10^3}{27.03} \times mg/l$$

$$mg/l = \frac{5.6 \times 10^4}{904.55}$$

$$mg/l = 61.9$$

If we wish to determine the upper concentration UEL for hydrogen cyanide, the UEL percent is substituted as above giving

$$mg/l = \frac{40 \times 10^4}{904.55}$$

$$mg/l = 442.2$$

Example 3--Does the concentration found in Example 1 represent a toxic hazard? The TLV for hydrogen cyanide is 11 mg/m^3.

Solution

The result obtained in Example 1 yielded 13.6 ppm. Converting the TLV to mg/l

$$mg/l = \frac{11\ mg}{m^3} \times \frac{1\ m^3}{1000\ liters}$$

$$mg/l = 0.011$$

This value can be converted to ppm by

$$ppm = \frac{24.45 \times 10^3}{27.03} \times .011$$

$$ppm = 9.95\ or\ 10$$

Thus the TLV for hydrogen cyanide (10 ppm) has been exceeded by the results obtained in Example 1 (13.6 ppm).

The above examples demonstrate the large concentration of a gas that is necessary to be combustible as compared to the TLV if the material is toxic.

For example in an environment where workers are present, the problem that is faced with hydrogen cyanide is not one of a potential fire hazard, but one of a potential toxic hazard.

Motion of Gases and Vapor. When a gas enters the air, a molecular mixture occurs as is predicted by Dalton's Law. One would expect that if the gas is much heavier than air, it would tend to settle out of the air. However, in terms of concentrations of interest to the industrial hygiene engineer, this fact is not true. In general, the mixture acts as if it were air alone. This can be predicted since the effect of gravity is on the average molecular weight of the mixture or the density of a mixture, not on the gas or vapor alone. Consider the following example to determine the specific gravity of a mixture of air and 1000 ppm vinyl chloride.

Molecular weight of vinyl chloride = 62.5

1000 ppm = 0.1%

so that
$$.001 \times 62.5 = 0.0625$$
$$.999 \times 28.94 = \underline{28.91}$$
$$\text{molecular wt. of mixture} = 28.9725$$

$$\frac{\text{MW mixture}}{\text{MW air}} = \frac{28.97}{28.94} = 1.001$$

even though

$$\frac{\text{MW vinyl chloride}}{\text{MW air}} = \frac{62.5}{28.94} = 2.16$$

In general, a mixture of a gas or vapor in air at the levels of concentration that are of significance to the industrial hygiene engineer will have a motion similar to the air alone. This can be shown by considering the velocity of a gas falling in air, using the familiar formula for a freely falling body:

(2.2.2) $v = \sqrt{2g(\sigma_g - \sigma_a)h/\sigma_g}$

where

g = acceleration due to force of gravity or 32.2 ft/sec^2
σ_g = specific gravity of the mixture
σ_a = specific gravity of the air
h = height of the fall in ft.

Hemeon, W. Plant and Process Ventilation, 2d. ed. New York: Industrial Press, 1963, p. 22.

Using this relationship, the velocity of a mixture of 2000 ppm butane and air can be calculated after falling 1 foot.

Molecular weight of mixture is calculated as:

$$.002 \times 58.12 = .12$$

$$.998 \times 28.94 = 28.88$$

$$\overline{29.00}$$

$$\sigma_a = \frac{29}{28.94} = 1.002$$

Substituting

$$v = \sqrt{2 \times 32.2(1.002 - 1.0)/1.002 \times 1}$$

$$v = .36 \text{ fps or } 21.6 \text{ fpm}$$

Since the minimum air velocities of 15 feet per minute are very likely to be found in almost any industrial area, the results obtained above indicate that any potential settling of the gas will be influenced by the motion of the air. In the above example, we have not considered the further diffusion of the gas within the air which in fact, as a result of Dalton's Law, does take place. Therefore, the velocity shown overstates significantly that which would actually occur.

In summary, then, in the design of an industrial ventilation system to handle gas and vapor contaminants, it is necessary only to control flow of air, since the contaminant gas or vapor will follow the pattern of air flow and thus can be controlled. One caution is necessary when considering a potential accidental contamination of air by large amounts of combustible gases or vapors with relatively high specific gravity. If the contamination results from a spill, it can easily be shown that this gas or vapor will tend to settle out and cause a large concentration to be present at floor level where the potential for an explosion can result. This, however, is a separate problem and should be handled apart from the need to control toxic materials at a level below the TLV.

Properties of Particulate Matter

Particulate matter includes dusts, fumes, smoke, and mists that are suspended in the air. This suspension is generally known as an aerosol. The presence of particulate matter in the air provides a major problem for the industrial hygiene engineer, particularly if this particulate matter includes toxic materials.

Dust particles that are present in the air are generally formed by a mechanical action. Dusts may be either solid organic or inorganic material. The size of the dust particles varies from the visible to the submicroscopic.

Dust is formed by grinding and crushing operations, movement of crushed materials, and air currents passing over settled dust, causing it to become airborne.

Figure 2.2.1

Particulates in air.

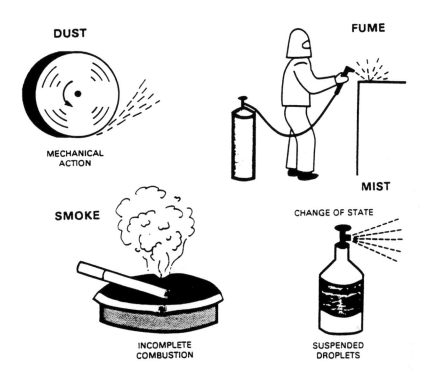

DUST

MECHANICAL
ACTION

FUME

MIST

SMOKE

CHANGE OF STATE

INCOMPLETE
COMBUSTION

SUSPENDED
DROPLETS

Fumes are formed by a chemical or physical process involving a <u>change of state</u>. Quite often the process requires high temperatures to create the fumes. Typical fumes include oxides of zinc, magnesium, iron, lead, and other metals. Some organic solids may also form fumes by the same processes. Fume particles are very small, normally in the range of 1 micrometer or less.

<u>Smoke</u> refers to airborne particulate matter resulting from <u>incomplete combustion</u> of organic materials. Smoke particles are usually less than one-half micrometer in size when they are produced. Soon after generation, many of the smoke particles will flocculate and form aggregates that appear to be larger particles but are, in fact, many small particles that have grouped together.

Fibers are a special type of particles in which one dimension is at least three times the length of the other dimension. Fibers can result from either natural fiber-forming materials such as asbestos or cotton or from synthetic materials such as fiberglass. In general, fibers are a special type of dust.

Mists are formed by <u>liquid droplets suspended in the air</u>. Mist may be formed by condensation of a vapor or by spraying which creates an atomized mist. In addition, air bubbles that form on the surface of a boiling liquid can collapse and result in a mist above the liquid. Fog and smog (a combination of smoke and fog) are special cases of a mist.

Particulate Size. Particles that are of interest to the industrial hygiene engineer are limited in size to those particles that are less than 10 micrometers in diameter. This is a result of the fact that particles of a diameter of more than 10 micrometers are not likely to be retained in the respiratory system of the worker. Particles of a size less than 1 micrometer may be retained in the alveoli of the lung. If a sample of air from a particular dust-producing operation is taken, it would be expected that a number of particles of each size would be normally distributed according to size. This is not the case. Since large particles tend to settle out of the air very quickly, the distribution of particles in the air follows what has been shown to be a log-normal distribution with the large number of particles being in the small size range.

Figure 2.2.2

Particle dispersion.

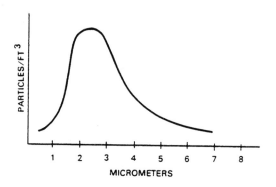

Measurement of particles to determine the number and distribution of size in a given sample is done in a number of ways. The standard method for sizing particles is by counting, using an optical microscope. Sizing is done by measuring using one of three methods:

A.   Projected Area Diameter--the diameter of a circle of area equal to the profile of the projected area of the particle.

B.   Feret's Diameter--the normal distance between two parallel targets to the extreme points of the particle.

C.   Martin's Diameter--The distance between opposite sides of a particle, measured in a consistent direction such that the diameter bisects the projected area.

Figure 2.2.3

Particle sizing.

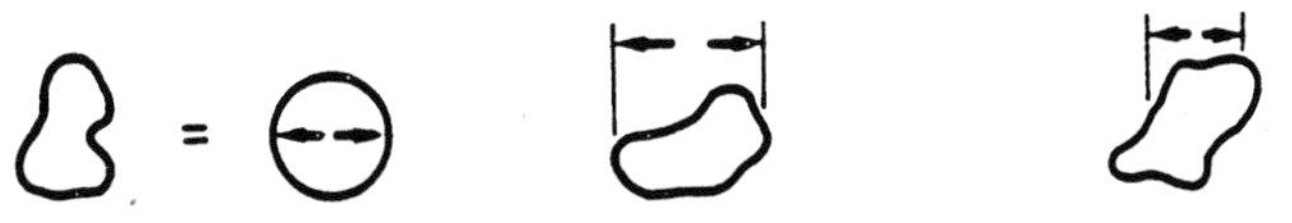

PROJECTED AREA   FERET'S   MARTIN'S
   DIAMETER   DIAMETER   DIAMETER

Other methods to measure and count particles are gaining in popularity. Such methods include the electron microscope, impaction with decreasing size orifices, light scattering, and electrostatic charging. However, the standard remains optical sizing because of the low cost and availability of the equipment involved.

Toxicity of Particulate Matter. Particulate matter may exhibit toxic properties. In general, this toxicity is through the respiration of particles. Examples of toxic particulate matter include silica dust, asbestos fibers, carbon tetrachloride mist, mercury mist, beryllium dust, and iron oxide fumes. The threshold limit value for particulate matter is expressed in milligrams per cubic meter. Thus, no conversion need be made to parts per million as in the case of gases and vapors.

Particulate matter has certain optical characteristics such that airborne particles will reflect and refract light. This fact can be easily observed by standing near a sunlit window where the dust particles are obvious as they float through the air. However, particles of the size of interest to the industrial hygiene engineer (10 micrometers or less) cannot be seen by the naked eye. In addition, hazardous concentrations of particulate matter regardless of size are visible in only a few cases and under the best conditions. Thus, observation does not indicate that a safe concentration is present. It is necessary to take samples of the air and analyze them before the safety of the air can be determined.

The Motion of Particulate Matter. The settling rate for dust that is dispersed in the air is determined by the gravitational force acting upon the dust and is a function of the size and specific gravity of the particles. Obviously particles of a larger size and higher specific gravity will tend to settle out of the air more quickly than those with a lower specific gravity.

As the particle settles out of the air, its velocity increases until such a time as it reaches a terminal velocity. As with any other falling body, the frictional force or turbulence that is created by the falling body acts as a frictional drag that tends to retard the acceleration of the body created by the gravitational force. The Reynolds number (R_e) is a dimensionless number that defines the amount of turbulence and the resultant frictional drag that is present. The Reynolds number becomes important in determining not only the frictional drag and terminal velocity of a falling particle but also the type of flow that will exist within a ventilation duct system. Two types of flow are defined by the Reynolds number. The first of these is <u>streamline flow</u> where there is no turbulence that might retard the flow of the particle or the air in a duct system. The second is <u>turbulent flow</u> where eddies of air are created that act as a frictional drag to retard the flow of the particle or the air. Between streamline flow and turbulent flow a transition flow area is present where the flow is neither entirely streamline nor turbulent.

The Reynolds number can be calculated to obtain a value that indicates in which area of flow the particle is at a given period of time. For a particle Reynolds number of less than or equal to 2, the particle is falling in streamline (laminar) motion. If the Reynolds number is greater than or equal to 2 but less than or equal to 500, the particle is falling in the transition area. Turbulent motion exists where the Reynolds number is calculated to be greater than 500.

The size limit of particles that will be confined to the streamline area can be determined by the following formula:

$$(2.2.3) \quad d_m = \sqrt[3]{103/z}$$

where

d_m = diameter of particle in micrometers
z = the specific gravity of the particle

For a specific gravity of 1, the size limit is 103 micrometers; and for a specific gravity of 3, the size limit is 70 micrometers. Therefore, for particles of industrial hygiene significance, that is, where d_m is less than or equal to 10 micrometers, only streamline motion need be considered.

The terminal velocity of a particle falling in the air in streamline flow can be found by the following equation: (Hemeon, <u>Plant and Process Ventilation</u>, p. 31)

$$(2.2.4) \quad u_t = 9.23 \times 10^{-5} z d_m^2$$

where

u_t = terminal velocity in feet per second
z = specific gravity of the particle
d_m = the diameter of the particle in micrometers

Using the above formula, the terminal velocity of a 10-micrometer particle of specific gravity = 3 when falling through the air can be calculated as follows:

$u_t = 9.23 \times 10^{-5} z d_m^2$
$u_t = 9.23 \times 10^{-5} \times 3 \times 10^2$
$u_t = .0277$ ft/sec or 1.66 ft/min

It is obvious that the velocity obtained by the particle is very small when compared to random air currents of at least 15 ft/min that occur in an industrial environment. Given this fact, it is unlikely that particles of the size of interest to the industrial hygiene engineer will settle out of the air. These particles will travel with the air currents and can be controlled by controlling the air itself.

Dust That Is Projected. Many mechanical actions that produce dust also cause the dust to be projected at some speed into the air. For example, a grinding operation will project dust particles in a direction that is tangential to the grinding wheel at the point of contact. Large particles with high velocities will result in large Reynolds numbers indicating high turbulence. As the particle slows down, it will go through a transition state and finally will enter streamline flow. Small particles, because of their small mass, will be projected only a small distance. This projection will occur in streamline flow alone because of the low velocities that are attained. Small particles will be carried in the turbulent motion of the air created by large particles. Small particles that are projected will follow the path of air currents rather than the projected path and, as a result, can be controlled by controlling the air at the source.

Brownian Motion. One final cause of particulate motion in the air, that of Brownian motion, should be briefly discussed. The molecules of air are in constant movement. During this movement, the molecules collide with particles suspended in the air, thus causing a constant random movement of the particle about a point. Small particles are affected greatly by this molecular motion. Brownian motion tends to keep small particles of less than .25 micrometers in diameter in the air. In fact, particles of the .25 micrometer size show a minimum amount of movement because the Brownian motion exactly offsets the gravitational attraction for particles of this size. Therefore, this size particle becomes extremely difficult to remove from the air. However, this fact also makes it difficult for these particles to be retained by the lungs. Particles smaller than 1 micrometer are too small to be affected by molecular action and thus are easily deposited.

Causes of Initial Dispersion of Particulates in the Air

During the previous discussion, the motion of particles after entering the air was investigated. It is of interest to determine what causes the particles to enter the air in the first place. There are a number of causes of particulate dispersion in the air, some of which have been alluded to in the earlier discussion.

The first cause of particulate dispersion is a mechanical cause resulting from grinding or cutting of a material. The grinding wheel or saw, as it cuts through the material, projects particles in a line tangent to the point of contact between the material and the mechanical wheel or saw. The smaller particles are picked up by air currents and carried through the air to other locations. Other examples of this type of mechanical action include drill presses, lathes, and sanders.

A second cause of dispersion is shattering. Consider hitting a rock with a hammer. Small chips and particles are broken away from the rock; and, if these particles are small enough, they will remain in the air and follow existing air currents.

Falling particles create a <u>splash</u> when they impinge upon a surface. This splash can be likened to an explosion where the particles tend to be pushed outward and upward away from the point of contact. At this point, passing air currents can hold the smaller particles in suspension.

Prior to impinging upon a surface, a stream of falling particles will create <u>turbulence</u>. Air currents resulting from the turbulence will carry small particles outward from the falling particulate stream. These small particles can then be dispersed in the air.

<u>Thermal convection</u> provides another method wherein particulate matter can become dispersed in the air. As hot air rises, it can carry with it fumes, mists, or particulate matter. These contaminants can then become further dispersed in the air as cooling and mixing in the atmosphere occurs.

The final method by which particulate matter can become dispersed in the air is by a <u>secondary air movement</u>. Consider a passing automobile. Turbulence created by the automobile causes swirls of dust and loose papers to become airborne. The papers will settle out quickly; however, the small dust particles may remain airborne for long periods of time as a result of this turbulent action. Certain types of machines produce a fan action that results in air currents about the machine. These air currents can cause particulates to be carried away from the source where the smaller particles will be subjected to further dispersion by the random air currents in the work environment.

Summary

From the preceding discussion, it can be seen that gases, vapors, and particulate matter of interest to the industrial hygiene engineer can be controlled by controlling the air in which they are suspended. This is an important fact to remember when designing an industrial ventilation system. Certain special operations require that larger particles be captured that have projected motion or that tend to settle quickly. The design of such a system involves different considerations from those that are necessary to control toxic contaminants in the air. The fact that the particles, gases, and vapors present in the air can be controlled by controlling the air tends to simplify the design of industrial ventilation systems. However, quite often this characteristic is not taken advantage of in the system design. As a result, the system may be over-designed for the job that is required.

3. Principles of Air Movement

Industrial ventilation is perhaps the most powerful tool that is available to the industrial hygiene engineer for use in controlling the work environment. The proper use of ventilation as a control can assure that the workroom air remains free of potentially hazardous levels of airborne contaminants. Through the use of ventilation, airborne contaminants can be removed from the workplace air or diluted by incoming air to a level that is not hazardous. However, just as a properly designed ventilation system can act as a powerful control, so can an improperly designed ventilation system act as a potential hazard. In fact, an improperly designed ventilation system may be more dangerous than no ventilation system at all, because of the false sense of security that the presence of such a system gives to the workers and management of the organization.

Because of the importance of proper design for ventilation systems, it is desirable that the industrial hygiene engineer possess the skill and knowledge that is necessary to evaluate existing systems and design new systems for control of the workroom environment. In the next few chapters, the general principles and concepts of ventilation system design and evaluation will be presented. This material should give the reader the basic concepts and principles that are necessary for the proper application of industrial ventilation systems.

General Concepts of Ventilation

The earth possesses a natural ventilation system that acts to remove pollutants and heat from the local environment and disperse them throughout the atmosphere. When the natural ventilation system fails, as it does when an inversion occurs in the Los Angeles area, pollutants can reach a level that is hazardous to the inhabitants of the area. In addition to the dispersion of pollutants, natural ventilation provides for the weather patterns at a particular time of year within a given region.

What causes air movement and forms the natural ventilation system for the earth? In general, air movement results from differences in pressure. Air moves from high pressure areas to low pressure areas. This difference in pressure is the result of thermal conditions. We know that hot air rises. Rising hot air allows smoke to escape from the chimney in a fireplace rather than be dispersed into the room. Hot air rises because air expands as it is heated and thus becomes lighter. The same principle is in effect when air in the atmosphere becomes heated. The air rises and is replaced by air from a higher pressure area. Thus, convection currents cause a natural ventilation effect through the resulting winds.

The <u>purpose of industrial ventilation</u> is essentially the same as that which occurs in natural ventilation. Simply stated, the purpose is <u>to circulate the air within an area so as to provide a supply of fresh air to replace air with undesirable characteristics</u>. One potential method for accomplishing this is to heat the air in the area, thus causing it to rise and escape through vents in the roof. This air is then replaced by fresh air that enters through openings in the building. However, quite often such a system does not circulate air fast enough to remove the contaminant before a hazardous level has been reached. Thus, it is necessary to provide an artificial means for moving the air. The mechanical fan provides such an artificial means.

There are a number of reasons ventilation systems should be used in a given work environment. First, ventilation can be used to maintain an adequate oxygen supply in the area. In the industrial environment, this reason is seldom of great importance because oxygen is replaced through natural ventilation at the rate which is required. However, in certain applications such as deep mining, workers at high altitudes, and space travel, the need for oxygen can become the major reason for a ventilation system.

A second reason for installing a ventilation system, and one that is of significant importance to the industrial hygiene engineer, is to control hazardous concentrations of toxic materials in the air. Airborne contaminants in the forms of particulate matter and gases must be kept below the threshold limit value in order to assure that the workplace is safe for the worker. Various methods of ventilation are available to accomplish this.

Another reason for providing a ventilation system is to remove odors from a given area. This type of system is found in locker rooms, rest rooms, and kitchens. The desired effect is accomplished either by removing the noxious air and replacing it with fresh air or by supplying air with a masking element.

Another reason for the use of ventilation with which we are all familiar is to control temperature and humidity. In the winter, heat can be added to the air space through a ventilation system. In the summer, chilled air can be added to the air space to provide cooling. Quite often humidity control is an integral part of such a system.

A final reason for a ventilation system, and one that is also of major importance to the industrial hygiene engineer, is the removal of undesirable contaminants at their source before they enter the workplace air. When dealing with highly toxic materials, this is the most effective control. If the contaminant never enters the breathing zone of the worker, then no danger to the worker will exist from the contaminant.

Components of a Ventilation System

There are four major components required for a ventilation system. First, there must be a <u>force that moves the air</u>. Second, there must be <u>an inlet or opening for air to enter the system</u>. Third, <u>an outlet must be present for air to leave the system</u>. Finally, there must be a <u>pathway or enclosure that limits the flow of air in the desired direction</u>.

The force causing the air to move may be natural, as in the case of the natural draft caused by prevailing winds, or it may be thermal draft caused by changes in temperature, or it may be mechanical. Natural draft can be very effective on a windy day. However, generally the moving force or wind is not constant and cannot be depended upon to provide the reliable force necessary to move the air in a system. Where large differences in temperature exist, thermal draft can provide adequate air movement for removal of contaminants. However, in most situations a mechanical air mover (fan) is required to provide the constant flow to operate the ventilation system.

All the above components are required for a ventilation system. However, some of the components are not obvious. For example, the inlets and outlets may be open windows. The pathway or enclosure that limits the flow may be the room itself with the location of the inlet and outlet being relative to the desired direction of flow of the air. However, for the most part, discussion of ventilation systems will be limited to those systems in which the components are found in the traditional form (i.e., a fan, a hood, a vent, and a duct).

One other general concept regarding ventilation systems that should be discussed is the difference between exhaust systems and supply systems. An exhaust ventilation system removes the air and airborne contaminants from the workplace. Such a system may exhaust the entire work area, or it may be placed at the source to remove the contaminant prior to the contaminant entering the workplace air. The second type of system is the supply system which adds air to the workroom. This system may be used to dilute contaminants in the work environment so as to lower the concentration of these contaminants. Supply systems can be used to provide motion to contaminated air to move it in the desired direction. Supply systems are also used to provide air to replace air that has been removed using an exhaust system. It is generally the case that if an exhaust system is present, some supply system must also be present.

Pressure in a Ventilation System

It was previously stated that air movement in a ventilation system is a result of differences in pressure. Pressures in a ventilation system are measured in relation to atmospheric pressure. The existing atmospheric pressure in the workplace is assumed to be the zero point. In the supply system, the pressure created by the system is in addition to the atmospheric pressure that exists in the workplace. In an exhaust system, the objective is to lower the pressure in the system below the atmospheric pressure.

The differences in pressure that exist within the ventilation system itself are small when compared to the atmospheric pressure of the room. For this reason, these differences are measured in terms of inches of water, or water gauge, which results in the desired sensitivity of measurement. Because of the small differences in pressure, air can be assumed to be incompressible. Since one pound per square inch of pressure is equal to 27 inches of water, one inch of water is equal to 0.036 pounds pressure or 0.24% of standard atmospheric pressure. Thus the potential error that is introduced by considering air to be incompressible is very small at pressures that exist within a ventilation system.

Three pressures are of importance in ventilation work; the velocity pressure, the static pressure, and the total pressure. The following discussion should help the reader to understand the characteristics of these three pressures.

Before discussing the three pressures, it is important that the reader be familiar with pressure itself. The energy of a fluid (in this case, air) that is flowing is termed "head" in fluid mechanics. Head is measured in terms of unit weight of the fluid or in foot-pounds/pound of fluid flowing. The usual convention is to describe head in terms of feet of fluid that is flowing.

Pressure is the force per unit area exerted by the fluid. This force is measured in lbs/ft^2 in the English system of measurement. When the fluid of concern is incompressible, as is assumed with air in ventilation systems, the pressure of a fluid is equal to the head.

As air travels at a given velocity through a ventilation system, a pressure is created. This pressure is called the velocity pressure of the system. Velocity pressure is always positive; that is, above atmospheric pressure. This is obvious when one considers that velocity must always be positive, and thus the pressure that causes it must be positive.

There is a direct relationship between the velocity of air moving within a ventilation system and the velocity pressure of the system. This relationship can be derived as follows:

The equation for a freely falling body is given as:

$$v = \sqrt{2gh}$$

where
   v = velocity in feet per second
   g = acceleration (32.2 ft/sec^2)
   h = head in feet

converting to feet per minute yields

$$v = 60 \sqrt{2gh}$$

To express head in inches of H_2O

$$h = \frac{1}{12} \, VP \times \frac{62.4}{\rho}$$

where

   VP = velocity pressure in inches of H_2O
   ρ = density of air in pounds/ft^3
   62.4 = density of H_2O in pounds/ft^3

Substituting

$$v = 60 \sqrt{2gVP \times 62.4/12\rho}$$

or

(2.3.1) $v = 1097 \sqrt{VP/\rho}$

For standard air where $\rho = 0.075$ pounds/ft^3

(2.3.2) $v = 4005 \sqrt{VP}$

The second important pressure within a ventilation system is the static pressure. <u>Static pressure</u> is the pressure that is exerted in all directions by the air within the system. Some commonplace examples might help the reader to grasp the concept of static pressure. Consider an automobile tire that is inflated to a given pressure. The pressure within the tire is exerted equally on all sides of the tire. This pressure is greater than atmospheric pressure; thus the tire will expand and support weight. However, no air velocity is present within the tire itself. The pressure in the tire is totally a result of static pressure. For another example of static pressure, take a common soda straw and put it in your mouth. Close one end with your finger and blow very hard. You have created a positive static pressure. This pressure does not result in movement of the air through the straw. However, as soon as you remove your finger from the end of the straw, the air begins to move outward away from the straw. The static pressure has been transformed into velocity pressure. The opposite effect can be demonstrated by sucking inward on the straw while holding the end of the straw. When you remove your finger from the end of the straw, the air will rush in as a result of the negative pressure that has been created in your mouth.

As demonstrated above, static pressure can be either positive or negative. Positive static pressure results in the tendency of the air to expand. Negative static pressure results in the tendency of the air to contract. In the example above using the straw, if one could blow hard enough while holding the end of the straw, it is possible that the straw could be blown apart. On the other hand, if one draws in air with enough force, the straw can collapse. This particular occurrence is one of the hazards that we all face when drinking a very thick milkshake (fluid with high viscosity).

<u>Static pressure within a ventilation system is the pressure that is required to accelerate the air to its velocity and to overcome frictional forces in the system.</u> These concepts will be discussed in more detail later in this chapter.

Bernoulli's Theorem, which is related to fluid energy, states that the total energy in a system remains constant if friction is ignored. This concept can be applied to the pressures within a ventilation system. Static pressure represents the potential energy that exists within a system. Velocity pressure represents the kinetic energy within a system. From elementary physics, we all know that the sum of the potential energy and kinetic energy in a system represents the total energy of that system. Transformed into ventilation systems, this means that the sum of the velocity pressure and the static pressure at a given point within a ventilation system is equal to the total pressure within the system. If all losses resulting from friction are ignored, this total pressure will remain constant over the entire system. Thus, a change in velocity pressure must be reflected by an opposite change in static pressure. The total pressure of a ventilation system can be either positive or negative; that is, above or below atmospheric pressure. In general, the total pressure is positive for a supply system while it is negative for an exhaust system. The pressure relationship is given as:

(2.3.3)   TP = VP + SP

Measurement of Pressures in a Ventilation System

Manometer. The manometer is used to obtain a measure of the static pressure in a ventilation system. The manometer is a simple, U-shaped tube that is open at both ends and is clear (usually constructed of glass) in order that the fluid level within can be observed. A graduated scale is usually present on the surface of the manometer so that measurements can be obtained. The manometer is filled with water, mercury, or light oil. For field measurement, one leg of the manometer is furnished with flexible tubing, and the other end of the tube is held flush and tight against a small static pressure opening in the side of the duct. Special fittings may be used if desired. The pressure exerted from the ventilation system on the liquid within the manometer will cause the level of liquid to change as it relates to the atmospheric pressure external to the ventilation system. Thus, the pressure measured is relative to atmospheric pressure as the zero point. The scale on the manometer is calibrated for use of one liquid, usually water. If other liquids are used in the manometer, correction for differing specific gravities must be made.

Figure 2.3.1

U-tube manometer.

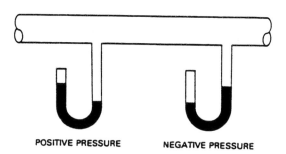

POSITIVE PRESSURE   NEGATIVE PRESSURE

When manometer measurements are used to obtain positive pressure readings in a ventilation system, the leg of the manometer that opens to the atmosphere will contain the higher level of fluid. When a negative pressure is being read, the leg of the tube open to the atmosphere will be lower, thus indicating the difference between the atmospheric pressure and the pressure within the system.

Inclined Manometer. Quite often it is necessary to obtain measurements of small pressure differences. The U-tube manometer does not provide the sensitivity necessary to obtain such measurements. For this purpose, an inclined manometer is used. In the inclined manometer, the leg that opens to the atmosphere is inclined at an angle to provide for the sensitivity required. The principles of use of the inclined manometer are the same as those for the normal U-tube manometer. Generally, the manometer is inclined at a ratio of 10:1. However, when greater sensitivity is required, special designs are available with a ratio of 20:1.

Figure 2.3.2

Inclined manometer.

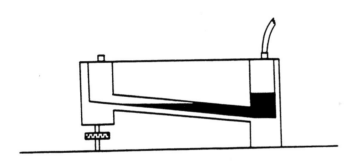

The Impact Tube. The impact tube is used to measure total pressure in a ventilation system. Generally the impact tube is an L-shaped tube made of material stiff enough to eliminate vibrations of the tube when placed within the ventilation system. The impact tube is placed in such a manner as to have the opening point upstream in the air current. A manometer filled with liquid is attached to the impact tube. The resulting positive or negative pressure is indicated on the manometer in the same manner as when using a manometer alone to measure static pressure.

The use of a manometer and an impact tube to obtain two measurements, i.e., the static pressure and the total pressure, will also result indirectly in a measurement of the velocity pressure of the system. The difference between the impact tube measurement and the manometer measurement will yield the velocity pressure present within the system. Should it be necessary to obtain more sensitive measurements, the impact tube can be connected to an inclined manometer with the resulting sensitivity of the inclined manometer being obtained.

The Pitot Tube. The Pitot tube combines the impact tube with a method for measuring static pressure directly. The Pitot tube is constructed of two concentric tubes. The inner tube forms the impact portion, while the outer tube is closed at the end and has static pressure holes normal to the surface of the tube. When the inner and outer tubes are connected to opposite legs of a single manometer, the velocity pressure is obtained directly. Two manometers can be used if it is desired to measure static pressure separately. Positive and negative pressure measurements are indicated on the manometer as was previously discussed for static pressure.

Figure 2.3.3

Pitot tube.

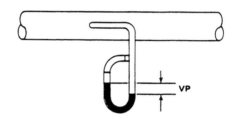

Flow in a Ventilation System

As was discussed above, the air flow in a ventilation system is caused by differences in pressure. These differences in pressure are reflected in the total pressure of the system. For a supply system, the total pressure of the system is positive; that is, above atmospheric pressure. In an exhaust system, the total pressure is negative or below atmospheric pressure. It will be remembered that the total pressure is composed of the velocity pressure and static pressure of the system. Velocity pressure within a system is always positive. Static pressure, therefore, is positive in a supply system and negative in an exhaust system. This is as would be expected since static pressure is the initial pressure necessary to accelerate the air from a point of no movement to the velocity within the system. Obviously, in an exhaust system the air must be moving from the room into the system; and, therefore, the static pressure within the system must be less than atmospheric. The opposite situation occurs for a supply system.

The concept of positive and negative pressure is important when designing a ventilation system. The designer must be careful to use the appropriate sign (for the pressure which exists). The normal convention of plus and minus for the signs is used. Thus, a static pressure in an exhaust system would be represented as a negative value, while a velocity pressure in either an exhaust or supply system will be represented by a positive or plus value. For example, if an exhaust system has a total pressure measured as -2 inches of

water and the velocity pressure is calculated as 1 inch of water, then the
static pressure would be:

$$TP = VP + SP$$
$$-2 = 1 + SP$$
$$SP = -3 \text{ inches of } H_2O$$

How Air Flows in a Ventilation System. Let us investigate the principles
involving the operation of an exhaust system. When the air mover or fan for
the system is turned on, energy is required to accelerate the air outside of
the system to a given velocity to be maintained within the system. This
energy is stated in inches of water static pressure. Once the air reaches the
design velocity, this velocity will remain constant for a given duct size
throughout the system. Thus, the velocity pressure will also remain constant
because of the direct relationship:

$$v = 4005 \sqrt{VP} \quad \text{(for standard air only)}.$$

The rate at which air is captured and flows through an exhaust system is
stated in cubic feet of air per minute. This rate of flow will also remain
constant throughout the total system. The general terms used to describe the
rate of flow are as follows:

If Q denotes the rate of flow within the system in cubic feet per minute
(cfm), then
$$Q = vA \quad (2.3.4)$$
where
$\quad$ v is the velocity of air in feet per minute, and
$\quad$ A is the cross-sectional area of the duct in square feet.

The following example is given to illustrate the use of this formula:

Example

Find the rate of flow in cubic feet per minute (cfm) of air traveling
at 4000 feet per minute (fpm) in a circular duct of 4 inches in
diameter.

Using the formula stated above

$$Q = vA \quad (2.3.4)$$

the area of the circle can be calculated by

$$A = \frac{\pi r^2}{144}$$

$$A = \frac{3.14 \times (2)^2}{144} = 0.087 \text{ ft}^2$$

Substituting in the equation

Q = 4000 fpm x 0.087 ft^2
Q = 348 cfm

The Effect of Friction on Air Flow. As air flows through the system, frictional forces (or drag) act to retard the flow as a result of turbulence within the duct. That turbulence is related to the Reynolds number. The Reynolds number, which was briefly presented in the discussion of the motion of particulate matter, is a result of experimental work done by the British scientist, Osborne Reynolds. The experiments involved the use of a thin filament of dye entering a clear glass tank containing water. The rate of entry of the dye was varied and the effect of the velocity of the water on the flow of dye was noted. At low velocities, the dye appeared as a thin filament extending the full length of the flow and was sharply defined. As the velocity increased, small eddies began to become apparent until the velocity was at such a rate that the entire stream appeared to be in violent motion.

The results of these experiments indicated the relationship between velocity and type of flow in a given fluid. The work of Reynolds has been applied to ventilation systems in that the flow Reynolds number is a function of pipe diameter, average velocity, fluid density, and fluid viscosity. This relationship is stated as follows:

$$R_e = f(D, v_{avg}, \rho, \mu)$$

(2.3.5) $$R_e = \frac{D v_{avg} \, \rho}{\mu}$$

where

D = duct diameter in feet
v_{avg} = average linear velocity (ft/sec) of the fluid
ρ = fluid density (lbs/ft^3)
μ = fluid viscosity (lbs/ft-sec)

As can be seen, R_e is dimensionless.

The criteria for the type of flow that can be expected within a ventilation system can be related to a given value for the Reynolds number:

For streamline flow (laminar) the Reynolds number is $R_e < 2100$.

The transition region between streamline and turbulent flow exists where the Reynolds number has values $2100 \leq R_e \leq 4000$.

Turbulent flow exists for Reynolds number values $R_e > 4000$.

Using the above information, let us now determine the characteristics of flow that can be expected within a ventilation system.

Example

Assume a ventilation system is operating with a 4-inch diameter duct. At what rate of flow (cfm) will the upper limit of streamline flow be reached?

Solution

$$R_e = \frac{D v_{avg}\, \rho}{\mu} \qquad (2.3.5)$$

R_e = 2100

D = 4 inches or 0.333 ft

ρ = 0.075 lbs/cu ft for air

μ = 0.0178 centipoise at 70°F

Since

μ = 0.0178 cP(6.719 x 10^{-4} lb/ft-sec/cP)

μ = 1.2 x 10^{-5} lb/ft-sec

Substituting in the formula for R_e gives

$$2100 = \frac{0.333 \text{ ft x v ft/sec x } 0.075 \text{ lbs/ft}^3}{1.2 \text{ x } 10^{-5} \text{ lbs/ft-sec}}$$

$$v = \frac{2100 \text{ x } (1.2 \text{ x } 10^{-5}) \text{ ft/sec}}{0.333 \text{ x } 0.075}$$

v = 1.01 fps or 60.6 fpm

Then

Q = vA   (2.3.4)
Q = 60.6 ft/min x 0.087 ft^2
Q = 5.27 cfm

Thus, for ventilation systems of interest, the flow will always be turbulent.

Now let us look further to determine the effect of this turbulent flow and the resulting frictional drag upon the operation of a ventilation system. Since the rate of flow (Q) remains constant for a system, if the cross-sectional area of the duct remains constant, then the velocity will remain constant throughout the system. This can be stated as

Q = Constant = vA

thus, for a given cross-sectional area

v = Constant

since

$$v = 4005 \sqrt{VP}$$
VP = Constant

When frictional losses occur in the system, the velocity pressure remains constant as shown above. The total pressure must change to overcome the losses within the system from the following:

TP = VP + SP + losses

The losses will then be reflected in the static pressure of the system, since the velocity pressure is constant. Thus, static pressure can be though of as being composed of two components. These components are:

1.   The pressure to accelerate air from rest to a given velocity.

2.   The pressure necessary to keep air moving at this velocity by overcoming frictional forces.

The following example is given to illustrate the change in static pressure to overcome the losses within a ventilation system.

Example

Assume a ventilation system is designed to exhaust air at a rate of 200 cfm through a 4-inch diameter duct. If the duct is 40 feet long and no losses occur at the inlet or hood, what are the two components of static pressure (the static pressure necessary to accelerate the air to a given velocity and the static pressure necessary to overcome losses)?

Solution

To obtain v, substitute in the formula
            Q = vA   (2.3.4)

obtaining
200 cfm = v x 0.087 ft^2
            v = 2300 fpm

Friction of air in straight ducts for volumes of 10 to 2000 cfm. (Based on standard air of 0.075 lb per ft^3 density flowing through average, clean, round galvanized metal ducts having approximately 40 joints per 100 feet.) Caution: Do not extrapolate below chart.

Source: The Industrial Environment: Its Evaluation and Control

Figure 2.3.4

Friction loss in inches of water per 100 ft.

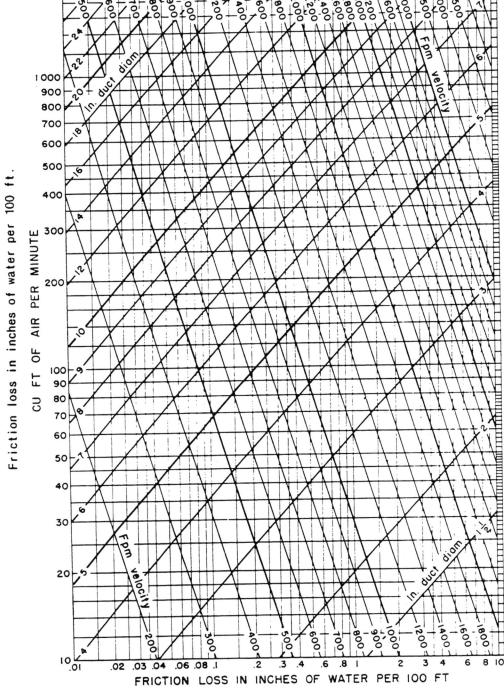

CU FT OF AIR PER MINUTE

FRICTION LOSS IN INCHES OF WATER PER 100 FT

The velocity pressure (VP) can be obtained from the relationship

$$v = 4005 \sqrt{VP} \quad (2.3.2)$$

$$VP = (2300/4500)^2$$

$$VP = 0.33 \text{ inches of } H_2O$$

To accelerate air to the velocity of 2300 fpm from rest and assuming no losses occur at the inlet, the following is obtained:

$$TP = SP + VP \quad (2.3.3)$$

but air at rest has TP = 0, so that

$$0 = SP + VP$$
$$SP = -VP$$
$$SP = -0.33 \text{ inches of } H_2O$$

To find frictional losses for straight duct, refer to Figure 2.3.4. Reading the intersection of Q and D or 200 cfm and 4 inches in diameter, we obtain

Loss = 2.5 inches of H_2O per 100 feet

Thus, the loss will be

$$SP = -2.5 \times \frac{40}{100}$$

$$SP = -1 \text{ inches of } H_2O \text{ to overcome losses.}$$

The profile of the pressures for this situation is given in Figure 2.3.5 below

Figure 2.3.5

Pressure profile.

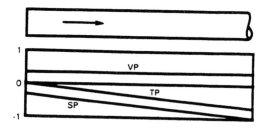

The Effect of Changes in Duct Diameter. As stated previously, the rate of flow (Q) remains constant throughout the system. Since Q = Constant = vA, then V must vary inversely with the area change. Since

$$v = 4005 \sqrt{VP},$$

the velocity pressure will vary directly with the square of the change in velocity. From the total pressure equation

TP = VP + SP

the total pressure will remain constant (ignoring any losses). Therefore, if a change in velocity occurs without loss of energy, the static pressure will reflect the change in velocity pressure in order that TP will remain constant.

However, when this change in velocity occurs, energy is lost. The transformation of static pressure to velocity pressure or vice versa does not occur at 100% efficiency. Turbulence at the contraction or expansion causes a loss to occur. This loss must be reflected in the static pressure as it was in the previous illustration. The following example is presented to illustrate the effect of changes in duct diameter on the pressure components within the system.

Example

A 4-inch duct exhausts air from a source at a rate of 300 cfm to a point 60 feet downstream where a 30° taper exists that reduces the duct diameter to 2 inches. Assuming 100% capture efficiency at the hood, what will be the static pressure, velocity pressure, and total pressure after the contraction?

Solution

At the beginning of the duct
$$Q = vA \qquad (2.3.4)$$
300 cfm = v × 0.087 ft^2
v = 3450 fpm
from

$$v = 4005 \sqrt{VP} \qquad (2.3.2)$$
$$VP = (3450/4005)^2$$
$$VP = 0.74 \text{ inches of } H_2O$$

If the inlet (hood) is assumed to be 100% efficient

$$SP = -VP = -0.74$$

The loss obtained over the 60 ft. in length is found by consulting Figure 2.3.4 for Q = 300 cfm and D = 4 inches

Loss = 5.3 inches of H_2O

for 60 feet

$$SP = -5.3 \times \frac{60}{100}$$

SP = -3.18 inches of H_2O

The total SP before the contraction is

SP = -3.18 + (-0.74)
SP = -3.92

For the loss and change in SP that is obtained for a 30° contraction, refer to Figure 2.3.6.

The formula presented is

(2.3.6) $SP_2 = SP_1 -(VP_2 -VP_1) -L(VP_2 - VP_1)$

To find VP_2 for a 2-inch duct, consult Figure 2.3.6.

Q = vA   (2.3.4)
300 cfm = v × 0.0218 ft^2
v = 13,761 fpm

To find VP_2

$$v = 4005 \sqrt{VP} \quad (2.3.2)$$

$VP_2 = (13,761/4005)^2$

VP_2 = 11.8 inches of H_2O

To obtain SP_2, substitute the loss factor of 0.13 from the table and the above value.

SP_2 = -3.92 - (11.8 - 0.74) - 0.13(11.8 - 0.74)   (2.3.6)
SP_2 = -3.92 - 11.06 - 1.44
SP_2 = -16.42 inches of H_2O

Thus, in this example VP increases from 0.74 to 11.8, and SP decreases from -3.92 to -16.42.

The pressure profile for the above situation is presented in Figure 2.3.7.

    The Effect of Changes in Direction of Airflow. When it is necessary for air to change direction while flowing through a ventilation duct system, this change of direction results in turbulence. The turbulence causes a loss that is reflected by the static pressure necessary to overcome the loss.

    Figure 2.3.8 is a chart that can be used to calculate the losses resultin from various changes in direction of air in a given duct system. The chart i

Figure 2.3.6

Losses at expansion or contraction.

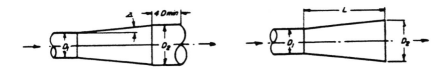

Within duct

Taper angle degrees	Regain (R), fraction of VP difference				
	Diameter ratios D_2/D_1				
	1.25:1	1.5:1	1.75:1	2:1	2.5:1
3 1/2	0.92	0.88	0.84	0.81	0.75
5	0.88	0.84	0.80	0.76	0.68
10	0.85	0.76	0.70	0.63	0.53
15	0.83	0.70	0.62	0.55	0.43
20	0.81	0.67	0.57	0.48	0.43
25	0.80	0.65	0.53	0.44	0.28
30	0.79	0.63	0.51	0.41	0.25
Abrupt 90	0.77	0.62	0.50	0.40	0.25

Where: $SP_2 = SP_1 + R(VP_1 - VP_2)$

At end of duct

Taper length to inlet diam L/D	Regain (R), fraction of inlet VP					
	Diameter ratios D_2/D_1					
	1.2:1	1.3:1	1.4:1	1.5:1	1.6:1	1.7:1
1.0:1	0.37	0.39	0.38	0.35	0.31	0.27
1.5:1	0.39	0.46	0.47	0.46	0.44	0.41
2.0:1	0.42	0.49	0.52	0.52	0.51	0.49
3.0:1	0.44	0.52	0.57	0.59	0.60	0.59
4.0:1	0.45	0.55	0.60	0.63	0.63	0.64
5.0:1	0.47	0.56	0.62	0.65	0.66	0.68
7.5:1	0.48	0.58	0.64	0.68	0.70	0.72

Where: $SP_1 = SP_2 - R(VP_1)$*

* When $SP_2 = 0$ (atmosphere) SP_1 will be (-)

The regain (R) will only be 70% of value shown above when expansion follows a disturbance or elbow (including a fan) by less than 5 duct diameters.

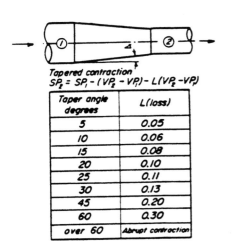

Tapered contraction
$$SP_2 = SP_1 - (VP_2 - VP_1) - L(VP_2 - VP_1)$$

Taper angle degrees	L (loss)
5	0.05
10	0.06
15	0.08
20	0.10
25	0.11
30	0.13
45	0.20
60	0.30
over 60	Abrupt contraction

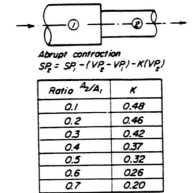

Abrupt contraction
$$SP_2 = SP_1 - (VP_2 - VP_1) - K(VP_2)$$

Ratio A_2/A_1	K
0.1	0.48
0.2	0.46
0.3	0.42
0.4	0.37
0.5	0.32
0.6	0.26
0.7	0.20

A = duct area, sq ft

Note:
In calculating SP for expansion or contraction use algebraic signs:
VP is (+)
and usually
SP is (+) in discharge duct from fan
SP is (-) in inlet duct to fan

Figure 2.3.7

Pressure profile.

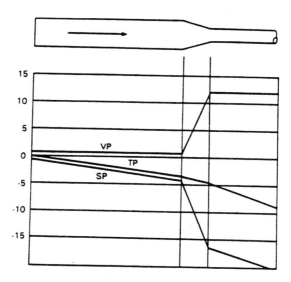

presented in equivalent feet of straight pipe. The loss as a result of
turbulence is related to the pipe diameter, degree of turn, and the radius of
the turn, such that

Loss = f(R,D,Angle,v)

   To illustrate the effect of a change in direction of airflow, an example
is presented below.

Example

What loss, in terms of static pressure, will occur for a pipe of a
diameter of 6 inches, turning the air $90°$ on a radius of 2.5D?
Assume the rate of flow in the system is 200 cfm.

Solution

From Figure 2.3.8
   Loss = 6 equivalent feet of straight pipe

From Figure 2.3.4
   Q = 200 cfm and D = 6 inches
   SP (loss) = $\pm$0.3 inches of. H_2O/100 feet

   Loss is then
   SP = $\pm$0.3 x .06
   SP = $\pm$0.018 inches of H_2O

Figure 2.3.8

Losses at elbows and branches.

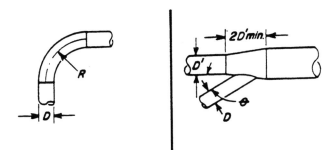

Pipe D	90° Elbow * Centerline Radius			Angle of Entry	
	1.5 D	2.0 D	2.5 D	30°	45°
3"	5	3	3	2	3
4"	6	4	4	3	5
5"	9	6	5	4	6
6"	12	7	6	5	7
7"	13	9	7	6	9
8"	15	10	8	7	11
10"	20	14	11	9	14
12"	25	17	14	11	17
14"	30	21	17	13	21
16"	36	24	20	16	25
18"	41	28	23	18	28
20"	46	32	26	20	32
24"	57	40	32		
30"	74	51	41		
36"	93	64	52		
40"	105	72	59		
48"	130	89	73		

* For 60° elbows —— 0.67 x loss for 90°
45° elbows —— 0.5 x loss for 90°
30° elbows —— 0.33 x loss for 90°

Since the example given did not specify whether the system is a supply system or an exhaust system, the sign for the static pressure is undetermined

Summary

The preceding discussion has presented the fundamental principles of air flow within a ventilation system. The effects of friction, changes in duct size, and changes in the direction of flow have been examined. In addition, the relationships relating to flow rate (Q), the velocity of the air (v), and the pressure in the system (TP, SP, and VP) have been discussed. This information will be used in designing ventilation systems and exhaust hoods in later chapters.

The following table summarizes the important relationships given in the chapter.

REFERENCE	RELATIONSHIP	FORMULA
2.3.1	Relationship between velocity and velocity pressure for any fluid	$v = 1096.2 \sqrt{VP/w}$
2.3.2	Relationship between velocity and velocity of air at standard conditions	$v = 4005 \sqrt{VP}$
2.3.3	Bernoulli's Theorem	$TP = VP + SP$
2.3.4	Rate of flow of air in a ventilation system	$Q = vA$
2.3.5	Reynolds number for flow in a ventilation system	$R_e = \dfrac{D v_{avg} \rho}{\mu}$
2.3.6	Static pressure at a point after a contraction in duct	$SP_2 = SP_1 - (VP_2 - VP_1) - L(VP_2 - VP_1)$

4. Dilution Ventilation

There are three major categories of ventilation systems that are used in modern industry: general ventilation systems, dilution ventilation systems, and local exhaust ventilation systems. Each of these systems has a specific purpose, and it is not uncommon to find all three types of systems present in a given plant location.

General ventilation systems are used to control the comfort level of the worker in the environment. These systems may involve the removal of air that has become heated by the process beyond a desired temperature level. In addition, a general ventilation system supplies air to the work area to condition the air in the work area or to make up for the air that has been exhausted by a dilution ventilation system or a local exhaust ventilation system. The air that is supplied to the area may or may not be conditioned by heating or cooling the air.

The purpose of a dilution ventilation system is to dilute the concentration of contaminants in the air with uncontaminated air so as to reduce the concentration below a given level, usually the threshold limit value (TLV) of the contaminant. This is accomplished by removing or supplying air so as to cause the air in the workplace to move and, as a result, mix the contaminated air with incoming uncontaminated air.

The third major category of ventilation systems is the local exhaust ventilation system. The purpose of a local exhaust ventilation system is to remove the contaminated air at its source before it is allowed to escape into the workroom. Contaminated air is captured and removed from the source through a hood and duct with no potential for escape of the contaminated air into the workplace environment.

In the following chapters, the subject of local exhaust ventilation and make-up air will be discussed in more detail. This chapter will discuss the subject of dilution ventilation.

Principles of Dilution Ventilation

In order to accomplish the objective of a dilution ventilation system, it is necessary that air movement be present. If the air is stagnant, the contaminant will move slowly within the workroom atmosphere. Thus, the highest concentration will be present near the source and, as a result, in the worker's breathing zone. In a typical workplace, some natural mixing will occur as a result of air currents. These currents may be caused by thermal draft or by the movement of people and equipment within the workplace. Air velocities of at least 50 feet per minute may be found in the workplace as a result of these causes. However, these air currents are not sufficient to provide the necessary mixing to dilute high concentrations of a toxic materia If the air is caused to move, the concentration of hazardous material will be mixed with the surrounding uncontaminated air in the workplace, resulting in lower concentration of contaminant for a given area. If the mixed air is the removed from the workplace and replaced by uncontaminated air, the level of contaminant can be controlled in the entire work area. The objective of dilution ventilation is to mix the contaminated air thoroughly with a large volume of uncontaminated air in the workplace and then to remove the mixture at a rate such that a buildup of contamination will not occur.

There are three major sources of air movement that can be used to mix the air in a dilution ventilation system. The first of these is the natural draf caused by prevailing winds moving through open doors and windows of the work area. However, this method of moving the air does not provide a satisfactory source for most dilution ventilation systems. If the outside ambient temperature is cold, the use of natural forces will induce a cold draft near doors and windows, thus making these areas uncomfortable for the workers. In addition, the wind provides neither a constant force nor a constant direction that can be used to assure adequate dilution.

Figure 2.4.1

Dilution of contaminants.

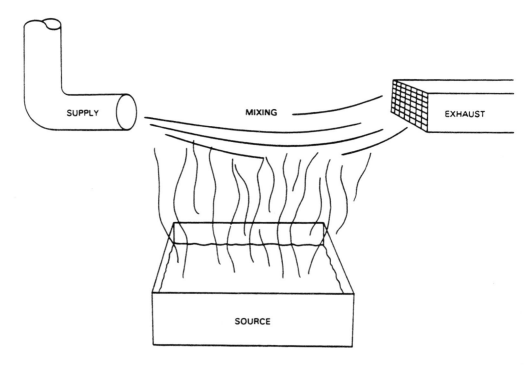

The second method for moving air is the use of thermal draft. Thermal draft may be the result of natural causes, or it may be generated from process heat. In either case, as the air is heated, it expands in volume and becomes lighter. The heated air rises, carrying any contaminant that is present upward with it. Vents in the roof allow this air to escape into the atmosphere. The supply of fresh air will enter the work area through doors and windows to replace the air that has escaped through the roof vents. In many cases, thermal draft is not sufficient to provide the air movement necessary to dilute the contaminant. However, in those cases where an extremely hot process is present, the draft caused may be sufficient to cause the contaminant to be carried upward through roof vents.

In cold temperatures, a natural thermal draft occurs because the work environment of the plant is at a higher temperature than the outside air. This results in a pressure difference between the building and the outside. The heated air escapes through roof vents and is replaced by the colder, fresh air from the outside. Such a system is not normally satisfactory for dilution ventilation because of the cold drafts that are induced and the potential for stratification of the air at different temperature levels within the building, thus creating in effect a barrier to the escape of the contaminated air.

The most reliable source for air movement in a dilution ventilation system is provided by a mechanical air mover. Such a system provides a constant source of air movement for mixing. Mechanical methods can be used to supply air to the work area, remove or exhaust air from the work area, or to supply and exhaust air at the same time. Mechanical methods may also be used to supplement natural or thermal sources of air movement. As a general rule, a dilution ventilation system will require a mechanical air mover to provide the air movement necessary for the system to operate effectively.

Components of a Dilution Ventilation System

A dilution ventilation system is a simple system. It requires a source of exhaust for contaminated air. This may involve vents through which the contaminated air will escape and a mechanical air mover to exhaust the contaminated air. A source of air supply is necessary to replace the air mixture that has been removed with uncontaminated air. This can involve an inlet for uncontaminated air, such as doors, windows, or vents; or it may involve a mechanical fan to supply the necessary air.

In most cases, since it is desirable that a complete mixing of the entire workroom air occur, a duct system is required to supply or remove air throughout the work area. The necessary duct is used to distribute the supply air and remove the contaminated air to assure that small pockets of low air flow do not exist where contamination buildup can occur. Because of this minimum duct requirement, the cost of installing a dilution ventilation system is often relatively low, even though the air mover required to operate the system is itself large and expensive.

Finally, the dilution ventilation system often requires a method to filter and temper the incoming air. Filtering is used to remove any particulate contamination in the air being supplied. Tempering of the supply air is required when the outside air temperature is so low or so high as to cause uncomfortable conditions in the work area. Most often tempering involves heating cold air before it enters the work environment.

Contamination Generation

In order to better understand the process that occurs in a dilution ventilation system, it is desirable to investigate in some detail the process of contaminant generation that can occur for a given industrial process. The objective of this investigation is to develop a formula that can be used to ascertain the volume of dilution ventilation that is required in a particular process.

If a process generates a contaminant, this contaminant will build up over time unless it is removed at a rate equal to or greater than that at which the buildup occurs. Should the rate of removal be less than the generation rate, the contaminant will build up. This relationship between generation and removal can be stated as:

Accumulation rate = Generation rate - Removal rate

Calculus can be utilized to state the above in a more rigorous form. The presentation given below is adapted from discussions presented in The Industrial Environment: Its Evaluation and Control, pages 579-580, and Hemeon's Plant and Process Ventilation, pages 228-230. Stated mathematically, the above formula is given as:

(2.4.1) $VdC = Gdt - Q'Cdt$

where

C = the concentration of gas or vapor at time t, ppm
G = the rate of generation of contaminant, cfm
Q = the rate of ventilation, cfm
K = design distribution constant to allow for incomplete mixing of contaminant and air
$Q' = \dfrac{Q}{K}$ = the effective rate of ventilation corrected for incomplete mixing, cfm
V = the volume of the room or enclosure, ft^3

To determine the concentration buildup that will occur over a given period of time, the above equation is rearranged for integration as follows:

$$\int_{C_1}^{C_2} \frac{dC}{G-Q'C} = \frac{Q'}{V} \int_{t_1}^{t_2} dt = \frac{1}{V} \int_{t_1}^{t_2} dt$$

Integrating the above gives:

$$\ln \frac{G - Q'C_2}{G - Q'C_1} = \frac{Q'}{V} (t_2 - t_1)$$

or since

$$\ln x = 2.303 \log x$$

$$(2.4.2) \quad \log \frac{G - Q'C_2}{G - Q'C_1} = -\frac{1}{2.303} \frac{Q'}{V} (t_2 - t_1)$$

Example

Consider a room that is 30 ft by 60 ft by 20 ft high where a contaminant is being generated at a rate of 2 cubic feet per minute. The room is being supplied with fresh air at a rate of 7,200 cubic feet per minute. If the room initially contains no concentration of contaminant, how long will it take for the concentration of contaminant in the room to reach 500 ppm? Assume a factor of 5 for incomplete mixing.

Solution

Rearranging the formula (2.4.2) where:

$$C_1 = 0 \text{ at } t_1, \quad t_1 = 0$$

$$t_2 = -2.303 \frac{V}{Q'} \log \frac{G - Q'C_2}{G - Q'C_1} \quad (2.4.2)$$

if

$$Q' = \frac{7200}{5} = 1440 \text{ cfm}$$

$$t_2 = -2.303 \times \frac{36000}{1440} \log \frac{2 - (1440 \times 500 \times 10^{-6})}{2}$$

$$t_2 = -57.6 \log \frac{2 - 0.72}{2}$$

$$t_2 = -57.6(-0.194)$$

$$t_2 = 11.17 \text{ min}$$

Purging of a Concentration Buildup

In the previous discussion, we looked at how a concentration of contaminant builds up in an area. Now assume a volume of contaminated air exists in a room with no additional contaminant being added. What will be the effect of a supply of fresh air being introduced into the room in order to purge the room of the contaminant?

Going back to the original relationship:
Accumulation rate = 0 - Removal rate
where
Purging rate = -Accumulation rate

Using calculus to state this relationship, the following is obtained:

$$VdC = -Q'Cdt$$

where the same notation as above applies.

$$\int_{C_1}^{C_2} \frac{dC}{C} = -\frac{Q'}{V} \int_{t_1}^{t_2} dt$$

(2.4.3) $$\log \frac{C_2}{C_1} = -\frac{1}{2.303} \times \frac{Q'}{V} (t_2 - t_1)$$

Example

Referring to the situation presented in the preceding discussion, how much time will be required to reduce the concentration from 500 ppm to 50 ppm at the same ventilation rate as was used previously?

Solution

If C_1 = 50 ppm

C_2 = 500 ppm

$\Delta t = t_2 - t_1$

then

$$\Delta t = \frac{2.303V}{Q'} \log \frac{C_2}{C_1} \quad (2.4.3)$$

$$\Delta t = \frac{2.303 \times 36,000}{1440} \log \frac{500}{50}$$

$$\Delta t = 57.58 \text{ min}$$

Maintaining a Steady State Concentration

The objective of a dilution ventilation system is to maintain a steady state concentration wherein the change in concentration or dC = 0. The desired steady state concentration is a value which is less than the threshold limit value for the contaminant of concern. Thus, if a source of fresh air can be introduced into the workroom atmosphere at a rate that will dilute any contaminant generated to a level below that of the threshold limit value, a potentially hazardous concentration will be controlled.

Again, using the original relationship,

Accumulation rate = Generation rate - Removal rate

and controlling the process to assure that the accumulation rate is equal to 0, the relationship becomes

0 = Generation rate - Removal rate

where

Generation rate = Removal rate

Again returning to calculus to develop the mathematical relationships involved, we have

$$Gdt = Q'Cdt$$

or

$$\int_{t_1}^{t_2} Gdt = \int_{t_1}^{t_2} Q'Cdt$$

Integrating, we obtain

$$G(t_2 - t_1) = Q'C(t_2 - t_1)$$

or

$$Q' = \frac{G}{C}$$

since

$$Q' = \frac{Q}{K}$$

(2.4.4) $$Q = \frac{KG}{C}$$

Example

Referring to the preceding example, determine the ventilation rate that is required to obtain a steady state concentration of 200 ppm of the contaminant.

Solution

Using the relationship developed above, the following result will be obtained:

If

K = 5
G = 2 cfm
C = 200 ppm

then

$$Q = \frac{KG}{C} \quad (2.4.4)$$

$$Q = \frac{5 \times 2 \text{ cfm} \times 10^6}{200}$$

$$Q = 50,000 \text{ cfm}$$

The above examples are somewhat artificial because the generation rate (G) is not obtainable in cfm in most situations. Most often the generation rate is obtained as an evaporation rate (ER) in pounds per hour or pints per hour. Thus, it is necessary to convert the generation rate to reflect these units in order that a useful relationship can be developed.

From Avogadro's hypothesis, we know that equal volumes of all gases under the same conditions of temperature and pressure contain the same number of molecules. Thus, one pound-mole of any gas will occupy the same volume as one pound-mole of any other gas if it is at the same temperature and pressure. A standard conditions of 70°F and 14.7 psia (29.92 inches of Hg), the mole-volume of a gas is 386.7 cubic feet per pound-mole. Thus, to determine the cubic feet of gas per pound-mole evaporated, the following relationship is developed:

$$\text{Cubic feet of gas per pound evaporated} = \frac{386.7}{\text{molecular weight}}$$

If the evaporation rate is in pints

   1 gallon = 8 pints = 8.345 pounds H_2O

      1 pint = 1.0432 pounds H_2O

or

$$\frac{386.7}{MW} \text{ ft}^3/\text{lb} \times 1.0432 \text{ lb/pt} = \frac{403.4}{MW} \text{ ft}^3/\text{pt}$$

which is the constant for any liquid. The volume is stated as

$$\frac{403}{\text{Molecular Weight}} \times \text{Specific Gravity}$$

Then, to determine the steady-state ventilation rate for a vapor at standard conditions if the evaporation rate is known in pints, the following is developed:

$$\text{From} \quad Q = \frac{KG}{C}$$

we obtain

$$Q = K \times ER \frac{403}{MW} \times \alpha \times \frac{10^6}{TLV}$$

(2.4.5) $$Q = \frac{403 \times \alpha \times 10^6 \times K}{MW \times TLV} \times ER$$

where

α = specific gravity of contaminant
K = safety factor
ER = evaporation rate of contaminant, pt/min
MW = molecular weight of contaminant
TLV = threshold limit value for the contaminant

If the ER is known in pounds, the above can be converted to:

(2.4.5) $$Q = \frac{386.7 \times \alpha \times 10^6 \times K}{MW \times TLV} \times ER$$

Example. As an illustration, let us apply the formula derived to determine the dilution ventilation rate which is required in a given situation. Assume a manual degreasing operation is being performed in which perchloroethylene (or tetrachloroethylene) is used at a rate of one-half pint per hour. The room in which the degreasing is being performed is 20 ft. long by 20 ft. wide by 15 ft. high. Assuming a K value of 6 for this operation, the following can be calculated:

$$Q = \frac{403 \times \alpha \times 10^6 \times K}{MW \times TLV} \times \frac{.5}{60} \quad (2.4.5)$$

$$Q = \frac{403 \times 1.62 \times 10^6 \times 6 \times .5}{166 \times 50 \times 60} \qquad \text{(Note: 1985-86 TLV used.)}$$

$$Q = 3932 \text{ cfm}$$

To determine the velocity of air in the room, assume the supply is at one end of the room.

$$Q = vA \quad (2.3.4)$$
$$3932 = v \times (20 \times 15)$$
$$v = 13 \text{ fpm}$$

From the above, it can be seen that dilution ventilation provides a reasonable control method to be used. Neither the rate of flow nor the velocity is excessive.

Determination of the Safety Factor (K)

The K value that has been introduced in the previous calculations represents a safety factor that is used in calculating the dilution ventilation rate. There are a number of considerations that go into the determination of the safety factor that should be used in calculating a given dilution ventilation rate. The safety factor, K, will generally range in the area of $3 \leq K \leq 10$ based upon the judgment of the industrial hygiene engineer. Consideration should be given to the following in the determination of the value to be used for K:

1.   Efficiency of mixing as a result of the distribution of supply air. If inefficiency is expected in the mixing, K will be increased to reflect this inefficiency.

2.   The toxicity of the contaminant involved. The following categories of toxicity are considered:

Slightly toxic--TLV $>$ 500 ppm
Moderately toxic--100 ppm $\leq$ TLV $\leq$ 500 ppm
Highly toxic--TLV $<$ 100 ppm

For highly toxic materials, the K value will take on the upper limit values.

3.   Other factors are important in determination of the K value to be used. Some of these factors are:

-Seasonal changes in natural ventilation.
-Reduction in operating efficiency of air movers because of age.
-The process cycle and its duration.
-The worker's location relative to the process.
-The number and location of the points of generation of the contaminant.

Substitution of Materials

When a material that has a high toxicity is used in the process, it requires excessive dilution rates for control. It may be possible to substitute a material of lower toxicity. The evaporation rate of the original material will be known. To determine the dilution ventilation rate required for the substitute material, it will be necessary to determine the evaporation rate for the substitute. To make this determination, n-butyl acetate is used as a standard since it has an ER of 100. The evaporation rate of the substitute material can then be calculated by

$$ER = f(MW, vp)$$

(2.4.7) $$ER = \frac{MW \times vapor\ pressure\ (mm\ Hg)}{11}$$

Once the evaporation rate for the substitute has been established, the amount that will be evaporated can be calculated by the ratio:

$$\frac{ER_1}{ER_2} = \frac{\text{pints per hour}_1}{\text{pints per hour}_2}$$

Example. As an example of such a substitution, consider the previous example using perchloroethylene. If it is desired to substitute trichloroethylene (vapor pressure = 62 mm Hg) for perchloroethylene (vapor pressure = 23 mm Hg), the following calculations of the ER for each solvent are given:

To calculate the ER for each solvent, formula 2.4.7 is used.
Perchloroethylene

$$ER = \frac{166 \times 23}{11} = 347$$

Trichloroethylene

$$ER = \frac{131 \times 62}{11} = 738$$

To determine the pints/hour evaporated for trichloroethylene:

$$\frac{ER_1}{ER_2} = \frac{\text{pints per hour}_1}{\text{pints per hour}_2}$$

$$\frac{347}{748} = \frac{0.5}{x}$$

$$x = 1.08 \text{ pints/hour}$$

To determine the new dilution rate, use formula 2.4.5.

$$Q = \frac{403 \times 1.46 \times 10^6 \times 6 \times 1.08}{131 \times 50 \times 60} \qquad \text{(Note: 1985–86 TLV used.)}$$

$$Q = 9700 \text{ cfm}$$

Dilution Ventilation for Mixtures

Quite often a process involves the use of two or more toxic materials. In the absence of any information concerning the hazardous effects of these materials, the effects should be considered as additive. Thus, the sum of the ratios of the concentration to TLV should be less than 1 for the mixture of materials in the atmosphere. This can be stated as:

$$(2.4.8) \qquad \frac{C_1}{TLV_1} + \frac{C_2}{TLV_2} + \ldots \frac{C_n}{TLV_n} < 1$$

If there is reason to believe that the effects are not additive, that is, the toxic materials affect different parts of the human system, then the individual concentration to TLV ratios should each be less than 1. This can be stated as follows:

$$(2.4.9) \quad \frac{C_1}{TLV_1} < 1, \quad \frac{C_2}{TLV_2} < 1 \ldots \frac{C_n}{TLV_n} < 1$$

If the effects are assumed to be additive, then the dilution ventilation rate (Q') is calculated by summing the dilution ventilation rates required for each toxic material alone. This is given as:

$$(2.4.10) \quad Q' = Q'_1 + Q'_2 + \ldots Q'_n$$

where

$$Q' = \frac{Q}{K}$$

If the effects are independent, then the required dilution rate for the mixture (Q') is given as

$(2.4.11)$ Q' = the largest Q' for contaminants in the mixture.

Dilution Ventilation for Fire and Explosion Control

The purpose of dilution ventilation for fire and explosion control is to reduce the concentration of vapors within an enclosure below the lower explosive limit (LEL). The approach used is not applicable where workers are present since the TLV for a given material is generally significantly less than the LEL and, as a result, becomes the controlling factor.

The formula for calculating the dilution ventilation rates for explosive materials is derived from the previous formula applied to hazardous concentrations. The formula can be stated as:

$$(2.4.12) \quad Q = \frac{403 \times \alpha \times 100 \times K'}{MW \times LEL \times B} \times ER$$

where
  100 = the factor for LEL that is given in percent (parts per hundred) rather than ppm as specified for a TLV
  LEL = the lower explosive limit
  K' = the safety factor
  B = the factor for a change in LEL with increasing temperature
  B = 1 for temperatures < 250°
  B = 0.7 for temperatures > 250°
  ER = evaporation rate, pt/min
  MW = molecular weight of the contaminant
  α = specific gravity of the contaminant

As in the case of applying dilution ventilation for hazardous substances, the safety factor is based upon the characteristics of the area being ventilated. In a continuous oven or a drying enclosure, K' = 4 or a vapor level of 25% of the LEL. In batch ovens with good air distribution, the safety factor may be K' = 10-12. In batch or continuous ovens with poor air circulation, the safety factor is given as K' > 12.

Care should be taken to be sure that corrections for high temperatures are made when calculating the dilution ventilation rate, Q. This precaution must be taken whether the contaminant is being controlled for fire and explosion control or for health reasons. However, correction becomes much more critical in fire and explosion control in drying ovens because of their high temperatures.

Example. To illustrate the application of the preceding to the control of a potential fire and explosion hazard, consider a batch oven with good air circulation that is operated at 325° for two hours to bake enamel pots. Xylol in the amount of 1 1/2 pints is evaporated during the process. Determine the ventilation rate in cfm required to maintain a safe concentration of xylol.

For xylol
$$LEL = 1\%$$
$$\alpha = 0.88$$
$$MW = 106$$

Since a batch oven is being used
$$K = 10$$
at 325°
$$B = 0.7$$
$$ER = 0.75 \text{ pt/hr}$$

Then from 2.4.12

$$Q = \frac{403 \times 0.88 \times 100 \times 10}{106 \times 1 \times 0.7} \times \frac{0.75}{60}$$

$$Q = 60 \text{ cfm}$$

Using 2.1.5 to correct for temperature:

$$Q_c = Q \times \frac{T_2 + 460°F}{T_1 + 460°F}$$

$$Q_c = 60 \times \frac{325°F + 460°F}{70°F + 460°F}$$

$$Q_c = 89 \text{ cfm}$$

Thermal Ventilation for Dilution

Consider the case where a process exists inside a plant that is heated continuously. The outdoor air is slightly colder than the air inside the plant. Because of this, a thermal draft in the plant will exist wherein the heated air with reduced density will rise and ventilate through roof openings. This will create an upward thermal draft that will cause air from the outside to enter the building at lower levels and, as it becomes heated, rise to the upper levels and exit. This draft will provide a rate of ventilation that will dilute any toxic materials present in the workplace. It is desirable to determine what effect this thermal draft will have in diluting the hazardous materials. The density of air can be given as

$$d_h = 0.075 \times \frac{460°F + 70°F}{460°F + t°F}$$

where

d_h = the density of the heated air
t = the temperature of the heated air

To determine the ventilation rate due to thermal draft, the following formula is given:

(2.4.13) $Q = 9.4A \sqrt{H(T_i - T_o)}$

where

Q = cfm rate of air flow
A = the area of the inlet or outlet, whichever is smaller, ft^2
H = the height in feet between the inlet and outlet, ft.
T_i = the average indoor temperature, °F
T_o = the temperature of the outdoor air, °F

Example. If the temperature difference $(T_i - T_o)$ is very large, the thermal draft that results can be significant. Consider a work area that has roof ventilation openings of 30 square feet and ground level openings of 40 square feet. The indoors is 80°F while the temperature outdoors is 45°F. To calculate the air flow which will result from the thermal draft caused by this temperature difference, the following is given:

$Q = 9.4A \sqrt{H(T_i - T_o)}$ (2.4.13)

$Q = 9.4 \times 30 \sqrt{20(80 - 45)}$

$Q = 7461 \ cfm$

As can be seen from the above, the ventilation rate obtained is significant and should be considered as a potential source for dilution ventilation.

General Rules for Application of Dilution Ventilation

Dilution ventilation for the control of toxic substances is normally applicable for substances with high TLV's: that is, low toxicity. Substances with moderate or low toxicity (TLV > 100) can be handled in many cases using dilution ventilation. However, it is important to remember that even with low toxicity substances, the breathing zone of the worker must be controlled below the TLV. The dilution ventilation system must be such as to carry away the high concentrations of contaminant before they reach the breathing zone of the worker.

Dilution ventilation is generally not applicable for fumes or dust since these materials are often highly toxic, and the velocity and rate of evolution are high. Data on the evolution rate of fumes and dust are difficult to obtain, and reliance on dilution ventilation without adequate evolution rate data is risky.

It is important, regardless of the level of toxicity of the contaminant, that the evolution occur at a reasonably uniform rate. Cyclical buildup of contaminant at levels higher than the design of the dilution ventilation system can produce airborne contaminant concentrations at higher than the TLV. In addition, the quantity of contaminant being released should be relatively small so as not to require high dilution rates. This is often the case for organic solvent vapors; and thus, dilution ventilation may be satisfactory for these vapors.

Often the design of the equipment or process involved eliminates the use of local exhaust ventilation equipment. In such cases, dilution ventilation becomes the only viable alternative that can be applied.

Economics is a major factor in considering dilution ventilation. The initial cost of a dilution ventilation system is generally much less than that of a local exhaust system. However, the operating cost may be high as a result of the large volumes of air that are exhausted, requiring tempered air to be introduced into the work environment to replace the exhausted air. The cost of heating or cooling the air can become excessive if the rate of flow is significant.

When applying dilution ventilation, a combined supply and exhaust system is usually the most appropriate. In such a system, an excess of exhaust is desirable if there are adjoining work areas. This will assure that contaminant released in the work area does not enter adjoining work areas through open doors or cracks. If only one work area is involved, an excess of supply air is desirable to force the contaminated air out of the work area as quickly as possible. In either case, it is important to take care in locating the exhaust outlets in order to avoid re-entry into the work area or other work areas. The exhaust outlets should be located as close to the source as possible so that the major contaminant will exit the work area quickly.

Dilution ventilation is applicable to the control of fire and explosion where workers are not present. Dilution ventilation is also useful in the control of odor and the general air quality of the work area in the absence of

Figure 2.4.2

Supply--exhaust location.

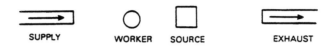

SUPPLY   WORKER   SOURCE   EXHAUST

hazardous substances. With appropriate air conditioning, the dilution ventilation system can also be of value in controlling the ambient temperature and humidity within the work area itself.

Problems Related to the Use of Dilution Ventilation

There are a number of problems that are related to the use of dilution ventilation. Among the most important of these are the following:

1. The high operating cost to condition air supplied to the workroom.
2. The requirement for high volumes of air to be moved through the workroom.
3. The dilution system does not remove the contaminant from the work area; it only lowers its concentration level.
4. Dilution ventilation is not applicable to particulate contamination.
5. Dilution ventilation is not applicable where high rates of evolution of toxic substances are present.

Summary

The following table summarizes the important formulas presented in the chapter.

REFERENCE	RELATIONSHIP	FORMULA
2.4.1	Accumulation rate as a function of generation and removal rate.	$VdC = Gdt - Q'Cdt$
2.4.2	Buildup of a contaminant with constant generation rate.	$\log \dfrac{G - Q'C_2}{G - Q'C_1} = -\dfrac{1}{2.303}\dfrac{Q'}{V}(t_2 - t_1)$
2.4.3	Purging of a contaminant with no generartion of new contaminant.	$\log \dfrac{C_2}{C_1} = -\dfrac{1}{2.303}\dfrac{Q'}{V}(t_2 - t_1)$

REFERENCE	RELATIONSHIP	FORMULA
2.4.4	Rate of dilution to obtain steady state contaminant generation.	$Q = \dfrac{KG}{C}$
2.4.5	Rate of dilution necessary to control concentration of contaminant with ER known in pints.	$Q = \dfrac{403 \times \alpha \times 10^6 \times K \times ER}{MW \times TLV}$
2.4.6	Rate of dilution necessary to control concentration of contaminant with ER known in pints.	$Q = \dfrac{386.7 \times \alpha \times 10^6 \times K \times ER}{MW \times TLV}$
2.4.7	Calculate evaporation rate of a given substance.	$ER = \dfrac{MW \times vapor\ pressure}{11}$
2.4.8	Concentration level for contaminant with additive effects.	$\dfrac{C_1}{TLV_1} + \dfrac{C_2}{TLV_2} + \ldots \dfrac{C_n}{TLV_n} < 1$
2.4.9	Concentration level for contaminant with nonadditive or unknown effects.	$\dfrac{C_1}{TLV_1} < 1, \dfrac{C_2}{TLV_2} < 1 \ldots \dfrac{C_n}{TLV_n} < 1$
2.4.10	Rate of dilution for contaminants with additive effects.	$Q' = Q'_1 + Q'_2 + \ldots Q'_n$
2.4.11	Rate of dilution for contaminants with nonadditive or unknown effects.	$Q' = Largest\ Q'$
2.4.12	Dilution rate for control of fire and explosion.	$Q = \dfrac{403 \times \alpha \times 100 \times K'}{MW \times LEL \times B} \times ER$
2.4.13	Ventilation rate due to thermal draft.	$Q = 9.4A\sqrt{H(T_i - T_o)}$

5. Local Exhaust Ventilation

The objective of a local exhaust ventilation system is to remove the
contaminant as it is generated at the source. Gases and vapors are controlled
by controlling the air in which they are contained. Particulates of
industrial hygiene significance (i.e., $d < 10\mu m$) are controlled by
controlling the air in which they exist. These factors were illustrated in
some detail in Chapter 2 of this section. Special procedures are required to
control large particles that are generated at the source. These particles are
controlled for other than health purposes.

Components of a Local Exhaust System

The initial opening through which contaminated air enters a local exhaust
system is called the hood. The term hood is used generically for any opening
whether it is specifically designed or consists of simply the open end of a
round or rectangular duct section. Many hoods are specifically designed and
located to meet the requirements of the operation and the contaminant being
generated. Later in this chapter, the general design characteristics that
describe different types of specially constructed hoods will be discussed.

After the contaminated air has entered the hood, it flows through a duct
system which directs the flow of contaminated air and prevents mixing of this
air with the workroom atmosphere. Branches may exist within the duct to join
separate local systems into one single exhaust system.

The third component of a local exhaust system is a method for cleaning the
air. It is often necessary to remove the contaminant from the air before
exhausting the air into the atmosphere to prevent hazardous materials from
entering the breathing zone of individuals in the community surrounding the

Figure 2.5.1

Local exhaust system components.

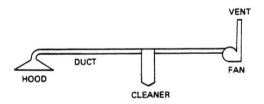

152

plant. Various types of air cleaners are used: filters, precipitators, and cyclones, among others. The type of cleaner used is selected for the particular characteristics of the contaminant that is being controlled. The design and operation of air cleaners will be covered in a later chapter.

The next component of a local exhaust system is the <u>air mover or fan</u>. The fan provides a source of air movement in a local exhaust system. Infrequently, natural draft is used as a source of air movement. This is particularly the case in hot processes that exhaust upward through a hood and outside the work area through vents on the roof. The fan to be used in a local exhaust system is sized to meet the specific air movement characteristics of the exhaust system. The desired rate of flow in cubic feet per minute and the system's static pressure are the major considerations when determining the size of fan to be used. A more complete discussion of the various types of air movers that are available and the appropriate methods for sizing these air movers will be discussed in a later chapter.

The final component of a local exhaust system is the <u>outlet or vent</u>. Often the outlet or vent for contaminated air is on the roof or through exterior stacks. In either case, care must be taken to avoid locating the outlet near any potential re-entry point to the plant to avoid recontamination of the workplace air. If an air cleaner is present, it is desirable to attach monitoring devices to assure operation of the air cleaner so that contaminated air is not exhausted in the case of equipment failure.

Blow Versus Exhaust

It is important that the reader understand the difference between the effects of blowing air from a supply system and removing air through an exhaust system. When air is supplied through a duct, it retains its directional effect for some distance beyond the end of the duct itself. At a distance of 30 diameters from the outlet, the velocity of the air is 10% of

Figure 2.5.2

Blowing air.

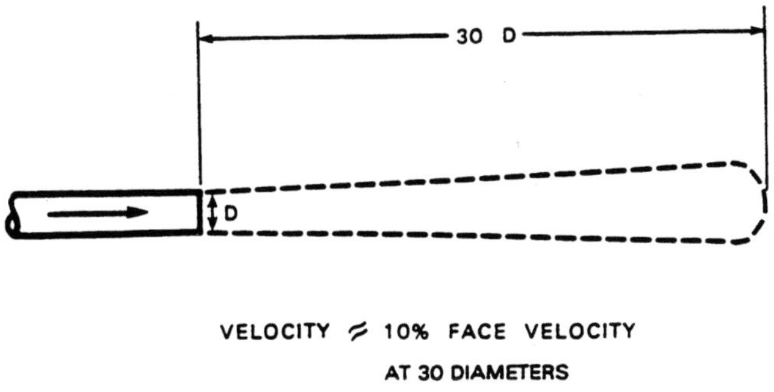

VELOCITY ≳ 10% FACE VELOCITY
AT 30 DIAMETERS

the velocity at the outlet. The diameter of the air jet increases with increasing distance from the nozzle but still retains essentially the same form for a significant distance.

As an illustration of this effect, consider the use of a common garden hose squirting water. Depending on the force of water pressure at the hose and the orifice for which the hose nozzle is set, water can be caused to travel for a significant distance from the nozzle. The water spray at a distance away from the nozzle is obviously wider than it is immediately after leaving the nozzle. However, the directional effect and the cross-sectional shape of the spray remain essentially the same.

On the other hand, consider what happens when water is collected using a wet vacuum cleaner. If a small piece of paper is placed a short distance away from the suction end of the wet vacuum, it will not be very easily gathered with the water. The same thing happens when air is exhausted through a local exhaust system. By changing the direction of the air flow through the system, we do not obtain similar velocity patterns. The velocity of the air through a local exhaust system is 10% of the inlet velocity at a distance of only one diameter from the inlet. This is illustrated by looking at the air contours that are involved in exhaust through an opening.

Figure 2.5.3

Exhausting air.

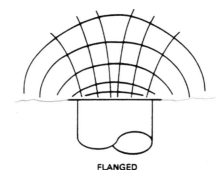

FLANGED

UNFLANGED

When air is exhausted through an opening, it is gathered equally from all directions around the opening. This includes the area behind the opening itself. Thus, the cross-sectional area of air flow approximates a spherical form rather than the conical form that is obtained when air is blown out of a supply system. By placing a flange around the exhaust opening, it is possible to reduce the air contour from the large spherical contour to that of a hemisphere and, as a result, increase the velocity of air at a given distance from the opening. This basic principle is used in designing exhaust hoods. The closer the exhaust hood is to the source and the less uncontaminated air it gathers, the more efficient the capture of the hood will be.

Rate of Flow in a Hood

Air that enters a local exhaust system enters at the hood face (the cross-sectional area of the hood at its opening). At this point, air has a given velocity that is called the _face velocity_. The face velocity is approximately equal over all points on the face of the hood if the hood has been properly designed. The rate of flow for a hood is given as the face velocity times the cross-sectional area of the hood opening.

$$Q = vA \quad (2.3.4)$$

where
   Q = the rate of flow in cfm
   v = the face velocity of the hood in fpm
   A = the area of the hood face in ft^2

Example. To illustrate the use of this formula, assume a face velocity is measured at 300 fpm on a circular flanged hood of diameter 10 inches. The rate of air flow in cubic feet per minute that is present in this system, assuming standard conditions, can be calculated as follows:

$$Q = vA \quad (2.3.4)$$
$$Q = 300 \text{ fpm} \times 0.5454 \text{ ft}^2$$
$$Q = 164 \text{ cfm}$$

The Application and Advantage of Local Exhaust Ventilation

One of the major advantages of a local exhaust system is the fact that the contaminant is removed at the source. This removal is necessary when working in areas where highly toxic contaminants are present. Though dilution ventilation can be used to control such contaminants, quite often the rate of flow that is required is too high to be practical as a method of control. In these cases, local exhaust ventilation systems are most appropriate.

Local exhaust ventilation systems require lower air volumes than are required for dilution ventilation. As a result, a lower cost of operation in terms of tempering the workplace air is experienced. Lower air cleaning costs are also encountered. The initial expense in installing the necessary duct can be partially offset by the fact that the air moving devices can be sized smaller to move the lower air volume required.

The air volume that is moved through the local exhaust ventilation system is dependent upon the required capture velocity for the contaminant. <u>Capture velocity</u> is the velocity that is necessary to capture the contaminant at its farthest possible distance from the hood. From the previous discussions concerning the characteristics of exhaust air contours, it is obvious that this distance cannot be very great. As the distance from the source to the hood is increased, the rate of flow of the system must also be increased in order to obtain the desired capture velocity at the source.

When designing and installing a local exhaust ventilation system, it is important to consider the presence of any air currents that might cause the contaminant to be moved away from the hood. Potential sources of external air motion that can result in inadequate contaminant capture in a local exhaust system include:

1. Currents caused by motion in the plant.
2. Currents caused by general ventilation systems.
3. Thermal draft.
4. Motion imparted to the contaminant air by the process.
5. Entrainment of contaminated air by motion of large particles that are also generated by the process.
6. Motion of the air caused by indirect mechanical action of the processing equipment.

The reader should remember that gases, vapors, and particulates that are of industrial hygiene significance follow the air currents and tend not to settle out or have projected motion. Thus, to remove these contaminants, control of the air flow is necessary.

General Categories of Local Exhaust Ventilation Hoods

<u>Enclosing Hoods--Total Enclosures</u>. The most efficient type of exhaust ventilation hood that can be constructed is a hood that encloses the entire operation. Openings in this enclosure are minimized with doors being used for access to the contaminant generation zone. Obviously, if no openings are required, and the enclosure can be made air-tight, then exhaust of this area is not necessary since there is no chance for the contaminant to escape into the workroom atmosphere.

The enclosing hood should be kept under negative pressure to create an inflow of air from the workroom atmosphere into the contamination zone through any openings that do exist. The capture velocity at the source of contaminant generation must be sufficient to overcome any air movement inside the enclosure itself. The effect of outside air movement is minimized in a total enclosure.

Generally, an enclosing hood is used where the process does not require that workers be present within the contaminant generation zone. Process and equipment limitations do not always allow for use of an enclosing hood. Openings may be necessary for material to enter and exit the process or

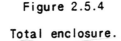

Figure 2.5.4

Total enclosure.

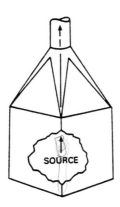

machinery. In some cases, it may be necessary for the worker to interact continuously or at intervals with the process. In these cases, openings are required for the worker's access, and a total enclosing hood cannot be applied.

Enclosing hoods have been applied in many situations. Some examples of enclosing hoods are presented in the Industrial Ventilation Manual, Section 5. If it is necessary to design a total enclosure for an exhaust ventilation system, these examples should be studied. Empirical data for the designs presented have been gathered for such things as the location of supply and exhaust vents, the velocity of the air, and the rate of flow that is necessary to control a given contaminant. Enclosing hoods have been used in such areas as abrasive blasting, crucible melting furnaces, foundry shakeouts, mixing and mulling machines, processes generating highly toxic contaminants, and screening applications. Wherever possible, the enclosing hood is the most appropriate type of exhaust hood to apply because of its inherent efficiency in capturing generated contaminants.

Enclosing Hoods--Booths and Tunnels. Where there is a necessity for access either on one side or two sides of a process, the most desirable type of enclosing hood to use is the booth or tunnel.

The face velocity of such an enclosure is determined at the opening of the tunnel or booth. The face velocity must be sufficient to eliminate the escape of air from the enclosure and to eliminate effects of external movement on the process within the enclosure.

The worker may work either inside or outside the booth. If the worker is internal, the work position should be located between the face of the booth and the exhaust inlet.

It is obvious that a booth or tunnel will require higher exhaust rates than will a total enclosure. Thus, the booth or tunnel is less efficient.

Figure 2.5.5

Booth and tunnel hoods.

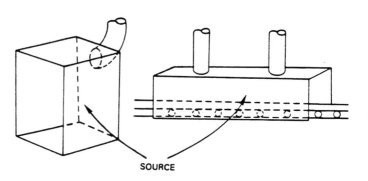

SOURCE

However, certain applications require the use of such an exhaust hood. Examples of the applications of the booth or tunnel include laboratory hoods, abrasive cut-off saws, continuous buffing where a tunnel is used, material movement where entry and exit points are necessary, grinding, paint spraying, and welding.

Rate of Flow for Enclosing Hoods. The air flow rate for an enclosing hood is determined by the required face velocity at any of the openings that are necessary to control for such things as internally induced air movement--including thermal effects, mechanical movements, process material movement, and worker movement--and externally induced air movement that may be caused by general ventilation systems, natural air currents, and movement of equipment and workers external to the process. The face velocity at any opening must be sufficient to overcome both the internal and external air movement. Thus, to determine the air flow rate for an enclosing hood, one should determine the velocity that is necessary at the face of the hood. The area of opening in square feet comprises the face area of the hood. Then, using $Q = vA$, the required rate of flow in cfm can be calculated.

Exterior Hoods. Where it is not possible to use a total enclosure or a partial enclosure such as a booth or tunnel, the exterior hood can be applied. Exterior hoods are hoods that are adjacent to the sources of contamination. The operation itself is exterior to the boundary of the hood face. For such a hood, the capture velocity is created at the source to overcome any movement and capture the contaminant. Capture velocity must be such as to overcome any exterior air currents, overcome any process-induced motion such as projected motion, and move the contaminant from its most distant location to the hood face.

Exterior hoods are inefficient when compared to enclosure-type hoods. Air enters the hood from all directions, and the area between the source and hood is subject to the effects of external air movement. External hoods are applied where it is not possible to use the more efficient type of hoods.

Figure 2.5.6

Exterior hood.

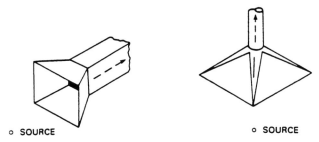

○ SOURCE   ○ SOURCE

The hood itself may be located in the path of contaminant generation in order to improve the capture of contaminants.

There are four general categories of exterior hoods. Two categories are by type of face opening, and two are by location of the hood relative to the source.

1. Type of Opening
    A.   Round or rectangular duct openings
    B.   Slot openings

2. Location Relative to Source
    A.   Canopy hoods
    B.   Receiving hoods

The round or rectangular duct opening is the simplest type of hood. It is also one of the most inefficient. The operation generating the contaminant must be close to the hood face in order to provide adequate capture velocity. The hood itself can be attached to a flexible duct so that it can be moved to capture sources of contamination that may be generated at different locations in the work area. As has been previously discussed, a flange or taper can be added to the round or rectangular opening hood to increase its efficiency.

Figure 2.5.7

Round or rectangular hoods.

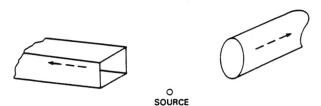

○
SOURCE

The round or rectangular duct opening hood can be used in many applications. Examples of its use include welding benches, surface grinding, and hand saws. In addition, it can be applied to various portable and hand tools when flexible duct or rubber hose is used.

The second category of exterior hood is the slot hood (Figure 2.5.8). Slot hoods are defined as hoods with openings whose width-to-length ratio is less than 0.2. The advantage of the slot hood is that it maintains an air flow over a large surface plane. Quite often the slot hood is used along the sides of large open tanks. If the distance for capture is great (the width o the tank is too large to apply adequate velocity at the midpoint of the tank) the slot opening is used in combination with a blowing supply slot. This typ of ventilation system is called a "push-pull" ventilation system and creates plane of air that acts as a barrier to any contaminant generated in the tank.

The slot hood is less efficient than a round or rectangular opening when it is necessary to remove air from a given point. Obviously, a series of discrete points of contamination would best be exhausted (not considering economic circumstances) by applying a series of round or rectangular hoods at each point source. Where the source of contamination is continuous over the entire length of the slot, this method is best.

The slot hood has been applied in a number of areas. There are slot hood for belt wiping, slot hoods on welding benches where any point may be used fo the actual weld, and slot hoods on degreasing tanks, other open surface tanks and process tables where any point may be used for the process.

The third type of exterior hood is the canopy hood. Canopy hoods are overhead openings that are generally used for hot processes which cause thermal draft. Canopy hoods can also be used for cold processes where, for example, it is necessary to control evaporation from an open tank. Sides or baffles can improve the operation of a canopy hood by approximating the design of an enclosed hood or booth.

<table>
<tr><td>Figure 2.5.8</td><td>Figure 2.5.9</td></tr>
<tr><td>Slot hood.</td><td>Canopy hood.</td></tr>
</table>

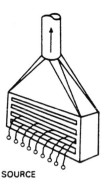

SOURCE

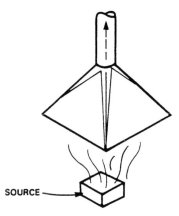

SOURCE

Applications of the canopy hood include die casting melting furnaces and the open surface tank.

The fourth type of external exhaust hood is the <u>receiving hood</u>. The receiving hood is actually one of the above types of hoods where the exhaust port itself is located in the path of contaminant generation. Thus, it is located at a point that receives any process-induced contamination. The canopy hood is a type of receiving hood where the process-induced motion caused by thermal effects is upward. The receiving hood takes advantage of any directional inertia of the contaminant, thus lowering the necessary capture velocity that must be applied. Examples of receiving hoods include hoods used for grinding wheels, polishing wheels, and hoods used for various types of table saws or band saws.

Figure 2.5.10

Receiving hood.

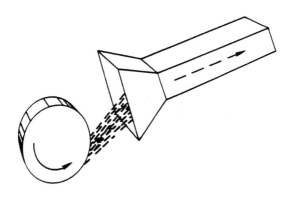

Summary

Local exhaust systems are used to capture the contaminant at the source before entry into the workroom air. Local exhaust systems generally include as components the hood, duct, an air cleaner, an air mover, and a vent or outlet. Local exhaust systems must provide the necessary control of the contaminant-laden air at the source. Because air is drawn into the hood from all points around the hood face, the hood must be relatively close to the source. In addition, the hood must be designed to be as efficient as possible. This involves enclosing as much of the source of the contamination as is possible without affecting the process operation. The major categories of hoods are the enclosing hood, partial enclosing hoods (booth or tunnel), and the exterior hood.

6. Make-Up Air

When a local exhaust system is operating, significant amounts of air can be removed from the workplace. In order to assure proper operation of local exhaust systems, the air that is removed from the workplace must be replaced. This supply of air is commonly called "make-up air." Make-up air is introduced into the work area from another area or from the outside to replace air that is removed by exhaust systems and the process itself.

Unless air is introduced to replace the air lost by exhaust systems and the process-generated air flow, the work area will develop a negative pressure. This pressure will cause problems in the operation of the ventilation system. Down drafts in stacks and flues will result from the air flowing from the higher pressure outside to the lower pressure in the work area. A reduced air flow will be obtained in local and dilution exhaust systems because of the increased static pressure against which the fan must operate.

Negative pressures within the work area will cause air to enter through cracks in the doors and windows of the building. Air entering in this manner can cause high-velocity cross drafts that will impair the operation of the local exhaust system. In addition, the workers will notice cold drafts during the winter, especially near the perimeter of the building.

Insufficient make-up air can cause potential hazards in the workplace. The improper operation of local exhaust and dilution systems because of inadequate make-up air can cause a hazardous buildup of contaminants. Cross drafts can cause contaminants to be carried away from hoods into the surrounding work environment. Carbon monoxide from back draft on heaters can also accumulate. The negative pressure present in the area will cause outward-opening doors to be difficult to open and result in these doors slamming shut quickly. This can present a potential safety hazard to the workers. Increased thermal loading in hot process areas as the result of inadequate exhaust can also result in a potential hazard to the worker.

General Principles of Make-Up Air

Volume Requirements. The volume of air supplied in a make-up air system should equal the volume of air exhausted from the area. In many situations, it is desirable to have a slight positive pressure in the work area to push contaminants out of the area. When determining the exhaust air volume, it is also important to consider any natural ventilation leakage that results from pressure differences caused by the winds or thermal draft.

The determination of the volume requirements is a relatively simple process: sum the total cfm being removed by the processes and ventilation systems operating in the work area. This total along with an estimate of any natural exhaust is the basis for sizing the make-up air system required.

Location. Certain general principles should be applied in locating the air supply for a make-up air system. The supply of air should flow past the worker, through the source of contamination, to the exhaust hood. This will cause the contaminant to move away from the worker and lower any potential concentration in the worker's breathing zone.

The air supply, if it is a result of recirculation from other plant areas, should flow from cleaner areas of the plant to those areas where higher concentrations of contaminant exist. For example, recirculating air from offices to process areas is desirable; the opposite flow is not. In any case, supply air should be delivered at multiple points throughout the work area in order to eliminate high-velocity air streams from one or two supply points with high rates of flow. The delivery points should be located 8 to 10 feet from the floor to obtain maximum air flow in the worker's environmental area. Diffusers can be installed on the outlets to allow for nondirectional supply to avoid drafts. It may be necessary to provide different distribution systems for make-up air to be used during the summer and winter.

The inlet of a make-up air system should be located in an area that is free from any potential for re-entry of the contaminants. When locating the inlet, potential contaminant entry from work processes in other areas of the plant or nearby plants should also be considered. Locating a make-up air inlet downwind from a contaminant exhaust can introduce a potential hazard that may be worse than that presented by the original contaminants.

Conditioning of the Air. The make-up air supplied to the work area often requires conditioning before entering the area. During the winter, it may be necessary to heat the outside air to raise the temperature to a level adequate for the comfort of the worker. On the other hand, during the summer it may be necessary to cool outside air before introducing it to the work area. In certain situations, humidification or dehumidification may also be required, depending upon the environmental conditions that exist in the geographic location of the plant and upon the particular processes involved. For example, low humidity can lead to a static electricity buildup, causing a potential fire and explosion hazard in particular processes. Conversely, high humidity can cause mechanical damage to equipment as a result of rusting.

Signs of Inadequate Make-Up Air

The trained observer can easily identify the signs of inadequate make-up air. Doors opening outward from the work area are difficult to open because of the high outside pressure. In such cases, these doors also tend to slam shut quickly. When the door is open, outside air rushes into the work area.

Quite often in cold weather workers will complain of drafts near windows and outside walls of the work area. This draft is caused by a negative pressure in the work area as a result of inadequate make-up air and can lead to excessive absence of workers due to colds, sore muscles, etc.

Another sign of inadequate make-up air is debris entering the plant work area and gathering near windows and under doors. In addition, one less obvious sign that has a more far-reaching hazardous effect on the worker is the fact that local exhaust systems will not be operating to the designed criteria. It is unlikely that sufficient buildup of contaminant will occur be visually evident. However, velocity and rate of flow tests on the exhaust systems and monitoring of contaminants in the air may indicate that the system is operating at less than design capacity.

Components of a Make-Up Air System

The first requirement of the make-up air system is an adequate <u>air mover or fan</u> to supply the required air. Make-up air should never depend upon the passive approach such as open windows or doors. An adequate make-up air supply should be positively provided to the work area. In order to size the fan for the required make-up air system, it is necessary to determine the rate of flow of air being exhausted from the work area. Where the potential for expansion exists in the work area, the fan can be sized to meet future requirements and geared down for present operations.

The second component of a make-up air system is a <u>method for filtering the outside air</u> prior to distribution. Often outside air entering the plant is not clean and should be filtered before being distributed to the work area. In situations where recirculation air is being used, this filtering or cleaning will normally be required.

The third component is that of providing a <u>method for tempering the air</u>. As previously discussed, this can include heating, cooling, humidifying, or dehumidifying the air. The particular requirements depend upon the geographical location of the plant, time of year, and the process involved.

In addition to providing a method for tempering the air, it is desirable to provide a <u>method for bypassing</u> this tempering when it is not required. The necessary ducts and bypass dampers must be included to meet this condition. Usually bypass systems operate automatically and depend upon the condition of the entering air and the desired exit condition for make-up air.

The final component for a make-up air system is the <u>distribution system</u>. This distribution system includes ducts to each of the multiple distribution points, the grille, directional louvers, and diffusers necessary to prevent high velocity air flow. The directional louvers should be designed to allow workers in any given area to adjust air flow patterns as their needs dictate.

Methods of Tempering the Air

As discussed above, the air often has to be tempered before entry into the work area to provide for the comfort of the worker. This tempering can include humidifying, dehumidifying, cooling, or heating the air. The following discussion will be limited to methods for heating the supply air. Methods for cooling, humidifying, and dehumidifying the air will be discussed in a later section, as these relate to the control of thermal hazards.

Steam Coil. One potential source for tempering the make-up air is through the use of a steam coil. Steam is supplied by a boiler installation within the plant. The steam travels under pressure to a coil in the intake duct of the make-up air system. As the air passes over the coil, heat from the coil is transferred to the air. The steam within the coil condenses as the heat is transferred to the air stream. The condensate travels back to the boiler to be reheated and supplied to the steam distribution system.   Because of the potential vacuum that can be caused when the steam condenses, vents must be present in the steam piping to relieve this vacuum.

Figure 2.6.1

Steam coil tempering.

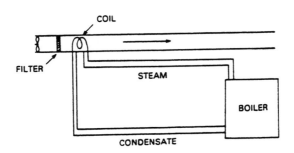

If a steam supply is present within the plant, a relatively low operating cost will be incurred to heat the incoming air. The steam coil can provide for a safe operation if the proper venting is provided. Steam coils can be used on recirculated air with excellent results.

However, steam coil heating does have certain disadvantages. The installation cost for a steam coil system is high because of the amount of plumbing involved. Steam coil heating does not provide for control of the temperature over the close range that may be necessary. Normal throttling using valves is not the best method for temperature control because of the pressure drop through the valves which can cause water hammer and its resulting damage. A bypass arrangement to mix untempered air with the tempered air can be helpful in providing more sensitive control of the air temperature. A steam coil heater requires safety controls to assure that condensate freeze-up does not occur. One method that has been used to eliminate condensate freeze-up and improve temperature control is that of providing multiple coils for preheat along with the use of bypass dampers. Although it is difficult to maintain the desired volume of air through the bypass, proper design can lead to adequate results.

Direct-Fired Heaters. The direct-fired heater involves a burner that is located in the duct. These burners operate on natural gas or liquid propane gas (LPG). The heat generated during the burning of the gas is transferred directly to the air. No outside venting is provided in a direct-fired gas heater.

Figure 2.6.2

Direct-fired tempering.

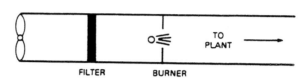

FILTER   BURNER

The direct-fired heater provides nearly 100% efficiency in heating the air. Thus the operating cost for such a system is relatively low as compared to other methods of heating the air. The installation cost is also low, particularly for larger systems. The direct-fired gas heater can provide temperature control within a very narrow range, thus leading to simplicity of operation. Because no venting is required, such a system can be easy to install.

However, there are certain problems inherent with the operation of a direct-fired heater. The products of combustion from the heater enter the air stream and are distributed to the workplace. As a result, certain safety controls are necessary to assure that improper operation does not cause a hazard. These safety controls can increase the equipment cost for small units and make such a unit impractical for installation. Care must be taken to assure that no chlorinated hydrocarbons are present in the intake air since heat can cause these materials to break down into toxic substances. The direct-fired heater is not normally permitted for use on recirculated make-up air systems.

Indirect-Fired Heaters. The indirect-fired heater involves a burner located in a combustion chamber in the duct. The combustion chamber is separated from the air stream by heat exchangers. In such a system, the products of combustion do not enter the air stream but are positively vented to the outside air by induced draft fans. The air in the duct flows by the heat exchanger where the heat is transferred to the air stream. The burner in an indirect-fired heater can operate using oil, natural gas, or LPG as a fuel.

The indirect-fired heater provides certain advantages over other methods of tempering the air. Because of the existence of a combustion chamber, no products of combustion enter the air supply. As a result, the heater can burn oil as well as gas. Small units are relatively inexpensive to install since the need for safety controls is not as great. Chlorinated hydrocarbons in the intake air will not break down in the heat exchanger. In addition, indirect-fired heaters may be used with recirculated air.

Figure 2.6.3

Indirect-fired tempering.

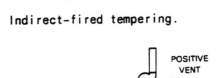
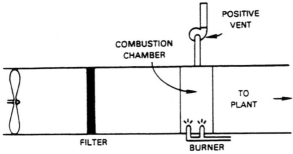

The indirect-fired heater is not as efficient as the direct-fired heater and thus results in a higher operating cost. In addition, the temperature control range for the indirect-fired heater is small, often requiring the installation of a bypass to obtain the desired temperature range. Offsetting the lower cost of the unit is the fact that a flue or chimney must be used to vent the gases from the combustion chamber. Wear on the heat exchanger can result in high maintenance costs for an indirect-fired unit.

Recirculated Air. Air that has been heated and removed from a given plant area can be recirculated to another area of the plant. This will result in a lower heating cost since the air will enter at a temperature higher than the outside temperature. It may be necessary to clean and filter the air prior to its reuse because of the potential contaminants that have been picked up in the process area.

Recirculated air may be used to lower the cost of heating make-up air. This is particularly the case where air can be recirculated from noncontaminated areas such as plant offices. If the recirculated air contains a toxic contaminant, an effective cleaning and monitoring system must be installed for reuse of this air. Such a system must include either redundant cleaning mechanisms or warning devices to alert the workers when the cleaning equipment is not working properly. For this reason, it is not generally recommended that air which has been exposed to a toxic contaminant be recirculated as make-up air. Further discussion of this topic can be found in Chapter 15 of this section.

Most states do not permit recirculated air to be tempered by direct-fired heating units. Thus, it may be necessary to install higher cost heating units if recirculated air is to be used. Whether the installation costs of these units will be offset by the lower operating cost obtained from using already tempered air must be investigated thoroughly before a decision is made.

Heat Recovery. In those cases where recirculation of exhaust air is not feasible, but where it is desirable to recover heat energy from the exhaust air, a possible approach is through the use of heat exchanger units. The general principle of operation is to pass the hot exhaust gas through a heat exchanger in some manner where the heat can be recovered and transferred to the incoming air.

One method for accomplishing this transfer is to install the incoming air duct parallel and adjacent to the exhaust duct. In such a system, the wall between the ducts can act as a heat exchanger, transferring the heat energy to the incoming cold air.

A second approach is to use the rotary heat exchanger. Such heat exchangers can be obtained in a package form for installation in the make-up and exhaust ducts. The heat exchanger acts to transfer the heat from the exhaust air to the incoming make-up air while at the same time separating the two in order to prevent contamination of the incoming air supply.

Figure 2.6.4

Rotary heat exchanger.

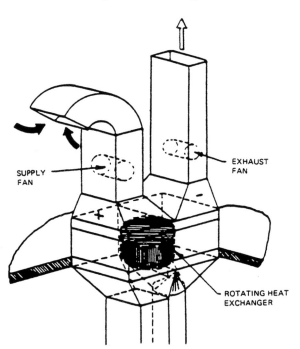

Determining the Amount and Cost of Tempering the Required Make-Up Air

In order to determine the amount of tempering that is required for a given make-up air system, the BTU's per hour output is calculated. The formula for calculating this is given below.

$$(2.6.1) \quad BTU = \frac{Q \times 1.08 \, (T_i - T_o)}{E}$$

where

BTU = BTU's per hour output
Q = cfm of air handled at standard conditions
1.08 = heat capacity of dry air
T_i = the indoor air discharge temperature desired
T_o = the outdoor air temperature for which the system is designed
E = the efficiency of the burner,
  Indirect fired
    Oil = .75
    Gas = .80
  Direct fired
    Gas = .90

Using the above formula, it is possible to estimate the cost of heating make-up air. The costs are given as:

$$(2.6.2) \quad \text{Hourly cost} = \frac{0.001 \, QN}{q} C$$

$$(2.6.3) \quad \text{Yearly cost} = \frac{0.154 \, QD \, dg}{q} C$$

where

Q = the air volume exhausted in cfm
N = the required heat in BTU's per hour per thousand cubic feet
D = the operating time in hours per week
q = the available heat per unit of fuel
dg = annual degree-days
C = the cost of fuel in dollars per unit

Example. As an example of how these formulas might be applied, consider a plant located in Cleveland, Ohio, that operates 16 hours per day, 5 days a week, and exhausts 120,000 cfm. Direct-fired gas burners are to be used to temper the air to a discharge temperature of 72°F. What total capacity of burners should be installed, and what yearly cost will be required to operate the heating system? Assume the cost of gas is $1.60 per thousand cubic feet.

Solution. Consulting temperature tables yields the fact that a low temperature of 7°F will be exceeded only 2 1/2% of the time in the Cleveland area. Using this as the design temperature, the sizing of the unit to meet the desired indoor temperature of 72°F is given by:

$$BTU = \frac{Q \times 1.08(T_i - T_o)}{E} \qquad (2.6.1)$$

$$BTU = \frac{120,000 \text{ cfm} \times 1.08(72°F - 7°F)}{0.90}$$

$$BTU/hr = 9,360,000$$

To obtain the yearly cost per year, the following formula is used:

$$\text{Yearly cost} = \frac{0.154 \text{ QD dg}}{q} C \qquad (2.6.3)$$

The degree-days and heat per unit to be used are found by consulting either the Heating, Ventilation, and Air-Conditioning Guide, ASHRAE, or the Industrial Ventilation Manual, Table 7-6, 7-7.

Using the formula:

$$\text{Yearly cost} = \frac{0.154 \times 120,000 \text{ cfm} \times 80 \text{ hrs} \times 8567 \text{ dg}}{900 \text{ BTU/ft}^3} \times \$0.00160/\text{ft}^3$$

Yearly cost = $22,516

7. Design of Exhaust Hoods

The purpose of a local exhaust ventilation system is to capture the contaminants in the air, at or near their source of generation. In this way the contaminant is prevented from entering the breathing zone of the worker.

The initial point of entry of the contaminant into the local exhaust ventilation system is at the hood. The exhaust hood, which may consist of only a simple round or rectangular opening or which may be specially designed for the process, is designed to provide the necessary velocity of air at the point of contamination to control the contaminant and draw it into the system. Proper design of the exhaust hood is crucial in the operation of a local exhaust ventilation system. If the contaminant is not initially controlled, then the local exhaust system will not perform its desired function.

There are basically three types of exhaust hoods that can be installed (See Figure 2.7.1).

Figure 2.7.1

Hood types.

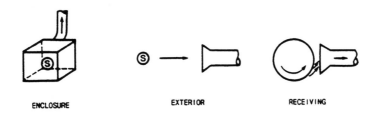

ENCLOSURE   EXTERIOR   RECEIVING

1. Enclosed hood--The source is enclosed either totally or partially, and adequate velocity is supplied to prevent the escape of the contaminant from the enclosure.

2. Exterior hood--The hood is installed exterior to and away from the source of contaminant. Adequate velocity is provided to capture the contaminant at its farthest distance from the hood and draw the contaminant into the hood. This velocity is called the "capture velocity" of the hood.

3.   Receiving hood--As the name implies, the receiving hood receives the contaminant that is generated at the source. This contaminant has a motion that has been imparted upon it by the process. In order for the receiving hood to function properly, it must provide an adequate rate of flow to remove the contaminant from the hood as it is received to assure that spillover of the contaminant does not occur. In addition, a receiving hood must also provide the capture velocity that is required to control contaminants not directed at the hood itself.

Determination of Capture or Control Velocity

The capture velocity that is necessary to control the contaminant at its farthest distance from the hood is determined by considering the following:

1.   The velocity and direction of release of the contaminant.
2.   The quantity of contaminant that is released in a given period of time.
3.   Secondary air currents that will affect the capture of the contaminant.
4.   The toxicity of the contaminant.
5.   The size of the exhaust hood that can be used.
6.   The potential points of contaminant escape.

Practical experience has identified certain guidelines that can be set for determining the capture velocity in a given situation. These guidelines, as presented in Table 4-1 of the Industrial Ventilation Manual, are summarized in Figure 2.7.2.

Capture Velocity for an Exterior Hood

When considering a total or partial enclosure, it is necessary to control the escape of contaminant from the enclosure itself. However in the case of an exterior hood, it is necessary that the hood be capable of reaching out and capturing the contaminant and drawing it into the hood. The following theoretical discussion will help to clarify the operation of an exterior hood in capturing the contaminant.

The reader will remember that the basic relationship for determining the rate of flow in a ventilation system is $Q = vA$. Assume a point source of exhaust. The term v is the capture velocity at the farthest point of dispersion of contaminant from the point source of exhaust. The pattern of flow for the air being drawn into this point source of exhaust can be visualized as that of a sphere. The velocity that is necessary to capture the contaminant must be provided at the intersection of the spherical contour and the farthest point of contaminant dispersion at a distance equal to r, the radius of the sphere.

Figure 2.7.2

Hood design data - range of capture velocities.

CONDITION OF DISPERSION OF CONTAMINANT	EXAMPLES	CAPTURE VELOCITY fpm
Released with practically no velocity into quiet air.	Evaporation from tanks, degreasing, etc.	50-100
Released at low velocity into moderately still air.	Spray booths; intermittent container filling; low-speed conveyor transfers; welding; plating; pickling	100-200
Active generation into zone of rapid air motion.	Spray painting in shallow booths; barrel filling; conveyor loading; crushers	200-500
Released at high initial velocity into zone of very rapid air motion.	Grinding; abrasive blasting; tumbling	500-2000

In each category above, a range of capture velocities is shown. The proper choice of values depends on several factors:

Lower End of Range
1. Room air currents minimal or favorable to capture.
2. Contaminants of low toxicity or of nuisance value only.
3. Intermittent, low production.
4. Large hood--large air mass in motion.

Upper End of Range
1. Disturbing room air currents.
2. Contaminants of high toxicity.
3. High production, heavy use.
4. Small hood--local control only.

Source: Industrial Ventilation Manual, ACGIH, 1974.

If a given rate of flow is assumed, it is possible to calculate the velocity of air moving at any distance, x, from the point source.

$$Q = vA   (2.3.4)$$
where
A = the surface area of the sphere = $4\pi r^2$
and
$r = x$, the distance from the point source
then
$$Q = v (4\pi x^2)$$

Figure 2.7.3

Point source exhaust.

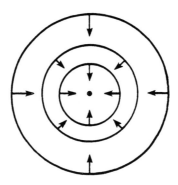

Example

Assume Q = 300 cfm, then

x	Q	÷	A	=	v
0.083 ft	300		0.087		3448
0.25 ft	300		0.785		382
0.5 ft	300		3.14		96
1.0 ft	300		12.57		24
1.5 ft	300		28.27		11
2.0 ft	300		50.26		6

The above example points out dramatically how exhaust velocities rapidly decrease at a distance from the hood. This illustrates the necessity of locating the exhaust hood close to the source of contamination to minimize the rate of flow required.

Example. In the above example, assume a capture velocity of 50 feet per minute. At what distance should the exhaust hood be located from the source or at its farthest point of contamination to capture the contaminant?

$$Q = vA \quad (2.3.4)$$
$$300 \text{ cfm} = 50 \ (4\pi x^2)$$
$$x^2 = 0.47 \text{ ft}^2$$
$$x = 0.69 \text{ ft}$$

Similar methods can be used for other geometric contours. For example, consider a point source of exhaust on a wall. The resulting geometric contours would assume the shape of a hemisphere. If an adjacent plane existed perpendicular to the wall at the point source of exhaust, a quartersphere would result. For a slot located on a plane, a hemicylinder and hemisphere result. In a like manner, other contours can be visualized.

Figure 2.7.4

Other theoretical contours.

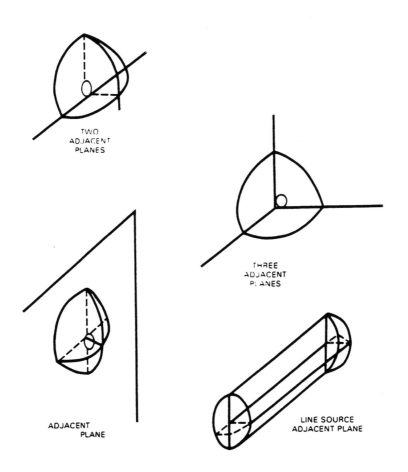

TWO
ADJACENT
PLANES

THREE
ADJACENT
PLANES

ADJACENT
PLANE

LINE SOURCE
ADJACENT PLANE

Limitations of Theoretical Model

In the above theoretical model, a point source of exhaust was assumed. However, in actual practice the diameter of the duct is large as compared to the x distance from the source of contaminant. Thus, the use of a spherical contour overstates the volume of air that will be moved at any distance away from the exhaust opening. This can be shown by assuming reasonable values for the face velocity and capture of a system and determining the ratio of the diameter to the distance of the exhaust from the source.

Example. Assuming a relatively high face velocity of 3000 feet per minute and the lower limit of capture velocity of 50 feet per minute, the following is developed:

$$Q_{face} = Q_x$$

where
        face velocity = 3000 fpm
    capture velocity = 50 fpm

Substituting in 2.3.4, we obtain

$$Q = \frac{\pi}{4} D^2 v_f = 4\pi x^2 v_x$$

$$Q = \frac{\pi}{4} D^2 (3000) = 4\pi x^2 (50)$$

$$x = 1.94 \, D$$

The above shows that, in general, the distance from the source is less than 2.0 times the diameter of the exhaust hood. In this case, the diameter is sufficiently large as compared to the x distance to prevent the use of spherical contours that assume a point source. Similar calculations can be performed for other geometric shapes.

Figure 2.7.5

Effect of hood on contours.

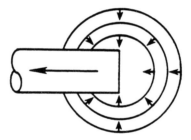

Experimental Determination of Contours

Although in practice the above discussion cannot be applied to determine the velocity contours that exist around an exhaust hood, it does provide a basis for the understanding of general principles of air flow into an exhaust hood. In order to describe the actual velocity contours that exist around a given exhaust hood, it is necessary that empirical data be gathered. Experiments to gather such data have been conducted by a number of individuals for various exhaust hood configurations. The work of Dalla Valle in this area is significant. Dalla Valle conducted experiments of velocity patterns resulting from both rectangular and round, flanged and unflanged, exhaust hoods. As a result of Dalla Valle's experiments, the following was developed to describe the velocity patterns that exist.

Velocity patterns for an unflanged exhaust hood:

(2.7.1) $v = \dfrac{Q}{10x^2 + A}$

Velocity patterns for a flanged exhaust hood:

(2.7.2) $v = \dfrac{Q}{0.75(10x^2 + A)}$

From the above it can be seen that the addition of a flange serves to increase the velocity at a given distance, x, from the exhaust hood. In addition, the velocity that results is a function of the distance from the hood to the source and the face area of the source (A). From the mathematical relationship, it is clear that the distance from the source to the exhaust hood has a greater effect upon the velocity at any given point than does the area of the hood face.

Other experiments conducted have established flow-velocity relationships. These relationships are summarized in Figure 2.7.6.

Example

A process requires a capture velocity of 200 feet per minute. A plain, round, flanged hood (D = 8 inches) is located at a point 14 inches from the farthest dispersion of contaminant. What exhaust rate is required to control the contaminant?

Solution

For a plain, flanged hood

$Q = 0.75v \, (10x^2 + A)$ (2.7.2)

Substituting

$Q = 0.75(200)[10(14/12)^2 + \pi(4/12)^2]$

$Q = 2094 \ cfm$

If an unflanged opening were to be used, the resulting rate of flow would be Q = 2792 cfm. By comparing these figures, the effect of a flange on a given opening is evident.

Efficiency of Exhaust Hoods

The previous discussion has been directed toward determining the capture velocity and rate of flow necessary to capture a contaminant exterior to the hood and draw it into the hood. In the following, what happens to the air once it crosses the face of the hood itself and enters the system will be determined.

Figure 2.7.6

Various hood volumes.

HOOD EXHAUST VS. CAPTURE VELOCITY

HOOD TYPE	DESCRIPTION	ASPECT RATIO $\frac{W}{L}$	AIR VOLUME
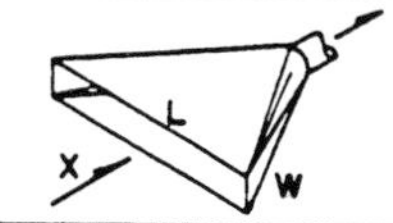	SLOT	0.2 OR LESS	Q=3.7 LVX
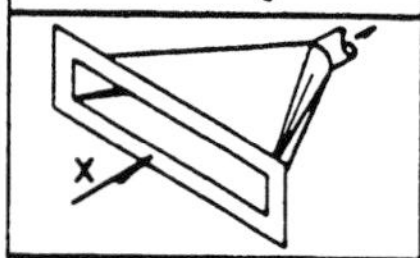	FLANGED SLOT	0.2 OR LESS	Q=2.8 LVX
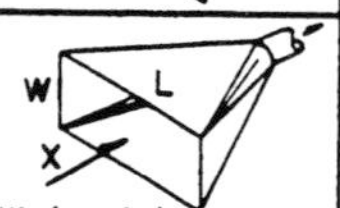 A=WL (sq.ft.)	PLAIN OPENING	0.2 OR GREATER AND ROUND	$Q=V(10 x^2 + A)$
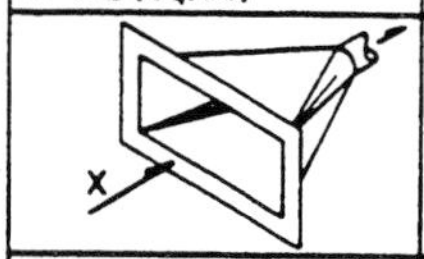	FLANGED OPENING	0.2 OR GREATER AND ROUND	$Q=0.75V(10X^2 + A)$
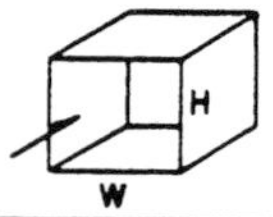	BOOTH	TO SUIT WORK	Q=VA= VWH
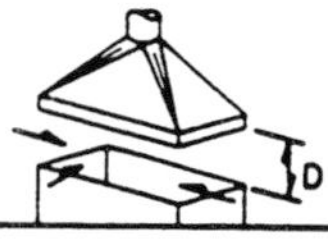	CANOPY	TO SUIT WORK	Q=1.4 PVD P=PERIMETER D= HEIGHT

Assume for the moment that a perfect hood has been designed. This perfect hood has no loss as air enters the exhaust system. This case was examined in the discussion of Principles of Ventilation where it was assumed that no loss occurred at the hood. Recall that in this case the static pressure necessary to accelerate the air to the velocity of the system would convert directly to velocity pressure. Thus,

(2.7.3) $SP = VP = (v/4005)^2$

However, such a perfect hood does not exist. As air enters the exhaust system through the hood, frictional and dynamic losses occur. Let us examine for a moment the reason for these losses.

As air enters the hood, the cross-sectional area of flow contracts and forms a stream with cross-sectional area less than that of the duct. This

contraction in the air stream is called the "vena contracta." During this
contraction, the velocity increases. From Bernoulli's theorem, TP = VP + SP
and the fact that if the velocity increases then the velocity pressure must
also increase, it is clear that some static pressure must be converted to
velocity pressure. During this conversion of static pressure to velocity
pressure, a loss of energy results. The energy loss is approximately 2% of
the static pressure.

Figure 2.7.7

Vena contracta.

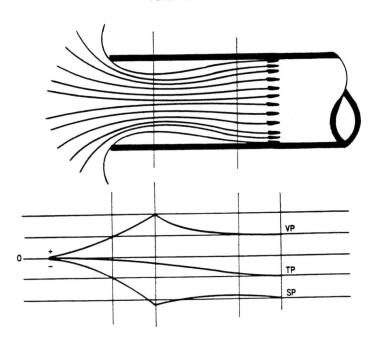

By permission of The Committee on Industrial Ventilation, Box 16153, Lansing,
MI   48901.

     As the air moves further into the system, it expands to fill the duct.
The velocity of the air decreases; thus, the VP is converted back to SP, and a
further loss of energy results. This energy loss is much greater than that
which occurred during the initial conversion because of the turbulence that
exists on the perimeter of the air flow. The result of the formation of the
vena contracta and the subsequent expansion of air to fill the duct is a loss
in energy of the total pressure of the system. An objective of exhaust hood
design is to design the hood to operate as efficiently as possible. This can
be accomplished by minimizing the loss that results from the vena contracta.

     Coefficient of Entry--C_e. One method for expressing the loss that
occurs in the exhaust hood is in terms of the coefficient of entry of the
hood. The coefficient of entry (C_e) is the ratio of the actual flow

obtained in a hood to that which theoretically could occur.   The theoretical flow is the flow that would be obtained in a perfect hood: that is, a hood where all the SP is converted with no losses.

$$Q = vA = 4005 \sqrt{SP_h} \times A$$

where

$$VP_h = SP_h$$

The actual flow that is obtained from an exhaust hood includes losses that are a result of the vena contracta.   Thus, the static pressure at the hood can be expressed as follows:

$$SP_h = VP + \text{loss at hood}$$

where

SP_h = hood static pressure in inches H_2O
VP = velocity pressure of hood duct in inches H_2O
loss at hood = h_e = hood entry loss in inches H_2O

The coefficient of entry (C_e) ratio can then be stated as:

$$C_e = \frac{Q_{actual}}{Q_{theoretical}}$$

$$C_e = \frac{4005 \sqrt{VP} \times A}{4005 \sqrt{SP_h} \times A}$$

(2.7.4) $C_e = \sqrt{VP/SP_h}$

Hood Entry Loss--h_e.   From previous discussions, we know that a loss in the system is reflected by a change in the static pressure and total pressure readings in inches of H_2O.   The hood entry loss (h_e) is the pressure drop in inches of H_2O that occurs as air enters the hood.   This pressure drop is the result of the losses that occur because of the vena contracta.   Hood entry loss can be determined by measuring the duct velocity and the hood static pressure three diameters downstream from the hood.   From the original relationship

(2.7.5) $SP_h = VP + h_e$

we obtain

$$h_e = SP_h - VP$$

Another convenient method for stating the hood entry loss is as a fraction of the duct velocity.   The relationship is as follows:

(2.7.6) $h_e = (F)VP$

where
$$F = \text{a dimensionless number}$$

Hood Design Relationships.   In the previous discussions, a number of relationships have been developed to describe the functioning of an exhaust hood. These relationships are summarized below.

1.   Rate of flow in a perfect hood, from 2.3.4

$$Q = 4005 \sqrt{VP} \times A$$

where

$$VP = SP_h$$

2.   Rate of actual flow in an exhaust hood

$$(2.7.7) \quad Q = 4005 \, C_e \sqrt{SP_h} \times A$$

3.   Hood entry loss

$$h_e = SP_h - VP$$

4.   Coefficient of entry

$$C_e = \sqrt{VP/SP_h}$$

In addition, the coefficient of entry and the hood entry loss can be related to one another. The following develops this relationship:

Relationship of C_e to h_e

$$C_e = \sqrt{VP/SP_h}$$

$$C_e = \sqrt{(h_e/F)/(h_e + VP)}$$

$$C_e = \sqrt{(h_e/F)/[h_e + (h_e/F)]}$$

$$(2.7.8) \quad C_e = \sqrt{1/(1 + F)}$$

Relationship of h_e to C_e

$$C_e = \sqrt{VP/SP_h}$$

$$C_e = \sqrt{VP/(h_e + VP)}$$

$$C_e^2 = \frac{VP}{h_e + VP}$$

$$(2.7.9) \quad h_e = \frac{(1 - C_e^2)}{C_e^2} VP$$

Some Problems. The following problems are presented to help the student to understand the relationships involved.

1.   Given a 6-inch round hood with a measured SP_h = 2 inches H_2O, find the flow into the hood, the duct velocity, the duct VP, the hood entry loss, and the hood entry factor (F).

Solution

To find the flow into the hood

$$Q = vA$$

$$= 4005 \sqrt{VP} \times A$$

$$= 4005 \, C_e \sqrt{SP_h} \times A \quad (2.7.7)$$

For a plain round hood, C_e = 0.72

$$Q = 4005(0.72) \sqrt{0.196}$$
$$Q = 800 \text{ cfm}$$

To find duct velocity

$$Q = vA$$

$$v = \frac{Q}{A}$$

$$v = \frac{800}{0.196}$$

$$v = 4082 \text{ fpm}$$

To find duct VP

$$v = 4005 \sqrt{VP}$$

$$VP = (v/4005)^2$$

$$VP = (4082/4005)^2$$

$$VP = 1.04 \text{ inches } H_2O$$

To find hood entry loss

$$SP_h = VP + h_e$$
$$h_e = SP_h - VP$$
$$h_e = 2 - 1.04$$
$$h_e = 0.96 \text{ inches } H_2O$$

To find hood-entry loss factor

$$h_e = (F)VP$$

$$F = \frac{h_e}{VP}$$

$$F = \frac{0.96}{1.04}$$

$$F = 0.92$$

2. In the above problem, determine the effect that a flange will have on each of the values calculated above.

    The reader is encouraged to work out this problem on his own. To facilitate checking, the following answers are given:

$$Q = 910 \text{ cfm}$$
$$v = 4643 \text{ fpm}$$
$$VP_d = 1.34 \text{ inches } H_2O$$
$$h_e = 0.66 \text{ inches } H_2O$$
$$F = 0.49$$

Hood Design

A summary of the hood entry loss, coefficient of entry, and flow rate for various simple exhaust openings is presented in Figure 2.7.8. In many cases, the data can be applied directly to the design of an exhaust hood. However, in certain cases, complex hoods are necessary. Complex hoods are made up of more than one of the basic designs; and, as a result, a synthetic coefficient of entry and entry loss must be developed. Consider a flanged hood with an adjacent plane perpendicular to the opening at the bottom of the hood. A special technique using Dalla Valle's half-hood formula can be used to determine the flow rate and velocity patterns for such a design. In this case, it is assumed that the hood is extended below the adjacent plane for an equal distance and, in fact, forms a hood of twice the size with a flange completely around the opening. The rate of flow is calculated for the whole hood and is then halved for the hood that actually exists.

Figure 2.7.8

Hood characteristics.

HOOD	h_e	C_e	FLOW RATE
PLAIN 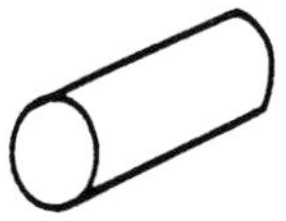	.93 VP	.72	$Q = V(10X^2+A)$
FLANGED 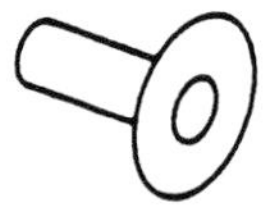	.49 VP	.82	$Q = .75V(10X^2+A)$
SLOT 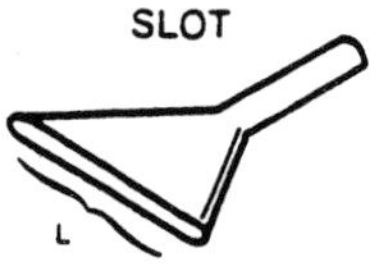	1.78 VP	.60	$Q = 3.7 LVX$
BOOTH. 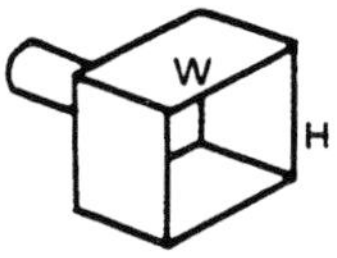	.50 VP	.82	$Q = VWH$
BELL 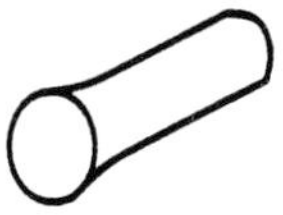	.04 VP	.98	$Q = V(10X^2+A)$

In the case of a slot hood with a plenum attached, the design can be treated as a combination of two simple hoods. The slot can be defined as a flanged duct. Losses can be estimated for each segment of the hood, and the total segment losses will be the loss for the complex hood. In a similar manner, synthetic entrance coefficients can be calculated for various other hood configurations.

Figure 2.7.9

Compound hoods.

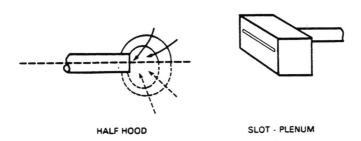

HALF HOOD   SLOT - PLENUM

Hood Design Procedure

Before designing an exhaust hood, it is important that the designer become
familiar with the operation involved. The characteristics of the contaminant
should be known. Is the contaminant a particulate, vapor, or gas? What is
the toxicity of the contaminant? Is the contaminant highly toxic, or is it
relatively low in toxicity? By what method is the contaminant
generated--evaporation, heat, splash, grinding, etc.? As a result of the
method of generation, how far is the contaminant dispersed? Is motion
imparted to the contaminant that causes it to travel great distances from the
source? Is the source relatively local, or is it a general source, generating
contaminant over a large area?

In addition, it is necessary to determine the location of the worker
relative to the source of the contaminant. Does the worker move about, or is
he stationary? What interaction is necessary between the worker and the
contaminant source? How does the contaminating source flow in production?
Does the process generate an air flow? Also, are there secondary air
movements around the process that will affect the capture velocity if an
exterior hood is used?

After the operation is thoroughly understood, the designer should
determine if hood designs have already been developed for the process. Many
processes are similar in nature. It is possible that a hood design has
already been developed and tested that will adequately meet the needs of the
process being studied. A number of such designs are presented in the Specific
Operations section (Section 5) of the Industrial Ventilation Manual.

If a specific design cannot be found to handle the problem being studied,
the designer should first consider the use of a total enclosure. The total
enclosure is the most efficient for capturing and controlling the contaminant
while using a relatively low rate of flow. If a total enclosure cannot be
applied, can a partial enclosure or booth meet the needs of the process?

If an enclosed hood cannot be used, then an exterior hood is required. It
is necessary to determine where the hood can be located in relation to the

source. The method of generation of contaminant may require that a receiving hood be used. In addition, if the contaminant is generated over a wide area, the use of a slot hood may be advisable. Heat-generated contaminant movement may require the application of a canopy-type hood above the process.

Next, it is necessary to design the actual hood to be used. The capture velocity that is required should be determined. In determining the capture velocity, it is important that the designer consider the existence of process-induced motion, the quantity of contaminant that is generated, any secondary air currents that may require baffles or shields around the process, the toxicity of the contaminant, the approximate size of the hood that can be used, and potential contaminant escape.

The designer then selects the hood that seems to best meet the needs of the system. The choice is not always clear cut, as it is necessary to give up certain operational advantages to obtain other operational advantages to meet the constraints of the process. Once the hood design has been chosen, the Q or rate of flow should be estimated based upon the capture velocity required and the location of the hood relative to the source. The size of the duct and hood face are then determined to provide the velocity that is desired. The designer should also estimate the effect of hood loss. This will be necessary when determining the size of air mover required or when adding a local exhaust system to a more general exhaust system.

Finally, after the hood has been designed, it is desirable to perform tests to determine if the installed hood meets the design criteria. Are the rate of flow and capture velocity adequate to capture and control the contaminant? Is the hood located in the appropriate place, and does the design prevent escape of the contaminant as a result of exterior air movement or process-induced movement?

Summary

The following table summarizes the important formulas presented in the chapter.

REFERENCE	RELATIONSHIP	FORMULA
2.7.1	The velocity at a point x distance from an unflanged exhaust hood. (Dalla Valle's formula)	$v = \dfrac{Q}{10x^2 + A}$
2.7.2	The velocity at a point x distance from a flanged exhaust hood	$v = \dfrac{Q}{0.75(10x^2 + A)}$
2.7.3	Theoretical static pressure of hood with no losses	$SP_h = VP = (v/4005)^2$
2.7.4	The coefficient of entry for a given hood--defined as ratio between actual flow and theoretical flow	$C_e = \sqrt{VP/SP_h}$
2.7.5	Relationship between the VP of the system, system, the hood entry loss, and the hood static pressure	$SP_h = VP + h_e$
2.7.6	The hood entry loss as a fraction of the duct VP	$h_e = (F)VP$
2.7.7	Actual rate of flow through a hood	$Q = 4005\ C_e \times \sqrt{SP_h} \times A$
2.7.8	The coefficient of entry as it relates to the hood entry loss	$C_e = \sqrt{1/(1+F)}$
2.7.9	The hood entry loss as it relates to the coefficient of entry	$h_e = \dfrac{(1 + C_e^2)}{C_e^2}$

8. Principles of Air Cleaning

It is necessary to dispose of the air that has been removed from the work environment. Often, depending upon the condition of the air exhausted, it is possible to introduce the contaminated air directly into the atmosphere through vents and stacks. In doing so, it is expected that the contaminant loading in the air will be sufficiently reduced by atmospheric dilution. However, in many cases the condition of the contaminated air is such that it must be treated before introduction into the atmosphere. The next two chapters will discuss in some detail the treatment of contaminated air prior to entry into the atmosphere.

The Reasons for Cleaning Air

1. <u>Remove hazardous contaminants</u>. One of the major reasons for an industrial exhaust system is to remove air containing potentially hazardous contaminants from the workplace. If the air is so contaminated that atmospheric dilution will not sufficiently reduce the contaminant level below that of a potential hazard, then the air must be treated in some manner before being vented into the atmosphere. Contaminants entering the atmosphere can cause a community hazard as well as a potential hazard for workers in plant areas adjacent to the contamination source. In determining the need for cleaning exhaust air, one should consider the possibility of an atmospheric inversion occurring which would limit the potential dilution rate that might normally occur. The air should enter the atmosphere in such a condition that under the worst possible case no potential hazard is present for those outside the facility.

2. <u>Remove nuisance contaminants</u>. Often, though no potentially hazardous contaminant exists in the exhausted air, a public nuisance may be created by the odor or amount of smoke present. The existence of such nuisance substances can cause community complaints and may detrimentally affect the public relations of the firm. Thus, although there may be no potential hazard from the air exhausted into the atmosphere, it may be necessary to clean the air of odors and smoke. This is particularly the case in areas where strict smoke control laws have been enacted.

3. <u>Protect air-moving equipment</u>. If the contamination in the air removed from the industrial environment contains abrasive or corrosive materials, it may be necessary to remove these materials from the air before passing it through the air-moving equipment (fans). If these contaminants are not removed, they can cause excessive wear from corrosion and abrasion on the air-moving equipment, thus necessitating costly repairs or frequent replacement.

4. <u>Recover valuable materials</u>. In some cases, the material contaminating the air has recovery value. If sufficient quantities of expensive materials are exhausted from the workroom atmosphere, the cost of air-cleaning equipment to remove these contaminants from the air may be partially or totally offset by the value of the materials that are recovered. These materials can then be recycled back through the production system.

5. <u>Enable recirculation</u>. Another reason for cleaning the air is to enable the recirculation of air removed from the work environment to other areas. Recirculation reduces the necessity for tempering the air (particularly heating in the winter). Although in the past recirculation was not widely used because of the problems inherent in cleaning the air and the potential for failure of the air-cleaning equipment (thus introducing a potentially hazardous contaminant into the work environment), more use of this method may be made in the future. As fuel costs rise, and the reliability and efficiency of equipment increases, recirculation may become feasible in terms of the savings generated.

6. <u>Meet environmental requirements</u>. One final reason for cleaning the exhaust air is to meet the environmental requirements in the area in which the plant is located. Environmental laws concerning air pollution have become stricter in the past few years, and it is likely that even more stringent laws will be introduced in the future. Thus, it may be necessary to install air-cleaning equipment in order to meet the requirements of environmental laws.

Factors Affecting Air Cleaning

When it becomes obvious that air-cleaning equipment is necessary in a particular industrial exhaust system, an engineering study must be conducted to determine the type and size of equipment to be installed. There are a number of factors that affect the type of equipment to be installed. These factors should be considered from the outset in order to implement the appropriate system. The major factors to be considered in such a study are:

a. Type of contaminant.
b. Size and shape of particulate contaminant.
c. The volume of air handled.
d. The degree of collection required.
e. The toxicity of the contaminant.
f. The radioactivity of the contaminant.
g. The heat and humidity of the carrier gas (air).
h. The corrosiveness of the contaminant material.
i. The presence of abrasive particulates.
j. The disposal methods for the collected contaminant.
k. The flammability of the carrier gas or the contaminant.
l. Chemical reactions that may occur.
m. Pressure loss in the cleaning mechanism.
n. The integrity of the air cleaner.
o. Variations in contaminant loading.
p. The necessary cleaning cycle.
q. The cost of cleaning the air.
r. The efficiency of the air cleaner to be installed.

The following discussion will briefly cover each of these factors.

The Type of Contaminant. The contaminant in the air may be either a particulate or a gas/vapor. Particulate matter includes dust, fumes, smoke, and mists. Different cleaning methods may be best for a given type of contaminant. For example, specific methods are most applicable for the removal of particulate matter, while other methods are more appropriate for the removal of gases and vapors.   The Size and Shape of Particulate Contamination. The size and shape of a particle will cause it to move through the air and to be acted upon by the air cleaner in different ways. This subject was discussed in some detail earlier when the properties of airborne contaminants were considered. The shape of an individual particle will influence its movement in the exhaust system and cleaning mechanism. The density will also be a factor in such a system. Obviously, from previous discussions, the size of particle has a major influence on its inertial and gravitational attraction. Particles less than 10 micrometers generally follow the movement of the air and are not materially affected by gravity or the inertia of the individual particle. A general rule is that the smaller and less dense the particle, the higher the cost required to remove it from the air. Certain air-cleaning methods are practical only for large particles, while others may be used to remove particles in the submicrometer range.

The Volume of Air Handled. For a given concentration, the larger the air volume handled, the greater the need for better air-cleaning equipment. Obviously, if a small amount of air is being exhausted, even though this air may have a high concentration of contaminant, the total amount of contaminant entering the environment is small. On the other hand, if a large volume of air is being exhausted with only a small percentage of contaminant, the total contaminant entering the atmosphere is significantly large and requires efficient air-cleaning equipment.

The Degree of Collection Required. The degree of collection of contaminant required will vary depending on a number of factors. The environmental laws may state the amount of contaminant that can be exhausted into the air. The potential hazard to the community will also be a factor. The location of the plant and the public relations image that is desired may also be considered when determining the degree of collection that is required. Many other factors are also important in this decision. Generally, it can be stated that the higher the degree of collection required, the higher the cost of the necessary air-cleaning equipment.

The Toxicity of the Contaminant. Toxic contaminants in the exhausted air can present potential hazards to the neighboring property and community. The presence of an atmospheric inversion may result in a potential hazard even though small quantities of the contaminant are released and normally diluted by air movement in the atmosphere. Generally, a toxic contaminant requires that the air cleaner efficiency be high. Other important factors to consider when working with toxic contaminants are the problems involved in disposing of the collected contaminant, and the special care that is required in the maintenance of the air cleaner and the duct leading to the air cleaner to remove any potential hazard to the maintenance worker.

Radioactivity of the Contaminant. Radioactive contaminants are highly toxic materials. Thus, they should be treated with the same care as is necessary for other toxic material. Additional precautions must be taken to assure that radioactive buildup does not occur within the air cleaner, resulting in a potential exposure of the workers.

Temperature and Humidity. In many cases, air removed from the workplace will be at a high temperature or may contain a high moisture content. These factors can affect the operation of certain types of air cleaners and must be considered when selecting the appropriate cleaner. High humidity can cause particulate matter to agglomerate and plug narrow sections of the air cleaner. Humidity in the exhausted air also may cause a vapor plume from the stacks which results in a possible community problem. The moisture in the air can also result in corrosion of the air-cleaning and air-moving equipment unless appropriate protective precautions are taken.

The Presence of Corrosive Contaminant Material. The air exhausted from the workplace may contain materials that are corrosive. These materials can affect the maintenance of the air-moving equipment. As such, it may be desirable to remove the materials before passing the air through the air mover. In addition, special consideration must be given to the type of air cleaner, since corrosive material can attack the cleaner and cause excessive wear.

The Presence of Abrasive Particulates. As in the case of corrosive contaminants, the presence of abrasive particulates in the air will cause damage to the air-moving and air-cleaning equipment. The type of equipment to be used must be specially designed to protect from this type of wear. In addition, abrasive particles can cause a buildup of dust within the system unless the appropriate transport velocities are present to prevent such a buildup.

Disposal of the Collected Contaminant. It is important to consider the methods of disposing of the collected contaminant during the design of the system. If the contaminant is toxic, it may present a danger to workers maintaining and/or cleaning the equipment in the exhaust system. In addition, if water is used to collect the contaminant, the engineer must consider how this water will be disposed of without causing a community water pollution problem. If the potential salvage value of the contaminant is high, a method must be devised to recover the contaminant for reuse.

Flammability of the Carrier Gas or the Contaminant. If the carrier gas or the contaminant is flammable, certain precautions must be taken. The concentration of the flammable material must be kept above the upper explosive limit (UEL) or below the lower explosive limit (LEL) to remove the potential for a fire or an explosion. In addition, the cleaning equipment and air-moving equipment must be designed to eliminate that potential for sparks which may ignite the flammable material.

Chemical Reactions. The carrier gas and the contaminant may react with each other, thus resulting in a material different from that which was originally produced. In addition, the contaminant may react with water vapor in the air, or the carrier gas may react with materials present in the cleaning mechanism. The potential for such reactions must be considered, since they may have a major effect on the type of cleaning that is necessary.

Pressure Losses. When air is passed through a cleaning device, it loses pressure because of turbulence and friction. These losses will be reflected in the static pressure of the system. Depending on the type of air-cleaning device used, the pressure loss will vary from a very small loss (one-half inch water gauge) to a very large pressure loss (20 inches water gauge or more). As the pressure loss in the system increases, the required size for the air-moving equipment will also increase. This will result in a higher initial cost for installation of air-moving equipment and also a higher operating cost for the system. These factors must be considered during the design of the air-cleaning system.

The Integrity of the Air Cleaner. The air-cleaning mechanism must be such that leaks do not occur. If leaks occur on the supply side of the fan, these leaks can cause the contaminant to be dispersed in the atmosphere. On the exhaust side of the fan, leaks in the air cleaner and duct will require larger volumes of air to be exhausted, thus requiring a larger air mover. In addition, there is a potential for re-entry of the contaminant that has been collected unless precautions are taken to prevent leakage between the cleaner and the collection hopper.

Variations in Contaminant Loading. Variations in the contaminant loading of the air may have an effect on the air-cleaning mechanism. Low loading may affect the efficiency of certain types of air cleaners. On the other hand, high loading may require a high frequency of cleaning for the air cleaner.

The Cycle for Cleaning. The method for cleaning the air cleaner must be considered. If the operation is continuous, it may be necessary to operate the air cleaner constantly. This will require either the use of redundant air cleaners or implementing some type of continuous cleaning mechanism so that the process does not need to be shut down to clean the air-cleaning mechanism.

The Cost of Cleaning the Air. When comparing methods of air cleaning, it is necessary to determine the costs that are incurred using various methods in order to choose the one that is the most cost effective. Three major factors are important in such a cost comparison:

a.   The initial installation cost of the air-cleaning equipment.
b.   The cost of the power necessary to operate the system (including the cost of the power to operate the air-moving equipment necessary to overcome pressure losses occurring within the air cleaner).
c.   The cost of maintenance and cleaning of the system.

Each of these factors must be considered in detail to determine the overall cost effectiveness of each system under consideration. It may be that to accomplish the job only one system can be used. However, even in this

:ase, it is desirable to determine the cost for operating the system to be
used.

The Efficiency of the Air Cleaner. The type of air cleaner that is used
will yield different results, depending upon the type of contaminant and the
size of the particles present in the contaminant. A common method for stating
the efficiency rating of a given air cleaner is

(2.8.1) $$\text{Efficiency} = 1 - \frac{\text{Contaminant discharge rate at outlet}}{\text{Contaminant discharge rate at inlet}}$$

Care must be exercised in the use of this expression since it is desirable
to consider the total contaminant that is exhausted into the atmosphere rather
than the percent or ratio that is volume-time related. For example, consider
an air cleaner that is rated at a 90 percent efficiency and operates to remove
silica dust that is generated at a rate of 12,000 pounds per hour. If the
above expression is used, the following is obtained:

$$\text{Efficiency} = 1 - \frac{\text{Contaminant discharge rate at outlet}}{\text{Contaminant discharge rate at inlet}}$$

$$0.90 = 1 - \frac{x}{12,000}$$

$$x = 1200 \text{ pounds per hour}$$

Thus at a 90 percent efficiency, a large quantity of dust is still being
exhausted into the atmosphere.

The effect of air cleaning on the quality of the vented air can be
obtained in a number of ways. Dust samples and counts may be taken at the
inlet and outlet of the air cleaner. The opacity of the plume at the stack
may be compared to existing standards. The weight of solids gathered per unit
of air handled may be obtained. Other standard air-quality tests may also be
used to determine the air-cleaner efficiency.

Characteristics of the Contaminant

Particulate contaminants include dust, fume, mist, and smoke. Small
particles will not settle from the air (particles that are of a diameter of
less than 30 to 40 micrometers). Large particles, on the other hand, will
settle from the air unless the transport velocity of the system overcomes the
gravitational attraction of these particles. The particles of interest to the
industrial hygiene engineer because of their respirability are those with a
diameter of less than 10 micrometers. The particle size in any given air
sample is distributed log-normally with most of the particles in the smaller
range. The problem of air cleaning, then, is to remove this large number of
small particles.

On the other hand, the problem may involve a gas or vapor. The gas or
vapor is mixed with the air and does not settle. Some method must be present

to remove this gas or vapor from the air which does not involve gravitational attraction.

In general, these two categories of contaminants (particulate and gas/vapor) will result in two different methods of air cleaning. In the following discussions, the general methods of air cleaning will be considered. Not all of these methods will be equally appropriate for particulates or gases and vapors.

General Methods of Air Cleaning

The basic law of air cleaning can be stated as follows:

The contaminant must be acted upon by a force which does not act on the carrier gas or acts with sufficient differential force to physically or chemically remove the contaminant.

The force must be great enough to overcome other forces within the air stream. If a particle exists in an air stream, it must be acted upon by a force that will cause it to travel across the air stream. The stream can be narrowed to decrease this distance of travel. In the following discussion, the basic methods for cleaning will be presented. The various types of air cleaners that are presented in the next chapter use one or more of these basic methods as the means for removing contaminants from the air. The basic methods of air cleaning are:

a. Gravitational force
b. Centrifugal force
c. Inertial impaction
d. Direct interception
e. Diffusion
f. Electrostatic precipitation
g. Adsorption
h. Absorption
i. Incineration
j. Catalytic combustion

Gravitational Force. As particles travel in the air stream, they are acted upon by gravitational force. If the force of gravity is larger than the force exerted on the particles to transport them with the air stream, the larger, more dense particles will settle from the air. This approach for cleaning air is generally useful only with particles that are large and dense. As has been previously discussed, small particles have a very slow terminal settling velocity; the force necessary to transport them is relatively small.

Centrifugal Force. If air is caused to rotate around a small diameter, a force much greater than that of gravity will act on the particles to remove them in a direction tangential to the direction of rotation. Thus, the particles will be projected across the rotating stream of air. If a barrier exists to halt the particles' tangential motion, these particles can then be captured on the outer edge of the rotating air stream. Such a method will

operate to capture particles much smaller than those that are normally
affected by gravitational force.

Figure 2.8.1

Gravitational attraction.

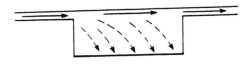

Figure 2.8.2

Centrifugal force.

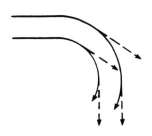

Inertial Impaction. As air flows, it diverges in order to pass around
objects present in the air stream. The inertia of each particle in the air
stream causes these particles to flow in a more nearly straight line. The
particles may then impact on the deflecting object. This method is more
effective for large particles that have an inertia apart from that which is
imparted by the air stream. In general, the higher the air velocity, the
higher the probability of impaction of particulate matter.

Figure 2.8.3

Inertial impaction.

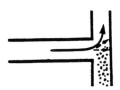

Direct Interception. As air passes around an object or series of objects
that are placed in the air (as in the case of inertial impaction), the
particles may strike or be intercepted by the object(s). The finite width of
the particle may cause the particle to be intercepted even though the
trajectory calculated at the center of the particle may pass through the
object. Thus, the larger the particle or the smaller the distance between the
objects, the greater the probability of interception. Interception is
independent of the velocity of the air.

Figure 2.8.4

Direct interception.

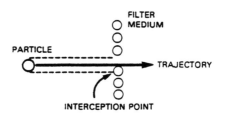

Diffusion. Small particles (those less than 0.5 micrometers) are caused
to separate from the air by Brownian motion (caused by molecular impact on the
small particle). The diffusion process is a slow process and requires the air
to remain in the area where cleaning takes place for a period of time. In
addition, low velocity air movement is required. Often, a filter medium is
used that then combines interception methods with diffusion methods.

Electrostatic Precipitation. In this method, the particle is given a
charge as it flows through an electrical field. A collector plate is given an
opposite charge. As the particle passes by the collector plate, it is
attracted to the oppositely charged plate. Some particles may have a natural
charge and, thus, do not require passing through an electrical field.

Figure 2.8.5

Electrostatic precipitation.

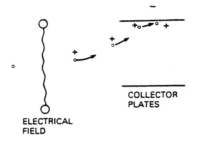

Adsorption. In the process of adsorption, a contaminant in the air passes through an adsorbing material. The molecules of the contaminant adhere to the surface of the adsorption medium. Adsorption is basically a physical process. The adsorbate-adsorbent relationship is generally a specific one with certain materials acting as adsorbents for other materials.

Absorption. In absorption, a soluble or chemically treated reactive contaminant in the air is caused to flow through water or a chemical medium. The contaminant is dissolved in the liquid or reacts with the medium in such a manner that its form is changed, and it is removed from the air.

Incineration. The contaminant-containing air is passed through an open flame. The combustible contaminant then burns off, producing only carbon dioxide and water.

Catalytic Combustion. In catalytic combustion, a catalyst is introduced to the contaminated air. This catalyst causes an oxidation of the contaminant to take place. The presence of the catalyst causes this oxidation to take place at a lower temperature than would occur in incineration, and no flame is present during the oxidation.

Summary

Among the many reasons for cleaning air exhausted from the workplace, perhaps the most important is the removal of potentially hazardous contaminants before they enter the atmosphere. Before selecting the air cleaner to be used, the industrial hygiene engineer must be familiar with the process and the contaminant of concern. Various methods of air cleaning are available, but not all are equally effective on all contaminants. The most common principles used in air cleaners are gravitational forces, centrifugal force, inertial impaction, direct interception, diffusion, electrostatic precipitation, adsorption, absorption, incineration, and catalytic combustion. It is not uncommon to find more than one of these principles utilized in a particular air cleaner design.

9. Air-Cleaning Devices

In the previous chapter, the general methods available for use in cleaning air were discussed. These methods have been applied by engineers to design specific air-cleaning equipment. Generally, a particular air-cleaning device will use more than one of the general methods for cleaning air. In this chapter, the various types of air-cleaning devices that are available will be discussed in some detail.

Air Cleaners for Particulate Contaminants--Mechanical Separators

Mechanical methods for separating particulate matter from the air primarily involve the use of the force of gravity, centrifugal force, and/or impaction. There are two factors that have a primary effect on the collection of particulate matter by mechanical means.

1. The force of gravity or particle inertia increases with the square of the particle diameter.
2. Since particles must travel across the air stream to be collected, the smaller the distance of travel across the air stream, the better the removal of the particles.

Thus, it is evident from the above that larger particles will be collected more easily by mechanical means. In addition, if the air stream can be made narrower, then the distance of travel for a particle will be less, and particles will be collected more easily.

Gravity Settling Chamber. The simplest type of air cleaner for particulates is the gravity settling chamber. The gravity settling chamber is simply a large settling container attached to the ventilation duct system. As the air enters the large chamber, the velocity slows to below the transport velocity for the particulate matter being carried in the air. Particles settle out of the air into the hopper as a result of the gravitational force acting on the particles. Theoretically, all particles except those affected by Brownian motion (approximately 0.5 micrometers) can be removed by gravity if the settling area can be made large enough. Practically, the settling chamber size must be limited; and, therefore, gravitational settling is effective only for relatively large particles.

Gravity settling chambers may include baffles upon which particulate matter with horizontal inertia will impact. The particles are then attracted by gravity downward into the collection hopper. After the particles are collected, removal may be accomplished by either intermittent cleaning of the hopper or a continuous cleanout using a conveyor system.

Figure 2.9.1

Settling chamber.

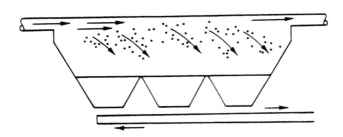

Certain hoods and ventilation duct systems have plenums that not only slow the air but also act as settling chambers. For this reason, it is necessary to provide a cleanout in any plenums to remove any settled particulates. In addition, long runs of ducts operating at less than the transport velocity of the particles also act as settling chambers and require the addition of cleanouts.

The efficiency of gravitational settling is difficult to determine because of the turbulence within the chamber. A theoretical formula has been developed to determine a theoretical efficiency for the chamber (Stokes Law). This formula can be useful in estimating the size chamber to be used for a particular minimum particle size. The formula is:

$$D_p = \frac{18\mu Hv}{gL(P_p - \rho)}$$

where

D_p = minimum particle size collected at 100% efficiency
μ = gas viscosity lb/ft-sec
H = chamber height in ft
v = gas velocity in ft/sec
g = 32.2 ft^2/sec
L = chamber length in ft
P_p = particle density in lbs/ft^3
ρ = gas density in lb/ft^3

In general, gravity settling chambers are used to collect large particles, normally in excess of 100 micrometers. They are often used as chip traps in conjunction with woodworking equipment; and in some cases, gravity settling chambers are attached to the system to act as a precleaner to remove large particles before further cleaning of the small particles by another method. Because of the required size and the lack of effectiveness of this method for removal of small particles, the gravity settling chamber is limited in its application as a primary cleaner.

Cyclone Cleaners. The cyclone cleaner represents a second type of
mechanical separator. In the cyclone cleaner, the air enters a circular or
conical chamber where it swirls around the outside perimeter of the chamber.
Particles in the air are acted upon by centrifugal force and forced to the
outside walls of the chamber. The particles follow the walls downward to the
point where the air reverses flow 180 degrees. At this point, the particles
fall into a hopper, and the clean air moves in a vortex upward inside the
outer vortex, exiting at the top of the chamber.

Figure 2.9.2

Cyclone.

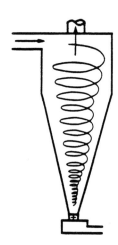

Cyclones have no moving parts. Special inlets are designed to eliminate
re-entrainment of dust from the entry air into that air which is exiting the
cyclone. Special materials can be used in a cyclone if the air contains
corrosive substances. Water may be sprayed along the wall of the cyclone to
increase the capture of particles. The design of a cyclone may or may not be
conical. In addition, the cyclone may be horizontal rather than vertical.
Also, varying inlet and outlet designs have been used by various cyclone
manufacturers.

Efficiency curves are developed by the manufacturers for a particular
cyclone. This efficiency is determined from performance tests on the
cyclone. There are a number of methods to increase the efficiency of a given
cyclone. A higher inlet velocity will increase efficiency since the particles
are subjected to a greater centrifugal force. The diameter of the cyclone
affects efficiency. The smaller the diameter, the higher the efficiency.
High-efficiency cyclones are designed around this principle and generally have
a diameter of less than or equal to 9 inches. High-efficiency cyclones often
use multiple tubes with the inlet air being split among the tubes. An
increase in the body length of a cyclone also increases the efficiency since

it allows for a longer separation time and lowers the possibility for re-entrainment of dust at the outlet. In addition, the inlet can be designed so that entering air is separated from the clean air being removed (shave off inlet); and directional elbows at entry will direct the contaminated air to the outside perimeter of the cyclone, thus separating the inlet and outlet streams.

Conventional cyclones are widely used for dust removal in industry. These cyclones have low pressure drops, in the neighborhood of 0.5 to 1.5 inches wg. Cyclones are inexpensive to install and operate; they are efficient for particles in the range of 20 to 40 micrometers; they can be used in high-temperature air streams. And cyclones are basically trouble free, with problems being encountered only where particularly corrosive materials are used or where plugging of the outlet or caking material on the walls result from handling air with a high moisture content.

Small high-efficiency cyclones exhibit pressure drops up to 6 inches of water. These cyclones are used for separation of particles with a diameter of 10 micrometers or more.

Impingement or Impaction Devices. In impingement or impaction devices, air is made to pass around or through specially shaped obstacles or openings. The openings or baffles are widely spaced (generally one inch or more). As the air passes around the obstacle, particle inertia causes the dust to travel in a straight line and hit the obstacle. The dust particles are deflected from the air path and into a dust collection hopper. The particles are then removed either intermittently or continuously from the hopper. The clean air flows out of the collector. There are a multitude of impaction cleaner designs. Some are simple zigzag baffle types, in which the air hits the zigzag baffles and passes upward vertically while the particles are directed downward by the force of gravity and their directional inertia. Another type is circular, with louvers to allow the air to pass through while the particles impact on the louvers and are directed away from the air flow. A third type uses a high-velocity jet caused by passing the air through perforations or nozzles. The air impinges on a plate which is placed in the path of the jet.

Figure 2.9.3

Impaction separator.

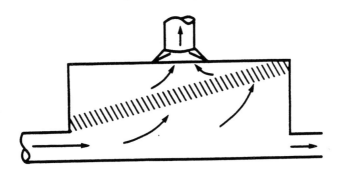

The high jet velocities increase the efficiency of such cleaners.   In some cases, impaction separators use water as the impingement medium.

Impaction separators generally operate at a low efficiency (50 to 80 percent).   The efficiency of an impaction separator can be increased by lengthening the baffles, increasing the airflow rate, or spacing the baffles closer together.   A limiting factor in increasing the efficiency is the potential plugging of the openings and the high pressure loss that may be encountered if small openings or nozzles are used.
Impactors generally have a pressure loss of from 0.5 inches wg to 3 inches wg.   They are effective in collecting particles of a diameter greater than 20 micrometers.   Other than the problem of plugging, impactors are generally trouble free and can be used in situations where cyclones are applicable.

Dynamic Collectors.   The dynamic collector utilizes a fan or impeller that operates in the air stream.   The blades gather the dust through centrifugal force, and the blade shape separates the particles from the air.

Figure 2.9.4

Dynamic precipitator.

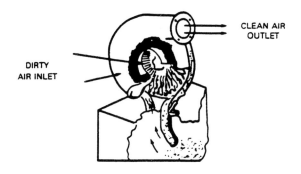

The efficiency of a dynamic collector is determined by performance tests. Generally, the efficiency falls between that of the conventional cyclone and the high-efficiency cyclone.   The efficiency of a dynamic collector remains essentially constant for a given collector over the entire range of operating velocities.

There is no pressure loss present when using a dynamic collector, since the collector acts in the same way as a fan.   The dynamic collector is effective for collecting particles of a diameter greater than 10 micrometers. In a corrosive or abrasive atmosphere, wear on the fan or impeller becomes a problem.   If the temperature of the carrier gas is in excess of 700°F, specially designed collectors must be used.

Air Cleaners for Particulate Contaminants--Filters

A filter is a porous material composed of granular or fibrous materials that removes particles from a fluid or gas which passes through it. As the fluid flows through the filter medium, particles impact or are intercepted by the filter fibers. Particles build up on the filter and fill void spaces. As the buildup occurs, resistance to the flow increases; and the filter can trap smaller particles. As the filter loads, the resistance increases, and it becomes necessary to replace or clean the filter to maintain the desired air flow. The best filter is one that can efficiently capture and hold particulates with a minimum resistance to flow.

Most filters utilize interception and impacting mechanisms in the filtering process. High-efficiency filters also utilize diffusion to remove particles. Depending upon the filter medium and the particulates involved, electrostatic attraction may also come into play. As the particles build up in the void spaces of the filter, a sieving action becomes important.

Deep-Bed or Mat Filters. Deep-bed or mat filters are made up of beds of granular or fibrous materials arranged to provide a porous cross section (90 to 99 percent void space). As a result, these filters have a low resistance and high dust load storage capacity. Generally such filters are cleaned by replacing.

These filters are inexpensive to buy and can be designed for high temperatures. In addition, such filters can be used where corrosive contaminants are present. However, this type filter is not widely used in air pollution control since most filters of this type cannot be cleaned. In some cases, mat filters have been used for filtration of sulfuric or phosphoric acid (coke-box type filters) and to collect dust and fumes from open-hearth furnaces. The deep-bed or mat filter can be graduated in order to obtain higher efficiencies with an accompanying increase in resistance to flow. Some special-design filters of this type have been used as moving filter beds or self-cleaning mat filters.

Fabric Filters--Bag Houses. In a bag house, the air flows into the bottom of a fabric tube; and, as it passes through the fabric, the particulate matter is removed and builds up on the fabric. Efficiency of such filters is high (up to 99 percent) for small particles of 0.25 micrometers or more. The particulate buildup (cake) provides a sieving action for particulate matter in subsequently cleaned air. As the cake forms, the resistance to flow increases, ultimately resulting in the need to clean the filter.

Typically, the resistance to flow encountered with the fabric type filter varies between 3 to 8 inches wg. Resistance to flow in excess of the upper limit for a particular filter indicates the need for cleaning.

There are three basic categories of bag houses being used in industry. These categories are based upon the method that is employed for cleaning the filters. The intermittently cleaned bag house is cleaned by shutting down the filtering operation and removing the cake buildup from the filters, generally

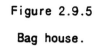

Figure 2.9.5

Bag house.

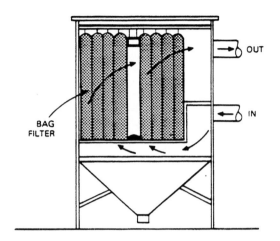

by shaking or rapping the filters. After the filters have been cleaned, the bag house can be put back into operation. Such a system requires either that the process be shut down while the cleaning takes place or that redundant cleaners be installed. Periodically cleaned equipment is constructed so that separate chambers within the bag house can be shut off from the process and the filters cleaned by rapping or shaking while the other chambers are operating to clean the air. The compartments of a periodically cleaned filter act as essentially separate air cleaners with varying efficiency, flow rate, and resistance. In continuously cleaned filters, the cleaning mechanism involves a continuously moving blow ring which directs a reverse flow of air through the filter to remove the cake. This ring moves up and down the filter tubes while the bag house remains in operation.

The use of a bag house is somewhat limited when high temperatures are encountered. Some fabrics are more heat resistant than others; but in general, the maximum air temperature for which a conventional bag house using cotton filters can be used is approximately 180°F.

Fabric filters are very widely used for many applications. This type filter is often used to remove dust, fly ash, and such things as electric-furnace fume emissions. However, certain problems can occur with the use of fabric filters. For example, excessive moisture in the air can make the cake difficult to remove. Also, fabric filters are subject to variations in flow between the filter immediately after cleaning and after some period of operation. Thus, a constant level of particulate removal is not likely to be obtained. In addition, fabric filters require large space allocations because of their size.

High-Efficiency Panel Filters. This type filter involves a continuous sheet of filter medium that is accordion folded, with or without separators

between the folds. The high-efficiency panel filter operates at low
velocities to capture very small particles in the range of 0.01 micrometers or
less by diffusion. In general, the efficiency of capture is in the range of
99.9 percent. The storage capacity of such filters is low because of the high
density of the filter medium. Filters of this type are rated by a military
standard (Department of Defense Smoke Penetration and Air Resistance Test).
The rated resistance for this type of filter is a maximum of 1 inches wg.

Figure 2.9.6

High efficiency filter.

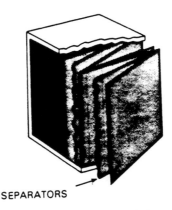

SEPARATORS

High-efficiency filters are most often used in such cases as clean rooms,
food processing plants, and hospitals. In these cases, the dirty filter is
disposed of rather than cleaned.

Air Cleaning for Particulate Contaminants--Wet Collectors

Wet collectors, often called scrubbers, involve the introduction of a
liquid to the air stream to remove particulate matter. Wet collectors employ
impaction as their primary method of air cleaning. The particles and the
water droplets collide, and the liquid condenses on the particle, increasing
its size and density. Small droplets provide a maximum area for impingement.
However, the impingement efficiency will fall off if the droplets become too
small, thus allowing the particle to pass between them. Small particles also
diffuse to the droplets within a wet scrubber. Humidification of the air may
cause some of the small particles to flocculate, thus increasing the
efficiency of a wet scrubber.

Wet scrubbers normally result in high-efficiency air cleaning with low
initial cost. In general, however, the efficiency obtained is directly
related to the resistance (pressure drop) encountered. Wet scrubbers are
effective in high temperatures or corrosive atmospheres. Removal of the waste
sludge from a wet scrubber can present a problem and must be considered in
their installation. The maintenance problems involved with wet scrubbing
vary, depending upon the type of scrubber and the design.

Chamber Scrubbers--Spray Towers. In a spray tower, water is sprayed into a chamber through which air is being passed. Baffles may be present to direct the air in order to increase the time within the chamber and, thus, the potential for contact between the particles and the water droplets. The spray tower is generally effective for particles of a diameter of 10 micrometers or more. High-pressure sprays can be used to capture particles in the one micrometer range.

The simplest spray tower design involves a gravity-chamber spray with the air being introduced at the bottom of the chamber. This design results in a very simple, trouble-free operation with water being introduced at line-pressure rates. In general, the spray tower operates with a low pressure drop of from 1 to 1.5 inches wg.

Figure 2.9.7

Spray tower.

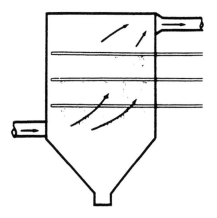

The conventional spray tower operates at a relatively low efficiency of collection. The high-efficiency type (fog tower) operates at a significantly higher efficiency and is, in fact, one of the most efficient of the wet collectors. However, the fog tower does require significant quantities of water and has an increased resistance to air flow of from 2 to 4 inches wg.

Cyclonic Scrubbers (Wet Cyclones). The cyclonic scrubber is similar to the normal dry cyclone with a water spray introduced tangential to the air entry. The cyclone action removes the particles that are wetted by the spray. This type cleaner is effective for particles of 5 micrometers with an efficiency of greater than 90 percent. The pressure drop is from 2 to 6 inches wg. Special designs have been used employing vanes and various nozzle arrangements to improve the efficiency of such scrubbers.

Self-Induced Spray Scrubbers. In this type of air cleaner, the air stream passes through constrictions or nozzles to increase its velocity. The

high-velocity air stream then impinges on a liquid. The liquid is fragmented
by the force of the air, and a spray is created. The droplets and particles
impact in the turbulent spray. The droplets and particles then impact on
baffles for removal. The efficiency of such a system is near 90 percent for
particles of 2 micrometers in diameter. The pressure drop of such a scrubber
is in the range of 3 to 6 inches wg.

Wet Impingement Scrubbers. In a wet impingement scrubber, the air enters
a spray area. The droplets in the spray capture the particles, which then
impact on the baffle plate. Small holes in the baffle plate allow the air to
pass. The efficiency of such a scrubber is approximately 90 percent for
particles with a diameter of 2 micrometers. The pressure drop in such systems
is from 1.5 to 8 inches of water, depending upon design.

Venturi Scrubber. In the venturi scrubber, air passes through a venturi
(constriction). Liquid is introduced perpendicular to the air flow at or
before the venturi. The liquid is atomized by the force of the air, and
turbulence causes a mixing of the particles and liquid. The particles impact
upon the spray drops and are separated from the air stream. The efficiency of
such scrubbers can be high (99 percent) for submicrometer particles. However,
for such units the pressure drop is also very high, with some scrubbers
operating at 60 to 100 inches wg.

Figure 2.9.8

Venturi scrubber.

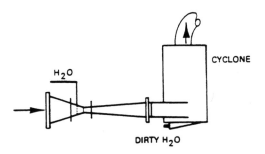

A venturi scrubber is often used in conjunction with a cyclone separator
which collects the droplets of water holding the particles. Small particles
passing through the venturi impact, impinge, or diffuse on the water droplets,
thus increasing the size of the particle (droplet and particle) to be
removed. The cyclone can then be effective in removing these larger particles
at relatively high efficiencies.

The effectiveness of the venturi for removing small particles at high
efficiency has led to its use in difficult air-cleaning jobs. However, as
with other cleaners, this increase in cleaning efficiency is not without
cost. The high pressure drop that occurs using a venturi results in the need
for large and costly air moving equipment.

Mechanical Scrubbers. The mechanical scrubber involves the use of a rotor propeller or fan to break up a liquid. The turbulence caused by the liquid breakup and the movement of the air enhance the potential contact of the particles and the droplets. The droplets and particles then fall into the liquid to be removed. This type of scrubber has an efficiency of approximately 90 percent for submicrometer particles. No resistance is present for this type of cleaner since the scrubber acts as a fan. However, the cost of operation can be high, because of the power requirements of the scrubber itself.

Air Cleaning for Particulates--Electrostatic Precipitators

Electrostatic precipitation involves charging the particles in the air with an electrical charge that is opposite to the charge applied to the plates where the particles are to be gathered. A high-voltage discharge electrode is placed opposite a grounded electrode. The gas passes through the electrodes and becomes ionized. (This is called the "corona.") The ions attach to the particles and are attracted to the oppositely charged plates, where they gather. The dust layer must not build up on the plates, or the efficiency of the precipitator will be affected. In some designs, the collector plates are shielded to prevent re-entrainment of the particles as air blows by the plates. The dust is cleaned from the plates by mechanical rapping or vibrating or by a liquid film on the plates themselves. Cleaning without re-entrainment of dust particles presents a difficult design problem. In some cases, shielded collector plates are used to lower the possibility of re-entrainment. Precipitators can also be sectionalized to facilitate cleaning without re-entry of dust. The liquid film type is particularly effective, as the dust is continuously washed from the plates with virtually no re-entrainment occurring.

Figure 2.9.9

Electrostatic precipitator.

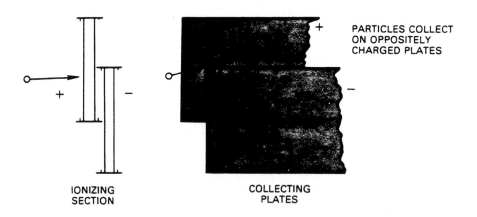

IONIZING
SECTION

COLLECTING
PLATES

PARTICLES COLLECT
ON OPPOSITELY
CHARGED PLATES

Once the plates have been cleaned, it is necessary to gather the removed dust and dispose of it. Baffled hoppers are used to collect the dust. The baffles act to prevent dirty air from bypassing the collection plates. The dust collected in the hopper can be removed intermittently by a conveying system.

There are basically two types of electrostatic precipitators. The first of these is a low-voltage precipitator that operates at approximately 12,000 volts. In low-voltage precipitators, the ionizer and collecting sections are separated. This type of precipitator is approximately 95 to 99 percent efficient in the removal of oil fumes. Except for this application, low-voltage precipitators are not widely installed in industry.

The second type of precipitator, the high-voltage precipitator, operates at up to 75,000 volts. The collector may be made up of tubes when a wet gas is being processed or plates for the cleaning of dry dust. The high-voltage precipitator is widely used for control of stack effluents from such operations as blast furnaces, power-generating stations, electric furnaces, and cement plants. A high-voltage precipitator is 95 to 99 percent efficient for 0.25 micrometer particles. Electrostatic precipitators exhibit low pressure drops from 0.5 to 1 inches wg. However, the cost of installation of precipitators is high, and space requirements for installation are large.

Air Cleaning for Gases--Adsorption

The previous discussion was limited to cleaning particulate matter from the air. The methods applied are not generally applicable to cleaning gases and vapors from the air. Special methods must be applied for this type of air cleaning.

Adsorption is a physical phenomenon in which the gas or liquid attaches or condenses on the surface of a solid (adsorbent). The forces that act to cause adsorption include van der Waal forces between the molecules and capillary condensation.

The general principles of adsorption involve the passage of air containing a gas or vapor to be removed through a bed of granulated adsorbent. The most common adsorbents are forms of activated carbon. Molecules of the gas attach to the granules of the adsorbent. The process is reversed to remove the adsorbate. Various adsorbents have specific applications for certain gases or vapors. For example, activated carbon has application with hydrocarbon vapors, while silica gel adsorbs water in preference to hydrocarbons.

The time the adsorbate spends in the adsorbent (dwell time) is important. If this time is not sufficient to allow the adsorbing action to take place, the efficiency of the system will suffer. Any velocity through the bed above the critical velocity will result in a decrease in the percentage of capture.

Some general principles apply to the process of adsorption. These principles are:

1.   Generally, adsorption varies directly with the vapor pressure of the adsorbate.

2. Adsorption varies inversely with the temperature and directly with the pressure of the system.
3. The more dense the adsorbate, the greater the quantity adsorbed.
4. When using activated carbon as an adsorbent, the material with the greatest surface area and the lowest bulk density for a given size (mesh) is the most efficient and holds the most adsorbate.
5. The ease of adsorption increases as the boiling point of the gas or vapor increases.
6. For organic vapors, a larger number of carbon atoms per molecule increases the ease of adsorption.
7. C_1 (carbon) and C_2 compounds (with one or two carbon atoms per molecule) do not adsorb.
8. Unsaturated compounds of carbon adsorb better than saturated compounds of carbon.
9. Synthetic hydrosilicates are more efficient in capture than activated carbon, but do not have the holding capacity.
    (Adapted from Air Pollution Manual, Part II, AIHA, 1968.)

Recirculating Adsorbing Systems. Recirculating adsorbing systems consist of a thin, loosely compacted bed approximately one-half inch in depth. The dwell time in such a bed is generally 0.05 seconds or less. The resistance to flow is less than 0.25 inches wg. The retention of such beds is between 5 and 50 percent. Generally such systems operate as one-pass systems and are used most often in room air conditioning. These systems are not suitable for general air pollution work.

One-Pass Nonregenerative Systems. These systems are made up of beds of three-quarters to several inches thick. Dwell time varies from 0.075 to 0.5 seconds. Such systems operate effectively on concentrations of a few parts per million. The pressure drop through such a bed is generally 0.5 inches wg. These systems are used where a small amount of contaminant is present.

One-Pass Regenerative Systems. The one-pass regenerative system is used when the contaminant exceeds a few parts per million. Two adsorber beds are used; one operates while the other is being regenerated. The beds in such systems are generally one to three feet in depth with a dwell time of 0.6 to 6.0 seconds. The pressure drop experienced in such a system is from 3 to 15 inches wg. Regeneration is accomplished by applying low pressure steam to raise the bed temperature and drive out the adsorbent. This type of system is widely used in industry.

Air Cleaning for Gases--Absorption

In the process of absorption, gas is dissolved in a liquid that is mixed with the gas. This process is commonly called "gas scrubbing" in the air pollution control industry.

In absorption, the air containing the contaminant gas or vapor is introduced to a liquid. The liquid dissolves the gas or vapor. The combined liquid-contaminant waste is then removed. Turbulent mixing of the liquid and gas increases the possibility of dissolving the gas in the liquid.

Among the types of absorption cleaners currently used in industry are packed towers, plate towers, and spray towers. A packed tower is filled with various shaped metals or crushed rock. Air enters the tower at the bottom, and liquid enters at the top. The liquid normally used is water, though other special liquids may be used for removal of a particular gas or vapor. The gas to be removed is dissolved in the liquid and flows out at the bottom of the tower. Air velocities are normally in the range of one foot per second for a packed tower. Packed towers can present problems with flooding when the air velocity is significantly greater and causes the liquid to bubble up. Particles can clog the packing medium. Generally, packed towers are used in small installations where corrosive materials exist.

Plate towers have plates with holes or slots in them. Air bubbles up in the down-flowing liquid, and the contaminating gas is absorbed. Air velocities in plate towers generally are in the area of one to two feet per second. These towers are applicable where higher velocities of air are required and are less susceptible to flooding and plugging. Cooling coils can be installed to cool the liquid and thus cool the incoming air.

The spray tower is similar to the spray tower used in particulate removal. A downward spray of liquid interacts with the air moving upward through the tower. Often the air is moving in a cyclonic motion. Spray towers exhibit relatively low pressure drop and are best used with easily absorbed gases. Sometimes a venturi is included in such a tower to maximize the mixing. These towers are particularly useful where dust particles are to be removed in addition to a gas or vapor.

There are other special types of absorbing equipment available. These include jet scrubbers, wet cell washers, and wet scrubbers that are normally designed for particulates, but which can be used to remove gases or vapors.

Air Cleaning for Gases--Incinerators

Incineration is rapid high-temperature oxidation of a contaminant gas. Incomplete combustion will normally cause a problem; therefore, the incineration must be controlled and complete.

Combustion requires the following three "t's":

A.   Time (reaction time)
B.   Temperature (increases reaction rate)
C.   Turbulence (to mix oxygen, fuel, and contaminant).

Fuel and air are mixed and passed to a combustion chamber. The flame in the combustion chamber burns the contaminant. A high temperature is present as a result of the combustion (1500°F will destroy any odorous organic material or odorous aerosol). The range of concentration must be maintained outside the range of the LEL and UEL to avoid spontaneous explosions. In some cases, a waste liquid can be burned if it has been atomized by spraying prior to combustion.

Incineration can cause a number of problems and requires safety precautions. Excessive temperature of the air after burning can be controlled by adding dilution air downstream from the combustion. Flashback can be controlled by diluting the incoming gases below the LEL, increasing the velocity of incoming air to a velocity greater than the flame propagation rate, passing the air through plates with openings too small to permit backward flame propagation, or placing a water spray on the incoming side that will stop any combustion. An incineration unit must have an automatic fuel shutoff to prevent problems occurring because of flame failure.

Air Cleaning for Gases--Catalytic Combustion (Oxidation)

Often it is necessary to provide a high temperature for complete combustion of the contaminant. In such cases, excessive cost is experienced both in terms of fuel use and the precautions necessary to maintain the incinerator itself. This situation can be overcome by the use of catalytic combustion.

In catalytic combustion, the contaminated air is passed through a bed containing a catalyst. A commonly used catalyst is an alloy of platinum that is placed on wires to form a mesh, or rods, beads, pellets, etc. The catalyst bed must expose the maximum surface of the catalyst to the gas stream. Sufficient area must be present to complete the oxidation. Gases may be heated prior to the catalytic oxidation. Catalytic combustion results in a low pressure drop, usually 1/4 to 1/2 inches wg. Catalytic combustion is not suitable for air containing fly ash, inorganic solids, vaporized metals, and some halogenated hydrocarbons.

Summary

Cleaning contaminants from exhaust air involves the removal of particulate matter, gases, and vapors. General methods for cleaning the air of these contaminants differ from each contaminant type. Various types of air cleaners have been designed to accomplish the desired cleaning. The cleaners operate at different efficiencies in removing particular contaminants. In general, as the efficiency of the cleaner increases, the cost of installation and operation also increases. For particulate cleaners, the resistance to flow increases in direct relationship to an increased efficiency. This in turn necessitates the use of more powerful air movers, thus increasing the cost of operation. Before selecting the appropriate air cleaner, the industrial hygiene engineer must be familiar with the process requirements and the desired quality of the exit air.

Table 2.9.1 summarizes the most common types of air cleaners discussed in this chapter.

Table 2.5.1

Common types of air cleaners.

Type	Effective Range (micrometers)	Pressure Loss (in. wg.)	Space	Problems	Common Use Areas
Particulate Cleaners					
Dry Type					
Settling Chamber	>100	Varies with size and design	Large	Only useful as pre-cleaner to remove large particles	Woodworking chip traps
Dry Cyclone	20-40	1 - 1.5	Large	Corrosive or moisture-laden contaminants	Crushing and grinding, metal working, woodworking
High Efficiency Cyclone	≥10	3 - 6	Moderate	Corrosive or moisture-laden contaminants	Crushing and grinding, fly ash, drying, metal working
Impingement	>20	0.5 - 3	Small	Low efficiency; corrosive or moisture-laden air	Fly ash, crushing and grinding, cement clinker coolers
Dynamic Collectors	>10	None	Small	Corrosive or moisture-laden air	Metal working, woodworking
Mat Filters	4-20	2 - 8	Small	Noncleanable	Coke box, open hearth furnaces
Bag Houses	≥0.25	3 - 6	Large	High temperature, moisture, cleaning	Crushing and grinding, material handling, foundries, wood-working, fly ash
High Efficiency Filters	≥0.01	1	Small	Low velocity of air flow, low capacity	Clean rooms, food processing, hospitals
Electrostatic Precipitators	≥0.25	0.5 - 1	Large	Installation cost high	Fly ash, blast and open hearth furnaces
Wet Type					
Spray Towers	≥10	1 - 1.5	Large	Clogging, low efficiency	Crushing and grinding, material handling, foundries, drying, metal working

Table 2.9.1 (continued)

Type	Effective Range (micrometers)	Pressure Loss (in. wg.)	Space	Problems	Common Use Areas
Wet Type-Continued					
Wet Cyclone	≥5	2 - 6	Moderate	Water usage	Same as above
Self-Induced Spray	≥2	3 - 6	Small	Water usage	Same as above
Wet Impingement	≥2	1.5 - 8	Small	Water usage	Same as above
Venturi	≥0.5	60 - 100	Moderate	Water usage, high power requirements	Where high efficiency cleaning for small particles is required
Mechanical	≥0.5	None	Small	High power requirements	Same as venturi
Gases and Vapors					
Adsorption--One Pass Regenerative	--	3 - 15	Large	Contamination of adsorbent	Solvent recovery, odor control, chemical manufacturing
Absorption--(Spray and Packed Tower)	--	Varies	Large	Plugging and flooding	Chemical manufacturing
Incineration	--	--	Large	Safety, cost of fuel	Odor control, reducing plume opacity, removal of hydrocarbons
Catalytic Combustion	--	0.5	Moderate	Not applicable where certain types of particulates are present	Organic gases and vapors

10. Air-Moving Devices

In order for air to move within a ventilation system, a driving force must be present. Generally, the force is provided by a mechanical fan. A fan is a device used for moving air and other gases or vapors at pressures low enough that the compression of the air or gas can be ignored. Fans can be classified into two major categories: the <u>axial</u> flow fan, where the air moves in a direction perpendicular to the fan blade; and the <u>centrifugal fan</u>, where the air moves in the same direction as the blades rotate.

<u>Terminology Relating to Fan Operation</u>

A number of terms and concepts are important in the discussion of fans. These terms are summarized below.

1. RPM--The revolutions per minute which the fan blades make.

2. CFM--The cubic feet of air per minute moved by the fan.

3. FPM--The velocity of air in feet per minute moved by the fan.

4. Velocity Pressure of the Fan--The gauge pressure in inches of water which is created by the fan pushing air into the outlet. VP_i is used to designate the velocity pressure on the inlet side of the fan, while VP_o is used to designate the velocity pressure on the outlet side of the fan.

5. Fan Pressure--Fan pressure is the driving force developed by the fan to overcome losses in the system. Fans are rated in terms of the total pressure of the fan (TP_f) (which is the absolute pressure at the fan outlet minus the absolute pressure at fan inlet) or in terms of the static pressure of the fan (SP_f). The development of these two pressures is shown below.

    <u>Fan Total Pressure</u>

    The total pressure of the system (or total pressure against which the fan must operate) is

    $$(2.10.1) \quad TP_f = TP_{fan\ outlet} - TP_{fan\ inlet}$$

    Since these pressures are gauge pressures relative to atmospheric pressure, then from Bernoulli's theorem where $TP = SP + VP$

(2.10.2) $TP_{fo} = SP_o + VP_o + TP_{atmosphere}$

and

(2.10.3) $TP_{fi} = SP_i + VP_i + TP_{atmosphere}$

Substituting 2.10.2 and 2.10.3 in 2.10.1,

$$TP_f = (SP_o + VP_o + TP_a) - (SP_i + VP_i + TP_a)$$

(2.10.4) $TP_f = SP_o - SP_i + VP_o - VP_i$

The SP_i represents the static pressure in the exhaust section of a system and will take on a negative value. Thus the

$$TP_f = |SP_o| + |SP_i| + VP_o - VP_i$$

If $VP_o = VP_i$ as is often the case when the inlet and outlet diameters are equal, then

(2.10.5) $TP_f = SP_o - SP_i$

Figure 2.10.1

Fan pressures.

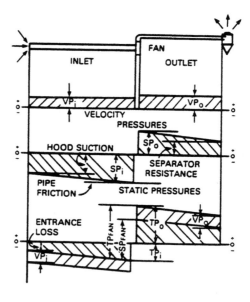

Fan Static Pressure

Most often fans are rated in terms of SP_f, which can be obtained from the relationship:

(2.10.6) $SP_f = TP_f - VP_o$

which can be written using the relationship developed in 2.10.4 as follows:

$$SP_f = (SP_o - SP_i + VP_o - VP_i) - VP_o$$

(2.10.7) $SP_f = SP_o - SP_i - VP_i$

The figure presented above illustrates the various pressures that would be encountered both before and after the fan in an industrial exhaust system. VP_i and VP_o are both positive. SP_i is negative on the inlet side, while SP_o is positive on the outlet side of the fan. The relationships developed in equation 2.10.4 and 2.10.7 can be determined by inspection of the bottom section of the graph.

6. Air Horsepower--Assuming 100 percent efficiency in transfer of power, the air horsepower is the horsepower necessary to move a given volume of air against a particular static pressure. If 1 inch of water equals 5.19 pounds per square foot, the fan working against 1 inch of water pressure must then produce 5.19 pounds per minute power.

    1 Horsepower = 33,000 foot-pounds per minute

Thus, to move 1 cubic foot per minute, with a total pressure of 1 inches wg:

$$AHP = \frac{5.19}{33,000} \times 1, \text{ or}$$

$$AHP = \frac{1}{6356}$$

For any pressure and volume, then, the air horsepower can be stated

(2.10.8) $$AHP = \frac{Q \text{ cfm} \times TP_f \text{ inches wg}}{6356}$$

7. Brake Horsepower--A fan does not normally operate at 100 percent efficiency, and brake horsepower takes this inefficiency into consideration. Brake horsepower is normally stated as

(2.10.9) $$BHP = \frac{HP}{\text{The efficiency of the fan}}$$

8. Efficiency--Efficiency is the relationship between the horsepower at 100 percent efficiency and the brake horsepower required to produce a given output.

$$\text{Efficiency} = \frac{AHP}{BHP}$$

(2.10.10) $$\text{Efficiency} = \frac{Q \times TP_f}{6356 \times BHP}$$

Static efficiency is obtained by substituting SP_f for TP_f.

Examples

1. Assuming a fan operates at 81% maximum efficiency and delivers 6,000 cfm of air against a total pressure of 2 inches wg. What horsepower is delivered, and what size motor is required?

    Solution

    Using 2.10.8 to calculate air horsepower (AHP):

    $$AHP = \frac{Q \times TP_f}{6356} \qquad (2.10.8)$$

    $$AHP = \frac{6000 \times 2}{6356}$$

    AHP = 1.89 HP

    Equation 2.10.9 can be utilized to obtain brake horsepower (BHP):

    $$BHP = \frac{HP}{\text{Efficiency}} \qquad (2.10.9)$$

    $$BHP = \frac{1.89}{0.81}$$

    BHP = 2.33 Horsepower

2. A system is designed with a 6-inch round duct. Air must move at a rate of 4000 feet per minute to transport particulates. The static pressure is calculated to be 5 inches wg at the inlet and 2 inches wg at the outlet. The outlet of the fan is constructed of 5-inch round duct. If a fan operates at a maximum efficiency of 85%, determine the size motor necessary to deliver the power required.

Solution

$$Q = vA \quad (2.3.4)$$
$$A = 0.1964 \text{ ft}^2$$
$$Q = 4000 \times 0.1964$$
$$Q = 786 \text{ cfm}$$

To calculate VP_i

$$VP = 4005 \sqrt{VP/2} \quad (2.3.2)$$
$$VP = (4000/4005)^2$$
$$VP = 1 \text{ inch wg}$$

To calculate VP_o

$$Q = vA$$
$$A = 0.1364 \text{ ft}^2$$

$$v = \frac{786}{0.1364}$$

$$v = 5762 \text{ fpm}$$

$$VP_o = (5762/4005)^2$$

$$VP_o = 2.1 \text{ inches wg}$$

From 2.10.4, the total pressure of the fan is then

$$TP_f = SP_o - SP_i + VP_o - VP_i \quad (2.10.4)$$
$$TP_f = 2 - (-5) + 2.1 - 1$$
$$TP_f = 8.1 \text{ inches wg}$$

Using 2.10.8 to calculate the horsepower required

$$AHP = \frac{Q \times TP_f}{6356} \quad (2.10.8)$$

$$AHP = \frac{786 \times 8.1}{6356}$$

$$AHP = 1.00 \text{ HP}$$

$$BHP = \frac{AHP}{E}$$

$$BHP = \frac{1.00}{0.85}$$

$$BHP = 1.18 \text{ HP}$$

Fan Laws

Any given fan can operate over a wide range. The CFM can vary, the outlet velocity can vary, the TP_f or SP_f can be different, the air horsepower required can vary, and the efficiency of the fan itself varies depending upon its point of operation. The rules governing the variance in these factors are called the "fan laws." Some, and only some, of the fan laws are summarized below. The fan laws apply to a family of fans of the same design type and manufacturer; they cannot be used for comparing fans of varying design or manufacture.

1. Variation in speed for a given fan size, duct system, and air density

   a. The CFM varies directly with the fan speed.

   $$(2.10.11) \quad \frac{Q_2}{Q_1} = \frac{RPM_2}{RPM_1}$$

   b. Static pressure varies as the square of the fan speed or rate.

   $$(2.10.12) \quad \frac{SP_2}{SP_1} = (RPM_2/RPM_1)^2$$

   c. Horsepower varies as the cube of the fan speed or rate.

   $$(2.10.13) \quad \frac{HP_2}{HP_1} = (RPM_2/RPM_1)^3$$

2. Variation in fan size--For a given speed (RPM), air density, fan proportions, and point of rating.

   a. Q varies as the cube of the wheel diameter.

   $$(2.10.14) \quad \frac{Q_2}{Q_1} = (D_2/D_1)^3$$

   b. Static pressure varies as the square of the wheel diameter.

   $$(2.10.15) \quad \frac{SP_2}{SP_1} = (D_2/D_1)^2$$

   c. Horsepower varies as the fifth power of the wheel diameter.

   $$(2.10.16) \quad \frac{HP_2}{HP_1} = (D_2/D_1)^5$$

   d. Tip speed of the blade varies as the wheel diameter.

$$(2.10.17) \quad \frac{TS_2}{TS_1} = \frac{D_2}{D_1}$$

3.   Variation in air density--For a given fan speed and system

   a.   Q is constant (assuming no compressibility).

$$(2.10.18) \quad \frac{Q_2}{Q_1} = 1$$

   b.   Static pressure varies as the density.

$$(2.10.19) \quad \frac{SP_2}{SP_1} = \frac{\rho_2}{\rho_1}$$

   c.   Horsepower varies as the density.

$$(2.10.20) \quad \frac{HP_2}{HP_1} = \frac{\rho_2}{\rho_1}$$

Fan Curves

In order to represent the operation of the fan laws in terms of the varying characteristics of a fan, curves are developed by the manufacturer for the operation of each specific fan at a given speed and air density. These curves indicate the relationship of power, pressure and efficiency of the fan. The first point to be considered on a fan curve is the static no delivery point (SND), which is the static pressure level at which no air is delivered from the fan when operating at a given RPM. This point is determined by shutting off either the inlet or the outlet of the fan and measuring the static pressure against which the fan operates.

The other extreme of the fan curve is the free delivery no pressure point (FDNP). At this point, the fan is operating at a given RPM against no static or total pressure other than that of the atmosphere. In this case, the fan is operating free of any inlet or outlet ducts.

Between these points, a characteristic curve is developed for a given fan at a number of RPM rates, using test procedures as prescribed by the Air Moving and Conditioning Association (AMCA). In general, the optimum area for the operation of a fan is in the middle one-third of the rate-of-flow curve. The point of operation for any given fan when attached to a system is the point of intersection between the pressure curve of the system and the fan curve. This point of intersection can be changed by moving upward through the family of RPM curves or by changing the pressure in the system. Such changes can result in more efficient operation of the fan.

Fan characteristic curves can provide useful information concerning the operation of a fan. Consider the curves illustrated in Figure 2.10.3. Quite often the design pressure is not obtained when the system is installed, or changes are made to the system which modify the pressure obtained. The effect of these changes in pressure can be observed on the fan characteristic curves illustrated.

Figure 2.10.2

Fan characteristic curve.

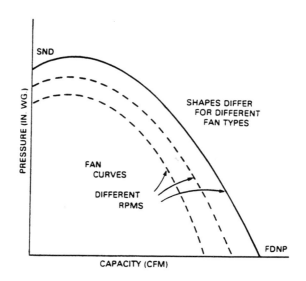

Figure 2.10.3

Variation in actual flow.

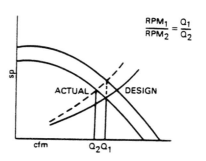

It can be seen that in both cases the change in pressure from design will result in a lower cfm being delivered by the system. However, the first case (a) will result in a smaller difference in cfm than will the second case (b).

When the above situation occurs, the designer has three alternatives available. First the fan speed (RPM) can be increased, resulting in the use of a higher fan curve as shown in Figure 2.10.4. The fan speed is increased by the ratio of the desired design flow to the actual flow (Q_1/Q_2) as presented in equation 2.10.11.

Figure 2.10.4

Change in RPM.

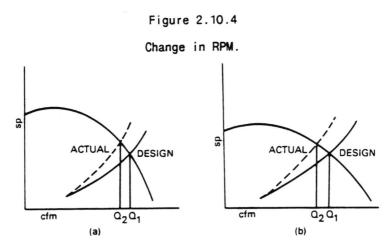

(a)   (b)

Another available alternative is to increase the static pressure of the
fan. To obtain the design flow in this case, the increase in static pressure
is made as the square of the rates of the desired to actual volume
$(Q_1/Q_2)^2$.

Finally, the designer can increase the fan BHP to obtain the desired flow
rates. The increase in BHP necessary is equal to the cube of the ratio of the
volumes or $(Q_1/Q_2)^3$. This and the above two relationships are derived
from the basic fan laws which have been stated for a given series of fans of a
similar design. (See previous discussion on fan laws for other laws.)

In order to simplify selection of fans, the manufacturers have constructed
rating tables for a given type fan. These tables relate Q to SP or TP,
depending upon the manufacturer. They indicate the RPM's and brake horsepower
required to obtain a given rate of flow against a particular static or total
pressure. Manufacturers' rating tables normally point out in some manner the
optimum area of operation for each fan.

To use such rating tables, it is necessary to determine the SP or TP
(depending upon the particular table) against which the fan is operating. The
rate of flow is then determined, and a look-up in the table is conducted to
determine the fan horsepower and RPM requirements. A sample section of a
table is presented in Table 2.10.1

Correcting for Nonstandard Conditions. Fan tables are based upon standard
conditions of 70°F and 29.9 inches Hg. In order to use these tables where
temperature and altitude are different from standard, the effect of changes in
the density of the air must be calculated to obtain the correct fan
performance. In such a situation, Q will remain constant as noted in the fan
laws (equation 2.10.18). The pressure at which the fan operates will vary as
will the pressure in the system (equation 2.10.19). The horsepower required
will also vary directly with the density (equation 2.10.20). In general, the
procedure used to correct for nonstandard conditions is as follows:

a. Design the system, using actual air volumes.
b. Determine SP as though the air were standard (SP_s).

Table 2.10.1

Fan rating table.

CAPACITY (CFM)	4" SP RPM	4" SP BHP	4.5" SP RPM	4.5" SP BHP	5" SP RPM	5" SP BHP	5.5" SP RPM	5.5" SP BHP	6" SP RPM	6" SP BHP
4500	789	4.36	832	4.90	873	5.47	912	6.04	950	6.63
5000	800	4.84	841	5.44	882	6.05	920	6.66	957	7.28
5500	811	5.38	852	5.99	892	6.66	930	7.31	967	7.98
6000	824	5.97	864	6.62	904	7.31	940	7.99	976	8.71
6500	838	6.63	878	7.32	915	8.01	952	8.75	988	9.49
7000	855	7.36	893	8.08	930	8.81	965	9.56	999	10.32

c.   Select the fan by correcting the fan static pressure using actual air volumes as follows (using equation 2.10.19):
     If SP_f denotes the corrected static pressure and SP_a denotes the static pressure calculated

$$SP_f = SP_a \times \frac{1}{\rho} \quad (2.10.19)$$

where

$$\rho = \frac{T_{std}}{T_{actual}} \times \frac{P_{actual}}{P_{std}}$$

or

$$\rho = \frac{460 + T_s}{460 + T_a} \times \frac{P_a}{P_s}$$

d.   Correct the horsepower on the table in the same manner as above (using equation 2.10.20) where BHP_s is the value obtained from the table for SP_f.

$$BHP = \rho \times BHP_s \quad (2.10.20)$$

The correction for BHP is seldom made because the load at cold start approximates BHP_s. If it is desired to use the calculated values, dampers can be installed to limit the volume until the system reaches operating conditions. Thus, a lower operating horsepower can be used

Example

Assume a fan is to operate against 4 inches static pressure at a rate of flow of 6000 cfm. The temperature and altitude for operation are 200°F and 4000 feet above sea level (25.84 inches Hg). What brake horsepower will be required to operate the fan under these conditions

Solution

Using the procedure outlined above

$$\rho = \frac{460 + 70}{460 + 200} \times \frac{25.84}{29.92}$$

$$\rho = 0.693$$

$$SP_f = 4 \times \frac{1}{0.693}$$

$$SP_f = 5.77 \text{ inches wg}$$

Looking up this figure on the sample table presented (Table 2.10.1) and interpolating between values, we obtain

RPM = 959
BHP = 8.38 HP

If the BHP is corrected and dampers installed until operating conditions are reached, the result will be

BHP = 0.693 x 8.38
BHP = 5.8

Categories of Fans

There are two major categories of fans--the axial-flow fan and the centrifugal fan. The axial-flow fan consists of a fan resembling a propeller where the flow of air is in the direction of the axis of rotation. This type fan is similar to the common table fan used in the household. The centrifugal fan is similar to a paddle wheel in design. The flow of air is perpendicular to the axis of rotation.

Figure 2.10.5

Types of fans.

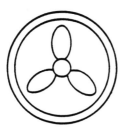 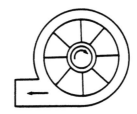

AXIAL FLOW   CENTRIFUGAL FLOW

Types of Axial Fans

The propeller fan--The propeller fan consists of two or more blades. Propeller fans operate against static pressures up to 2 inches wg. This type fan is used in general ventilation work or where very little resistance is present. The propeller fan tends to be noisy and inefficient because of the turbulence of the air leaving the fan and, as a result, is not widely used in industry where heavy air-moving loads are required.

Tube-axial fans--A tube-axial fan is fabricated within a duct section. This fan is basically the standard propeller fan fabricated in such a manner to allow for ease of installation. There are no significant performance differences between a tube-axial fan and a propeller fan.

Vane-axial fan--The vane-axial fan is a propeller within a cylinder in which the blades are short and the hub is large (one-half to two-thirds the diameter of the fan itself). Vanes are used to straighten the air flow and recover energy that is normally lost in turbulence with a standard axial fan. The vane-axial fan can operate against pressures in excess of 15 inches wg. This type fan is compact in design and can be easily installed.

Figure 2.10.6

Vane-axial fan.

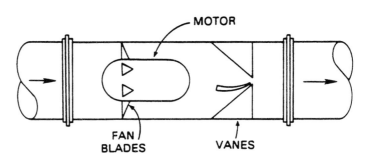

Types of Centrifugal Fans. The centrifugal fan differs in design by the type of blade curve that is present on the fan. The various types of blade curves are as follows:

1.   Radial or straight blade
2.   Forward curve blade
3.   Backward curve blade
4.   Special designs, such as air foils and variable pitch blades

As is evident from an analysis of the vectors for the different blade shapes, the resultant velocity varies between types of blades (Figure 2.10.7). Also illustrated in the figure are typical fan characteristic curves for the three major designs of centrifugal fans.

Figure 2.10.7

Centrifugal fan designs.

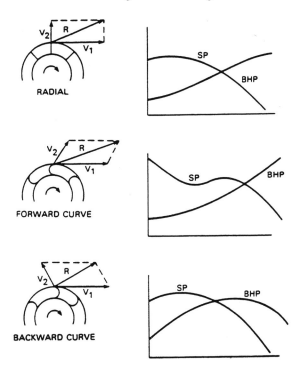

Selecting and Installing a Fan

There are a number of considerations when selecting and installing a fan into a ventilation system. These considerations are discussed below.

Type of Fan to Use

1. Axial Fans--Propeller and Axial-Tube Types
    a. Best used in general and dilution ventilation work.
    b. Best used when low static pressure is present.
    c. Used when particulate contamination is not present.
    d. Used where space is a consideration.

2. Centrifugal Fans--Radial Blades
    a. Most commonly used type in local exhaust ventilation systems.
    b. Particulate loading in the air is not a problem with radial type blades.
    c. High static pressures can be handled with this type fan.

3. Centrifugal Fans--Forward Curve Blades
    a. Quiet operation is a factor when this fan is installed.

b.   This fan operates against low to moderate static pressure.
c.   Must operate in relatively clean air because of the potential buildup of contaminant on the blades.
d.   Often used in heating and air-conditioning work.

4.   Centrifugal Fan--Backward Curve Blades
a.   This type fan results in high efficiency of operation.
b.   Relatively clean air is necessary for operation of this fan.
c.   The backward curve blade results in quiet operation.
d.   This type fan is often called a "limit loading fan" because of the backward curve characteristic of the blade.

5.   Vane-Axial Propeller Fan
a.   This type fan can be used in small areas.
b.   The vane-axial fan results in a high efficiency of operation.
c.   Where moderate noise levels are acceptable, the vane-axial fan can be used.
d.   It should be used in relatively clean air.
e.   The vane-axial fan is generally comparable to the centrifugal fan in terms of static pressure handled.
f.   The vane-axial fan is used extensively in mining and tunnel work.

The Type of Drive Mechanism

1.   Direct Drive
a.   Direct drive results in a more compact power drive system.
b.   Direct drive results in steady RPM.
c.   Variation in motor speed limits the variation in RPM which can be obtained using direct drive.
d.   Motor maintenance is difficult because of the location of the motor in the duct.
e.   Direct drive is most common on axial-flow type fans.

2.   Belt Driven
a.   A variable speed can be obtained using belt drive.
b.   Maintenance on the motor is simple.
c.   The speed can be changed to meet the system requirements.
d.   Belt wear and slippage can modify the RPM below that of the design.

The Direction of Rotation of the Fan. The direction of rotation of the fan is normally determined from the drive side. This direction of rotation can be either clockwise or counterclockwise, depending upon the manufacturer's design. The direction of rotation must be noted before installation; it is relatively simple to install a centrifugal fan backwards. Such a fan will operate and produce an air flow at less than the design of the system.

Duct Connections. When connecting a fan to a duct, it is desirable to use flexible duct connections in order to isolate vibration at the fan. It is important to avoid connections that produce unequal distribution at the inlet. In general, avoid abrupt changes in the direction of the air flow or the duct size at either the inlet or the outlet, since the turbulence they introduce will require the fan to work harder to produce the same air flow. A special case can be made for changing the direction of the air at inlet or outlet. This case is discussed in the next chapter.

Fan Installation. The fan should be mounted using vibration isolators on a sturdy support such as concrete or steel. The installation should take place downstream from any air cleaner to prevent abrasive material from damaging the fan. Various arrangements for discharge and drive are available, depending on the requirements of the installation and can be specified from the manufacturer.

Other Factors to be Considered in Installation. Nonseasonal operating conditions such as high temperatures require special bearings. When corrosive contaminants are present, special blade coating must be considered. In addition, if the contaminated air is explosive or flammable, nonsparking construction of the fan will be necessary.

Changing the Rate of Flow of the Fan. Once a fan is installed, it is sometimes necessary to change the rate of flow to balance the system or to allow for additional duct work to be installed. This can be accomplished in two ways. Dampers can be placed in the duct which increase the static pressure against which the fan must operate. A second method is to vary the speed of the fan, thus changing the relationship between the static pressure and the rate of flow.

Injectors

In some cases, injectors are used in place of fans to provide air movement. An injector operates by introducing a high-velocity air jet into the duct. As the air discharged from the jet expands, it entrains the surrounding air. After all the air in the duct is mixed with the supply, an abrupt expansion occurs. During this expansion, VP is transformed to SP. The SP causes the air to move forward and the upstream air to move through the duct. By adding a venturi, efficiency of this method can be increased. The venturi removes an abrupt expansion and makes additional static pressure available to overcome duct resistance.

Air injectors are used in place of fans where there are intermittent needs for exhaust air. Injectors are also used for handling highly corrosive or sticky materials which would tend to foul a mechanically operating fan.

Figure 2.10.8

Venturi injector.

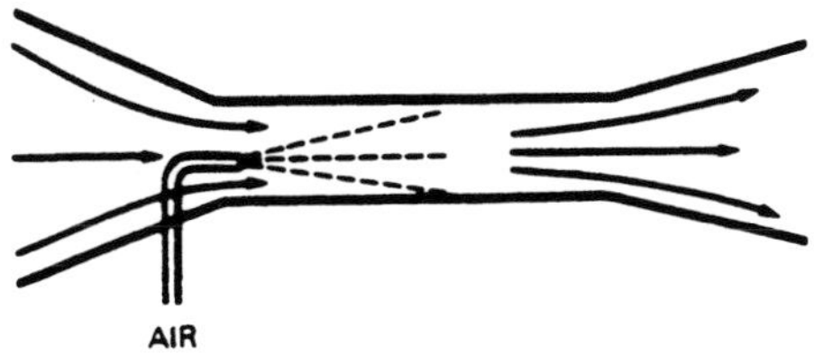

AIR

Summary

Two major designs of fans can be utilized as air movers in a ventilation system--the axial fan and the centrifugal fan. Various blade designs are utilized in centrifugal fans to obtain the desired operating characteristics.

Various formulas are utilized in selecting the appropriate size of fan fo a given system design. The major formulas are summarized below.

REFERENCE	RELATIONSHIP	FORMULA
2.10.4	The total pressure of a fan	$TP_f = SP_o - SP_i + VP_o - VP_i$
2.10.7	The static pressure of a fan	$SP_f = SP_o - SP_i - VP_i$
2.10.8	Air horsepower of a fan	$AHP = \dfrac{Q \times TP_f}{6356}$
2.10.9	Brake horsepower of fan	$BHP = \dfrac{HP}{Fan\ Efficiency}$
2.10.10	Efficiency of fan	$EFF = \dfrac{Q \times TP_f}{6356 \times BHP}$
2.10.11	Q related to RPM	$\dfrac{Q_2}{Q_1} = \dfrac{RPM_2}{RPM_1}$
2.10.12	Static pressure related to RPM	$\dfrac{SP_2}{SP_1} = (RPM_2/RPM_1)^2$
2.10.13	Horsepower related to RPM	$\dfrac{HP_2}{HP_1} = (RPM_2/RPM_1)^3$
2.10.18	Q related to density	$\dfrac{Q_2}{Q_1} = 1$
2.10.19	Static pressure related to density	$\dfrac{SP_2}{SP_1} = \dfrac{\rho_2}{\rho_1}$
2.10.20	Horsepower related to density	$\dfrac{HP_2}{HP_1} = \dfrac{\rho_2}{\rho_1}$

11. Design of Ducts

The final major component of a ventilation system is the duct. The purpose of a duct is to enclose and direct the flow of air in a ventilation system from one point to another point. In an exhaust system, the duct prevents the contaminated air from mixing with the workroom air as it is being removed. In a supply system, the duct serves to direct the supply air to the point where it is required. The duct, then, can be thought of as a pathway within which the air in a ventilation system travels.

The reader will remember from previous discussions that, as air travels through the duct, turbulence is caused by friction along the walls of the duct. Turbulence and friction cause a loss of energy within the ventilation system. In order that there be conservation of energy, Bernoulli's theorem must hold and can be written as:

$$TP = VP + SP + Losses$$

From this relationship, it can be seen that, if losses occur, the total pressure will change. If the total pressure changes and the velocity pressure remains constant, as it will within a given duct size, the change in total pressure to overcome the losses is reflected in the static pressure. Thus, as losses occur within the system, these losses will be reflected in the static pressure measurements obtained.

Losses occur within ventilation systems as the air passes through straight duct; as the air passes through a change in duct diameter (an expansion or contraction) with a resulting change in velocity pressure; as the air changes direction of flow when passing through an elbow; and at the intersection of two or more streams of air in branch connections.

Components of a Duct System

Straight Duct. The most common duct used in ventilation systems work has a round cross section. This is the case since round duct results in a more uniform velocity profile within the system. However in certain situations, conditions may require that other cross section configurations be used (e.g., rectangular or oval). If a rectangular duct is being used, it is necessary to determine its equivalent size of round duct in order to use the friction charts that have been developed for losses. There are two methods to accomplish this. The first of these methods is an estimated method that results in some error. The estimated method is based upon the formula

$$(2.11.1) \quad D = \frac{2WL}{W + L}$$

where

   D = the estimated equivalent diameter of round duct for a rectangular
       duct of dimensions W and L, inches
   W = the width of rectangular duct cross section, inches
   L = the length of rectangular duct cross section, inches

A more accurate conversion to equivalent diameter round duct can be made by
using empirical data. A chart providing such data can be found in the
Industrial Ventilation Manual (Figure 6-24, p. 6.41). A small section of this
chart has been reproduced in the accompanying table. By reading the
intersection of the column and row for the width and length of the rectangular
duct, the equivalent round diameter can be obtained directly.

   The following example illustrates the use of both methods to determine the
error that occurs between these methods.

   Example

       Determine the equivalent round diameter of a rectangular duct with
       dimensions 8 inches by 22 inches using both the estimated and
       accurate method.

   Estimated

$$D = \frac{2WL}{D + L} \quad (2.11.1)$$

$$D = \frac{2 \times 8 \times 22}{8 + 22}$$

$$D = 11.7 \text{ inches}$$

   Accurate

       Reading the chart for 8 inches in width and 22 inches in length,
       we obtain

       $D = 14.1$ inches

In this particular case, the error obtained using the estimated method is
significant, but because it results in a lower value, the result will
overstate the frictional losses. Thus, a safety factor is included when the
estimated conversion is used.

   The size of duct to be used in a given ventilation system is determined
based upon the velocity required to transport the contaminant and the economy
of the system construction. Transport velocity varies depending upon the

Table 2.11.1

Circular equivalents of rectangular ducts for equal friction and capacity.

Side Rectangular Duct	4.0	4.5	5.0	5.5	6.0	6.5	7.0	7.5	8.0	8.5	9.0	9.5	10.0	10.5	11.0	11.5	12.0	12.5	13.0	13.5
3.0	3.8	4.0	4.2	4.4	4.6	4.8	4.9	5.1	5.2	5.4	5.5	5.6	5.7	5.9	6.0	6.1	6.2	6.3	6.4	6.5
3.5	4.1	4.3	4.6	4.8	5.0	5.2	5.3	5.5	5.7	5.6	6.0	6.1	6.3	6.4	6.5	6.7	6.8	6.9	7.0	7.1
4.0	4.4	4.6	4.9	5.1	5.3	5.5	5.7	5.9	6.1	6.3	6.4	6.6	6.8	6.9	7.1	7.2	7.3	7.5	7.6	7.7
4.5	4.6	4.9	5.2	5.4	5.6	5.9	6.1	6.3	6.5	6.7	6.9	7.0	7.2	7.4	7.5	7.7	7.8	8.0	8.1	8.2
5.0	4.9	5.2	5.5	5.7	6.0	6.2	6.4	6.7	6.9	7.1	7.3	7.4	7.6	7.8	8.0	8.1	8.3	8.4	8.6	8.7
5.5	5.1	5.4	5.7	6.0	6.3	6.5	6.8	7.0	7.2	7.4	7.6	7.8	8.0	8.2	8.4	8.6	8.7	8.8	9.0	9.2

Side Rectangular Duct	6	7	8	9	10	11	12	13	14	15	16	17	18	19	20	22	24	26	28	30
6	6.6																			
7	7.1	7.7																		
8	7.5	8.2	8.8																	
9	8.0	8.6	9.3	9.9																
10	8.4	9.1	9.8	10.4	10.9															
11	8.8	9.5	10.2	10.8	11.4	12.0														
12	9.1	9.9	10.7	11.3	11.9	12.5	13.1													
13	9.5	10.3	11.1	11.8	12.4	13.0	13.6	14.2												
14	9.8	10.7	11.5	12.2	12.9	13.5	14.2	14.7	15.3											
15	10.1	11.0	11.8	12.6	13.3	14.0	14.6	15.3	15.8	16.4										
16	10.4	11.4	12.2	13.0	13.7	14.4	15.1	15.7	16.3	16.9	17.5									
17	10.7	11.7	12.5	13.4	14.1	14.9	15.5	16.1	16.8	17.4	18.0	18.6								
18	11.0	11.9	12.9	13.7	14.5	15.3	16.0	16.6	17.3	17.9	18.5	19.1	19.7							
19	11.2	12.2	13.2	14.1	14.9	15.6	16.4	17.1	17.8	18.4	19.0	19.6	20.2	20.8						
20	11.5	12.5	13.5	14.4	15.2	15.9	16.8	17.5	18.2	18.8	19.5	20.1	20.7	21.3	21.9					
22	12.0	13.1	14.1	15.0	15.9	16.7	17.6	18.3	19.1	19.7	20.4	21.0	21.7	22.3	22.9	24.1				
24	12.4	13.6	14.6	15.6	16.6	17.5	18.3	19.1	19.8	20.6	21.3	21.9	22.6	23.2	23.9	25.1	26.2			
26	12.8	14.1	15.2	16.2	17.2	18.1	19.0	19.8	20.6	21.4	22.1	22.8	23.5	24.1	24.8	26.1	27.2	28.4		
28	13.2	14.5	15.6	16.7	17.7	18.7	19.6	20.5	21.3	22.1	22.9	23.6	24.4	25.0	25.7	27.1	28.2	29.5	30.6	
30	13.6	14.9	16.1	17.2	18.3	19.3	20.2	21.1	22.0	22.9	23.7	24.4	25.2	25.9	26.7	28.0	29.3	30.5	31.6	32.8
32	14.0	15.3	16.5	17.7	18.8	19.8	20.8	21.8	22.7	23.6	24.4	25.2	26.0	26.7	27.5	28.9	30.1	31.4	32.6	33.8
34	14.4	15.7	17.0	18.2	19.3	20.4	21.4	22.4	23.3	24.2	25.1	25.9	26.7	27.5	28.3	29.7	31.0	32.3	33.6	34.8
36	14.7	16.1	17.4	18.6	19.8	20.9	21.9	23.0	23.9	24.8	25.8	26.6	27.4	28.3	29.0	30.5	32.0	33.0	34.6	35.8
38	15.0	16.4	17.8	19.0	20.3	21.4	22.5	23.5	24.5	25.4	26.4	27.3	28.1	29.0	29.8	31.4	32.8	34.2	35.5	36.7
40	15.3	16.8	18.2	19.4	20.7	21.9	23.0	24.0	25.1	26.0	27.0	27.9	28.8	29.7	30.5	32.1	33.6	35.1	36.4	37.6
42	15.6	17.1	18.5	19.8	21.1	22.3	23.4	24.5	25.6	26.6	27.6	28.5	29.4	30.4	31.2	32.8	34.4	35.9	37.3	38.6
44	15.9	17.5	18.9	20.2	21.5	22.7	23.9	25.0	26.1	27.2	28.2	29.1	30.0	31.0	31.9	33.5	35.2	36.7	38.1	39.5
46	16.2	17.8	19.2	20.6	21.9	23.2	24.3	25.5	26.7	27.7	28.7	29.7	30.6	31.6	32.5	34.2	35.9	37.4	38.9	40.3

characteristics of the contaminant that is present in the air. Specifically, when vapors are being transported, the transport velocity within the duct should be between 2000 to 3000 feet per minute; while particulate matter requires a transport velocity of about 3500 feet per minute in the main duct and 4500 feet per minute for any branch duct.

As duct size increases, the velocity of the air within the duct decreases. In addition, frictional losses decrease as the duct size increases. This results in a decrease in the required air-moving horsepower which must be used per equivalent cubic foot of air moved. Thus, it would appear that the larger the duct, the lower the operating cost of the system. This statement is offset by the fact that as the duct size increases, the material cost of construction of the duct and the required support for the heavier system increase. Thus, a break-even point must be determined that results in the lowest total cost per unit of air moved.

Another factor which must be considered when determining the size of the duct is that as friction loss increases, the noise level increases. This is because of the greater fan tip speed that is required to work against high friction loss. The most common source of noise in a ventilation system results from the fan blades compressing air. The greater the speed, the greater the number of compressions.

Duct sizes generally come in 1/2-inch increments through 5.5 inches; 1-inch increments through 20 inches; and 2-inch increments for 22 inch and larger diameters.

Duct is generally constructed from galvanized sheet steel or black iron. If galvanized sheet steel is used, the air being transported should be of a temperature less than 400°F. The longitudinal seams of the duct are welded if black iron is used or soldered and riveted if galvanized metal is used. As the duct diameter increases, it is necessary that the gauge of the sheet steel become heavier to provide the necessary structural strength in the duct wall. The accompanying table presents the recommended gauge which should be used in a given application for various duct sizes.

Table 2.11.2

Duct wall gauge.

Diameter	US Standard Gauge for Sheet Steel		
	Class		
	I	II	III
To 8"	24	22	20
Over 8" to 18"	22	20	18
Over 18" to 30"	20	18	16
Over 30"	18	16	14

Class I   Includes nonabrasive applications, such as paint spray, wood
             working, pharmaceutical and food products, discharge ducts from
             dust collectors.
Class II   Includes nonabrasive material in high concentration
             (low-pressure pneumatic conveying), moderately abrasive
             material; and highly abrasive material in light concentrations.
             Typical examples are conveying of chemicals and wood dust,
             exhaust of grain dusts, buffing and polishing.
Class III   Includes highly abrasive materials in moderate to heavy
             concentrations and moderately abrasive materials in heavy
             concentration such as low-pressure conveying of tobacco, exhaust
             systems from sand and grit blasting, abrasive cleaning
             operations, rock and ore screening, crushing, dryers, and kilns;
             fly ash from boiler stacks; foundry shakeouts and sand handling
             systems, coal crushing and screening, grinding.

(Industrial Ventilation Manual, page 8-1)

In certain cases, corrosive contaminants must pass through the ventilation
system. Where these contaminants may cause sweat on the duct system, special
coatings or alloys may be used in the construction of the duct.

The length of the duct section is normally equal to the width of the sheet
steel that can be obtained in the local area. A 36-inch width sheet is
commonly used; thus, the most common size for duct is 36 inches in length.
When the duct is constructed, a 1-inch lap is present along the longitudinal
seam. This lap is either welded or riveted on 3-inch centers. In special
cases where light particulate matter or relatively clean air is being handled,
a double lock seam can be used to form the duct. Each duct section is tapered
slightly to provide for the ability to join the duct sections. The small end
(which is the nominal diameter of the duct) is joined with the large end of
the next section downstream in the system. For diameters of duct up to 19
inches, a 1-inch lap is recommended at the joint. For diameters over
19 inches, a 1.25 inch lap is recommended.

Figure 2.11.1

Duct construction.

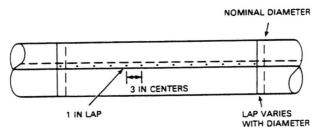

Expansions and Contractions. It is sometimes necessary to expand or
contract the cross-sectional area of air flow within a ventilation system.
This can be required when it is necessary to join a branch duct to a larger
main duct. In an exhaust system, this would result in the air passing through

Figure 2.11.2

Expansions.

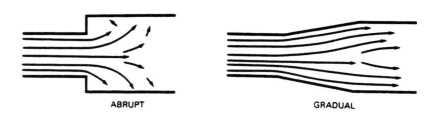

ABRUPT   GRADUAL

an expansion; while in a supply system, the air flowing in the opposite direction would be passing through a contraction. Another situation where an expansion or contraction may be required is to connect the duct system to an air cleaner, fan, or other type of equipment with a different inlet or outlet size.

As air passes through an expansion or contraction, the velocity pressure is converted to static pressure, or the static pressure is converted to velocity pressure, respectively. Losses result because of the turbulence at the vena contracta which forms during the expansion or contraction. If the velocity pressure can be gradually converted to or from the static pressure, the turbulence losses can be minimized. An abrupt change in duct diameter will result in the largest loss.

In order to assure a gradual transition from velocity pressure to static pressure or vice versa, a minimum taper from the expansion or contraction is given as

$$L = 5(D_1 - D_2)$$
where
    L = length of taper
    D_1 = largest diameter
    D_2 = smallest diameter

The general construction and materials specifications used for expansions and contractions are the same as those required for straight duct.

Elbows. The purpose of an elbow is to change the direction of air flow within the ventilation system. Such a change in direction may be necessary because of the layout of the ventilation system within the plant. In addition, certain advantages can be obtained by using elbows in a ventilation system. The appropriate elbow at the entry to an air cleaner, such as a cyclone, can help clean particulates from the air by applying a centrifugal force to the dust-laden air prior to entry to the cleaner. In addition, an elbow placed in the proper location at the exit of an air mover can aid in the reduction of losses experienced at this point of the ventilation system.

As air passes through an elbow, its velocity is less at the outside of the elbow than it is at the inner elbow radius. If air velocity across the duct

Figure 2.11.3

Discharge elbows.

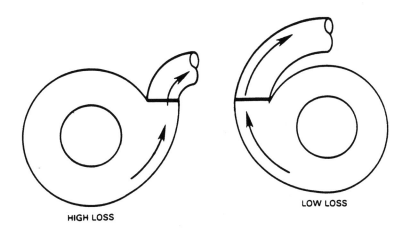

LOW LOSS

HIGH LOSS

at the entry to the elbow is higher at the inner radius of the elbow before the turn, losses will be higher in the system. It is desirable that the cross-sectional velocity pattern within the duct be such that the higher velocity occurs at the outer radius entry point to the elbow.

Where double elbows are used (such as a "U" or "S" elbow), the loss experienced is not necessarily proportional to the number of elbows being used. For example, the loss is higher for an "S" configuration of two elbows than would be expected for two separate elbows of the same radius and diameter. On the other hand, for the "U" configuration, the loss is lower than would be expected for two separate elbows.

Figure 2.11.4

Double elbows.

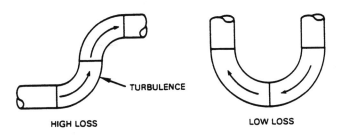

TURBULENCE

HIGH LOSS   LOW LOSS

One method to reduce losses in elbows is to construct a venturi-type elbow. The venturi elbow consists of an elbow with a constriction and a gradual expansion beyond the elbow to provide an area where the air flow can return to its normal cross section.

Figure 2.11.5

Venturi elbow.

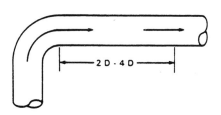

Construction materials for elbows should be a minimum of two gauges heavier than that which is required for the accompanying straight duct. The centerline radius of the elbow should be at least two diameters where possible. A larger radius is desirable for abrasive materials. Five-section construction is recommended for duct that is 6-inch diameter or less. Seven-section construction should be used where the diameter is greater than 6-inches.

Branch Connections. Branch connections are used to join ducts together to form a single ventilation system. As air enters the main duct from the branch at the tee intersection, turbulence occurs as the two air streams mix. This turbulence results in losses reflected in the static pressure. The losses are greatest in the branch; and, in general, losses in the main can be ignored in any duct design. At breaches or Y-shaped intersections of two ducts joining into one duct, lower losses are obtained than at a 90° (T) intersection. In some cases, it is desirable to increase the exhaust in the branch. To do this, vacuum boosters are used. These boosters increase the exhaust obtained in the branch at the expense of a greater pressure drop in the main duct system.

Figure 2.11.6

Vacuum booster.

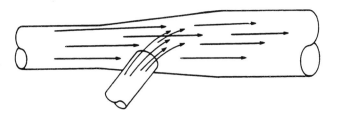

Branch connections are constructed of the same material as the straight duct. The angle of entry of the branch into the main should not be more than 45°. A 30° angle of entry is preferable if the duct structure can be made strong enough. Branches should be connected at only the top or side of the main duct.

Other Components of a Duct System. Other components that may be included in a ventilation system are discussed below.

Dampers. Dampers can be used to shut off the flow of air within the ventilation system. Dampers should be installed where there is a potential that a fire occurring in one area of the plant may be transmitted through the duct to other areas of the plant. This is particularly the case when a flammable substance is being transmitted by the ventilation system. Dampers should be installed according to the National Fire Protection Association code.

The second use of the damper is to protect against back pressure and loss of contaminants through the system from an air cleaner. Dampers automatically close when the system is turned off, thus preventing backflow.

Figure 2.11.7

Back pressure damper.

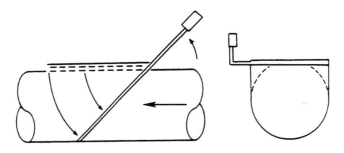

Dampers should not be used to adjust the flow to balance the system, since workers may modify or change the dampers and, as a result, affect the system operation.

Equalizer. An equalizer is a damper which is welded in place to balance the system. Equalizers are placed close to the branch connection and welded into place so that workers cannot affect the system by modifying the damper setting.

Switch. A switch is used where the duct is separated into two ducts, only one of which is active at any given time. Switches can be used when multiple air cleaners are installed, and one or more of them must go off line to be cleaned.

Figure 2.11.8

Switch.

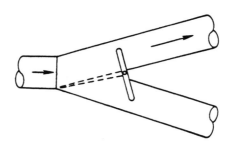

Slip Joints. Slip joints or ball joints are used to connect a movable hood to the duct. These joints provide the ability to move the hood around a small area in the workplace.

Cleanouts. If dust-laden air is being moved in a ventilation system, cleanouts should be provided at approximately 10-foot intervals. This gives the maintenance crew the ability to remove dust buildup before it affects the system operation.

Weather Cap or Stackhead. Where a vertical vent from an exhaust system to the outside atmosphere is present, it is necessary to protect the exhaust from entry of moisture from the atmosphere. This can be accomplished by various designs of weather caps or stackheads. Weather caps cause losses at the vent. Stackhead designs are generally superior to weather caps because they result in lower losses. For this reason, weather caps are not recommended. In some cases, a horizontal discharge may also require weather protection.

Supports. The ventilation system must be supported in some manner. Straps or hangers are often used to support the duct from the ceiling or walls of the plant. In some cases, floor mounted supports may be used. If long runs are necessary, tension rods may be required to avoid sagging of the duct system.

Transitions. Although such design is not recommended, it is sometimes necessary to use transitions to connect rectangular duct to round duct and vice versa. If it is possible, this change in shape should be avoided, since it results in significant static pressure loss.

Figure 2.11.9

Weather protection.

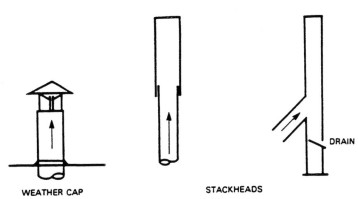

WEATHER CAP   STACKHEADS

(Not recommended.)

Summary

In the preceding chapter, various components of a duct system have been discussed. General design and structural characteristics of these components were presented. These characteristics are as important to the operation of a ventilation system as the selection of the appropriate hood. If improper duct construction is used, the system may leak. If elbows, expansions, and other components are improperly designed, significant losses can occur. These situations can result in the system operating at less than design. This in turn can present a hazard which, because of the fact it may go unrecognized, may be worse than the initial contaminant problem for which the system was designed.

12. Principles of System Design

Losses occur in a ventilation system because of turbulence and friction. The initial loss in an exhaust system occurs at the hood or entry to the system. Entry loss (h_e) depends upon the configuration of the hood. For example, a plain duct opening results in a loss of 0.93 velocity pressures while a flanged duct opening results in a loss of 0.49 velocity pressures. The most efficient hood is the tapered or bell-shaped hood which results in a loss of 0.04 velocity pressures. It is recommended that the losses for special design hoods be checked after construction to assure the losses are as expected.

Figure 2.12.1

Exhaust hoods.

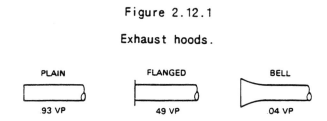

As air flows through a straight duct section, friction causes turbulence along the sides of the duct. In general, as the cross section of the duct increases, the friction loss decreases. Thus, the friction loss encountered in a given length of duct is inversely proportional to the diameter of the duct. On the other hand, as the velocity within the duct increases, the loss also increases. The losses in a given ventilation duct system can be estimated using friction loss charts that have been prepared for various velocities, rates of flow, and duct diameters. (See Figure 2.3.4.)

As the flow of air in a ventilation system is made to change direction by passing through an elbow, additional friction losses are incurred. These losses are dependent upon the diameter of the duct, the degree of turning, and the centerline radius of the elbow. As the diameter of the duct increases, the losses become proportionally smaller. Also, as the centerline radius diameter becomes larger, the losses become proportionally smaller. (See Figure 2.3.8.) The losses that occur as the air changes direction are generally stated in terms of a 90° change in direction. For changes other than this, the losses are directly proportional to the percentage relationship between the degree of turn and a 90° turn. For example, a 45° elbow will result in one-half the loss of a 90° elbow.

As the duct diameter changes (given a constant rate of flow), a dynamic change occurs between the static pressure and velocity pressure within a system in order that Bernoulli's theorem, TP = VP + SP, will hold. As the duct diameter increases, the velocity--and thus the velocity pressure--decreases. As a result, the static pressure of the system must increase. When the duct diameter decreases, the opposite effect will occur. During this dynamic change between velocity pressure and static pressure, a turbulence loss also occurs.

Figure 2.12.2

Losses experienced.

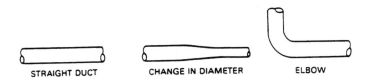

STRAIGHT DUCT   CHANGE IN DIAMETER   ELBOW

Losses can also occur at the outlet of the system, depending on the type of stackhead design which is used. For example, the weather cap design, which is not generally recommended, can result in significant losses because of the turbulence that occurs at the outlet.

Review Problem. Consider the following problems:

Figure 2.12.3

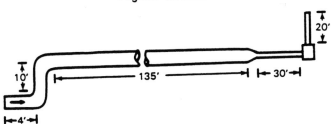

Assume

a. Plain end hood
b. Duct diameter 14"
c. Elbows 90° with radius 2D
d. 30° taper at contraction
e. Duct diameter after contraction 12"
f. Stack diameter 12"
g. A flow of 2780 cfm

Determine

a. The static pressure of the system.
b. The size fan to use for this system, including the RPM and BHP at which it should be operated.

Solution

a.   Static Pressure

1.   Loss at hood

Loss for plain hood = 0.93 VP
To determine the velocity and velocity pressure
   $Q = vA$ (2.3.4)
2780 = v x 1.069 ft^2
   v = 2600 fpm
   VP = 0.42 inches wg
Static pressure to accelerate air = 0.42 inches wg
Hood loss (h_e) = 0.93 x -0.42 = -0.39 inches wg

2.   Losses for straight duct of diameter 14"

Feet of 14" straight duct = 4 + 10 + 135 = 149 feet
   Loss from chart (Figure 2.3.4)
      -0.65 inches wg/100 ft
      149 x -0.65 inches wg/100 ft = -0.97 inches wg

3.   Losses from elbows

2-90° elbows of radius 2D
From Figure 2.3.8:
      Equivalent feet = 21 ft x 2 = 42 ft
      42 x.-0.65 inches wg/100 ft = -0.27 inches wg

4.   Contraction loss

$$v_2 = \frac{2780}{0.7854} = 3540 \text{ fpm}$$

VP$_2$ = 0.78 inches wg

Loss at contraction

From Figure 2.3.6

   SP = $-L(VP_2 - VP_1)$
   SP = -0.13(0.78 - 0.42)
   SP = -0.047 inches wg

Dynamic change in SP
   $-(VP_2 - VP_1)$
   -(0.78 - 0.42) = -0.36 inches wg

5. <u>Loss from straight duct diameter 12"</u>

From Figure 2.3.4, calculate the loss
30 ft x (-1.4 inches wg/100 ft) = - 0.42 inches wg

6. <u>Loss for outlet side of fan</u>

From Figure 2.3.4, assuming inlet and outlet duct are the same
diameter
20 ft x 1.4 inches wg/100 ft = 0.28 inches wg

7. <u>Stackhead</u>

No loss is encountered.

8. <u>Total Loss</u>

Inlet loss

SP_i = (-0.42) + (-0.39) + (-0.97) + (-0.27) + (-0.047)
       + (-0.36) + (-0.42)

SP_i = -2.877 inches wg

Outlet loss

SP_o = 0.28 inches wg

b. Fan Size and Operating Characteristics

Q = 2780 cfm
From 2.10.7
$SP_f = SP_o - SP_i - VP_i$ (2.10.7)
SP_f = 0.28 -(-2.877) - 0.78
SP_f = 2.377 or 2.38 inches wg

Using the following rating table for a particular size fan which seems to
fit the system requirements:

Static Pressure

Capacity cfm	2.0 inches wg RPM	BHP	2.5 inches wg. RPM	BHP
2550	1296	2.20	1364	2.44
2725	1327	2.46	1395	2.72
2900	1361	2.74	1426	3.02
3075	1393	3.03	1459	3.35
3250	1429	3.35	1492	3.68

In order to determine the operating characteristics for the fan given in the above table, it is necessary to interpolate between stated values in the table.

Interpolating between static pressure values

At 2725 cfm for 2.0 inches wg
    RPM = 1327   BHP = 2.46
At 2725 cfm for 2.5 inches wg
    RPM = 1395   BHP = 2.72

Thus at 2725 cfm for 2.38 inches wg determine RPM

$$\frac{(2.38 - 2.0)}{(2.5 - 2.0)} = \frac{(RPM - 1327)}{(1395 - 1327)}$$

RPM = 1379

determine BHP

$$\frac{(2.38 - 2.0)}{(2.5 - 2.0)} = \frac{(BHP - 2.46)}{(2.72 - 2.46)}$$

BHP = 2.66

Similarly, for 2900 cfm and 2.38 inches wg, RPM = 1410 and BHP = 2.95.

Now interpolating between the values obtained for Q = 2780 cfm determine RPM

$$\frac{(2780 - 2725)}{(2900 - 2725)} = \frac{(RPM - 1379)}{(1410 - 1879)}$$

RPM = 1389

determine BHP

$$\frac{(2780 - 2725)}{(2900 - 2725)} = \frac{(BHP - 2.66)}{(2.95 - 2.66)}$$

BHP = 2.75

Thus for the system shown, the fan will operate against a static pressure (SP_f) of 2.38 inches wg at an RPM of 1389 and a BHP of 2.75.

The Effect of Branches in a Ventilation System

To this point, the reader has been working with simple systems; i.e., systems composed of one continuous duct. In practice, systems are generally composed of a series of branches connected to an air cleaner and an air mover. Although each branch of the system can be thought of as a simple system, the need to balance the losses of the branches at the point of intersection makes the problem more complex. It is more important that the reader understand the results that are obtained when an unbalance in the system exists. Three basic methods for obtaining system balance during operation are available. These are the balanced-flow method, the blast-gate method, and the plenum-design method. The emphasis in this chapter is on the balanced flow method. The blast gate and plenum designs will be discussed in the next chapter.

In practice, ventilation systems of the simple design illustrated in the previous problem are not common. More often exhaust systems are made up of many small systems, each serving a given piece of equipment and connected to a main duct by a series of branches. This type of system provides a more complex problem. If the resistance in each of the branches entering the main duct is not the same, air within the system will flow through the path of least resistance (lowest static pressure measured in inches of water). As the air flow increases in the branch with the least resistance, the resistance in that branch will increase until a natural balance within the system will occur. However, such an occurrence can cause a major problem in the operation of a ventilation system. The balanced flow that results from this situation may not be sufficient to remove the hazardous material from the point of operation through branches with higher resistance. If both branches are designed to give the same flow rate but the resistance differs between the branches, the flow rate will adjust until the resistances are equal. Since Q = vA, if A is the same in both cases, then the velocity in the branch with the highest static pressure will decrease, causing a lower static pressure and resulting in a lower Q in this branch. At the point where the resistance in each of the branches is equal, the system will be operating in balance. In the branch with the lower resistance originally, the Q will be higher than that for which the system was designed. In the branch with the higher resistance originally, the Q will be lower than designed; and, as a result, the amount of air exhausted from that operation will be less than desired. Thus, the natural balance that occurs will result in an improperly operating ventilation system.

One solution to the above problem is to balance the branches during the design stage. There are three basic methods available to the design engineer to accomplish the necessary balance of the system. These methods are:

1. Decreasing the duct size in the branch with the lowest resistance. This results in an increased velocity and an increased friction loss for that branch.
2. Increasing the overall system flow which will increase the flow in each branch at a rate sufficient to overcome the change in flow which will occur in attaining natural balance and yet allow for a sufficient volume to be exhausted.
3. Installing dampers to increase the resistance in the branch with the lowest static pressure.

Some general rules have been developed for balancing branches when designing a ventilation system. These rules are:

1. If $SP_{larger}/SP_{smaller} \leq 1.05$, assume the system is in balance and ignore the difference in static pressure.

2. If $1.05 < (SP_{larger}/SP_{smaller}) \leq 1.20$, correct the overall system flow by increasing the Q for the smaller static pressure using the formula

    (2.12.1) $Q = Q_{smaller\ static\ pressure} \times \sqrt{SP_{larger}/SP_{smaller}}$

3. If $SP_{larger}/SP_{smaller} > 1.20$, the resistance of the branch with the smaller static pressure is increased by decreasing the duct size for that branch.

Sizing the Duct

Before balancing can be accomplished, it is necessary to determine the size of the duct that is required for each of the branches. The duct size is determined by considering the capture velocity at the hood, the transport velocity that must be maintained within the branch, and the required Q, or rate of flow which must be maintained. The size duct required is calculated from the formula, $Q = vA$, where the transport velocity is substituted for v and the required Q is used. Duct diameter is determined from the area which is obtained. Charts converting areas to duct diameters are available (see Table 2.12.1). Using the table value, the area in ft^2 nearest the calculated A from the formula is used and the appropriate duct diameter chosen.

Table 2.12.1

Relationship of duct diameter to duct area.

Duct Diameter in inches	Area in ft^2	Duct Diameter in inches	Area in ft^2
1	.0054	11	.6600
1.5	.0123	12	.7854
2	.0218	13	.9218
2.5	.0341	14	1.069
3	.0491	15	1.227
3.5	.0668	16	1.396
4	.0873	17	1.576
4.5	.1105	18	1.767
5	.1364	19	1.969
5.5	.1650	20	2.182
6	.1964	21	2.405
6.5	.2305	22	2.640
7	.2673	23	2.885
7.5	.3068	24	3.142
8	.3491	25	3.409
8.5	.3940	26	3.687
9	.4418	27	3.976
9.5	.4923	28	4.276
10	.5454	29	4.587

In sizing the duct for a complex system, it is advantageous to first size the branch that is assumed to have the highest resistance. However, if an inaccurate choice is made on the branch with the highest resistance, the balancing methods will point out this error, and recalculations can be made to determine the duct size.

Determining the SP$_f$

Once the branches have been balanced, it is necessary to determine SP$_f$ to select the appropriate fan and operating characteristics (BHP and RPM). This is accomplished by selecting the branch with the highest static pressure at each branch junction point, beginning at the farthest point from the fan. Even when the system is in balance, the branch static pressure may differ by as much as 5 percent since the difference is ignored. The largest static pressure becomes the governing static pressure to that point and is the base value that is added to further static pressure losses downstream. If two branches, each having a static pressure of 3 inches wg, come together at a point, the value used to determine the SP$_f$ is 3 inches wg, not 6 inches wg. The reader is cautioned to note this fact since the natural tendency is to add static pressures for two branches. To illustrate this point, consider the following:

Figure 2.12.4

Branch static pressure.

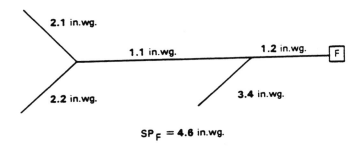

Now to illustrate the design procedure, consider the following problem and accompanying solution. The situation presented is for a simple exhaust system. However, the procedures used are the same as would be used for a complex system. The method presented is termed the equivalent foot method of balancing.

Example. The following problem is presented to illustrate the techniques used in balancing a simple ventilation system consisting of more than one branch. The objective is to determine the balanced design and required static pressure for the fan.

Figure 2.12.5

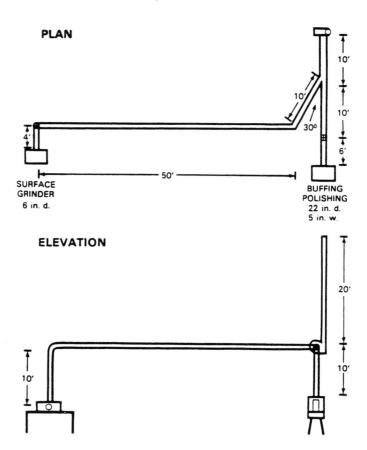

All elbows are 2D centerline radius.
What design is required for such a system?

Solution

A. Determine hood design.
    To determine the appropriate hood design, consult the Specific Operations
    section of the Industrial Ventilation Manual (Section 5).

        Surface Grinding
            Use VS-417
                    v = 3500 fpm minimum
                    Q = 300 cfm
                    h_e = 0.25 VP

Buffing and Polishing

Use VS-406
v = 4500 fpm for branch
Q = 740 cfm (assume good enclosure)
h_e = 0.40 VP using tapered takeoff.

B. Select branch of greatest resistance.
Assume surface grinding has greatest resistance. To size duct for surface grinding:

$$Q = v \times A$$

$$A = \frac{300}{3500}$$

$$A = 0.0857$$

Nearest duct diameter is 4 inches (Table 2.12.1). Calculating the velocity for a 4" duct:

$$v = \frac{300}{0.0873}$$

$$v = 3440 \text{ fpm}$$

C. Calculate losses in branch (surface grinding).

To calculate losses occurring in the branch, consider the following losses:

1. Loss as result of acceleration of air

$$3440 = 4005 \sqrt{VP}$$
VP = 0.74 inches wg
SP = -VP
SP = -0.74 inches wg

2. Loss occurring at hood
Loss = -0.25 VP
Loss = -0.19 inches wg

3. Loss for 74 ft of straight duct
From Figure 2.3.4, calculate the static pressure loss:
74 ft. x -5.3 inches wg/100 ft = -3.92 inches wg

4. Loss occurring at elbows:
From Figure 2.3.8, calculate the static pressure loss:
2-90° elbows = 4 equivalent ft/elbow x 2   = 8 ft
1-60° elbow = 4 equivalent ft/elbow x 0.67   = 2.67 ft
Total loss
10.67 ft x -5.3 inches wg/100 ft = -0.57 inches wg

5. Loss at branch entry:
From Figure 2.3.6, calculate the static pressure loss:
30° entry = 3 equivalent feet
3 ft x (-5.3 inches wg/100 ft) = -0.16 inches wg

6.   Total loss for branch:
     $(-0.76) + (-0.19) + (-3.92) + (-0.57) + (-0.16) = -5.6$ inches wg

Calculate losses occurring in branch (buffing and polishing). To
determine losses occurring in branch, consider:

1.   To size duct for buffing and polishing

$$A = \frac{740 \text{ cfm}}{4500 \text{ ft/min}}$$

$$A = 0.164 \text{ ft}^2$$

Using a duct diameter of 5.5" or 0.1650 ft^2 (Table 2.12.1)
     To calculate actual v

$$v = \frac{740}{0.165}$$

$$v = 4480 \text{ fpm}$$

2.   Loss as result of acceleration of air

$$4480 = 4005 \sqrt{VP}$$
$$VP = 1.25 \text{ inches wg}$$
$$SP = -1.25 \text{ inches wg}$$

3.   Losses occurring at hood
     Loss = -0.40 VP
     Loss = -0.50 inches wg

4.   Loss for 26 feet of straight duct
     From Figure 2.3.4, calculate the static pressure loss:
         26 ft. x -5.9 inches wg/100 ft = -1.53 inches wg

5.   Loss occurring at elbows
     From Figure 2.3.8, calculate the static pressure loss:
         2-90° elbows = 6.5 equivalent ft x 2 = 13 equivalent feet
         13 ft x -5.9 inches wg/100 ft. = -0.77 inches wg

6.   Total loss
     $(-1.25) + (-0.50) + (-1.53) + (-0.77) = -4.05$ inches wg

E. Determine if branches are in balance.

$$\text{Ratio of branch SP loss} = \frac{5.6}{4.05} = 1.38$$

Balance by raising SP loss in buffing and polishing. This can be
accomplished by decreasing the duct size to 5 inches which will increase

the velocity and also the loss that occurs. To recalculate this loss, the following is obtained:

1. Acceleration loss
$$Q = vA$$
$$740 = v \times 0.1364 \text{ ft}^2$$
$$v = 5425 \text{ fpm}$$
$$VP = 1.83 \text{ inches wg}$$
$$SP = -1.83 \text{ inches wg}$$

2. Hood loss
$$\text{Loss} = -0.40 \times 1.83 \text{ inches wg} = -0.73 \text{ inches wg}$$

3. Straight duct
From Figure 2.3.4, calculate the static pressure loss:
$$26 \text{ ft.} \times -9.6 \text{ inches wg}/100 \text{ ft} = -2.50 \text{ inches wg}$$

4. Elbow loss
From Figure 2.3.8, calculate the static pressure loss:
$$12 \text{ ft} \times -9.6 \text{ inches wg}/100 \text{ ft} = -1.15 \text{ inches wg}$$

5. Total loss
$$(-1.83) + (0.73) + (-2.50) + (-1.15) = -6.21 \text{ inches wg}$$

F. Determine ratio of balanced branches
$$\text{Ratio} = \frac{6.21}{5.6} = 1.11$$

Since
$$1.05 < \frac{SP_{larger}}{SP_{smaller}} < 1.20$$

Balance system Q for system by increasing flow in branch with lower resistance. To obtain corrected flow:

$$Q_{corrected} = Q_{calculated} \sqrt{SP_{larger}/SP_{smaller}}$$

$$Q_c = 300 \text{ cfm} \sqrt{6.21/5.6}$$

$$Q_c = 316 \text{ cfm}$$

G. To determine main duct size:
Total flow will be
$$316 \text{ cfm} + 740 \text{ cfm} = 1056 \text{ cfm}$$
To maintain v at 3500 and transport contaminant, then
$$1056 = 3500 \times A$$
$$A = 0.3017 \text{ ft}^2$$
Using nearest duct size of 7.5 inches diameter (0.3068 ft^2) and recalculating actual v, obtain

$$1056 = v \times 0.3068$$
$$v = 3440 \text{ fpm}$$
$$VP = 0.74 \text{ inches wg}$$

H. To calculate losses to fan from 7 1/2 inch duct
    From Figure 2.3.4, calculate the static pressure loss:
    10 ft x -2.5 inches wg/100 ft = -0.25 inches wg

I. Total loss on inlet of an (SP_i)
    Calculate loss by using governing SP and adding losses in main. The
    governing SP is the SP of the branch with greatest resistance.
    (-6.21) + (-0.25) = -6.46

J. To calculate loss at fan outlet (SP_o)
    Assume outlet diameter is same as inlet diameter. From Figure 2.3.4
    calculate the static pressure loss:
    20 ft x +2.5 inches wg/100 ft = +0.50 inches wg

K. To calculate SP_f
    $$SP_f = SP_o - SP_i - VP_i$$
    $$SP_f = (0.50) - (-6.46) - 0.74$$
    $$SP_f = 6.22 \text{ inches wg}$$

The Calculation Worksheet

In order to simplify the calculation necessary to design and balance an
industrial ventilation system, a calculation worksheet has been designed. The
use of this sheet will result in a systematic approach to the problem and
should help to eliminate errors that may occur in the calculations. The
worksheet also documents the design, which is helpful when reviewing an
already installed system to determine if the branches are operating properly.
The calculation worksheet is shown in Figure 2.12.6.

The following briefly explains the use of each of the columns of the
calculation worksheet.

Column 1--Duct Number or Name. A schematic drawing of the proposed
ventilation system is drawn, and each of the branches and sections of the main
duct is numbered and lettered. These designations are placed in Column 1; one
segment of the system per row on the calculation sheet.
Column 2--Design Q (cfm). The desired rate of flow.
Column 3--Minimum Transport Velocity (fpm). This is the minimum transport
velocity that must be maintained within the branch or segment of the duct
under construction.
Column 4--Duct Diameter in Inches. After the initial area has been
calculated using the transport velocity and design Q, it is necessary to
translate this into the actual duct diameter to be used, considering the fact
that ducts are generally sized in one-half inch increments up to six inches in
diameter and one-inch increments above six inches in diameter. The actual
diameter to be used is entered in this column.

Figure 2.12.6

Calculation sheet

Static pressure balance--equivalent length method.

#	Column heading
1	Duct number or name
2	Design Q, cfm
3	Min. tran. velocity, fpm
4	Duct diam., inches
5	Duct area, ft^2
6	Actual duct velocity, fpm
7	Actual duct velocity press in W.G.
8	SLOTS — Slot area ft^2
9	SLOTS — Slot velocity, fpm
10	SLOTS — Slot velocity press in W.G.
11	SLOTS — Slot entry loss factor
12	SLOTS — Accel. factor* (1.0 + col 11)
13	SLOTS — Slot entry loss in W.G. [(col 10 to col 11) or (col 10 x col 12)]
14	HOODS — Hood entry loss factor, VP
15	HOODS — Accel. factor* (1.0 + col 14)
16	HOODS — Hood entry loss in W.G. [(col 7 x col 15) or (col 7 x col 14)]
17	DUCT LOSSES — Length, ft
18	DUCT LOSSES — Friction loss per 100 ft in W.G.
19	DUCT LOSSES — Duct loss in W.G. (col 17 x col 18)/100
20	ELBOWS — Centerline rad./duct diam.
21	ELBOWS — Equiv. length per 90° elbow
22	ELBOWS — Number of 90° ells
23	ELBOWS — Equiv. lengths, ft
24	ELBOWS — Elbow loss in W.G. (col 18 x col 23)/100
25	ENTRIES — Angle of entry, deg.
26	ENTRIES — Equiv. length per entry, ft
27	ENTRIES — Entry loss in W.G. (col 18 x col 26)/100
28	MISCELLANEOUS CALCULATIONS
29	Total losses (SP) in W.G. (col 13 + 16 + 19 + 24 + 27)
30	Cumulative losses (SP) in W.G.
31	Governing SP in. W.G.
32	Balanced Q, cfm

(ENTRY LOSSES groups columns 8–16; FITTING LOSSES groups columns 20–27)

*This represents the amount of energy needed to get air to flow into the hood. NOTE: When dealing with hoods that also contain slots, add the acceleration factor to either the hood VP or slot VP, whichever has the higher value (usually the hood VP). This is only added one time, that is, only where air initially enters the duct (e.g., through a hood).

PLANT NAME _____ ELEVATION _____

LOCATION _____ TEMPERATURE _____

DEPARTMENT _____

CALCULATIONS BY _____

CHECKED BY _____

APPROVED BY _____ DATE _____

Column 5--Duct Area Square Feet. This is the area that results from the duct diameter indicated in column 4 and is obtained by using the formula, $A = \pi r^2$, or a chart indicating the relationship between area and diameter (Table 2.12.1).

Column 6--Actual Duct Velocity (fpm). The actual duct velocity that results as air passes through the duct of the diameter chosen in column 4 at the rate of flow designed in column 2 (i.e., column 2   column 5).

Column 7--Actual Duct Velocity Pressure in Inches Water Gauge. The translation of the duct velocity into velocity pressure, using the formula,

$$v = 4005 \sqrt{VP}.$$

Column 8--Slot Area Square Feet. The area of the slot when a slot hood i used which is obtained by multiplying the length times the width of the slot in feet.

Column 9--Slot Velocity (fpm). The slot velocity which is obtained as ai passes through the slot in the hood.

Column 10--Slot Velocity Pressure in Inches Water Gauge. The velocity pressure translation for the slot velocity entered in column 9 which is

calculated using $v = 4005 \sqrt{VP}.$

Column 11--Slot Entry-Loss Factor in Velocity Pressure. The loss factor that is obtained as air enters the slot. This loss factor can be found by consulting tables related to the design of various industrial hoods.

Column 12--Acceleration Factor. The acceleration factor represents the amount of energy required to accelerate air from rest to slot (or duct, colum 15) velocity; it is equal to 1 and is usually referred to as one velocity pressure or 1 VP. For the total energy required to overcome the losses upon entry into the hood and to accelerate the air to velocity, add 1 to the value in column 11. When dealing with hoods that also contain slots, the acceleration factor is added to either the hood VP or the slot VP, whichever is the higher. Thus, if the slot VP becomes higher, column 12 will include the acceleration factor; otherwise the factor will be added to column 15.

Column 13--The Slot Entry Loss in Inches Water Gauge. The value is obtained by multiplying either column 10 by column 11 or column 10 by column 12. If the slot VP loss is higher than the hood VP loss, then column 12 is used; otherwise, column 11 is used.

Column 14--Hood Entry Loss Factor in Velocity Pressure. The entry loss factor which occurs as air enters the hood.

Column 15--Acceleration Factor. 1 + entry loss factor. Where a slot is also involved, this value is used if the hood velocity pressure is higher than the slot velocity pressure, as is often the case.

Column 16--Hood Entry Loss in Inches Water Gauge. Column 7 x column 15, or column 7 x column 14, depending upon whether the hood velocity pressure or slot velocity pressure is higher.

Column 17--Length in Feet. The length of straight duct in feet.

Column 18--Friction Loss per Hundred Feet in Inches Water Gauge. Obtained directly from friction loss charts for the given size duct at the velocity and rate of flow (Figure 2.3.4) or by the equation:

$$2.74 \ (v/1000)^{1.9}/(D)^{1.22}$$

where v is in fpm and D is in inches.

Column 19--Duct Loss in Inches Water Gauge. Column 17/100 x column 18.

Column 20--Centerline Radius Duct Diameter. The centerline radius stated in the number of duct diameters for elbows in the system.

Column 21--Equivalent Length per 90° Elbow. Obtained directly from friction loss charts for elbows (Figure 2.3.8).

Column 22--Number of 90° Ells. The number of equivalent 90° elbows that are present in the branch or segment of the system (a 45° Ell = .5 x 90° Ells).

Column 23--Equivalent Length in Feet. Column 21 x column 22.

Column 24--Elbow Loss in Inches Water Gauge. Column 18 x column 23.

Column 25--Angle of Entry in Degrees. The branch entry angle in degrees.

Column 26--Equivalent Length per Entry in Feet. Obtain directly from charts indicating losses in equivalent feet for entries of a given duct diameter and angle of entry (Figure 2.3.8).

Column 27--Entry-Loss in Inches of Water Gauge. Column 18 x column 26/100.

Column 28--Miscellaneous Calculations. Any miscellaneous calculations that must be made such as may occur where contractions or expansions occur in the branch under consideration.

Column 29--Total Losses (SP) in Inches Water Gauge. The value is the total of the losses obtained in columns 13, 16, 19, 24, and 27.

Column 30--Cumulative Losses (SP) in Inches Water Gauge. The total of all values in column 29 for a given branch or segment of the system to that point in the system.

Column 31--Governing SP in Inches Water Gauge. The highest resistance or static pressure of a series of branches at the point where the branches meet.

Column 32--Balance Q (cfm). Where it is necessary to balance the system using a recalculated Q (i.e., where the ratio of the static pressures is between 1.05 and 1.20). The calculated Q from the formula,

$$Q_{balance} = Q_{smaller\ static\ pressure} \times \sqrt{SP_{larger}/SP_{smaller}}$$

Example Problem

The example problem presented below illustrates the use of the calculation worksheet.

Problem. Consider a shop layout as presented in Figure 2.12.7. It is desired to design a ventilation system to handle particulates from the 3 grinders operating in the locations shown in the figure. Provide the following:

a.   duct layout
b.   duct sizes
c. SP_f

Assume the duct will be supported two feet below the 15-foot ceiling. The fan must be located in the SE corner on a platform 12 feet high in order that the duct is level on entry to the fan. The fan outlet will penetrate the roof and extend 8 feet. There is an obstruction near the large grinder.

Figure 2.12.7

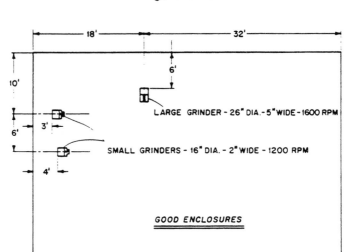

GOOD ENCLOSURES

Solution

In designing the system, the following can be determined:

1. Dimensions determined for layout (Figure 2.12.8) using trigonometric relations to obtain duct lengths. All branch entries at 30° angle.

2. Hoods used for small grinders from VS-411 since speed = 5027 sfm. Surface speed is (πD x rpm).
    For 16" D and 1200 rpm π(16"/12")(1200 rpm) = 5027 sfm.

3. Hood used for large grinders from VS-411.1 since speed = 10,891 sfm.

4. Required cfm and transport velocity.
        Small grinders--390 cfm each and 4500 fpm
        Large grinders--1200 cfm each and 4500 fpm

5. All elbows with 2D radius.

Some Final Comments on the Principles of System Design

When designing an industrial exhaust ventilation system, a multitude of layouts can be used. Experience, and in some cases recalculation using different designs, will provide the system that is most efficient for a given problem. In addition, structural problems in the plant location where the ventilation system must be placed will limit the number of options that may be considered in the design of the system.

Figure 2.12.8

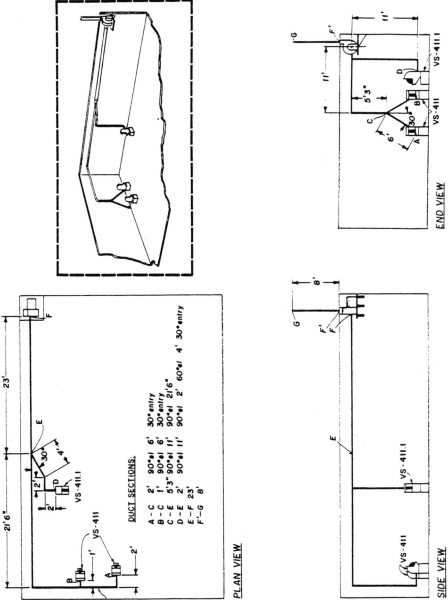

DUCT SECTIONS:

A - C   2'   90°el   6'   30° entry
B - C   1'   90°el   6'   30° entry
C - E   5'3" 90°el 11'   21'6"
D - E   2'   90°el   11'   90°el   2'   60°el   4'   30° entry
E - F   23'
F - G   8'

PLAN VIEW

END VIEW

SIDE VIEW

Figure 2.12.9

Calculation sheet
Static pressure balance--equivalent length method.

Duct number or name	Design Q, cfm	Min. tran. velocity, fpm	Duct diam. inches	Duct area, ft²	Actual duct velocity, fpm	Actual duct velocity press in W.G.	ENTRY LOSSES – SLOTS: Slot area ft²	Slot velocity, fpm	Slot velocity press in W.G.	Slot entry loss factor VP	Accel. factor* (1.0 + col 11)	Slot entry* loss in W.G. (col 10 x col 11) or (col 10 x col 12)	HOODS: Hood entry loss factor, VP	Accel. factor* (1.0 + col 14)	Hood entry* loss in W.G. (col 7 x col 15) or (col 7 x col 14)	DUCT LOSSES: Length, ft	Friction loss per 100 ft in W.G.	Duct loss in W.G. (col 17 x col 18)/100	FITTING LOSSES – ELBOWS: Centerline rad. duct diam.	Equiv. length per 90° elbow	Number of 90° ells	Equiv. lengths, ft	Elbow loss in W.G. (col 18 x col 23)/100	ENTRIES: Angle of entry, deg.	Equiv. length per entry, ft	Entry loss in W.G. (col 18 x col 26)/100	MISCELLANEOUS CALCULATIONS	Total losses (SP) in. W.G. (col 13 + 16 + 19 + 24 + 27)	Cumulative losses (SP) in W.G.	Governing SP in. W.G.	Balanced Q, cfm
1	2	3	4	5	6	7	8	9	10	11	12	13	14	15	16	17	18	19	20	21	22	23	24	25	26	27	28	29	30	31	32
A C	390	4500	4	.0873	4467	1.24							.40	1.40	-1.74	8	8.7	-.70	2	4	1	4	-.35	30	3	-.26		-3.06	-3.06	-3.05	390
B C	390	4500	4	.0873	4467	1.24							.40	1.40	-1.24	7	8.7	-.61	2	4	1	4	-.36	30	3	-.26	-3.05/-2.96 = 1.03	-2.96	-2.96	-3.06	390
	Ignore SP difference in branch B–C since ratio of SP's is less than or equal to 1.05																														
C																														-3.06	780
C E	780	3500	6	.1964	3971	0.98										37.8	4.2	-1.59	2	7	2	14	-.69					-2.18	-6.23		
D E	1200	4500	7	.2673	4489	1.26							.40	1.40	-1.76	19	4.4	-.84	2	9	2.67	24	-1.06	30	6	-.26	-6.23/-3.92 = 1.33	-3.92	-3.92		
	Recalculate branch D–E since ratio of SP's is greater than 1.20																														
D E	1200	4600	6	.1964	6110	2.33							.40	1.40	-3.26	19	9.6	-1.82	2	7	2.67	18.7	-1.80	30	6	-.48	-7.36/-6.23 = 1.41	-7.36	-7.36	-7.36	1200
	Recalculate branch C–E since ratio of SP's is greater than 1.20																														
C E	780	3500	6.5	.1650	4727	1.39										37.8	6.6	-2.46	2	6.5	2	13	-.85				-7.36/-6.36 = 1.18	-3.31	-6.36	-7.36	840
	Calculate balanced branch Q since ratio of SP's is between 1.05 and 1.20																														
	Multiply branch Q with smaller SP by square root of SP ratio																										$Q' = 780\sqrt{1.18} = 840$				
E																														-7.36	2040
E F	2040	3500	10	.5454	3740	0.87										23	2.0	-.46										-.46	-7.82	-7.82	2040
FAN																															
F G	2040	3500	10	.5454	3740	0.87										8	2.0	.16										.16	.16		
	Now, calculate fan SP: $SP_f = SP_o - SP_i - VP_i$ = (.16) − (−7.82) − (.87) = 7.11 in. w.g.																														

NOTE: In many cases, the inlet and outlet diameter of the fan which is selected will differ, requiring that the outlet branch be recalculated for the different diameter. In addition, it may also be necessary to use either an expansion or a contraction to match the inlet duct to the fan inlet size. This case will also necessitate recalculation of the SP for the change in diameter before sizing the actual fan.

*This represents the amount of energy needed to get air to flow into the hood. NOTE: When dealing with hoods that also contain slots, add the acceleration factor to either the hood VP or slot VP, whichever has the higher value (usually the hood VP). This is only added one time, that is, only where air initially enters the duct (e.g., through a hood).

PLANT NAME ______ CALCULATIONS BY ______ ELEVATION Standard: 0 1000 feet

LOCATION ______ CHECKED BY ______ TEMPERATURE Standard: (70 ± 30)°F

DEPARTMENT ______ APPROVED BY ______ DATE ______

Based on Industrial Ventilation, 13th edition, ACGIH, 1974.

In general, small losses which result from dynamic changes in pressures in the system are ignored as in the case where balance is assumed when less than a 5 percent difference between branch static pressures is obtained. However, an exception to this rule exists where the main duct velocity exceeds the higher of the branch velocities. If this is the case and the difference in velocity pressure is great, a correction must be made. This correction is made as follows:

1.   Calculate the VP_r or the resultant velocity pressure which would result from the volumes entering the new branch.

$$(2.12.2) \quad VP_r = [(Q_1 + Q_2)/4005(A_1 + A_2)]^2$$

where
Q_1 = the flow in branch #1
Q_2 = the flow in branch #2
A_1 = the area of branch duct #1
A_2 = the area of branch duct #2

2.   If $VP_m > 1.1 \times VP_r$, then the static pressure is corrected by the formula

$$(2.12.3) \quad SP_m = SP_b - (VP_m - VP_r)$$
where
SP_m = static pressure in main
SP_b = branch static pressure using the highest value after balancing

VP_r = the calculated VP_r from step 1
VP_m = the velocity pressure in the main duct and algebraic values of SP are negative.

Consider the following example:

Figure 2.12.10

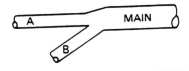

Section	Diam.	Area	Q	V	VP	SP
A	8	.3941	1200	3437	737	-2.40
B	4	.087	310	3563	792	-2.40
Main	8 1/2	.3940	1510	3832	916	- -

Section	Diam.	Area	Q	v	VP	SP
A	8	.3491	1200	3437	.74	-2.40
B	4	.0873	310	3551	.79	-2.40
Main	8	.3491	1510	4325	1.17	--

Since $VP_m > 1.1 \times VP_b$, it may be necessary to determine loss as a result of dynamic change in velocity. Using 2.12.2, we obtain

$$VP_r = [(1200 + 310)/4005(0.3491 + 0.087)]^2$$

$$VP_r = (0.864)^2$$
$$VP_r = 0.75$$

Since $VP_m > 1.1 \times VP_r$, then from 2.12.3, we obtain

$$SP_m = SP_b - (VP_m - VP_r)$$
$$SP_m = -2.40 - (1.17 - 0.75)$$
$$SP_m = -2.82$$

Thus, the corrected SP for the main is -2.82 to account for the dynamic change in VP which occurs.

Velocity Pressure Method of Calculation

The preceding problems were worked using the equivalent foot method of calculation. Another method that can be used and which obtains approximately the same result is the velocity pressure method. Space does not permit the explanation of the velocity pressure method of calculation in this book. However, an example of the velocity pressure method of calculation can be found in the Industrial Ventilation Manual, Section 6.

Summary

The procedure for designing a balanced ventilation system involves the following steps:

1. Determine the branch of greatest resistance; size the duct to obtain the desired flow rate and transport velocity.
2. Calculate all losses for the branch of concern. Include hood losses, acceleration losses, losses at elbows, and losses at branch connections.
3. Total the losses to obtain the static pressure of the branch.
4. If a static pressure value has been obtained for the connecting branches, go to step 5; otherwise, go to step 2 to calculate the other branch.
5. Compare the static pressure ratios for the two branches. If $SP_{larger}/SP_{smaller} \leq 1.05$, assume the system is in balance and go to step 8.

6. If $1.05 < (SP_{larger}/SP_{smaller}) \leq 1.20$, recalculate Q for the branch of least resistance from 2.12.1

   (2.12.1) $Q = Q_{smaller} SP \sqrt{SP_{larger}/SP_{smaller}}$

Use this value as the balanced Q.

7. If $SP_{larger}/SP_{smaller} > 1.20$, the branch with least resistance must be sizedto obtain a higher resistance. Choose a smaller duct size and go to step 2 to recalculate the branch resistance.

8. Choose the highest static pressure value for the two branches and calculate losses for any duct beyond the branch to the next branch point or the fan. Be sure that the connecting duct beyond the branch does not have a VP exceeding 1.1 x the resultant branch VP. If this is the case, a correction to account for this difference must be made using 2.12.2 and 2.12.3.

   (2.12.2) $VP_r = [(Q_1 + Q_2)/4005(A_1 + A_2]^2$

   (2.12.3) $SP_m = SP_b - (VP_m - VP_r)$

9. If another branch point has been reached, go to step 2.

10. Calculate the losses by adding the connecting duct losses to the governing static pressure at the last branch point.

11. Calculate any losses on the opposite side of the fan using the same method as in step 2.

12. Calculate the fan static pressure (SP_f) using 2.10.7.
    (2.10.7) $SP_f = SP_o - SP_i - VP_i$

13. Determine the fan to use from manufacturers' rating tables.

14. If inlet and outlet diameters for the fan differ from the size chosen, it will be necessary to use either expansions or contractions to resize the duct to fit the fan. This will require a recalculation of losses for the change in duct diameter.

15. Determine the fan operating characteristics using the rating table and interpolating as necessary.

13. Ventilation System Design

Introduction

In the previous chapter, the calculations necessary to design a ventilation system were introduced. These calculations provide the designer with the tools necessary to design a properly operating ventilation system. However, having the tools and knowing how to use them does not always result in a well-designed system. For example, the knowledge of electronic computers and computer language does not always result in a system that provides the results desired. How many times have we heard of people receiving incorrect bills or of reports generating unintelligible information for the user. The designer obviously knows how to use the computer and computer languages or else the bad information generated would not result. What is missing from such a situation is the proper design procedures that result in the total system operating as desired. It is to this point that the following is directed.

A Design Procedure for Ventilation Systems

Obviously, the first thing that must occur before a ventilation system design is begun is that a problem must be recognized. Though this is not a part of the system's design procedure, it is the necessary step that initiates action toward the design of a ventilation system. Someone must recognize the need for considering the use of a ventilation system as a control technique for a potential hazard in the workplace. In many cases, the problem will be recognized by someone other than the person who is responsible for the design of ventilation systems. In such cases, the individual recognizing the problem will come to the designer and indicate that a ventilation system is necessary for a given operation or operations. Now the design procedure can begin.

The first step is to gather the information regarding the design problem. Ideally, this information should be transmitted to the designer by the person who recognized the potential hazard. However, such is not normally the case. Thus, it becomes a responsibility of the designer to gather the necessary information.

The designer must obtain a layout of the work area and building showing the locations of existing equipment and ventilation systems. Obviously, the ventilation system to be designed must not interfere with other operations in the building or work area. In addition, it is possible that the new ventilation system may be tied into an existing system close to the problem area.

If existing ventilation systems may be considered for tie-in, the design specifications for these systems must be obtained. This includes the original design for the system, specifications on any air movers and cleaners within the existing system, and the rate of flow, transport velocity, and resistance of the existing system.

Specifications for the production equipment that is used in the problem operation must be obtained. These specifications should include mechanical drawings of the equipment that can be used as a basis for properly designing the exhaust hood. For example, such things as the wheel diameter, width, and revolutions per minute are important when designing an exhaust system for a grinder or polisher.

It is also necessary to determine the characteristics of the contaminant that is to be removed. Is it particulate, gas, or vapor? Is the carrier gas temperature or humidity significantly different from standard conditions? What is the toxicity or threshold limit value of the contaminant being handled and at what rate is the contaminant being generated? The above information will play an important role in calculating the necessary rate of flow, the required transport velocity, the need for air-cleaning devices, and any precautions that must be taken concerning maintenance and failure of the equipment.

It is also necessary to obtain information concerning the workers who are exposed to the potential hazard. Area work schedules are important; in addition, the methods and procedures used by the workers must be considered when designing the exhaust system and hood to assure that the ventilation system does not interfere with the workers' production.

After information concerning the problem has been gathered, the designer should <u>determine the general method</u> that will be used to control the contaminant. The designer has two major alternatives that can be used; <u>local exhaust</u> ventilation and <u>dilution</u> ventilation. It is important that each of these methods be investigated to assure that the appropriate approach is used. Often the designer may jump to the conclusion that a local exhaust system is necessary when a dilution system may provide equal results at a significantly lower installation cost. There is obviously a trade-off between the two systems. Though the installation cost of a local exhaust system is generally higher than that of a dilution system, the air-moving device must be larger for the dilution system and, as a result, will be more expensive. In addition, the dilution system will require a larger volume of make-up air that in many cases must be tempered, thus increasing the overall operating cost of the system.

The next step is to determine if an <u>air cleaner</u> is required and, if so, what <u>air-cleaning method</u> should be used. The various methods for cleaning air were presented in chapter 9. Not all methods are equally applicable for a given problem. Some methods work best with certain sizes of particulate matter, while others are more appropriately used when a gas or vapor is present. In addition, the various air-cleaning methods have different characteristics of operation. Resistance loss can vary widely between methods of cleaning, thus resulting in the necessity for more powerful air movers as the resistance increases. This adds to the cost of the system. The method for removing waste from the air cleaner is also important since it may result in down time that can be translated into a cost associated with the loss of production.

The next step that must be performed is to draw a line sketch of the layout showing the ductwork, fan, and cleaner. Both a plan and elevation view of the proposed system should be prepared. At this point the designer will have to consider existing equipment within the area as well as any obstructions such as columns, pipes, walls, and other ventilation ducts. Once the line sketch has been drawn, the appropriate measurements can be made to determine the lengths of duct that will be necessary for each section of the system.

Now the designer should consider the hood design that is to be used for the operation in question. Information gathered concerning work procedures, characteristics of the contaminant, process-induced motion of the contaminant, and other restrictions related to the production method itself must be considered in the design of the hood. It is important to determine if an existing hood can be used. This can save significant time on the part of the designer and is likely to result in a properly operating system. However, the situation may require a new hood design. If so, it will be necessary to test the design of the hood after construction to assure that the proper capture velocity and hood loss are being obtained. This may require that a prototype hood be constructed and installed before the rest of the ventilation system is completed.

Now the designer is ready to perform the calculations that are necessary to design the system. As has been mentioned, there are two primary calculation methods that are available: the equivalent-foot method and the velocity pressure method. The method used by the designer will not affect the overall design as each method results in basically the same product. The designer also has a choice of design methods that can be used. These methods are the balance system design, the blast-gate system design, and the plenum system design. The characteristics and advantages/disadvantages of each of these methods will be discussed later in this chapter.

After the system has been designed and the resistance known, it is necessary to select the type, size, and operating criteria for the air mover to be used. Fan selection involves more than determining the brake horsepower and RPM for a given size fan. Certain types of fans are better when handling particulate matter while others are better for handling gases and vapors. The designer must be sure that the appropriate type fan is specified.

Before moving ahead, the designer should check the calculations that have been made in the design and compare alternative designs to determine the design that results in the lowest cost. The layout can be modified to produce a different design that may result in a lower installation or operating cost. It is desirable that the designer consider the various alternative designs that are available and compare these alternatives in terms of both installation cost and operating cost before choosing the actual design to be implemented. Though the calculations may seem tedious and the time spent long, remember that once the system is installed, it will be very expensive to modify it.

After the appropriate design has been selected, <u>detailed shop drawings and specifications must be prepared</u> for the construction and installation of the system. As was mentioned in chapter 11, there are various duct characteristics which the design should reflect in order to provide for optimum operation. These characteristics should be specified by the designer in order to insure proper construction and installation of the system.

After the system has been installed, <u>testing of the system</u> should be conducted to determine if it is operating to specification. Periodically, after initial testing, further tests should be made and compared to the design calculation to assure that nothing has happened that affects the overall operation of the system. The subject of system testing will be discussed in a later section of this book.

Types of Ventilation System Design

There are three major types of designs for ventilation systems: the balanced-system design, the blast-gate design, and the plenum design. The characteristics of each of these designs will be discussed and the relative advantages and disadvantages of each will be presented in the following discussion.

The <u>balanced-system design</u> is the design that results from balancing all the branches to equivalent resistance levels. This is the method that has been used in working previous problems. In the balance system design, small variations in resistance between branches are ignored. A natural balance occurs to overcome the small variations; but the change in rate of flow which results from this natural balance is not significant enough to affect the designed operation of the system.

The second method of design, the <u>blast-gate design</u>, involves using blast gates within the branches to adjust the flow of the system after installation. Calculations are performed in the same manner as with the balance system design. However, when branches result in differences in resistance, no attempt is made to balance these by changing the duct size or varying the rate of flow. In order to obtain actual operating balance, a gate is indicated to be installed in the branch of least resistance. The air flow into the next section of the system is determined by combining the design air flow for each of the branches.

The blast-gate system design saves time and calculations, since it is not necessary to recalculate branches where a lower resistance has been obtained. Care must be taken to begin calculations with the highest resistance branches. This can present some problems, since the choice is not always obvious. A wrong choice will result in a poorly operating system. The safest method is to calculate all branches to be sure the branch with the greatest resistance is chosen. The system is balanced after installation by adjusting the gate to obtain the proper flow through each exhaust opening.

The third method of design is the <u>plenum design</u>. In the plenum design, branch ducts connect to a large plenum type duct. Minimum transport velocity must be maintained in the branches. However, a lower velocity and resistance are usually present within the plenum. The branches are balanced either by design or by blast-gate method to the branch of the greatest resistance. The plenum acts as a settling chamber for large particles. As such, it becomes necessary to provide some method for cleanout of particulate matter which gathers in the plenum. A manual drag chain or belt conveyor can be used.

Figure 2.13.1

Plenum design.

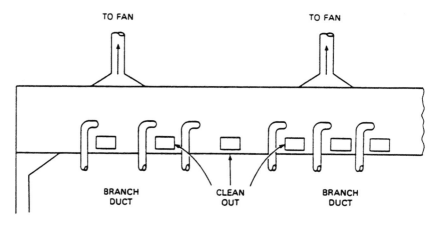

A plenum allows for duct sections to be added or deleted from the operation without materially affecting the overall result obtained. Thus, the plenum design provides a flexible design that can meet the needs of a growing plant or can be used where plant operations are intermittent.

Advantages and Disadvantages of the Three Methods of Design

The balanced-system design has a number of advantages.
Advantages of balanced-system design:

1.   The calculation results in the optimum design for a given individual operation or operations.
2.   This design assures constant operation at the proper volumes and velocities.
3.   No unusual accumulation of contaminant occurs within the duct system.
4.   This is the best method to use for highly toxic materials since it can result in complete removal of the toxic materials from the workplace and the duct system.

On the other hand, the balanced-system design has certain disadvantages.
Disadvantages of balanced-system design:

1.   The balanced system results in a somewhat inflexible system for future additions.

2. The choice of incorrect exhaust volume will result in improper operation and the possibility of major modifications to assure proper ventilation.
3. Balancing may require that higher air volumes be handled than with other methods, thus resulting in a higher operating cost.
4. Care must be taken in laying out the system to be sure that it is exact since differences in length of duct will result in differences of resistance.

There are several advantages to using the blast-gate design.
Advantages of blast-gate design:

1. The system that has been designed is relatively flexible for future additions since gates can be removed or changed.
2. An incorrect choice of exhaust volume can be corrected more easily within a certain range.
3. System balance is obtained within the prescribed design volumes, thus resulting in a lower operating cost than the balance system design.
4. Variation in duct layout can occur within limits since changes in resistance can be controlled by the blast gates.

On the other hand, this method does present certain disadvantages.
Disadvantages of the blast-gate design:

1. Blast gates present an obstruction within the duct system which can yield a buildup of contaminant.
2. The setting of the gates can be changed by personnel, thus causing the system to operate improperly.
3. An error in the choice of the branch of least resistance is serious and will result in improper operation of the system.
4. Turbulence is significant at gates.

The plenum system design has several advantages.
Advantages of plenum system design:

1. The plenum system is flexible, and additions to the system can be made with very little problems.
2. Branches of the plenum system can be closed off and the system will operate effectively. This allows for intermittent operations to be shut down for maintenance.
3. The plenum acts as a settling chamber which will remove large particles of dust, thus lowering the requirements upon an air cleaner.

The plenum system design does have some disadvantages.
Disadvantages of plenum system design:

1. The plenum can clog if sticky or linty materials are being handled in the system.
2. A plenum is not recommended for handling explosive materials since an explosive buildup can occur within the plenum as a result of settling.
3. A buildup of toxic materials which may have settled in the plenum can result in hazard during maintenance and cleanout.
4. The mechanism used to clean out the plenum is expensive.

5.   The overall installation of the plenum is more expensive than either of the other design methods.

Other Design Considerations

Transport Velocity. The concept of transport velocity has been discussed previously. However, it is of sufficient importance that it should be mentioned again. The minimum transport velocity is important to prevent settling of particles within the duct. Except for the plenum design, where such settling is expected and for which provision has been made, the settling of particles in a duct can cause clogging which will materially affect the operation of the system. In addition, if the materials are toxic, the removal of these materials from the duct becomes hazardous to the health of the maintenance workers involved in cleaning the ducts. Thus, it is important that a minimum transport velocity be maintained within the system. The reader will remember that this minimum transport velocity affects only the large particles since small particles follow the air movement and do not settle.

In some cases, a sloped duct is installed. If the slope of this duct is greater than 60 degrees, settling can be avoided regardless of the transport velocity of the system. The sloped duct will require a lower transport velocity, and thus the cost of installation and operation will be significantly lower. Where possible, such an approach should be used. However, it is important that cleanouts be present to remove the particulate matter which has been gathered.

Fire and Explosion Hazards. A ventilation system provides a clear pathway through which fire can spread within a building. In addition, the ventilation system can be a source for explosion and fire if the materials being exhausted are of an explosive or flammable nature. A number of steps should be taken to assure that the potential fire explosion hazard is controlled. Among these steps are:

1.   Some ventilation systems handle materials such as metal shavings which are capable of producing sparks as they pass through the ventilation system. Such systems should be separated from ventilation systems that handle combustible materials.
2.   In order to avoid generation of sparks, the system should allow for settling of large metallic particles near the source of exhaust.
3.   Where possible, ducts should not run through fire walls.
4.   Automatic fire dampers should be installed within the duct on both sides of any walls through which the duct passes.
5.   Duct joints and seams should be riveted. Solder does not provide the structural strength necessary to withstand an explosion within the system and may melt in the presence of a fire inside the duct.
6.   A clearance should be allowed between exhaust ducts and the walls, ceiling, and floors of the building to prevent the spread of fire should an explosion occur within the duct system.
7.   Fans, ducts, and cleaners should be grounded to prevent a static electricity buildup.
8.   Whenever a fine dust is being handled, it should be assumed to be explosive unless it is definitely known to be otherwise.

9. Locate cleaners for explosive contaminants in isolated places since a buildup will occur within the cleaner, and the potential for fire and explosion exists.
10. The use of nonsparking, nonmetallic blade fans when handling explosive contaminants is recommended.
11. Air cleaners and collectors should be vented for explosion if explosive contaminants are being handled.
12. Fan motors should be outside the actual duct.
13. Fire detection devices should be present in the duct. These devices may be connected to automatic shutdown and sprinkler systems in the duct.

Make-up Air. The subject of make-up air was discussed extensively in a previous chapter. However, it is important that it be mentioned again since the absence of make-up air can cause improper operation of the system. Whenever a system exhausts large volumes of air, a make-up system must be present to provide air at the source in order to maintain a positive pressure outside the exhaust system. Without adequate make-up air, the local exhaust system will work hard, but it will not operate at the design volume. Often problems encountered in the operation of a ventilation system result from an inadequate make-up air supply.

Maintenance. All mechanical systems, including a ventilation system, must be maintained. As a result, provision should be made for such maintenance. Cleanouts should be located in accessible areas to minimize the potential for accident or injury to the maintenance worker. In addition, if the cleanouts are in relatively inaccessible areas, the probability that a buildup will occur before cleaning will be enhanced. In addition, fans, motors, and air cleaners should also be located in accessible areas.

The system design should provide adequate protection to the maintenance worker from the hazardous effects of toxic materials that can settle in the system. It is foolhardy to design a system that removes the hazard from the workers in the production area at the expense of presenting a hazard to workers who are required to maintain the system.

It is important to keep a preventive maintenance schedule for the air-moving and air-cleaning equipment. This will assure that the system is maintained in proper operating condition and will do the job for which it was designed.

Noise. Noise within a ventilation system is generated by the fan, the air cleaner, and the high-volume and high-velocity air within the duct. Often this noise level can become a significant contributor to the overall noise level within the workplace.

The location and mounting of the fan and air cleaner should be considered, since this provides a potential noise hazard to the workers in the immediate area. In addition, the ducts themselves can be located away from the workers. Where noise levels exceed those which are desirable, the ducts can be lined with an acoustical absorbing material. It should be remembered by the designer that certain types of fans are less noisy and thus may be preferable for a given installation (e.g., backward curve blade, centrifugal fan). Where additional noise reduction is necessary, commercial silencers are available.

Summary

The designer of a ventilation system has essentially three methods that can be utilized to design the system. These methods are the

1. balanced-system design
2. blast-gate design
3. plenum design

In general, where a system is designed to remove toxic materials, the balanced system design is preferred. When additions and changes to an existing system are necessary, the blast gate design is used. In cases where significant growth is expected or when intermittent operations are attached to the system, the plenum design will be best.

When designing a ventilation system, the designer must approach the problem logically. This involves the following general steps:

1. Gather information to describe the problem and constraints.
2. Determine the design method to be used.
3. Select air cleaner to be used.
4. Lay out system.
5. Design hoods required.
6. Perform design calculations.
7. Select and size air mover.
8. Check calculations and compare alternatives.
9. Prepare detailed shop drawings and install system.
10. Perform checkout of system.

14. Recirculation of Exhaust Air

In order for a local exhaust system to operate according to specification, make-up air must be supplied to the work area to replace that air which has been exhausted. Air that is removed through the exhaust system contains a contaminant that is being removed to protect the workers' health. But this air also contains heat that has been provided in the workplace to assure the workers' comfort. When make-up air is supplied to replace the air removed, it must be heated to maintain a constant temperature within the workplace and to avoid drafts on the workers.

Energy is required to heat make-up air. If a large volume of air is exhausted from the workplace, then a large volume of make-up air must be supplied. If the make-up air must be tempered, a significant amount of energy will be consumed during the tempering process. In the past, energy has been readily available and low in cost; thus, little consideration was given to the cost and consumption of energy necessary to temper the incoming make-up air. However, the situation has drastically changed. Energy is in short supply, and its cost has become a major factor. Consideration must now be given to methods to reduce the consumption of energy necessary for tempering incoming make-up air.

One possible solution to this problem is the recirculation of exhaust air. In a recirculation system, exhaust air that is removed from the process is cleaned and recycled back to the workplace. This reduces the energy needed for tempering cold incoming air, since the recycled air contains the heat that was present in the workplace when it was removed. Thus, a lowering in the cost of energy is realized. An additional benefit is obtained from the lowering of the capacity requirements for the plant heating system.

Problems Relating to Recirculation

Though the benefits obtained by recirculating exhaust air can be great, the method is not a simple one, and it is not without problems. The air quality of the recirculated air must be such that the worker is not exposed to a potential health hazard. The air that has been exhausted contains contaminants. Before returning this air to the workplace, the contaminants must be removed.

Certain guidelines for the air quality of incoming recirculated air have been developed. One generally accepted guideline that is used by many health agencies at the state level is that the return air shall have a concentration of the contaminant $\leq$ 10 percent of the TLV for the given contaminant. This

273

guideline is subject to some interpretation. In some cases, it is assumed that the 10 percent level shall be maintained at the exhaust of the air cleaner prior to re-entry to the workplace; while in other situations, the 10 percent is assumed to be within the work area itself. Obviously, this results in a discrepancy concerning the quality of air that may be recirculated into the workplace.

The Industrial Ventilation Manual presents a formula that can be used to calculate the permissible concentration of the contaminant in recirculated air under equilibrium conditions. This formula is as follows:

$$C_r = (1/2)(TLV - C_o) \frac{Q_t}{Q_r} \times \frac{1}{K}$$

where

C_r = the concentration of contaminant in the <u>exit air from the collector</u> before mixing

Q_t = the total ventilation flow in the affected work space (cfm)

Q_r = the recirculation air flow (cfm)

K = the mixing effectiveness factor, usually from 3 to 10 where 3 is good mixing

TLV = the threshold limit value of the contaminant

C_o = the concentration of the contaminant in the worker's breathing zone without recirculation of exhaust

NOTE: In recirculating air containing a nuisance or inert contaminant, the factor in the above formula changes from 1/2 to 0.9.

As can be seen from the above formula, the basis for calculating the permissible concentration is at the exit of the air cleaner itself. The K factor for mixing of contaminant within the workroom air is then used. The specification of a K factor is somewhat arbitrary; and though it presents a safety factor, the value that should be used in a given situation is difficult to determine. In addition, the formula can best be applied after the recirculating system has been designed and built, since much of the information necessary is not available at the design stage. This fact presents a problem when using this approach.

Obtaining Clean Air to be Recirculated. The efficiency of any air cleaner in a recirculation system must be such that respirable particles or harmful gases or vapors are removed before the air re-enters the workroom. In addition, the cleaner must provide that the failure rate and down time for cleaning are minimal since, without additional precautions being taken, down time on the cleaner means down time in the production operation. This problem has been approached by specification of redundant air cleaners or a provision for bypass to the outside environment when a failure occurs. However, each of these methods results in a higher cost for installation of the system.

Necessity to Monitor Incoming Recirculated Air. If air is being recirculated back into the workplace, some method must be available to determine if the recirculated air is clean. In many cases, monitoring equipment that is specific to the particular contaminant involved is not available to provide continuous monitoring of the recirculated air. In addition, the cost of monitoring equipment is high. Certain difficulties result when determining where the monitoring equipment should be placed. As previously discussed, should the monitoring occur at the exit of the air cleaner, or should it occur within the worker's breathing zone? Also, standardized measurement techniques are not always available for a given contaminant.

The monitoring that does occur must occur on a real-time basis since to determine that an exposure has occurred after the fact does not provide adequate protection to the worker. Monitoring methods for particulate concentration on a continuous basis are currently feasible. In addition, hydrocarbon monitors are also available. If these nonspecific methods can be used to monitor in real time for contaminants lacking specific monitoring methods and if it is known that the exhaust air contains certain materials, then it is possible that adequate protection can be provided for the worker.

Contaminants Not to be Recirculated. Guidelines have been presented for certain contaminants that are not to be recirculated. For example, in a research report to NIOSH entitled "Recirculation of Exhaust Air," published in 1976, a list of contaminants that are not to be recirculated is presented. This list stated that those contaminants which

1. are carcinogenic,
2. have a maximum allowable concentration (MAC), or
3. produce neoplastic (tumor-producing) or systemic effects within permissible excursions

should not be recirculated.

Some controversy, however, may be generated if these guidelines are to be taken as fact. For example, a compound may be carcinogenic in large quantities or over a very long exposure. However, a short time excursion may not result in any particular hazard to the worker. On the other hand, certain noncarcinogenic compounds may present a hazard with a short exposure (for example, some of the halogenated hydrocarbons that can result in narcosis of the worker and increase the potential for an accident occurring).

The guidelines do indicate where extreme caution should be used in considering the recirculation of exhaust air containing contaminants falling within the classifications listed. However, this does not say that caution should not be exercised when considering certain other contaminants. Perhaps the best rule of thumb to use when considering recirculation of exhaust air is to consider each situation as presenting a danger to the worker should the air-cleaning equipment fail.

An Approach to Recirculation

The first major component that is present in a recirculation system is an air cleaner. The efficiency of the air cleaner must be adequate to remove the contaminant from the air to obtain the desirable concentration in the exit air from the cleaner. The cost of operation and maintenance of the equipment must be such that the savings generated justify the use of the air cleaner. For example, a combustion unit for cleaning air containing a given gas may use more energy than is saved through recirculation of the air back to the workplace.

The second major component of a recirculation system is a method with which to provide for fail-safe operation. Failure of the air cleaner results in a return of the contaminant to the workplace. Redundant air cleaners can be employed to protect against failure of one air cleaner and return of the contaminant to the workplace. (See Figure 2.14.1.) Another method is to monitor the air exiting the cleaner in order to provide for a warning when a failure in the air cleaner is indicated. (See Figure 2.14.2.) When such a failure occurs, the operation can be shut down, thus preventing further generation of the contaminant. If immediate shutdown of the operation is not desirable, or if such a shutdown results in a high cost, the system can be designed with a bypass to the outside environment. When the monitor senses a failure of the air cleaner, a damper can automatically switch the exhausted air and discharge it outside the plant. When this situation takes place, provision should be made for additional make-up air to enter the workplace to assure that the exhaust system operates properly in removing the contaminant at the source. One potential safeguard that can help to provide for fail-safe operation is adequate maintenance of equipment within the system. A preventive maintenance program should be instituted on any equipment present within the recirculation system.

The need for a fail-safe operation is a controversial subject. One could argue that the failure of the primary exhaust system results in a concentration of buildup of essentially the same magnitude as that which occurs during a failure of the recirculation system. Yet, no provision beyond shutdown of the operation is made for the failure of the primary exhaust system.   However, the other side of this controversy is that a failure of the recirculation system is not as evident as a failure of the primary exhaust system. Thus, the failure of air cleaners to adequately remove the contaminant may not be obvious and, as a result, may require precautions above and beyond those that are present to protect the worker in case of a primary exhaust system failure.

Some General Considerations in Designing a Recirculation System. General dilution ventilation should be provided in addition to that provided by recirculated air. This general dilution ventilation will further dilute the contaminant that is being introduced by the recirculation system. Thus, a safeguard will be present. In addition, the general dilution system can provide make-up air in place of that which has been lost when a failure of the recirculation system causes the exhausted air to be directed outside the plant.

The design should assure that methods for cleaning the air of all hazardous contaminants are provided. Even though a particulate contaminant may be present in the air and this contaminant is adequately removed, one must also consider the possibility that a gas or vapor is also present and must be removed before re-entry of the exhausted air. A complete analysis of the

Figure 2.14.1

Physical recirculation model for Case I:
redundant air cleaners.

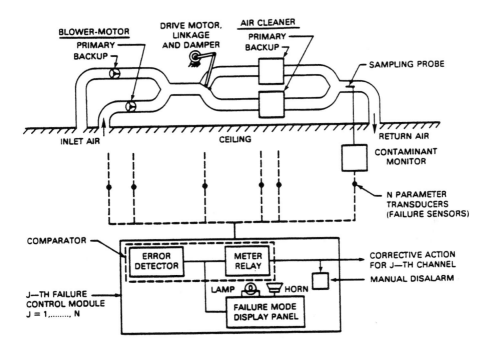

contaminated air should be made before designing and building a recirculation
system.

One safety precaution that can result in a lower potential for shutdown is
to recirculate exhaust air only when it is necessary to conserve energy. If
the air contains heat, it is desirable that the bypass be used during the
summer months since the additional heat is not required within the work area.

If a wet collector is being used to remove the contaminant from the air,
the excess humidity that may be present in the recirculated air must be
considered. The designer must make provision to remove this humidity from the
air before it is recirculated, since this excess humidity can cause worker
discomfort and also can cause condensation on equipment, resulting in damage.

Odors and nuisance contaminants should also be considered before
recirculating exhaust air. Though these may present no potential danger to
the worker, worker complaints and morale may be affected by recirculating air
containing noxious odors and other nuisance contaminants. These should be
removed before recirculating.

Figure 2.14.2

Physical recirculation model for Case II:
air cleaning with bypass.

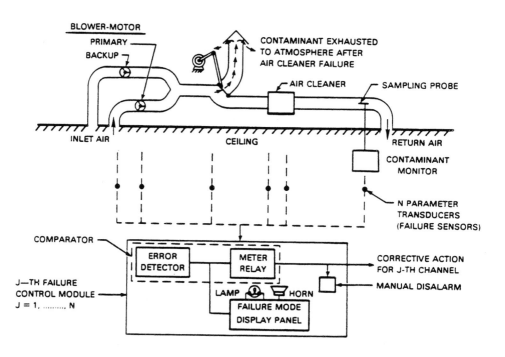

Provision for maintenance schedules on the recirculation equipment should be made. Assurance must also be made that these maintenance schedules are kept in order to provide continuous operation of the system.

The workroom air and the workers' breathing zone should be tested periodically to assure that all is working as planned. Quite often monitoring equipment is the least reliable link in the chain, and, as a result, this equipment should be checked periodically.

Other Alternatives to Conserve Energy Usage

The objective of recirculating air is to reduce the energy usage necessary for tempering make-up air. Other alternatives to recirculation of exhaust air exist. These alternatives should be considered before embarking on a recirculation design.

One obvious way to reduce energy costs is to reduce the need for tempered make-up air. The workplace should be surveyed to determine if the air volumes being exhausted are necessary. Can a lower volume of air be exhausted to obtain the desired results? Can push-pull ventilation lower the required volume exhausted? Can a slot hood be used to obtain a lower volume, high-velocity system? Can a local exhaust system replace a general dilution system which requires that large volumes of air be exhausted from the workplace? Can an enclosure or partial enclosure be used to reduce the air exhaust volume requirements at the source?

Another question that might be asked concerning the need for tempered air is whether the plant or process needs to be operated at the temperature being provided. Can a lower temperature within the work area be tolerated without detrimental effect to the production? Perhaps the workers can dress more warmly, thus requiring less heated air to be supplied to the workplace.

In certain situations, it may be possible to provide untempered make-up air to be used at the source of the exhaust, away from the worker. In this manner, the tempered air within the working area will not be removed in large volumes. Such a system would result in a push-pull type ventilation system such as is used over open surface tanks.

Another alternative that might be considered in reducing the energy costs is to recirculate the tempered exhaust air to locations where workers are not present. Thus, the hazard resulting from a failure of cleaning equipment will not be a problem. Such a system might recirculate heated exhaust air to drying ovens or be used to preheat parts before entering a process.

If it is not possible to recirculate the air through the work area, it may be possible to reclaim the heat from the exhausted air and to use this heat to temper the incoming make-up air. Heat exchangers of the coil type or rotating cylinder type might be used to heat the incoming air, using the heat present within the exhausted air. Another potential method is to parallel incoming and exhaust air ducts so that the duct wall acts as a heat exchange unit. Process generated heat might also be used to temper incoming make-up air.

Heat exchange itself generally results in losses and, thus, is less efficient than direct recirculation. However, it may be the best and cheapest alternative for a given situation.

Table 2.14.1

Alternatives to recirculation.

---

1. Reduce volume of air exhausted.
2. Lower temperature in workplace.
3. Provide untempered make-up air at the source.
4. Recirculate to unmanned areas.
5. Reclaim heat from exhaust area.

There are two other possibilities that may not be quite as obvious. One is to recycle hot water away from the cooling tower and pass it through coils in the incoming duct, thus obtaining both a cooling effect on the water and transferring the heat from the water to the incoming air. The second method is to use the heat generated from a combustion-type cleaner to heat the incoming air through the use of a heat exchanger.

Summary

The cost and availability of energy demand that energy conservation methods be considered. Recirculation of heated exhaust air can result in energy savings. In general, to obtain recirculation, it is necessary to identify the process exhausts that are recirculable, develop a system that adequately cleans the air to remove the contaminants, and establish a procedure to overcome failures and the resultant recirculation of contaminants. Much research is necessary before definite statements can be made concerning when and how best recirculation can be used.

Other alternatives should also be considered to conserve energy. These alternatives include such things as reduction of the air exhausted from the workplace, recycling of heat from exhausted air, lowering the temperature of make-up air required, and using process heat to temper make-up air.

Recirculation is currently a controversial subject. However, with increasing energy costs and diminishing energy supplies, recirculation may be used more in the future. As recirculation becomes more common, many of the problems that currently exist will be solved.

15. Correcting for Nonstandard Conditions

Standard Versus Nonstandard Conditions

Standard conditions for ventilation design are a temperature of 70°F and an atmospheric pressure of 14.7 pounds per square inch. These standard conditions are different than those that are presently used for industrial hygiene and chemistry work (i.e., 77°F and 20°C).

In the previous design problems, charts have been used that assume that standard air is being moved through the system. These charts are not applicable to nonstandard conditions without correction. The effect of heat, pressure, and moisture in the air will change the values that are obtained from these charts.

If heat is added to the air, the molecules become more active, and the heated air expands. This relationship is stated by Charles' Law. On the other hand, as the pressure increases, the volume decreases as presented in Boyle's Law.

These two laws have been combined to form the Perfect Gas law which is stated as

$$PV = WRT \quad (2.1.7)$$

where
- P = absolute pressure in pounds per square foot
- V = the total volume of gas in cubic feet
- W = the total mass of the gas in pounds
- R = the gas constant which has a value of 53.4 for air
- T = absolute temperature in °R (for temperatures in Fahrenheit (460 + F))

When humidity (water vapor) is present in the air, the partial pressures of the air and humidity together make up the total atmospheric pressure. The moisture content within the air exerts a partial pressure while the air itself exerts a partial pressure. The sum of these two partial pressures becomes the atmospheric pressure which is present for the mixture. Water vapor is then treated as a gas.

Need for Correction

Some generally accepted rules have been developed to determine when correction for temperature, pressure, and moisture content are necessary. In general, standard conditions are assumed when

1. the temperature range is between 40°F and 100°F.
2. the pressure range is equivalent to an altitude range of -1000 feet
    to +1000 feet.
3. moisture content is considered standard if the air temperature is
    less than 100°F. If the air temperature is greater than 100°F and
    the moisture content is greater than 0.02 pounds of water per pound
    of dry air, correction is required for the moisture in the air.

Corrections are made because of the effect which these factors have on the
volume of air being handled in a ventilation system. The volume of air itself
remains the same regardless of the density. The weight of air moved within a
ventilation system will be different and is a function of density. The
pressure developed in the system will differ; and the horsepower used, as well
as the rpm's at which a fan operates, will differ varying with the pressure
developed within the system. The simplest way to illustrate these varying
effects is to solve a problem involving nonstandard conditions.

Example Problem

A detergent manufacturer has a spray-drying operation that is used to
transform liquid droplets to detergent flakes. The operation involves the
upward flow of heated air at a temperature of 400°F dry bulb at a rate of
12,000 cfm. The droplets are sprayed downward through the upward flowing air,
and the dried flakes collect at the bottom for further processing. An exhaust
ventilation system is to be connected to the dryer to remove the moist, hot
air that also contains particles of the detergent. It is determined that a
high-efficiency centrifugal cleaner will be used to reclaim the particles that
are exhausted, followed by a wet scrubber for final cleaning. The following
presents a schematic of the required setup:

Detergent drying.

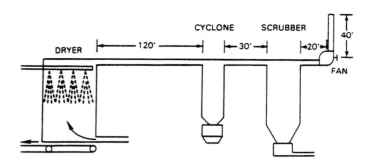

Given

Moisture removed--150 pounds/minute in dryer
At exit of wet scrubber, air is 90% saturated

Pressure drop--0.4 inches wg for dryer,
            8 inches wg for centrifugal cleaner, and
            15 inches wg for wet scrubber
Hood loss = 1.5 VP at entry to duct

Problem

Size duct and fan for the ventilation of the process, considering the effect of temperature and humidity.

Solution

1. To determine actual volume exhausted from spray dryer. Air exhausted contains moisture that must be considered because of the weight of the moisture and partial pressure exerted by the water vapor.

    ### Moisture exhausted

    150 lbs/minute of H_2O

    ### Dry air exhausted at standard conditions

    12,000 cfm at 400°F
    12,000 cfm x 0.075 lb/ft^3 = 900 pounds/minute dry air
                                        exhausted at standard conditions

    ### Water/pound dry air

    $$\frac{lbs\ H_2O}{lb\ dry\ air} = \frac{150\ lbs\ H_2O/min}{900\ lbs\ dry\ air/min} = 0.167\ lbs\ water/lb\ dry\ air$$

    To determine the characteristics of the air/water mixture, consult Psychrometric Chart for 400°F and 0.167 lbs H_2O.

    Dew Point = 142°F
    Wet bulb temperature = 153°F
    Humid volume = 27 ft^3/lb dry air
    Density factor = 0.57
    Enthalpy = 300 BTU/lb dry air

    ### To find actual volume of air/water mixture to be exhausted:

    Volume$_{actual}$ = Humid vol x weight of dry air/minute
                = 27 ft^3/lb dry air x 900 lbs dry air/minute
                = 24,300 cfm

2. Calculate resistance and hood loss from dryer to cyclone.

    ### Duct Size

    Assume minimum transport velocity to be 4500 fpm

$$A = \frac{Q}{v} = \frac{24{,}000}{4{,}500} = 5.4 \ ft^2$$

Using 32 inch duct (area 5.585 ft^2)

$$v = \frac{Q}{A} = \frac{24{,}300}{5.585} = 4351 \ fpm$$

Correcting for density to obtain VP:

$$v = 1096.2 \ \sqrt{VP/\rho} \quad (2.3.1)$$

where ρ = 0.075 x density factor = 0.075 (0.57)

VP = 0.67 inches wg

Hood Loss

Since H_e is given as 1.5 VP, the hood loss (corrected for density) is obtained from:

$$Loss_H = h_e \ x \ d$$
$$= 1.5 \ x \ 0.67 \ x \ 0.57$$
$$Loss = 0.57 \ inches \ wg$$

Acceleration Factor

One VP = 0.67 inches wg

Friction Loss--Dryer to cyclone

0.65 inches wg/100 ft x 120 ft x 0.57 = 0.44 inches wg

3. Calculate resistance within cyclone.

Cyclone Loss

8 inches wg at standard x 0.57 = 4.56 inches wg

4. Calculate resistance between cyclone and wet scrubber.

0.65/100 ft x 30 ft x 0.57 = 0.11 inches wg

5. Calculate air/water mixture at exit of scrubber.

At the point the air leaves the wet scrubber, it has a different set of characteristics than were previously calculated. This is because of the humidifying effect upon the air that occurs as the air passes through the wet scrubber.

"An important characteristic of wet collectors is their ability to humidify a gas stream. The humidification process is generally assumed to be adiabatic or without gain or loss of heat to the surroundings. Therefore, water vapor is added to the mixture, but

the enthalpy, BTU/lb dry air, remains unchanged. During the
humidification process, the point on the Psychrometric Chart that
describes the mixture moves to the left, along a line of constant
enthalpy, toward saturation where no more water vapor can be added.

"All wet collectors do not have the same ability to humidify. If a
wet collector is capable of taking an air stream to complete adiabatic saturation, it is said to have a humidifying efficiency of
100%. The efficiency of a given device to humidify may be expressed by

$$\text{Humidifying efficiency \% } = \frac{(t_i - t_o)}{(t_i - t_s)} \times 100$$

where

t_i = dry bulb temperature at inlet
t_o = dry bulb temperature at outlet
t_s = adiabatic saturation temperature

(Industrial Ventilation Manual, ACGIH, 1974, page 6-16)

To describe the characteristics of the air at the outlet of the scrubber,
the above formula is used to calculate the temperature.

$$0.90 = \frac{(400 - t_o)}{(400 - 153)}$$

$t_o = 178°F$

Since in previous reference to Psychometric Chart
        Enthalpy = 300 BTU/pound
and enthalpy remains constant, reading the Psychrometric Chart for the
characteristics of the new mixture yields

Dew point 151°F
Wet bulb temperature = 153°F
Humid volume = 21.8 ft^3/pound
Enthalpy = 300 BTU/pound dry air
Density factor = 0.74

Resistance loss for the scrubber is assumed to be 15 inches wg since
specifications of the manufacturer will include the effect of
humidification on the pressure loss.

Exhaust volume at collector outlet

Q = humid volume x weight dry air/min
Q = 21.8 ft^3/lb x 900 lbs/minute
Q = 19,620 cfm

6. Calculate losses between collector and fan

0.44 inches wg/100 ft x 20 ft x 0.74 = 0.07 inches wg

7. Fan

Generally, if static pressure losses are less than 20 inches wg, the effect of the lower pressure in the duct as compared to atmospheric pressure is ignored. However, if pressure decreases significantly below atmospheric pressure, the air within the duct will expand. If this effect is not considered when sizing the fan, the volume of air handled will not be sufficient.

Since the static pressure losses to point of fan = 21.42 inches wg (the total of the losses from entry to the fan), it will be necessary to make this correction.

To correct for low pressure using Boyle's Law (2.1.5)

$$\frac{P_1}{P_2} = \frac{V_2}{V_1}$$

Standard atmospheric pressure = 407 inches wg

$$\frac{407 \text{ inches wg}}{(407 - 21.42) \text{ inches wg}} = \frac{Q_2}{19,620}$$

$$Q_2 = 20,710 \text{ cfm}$$

The change in pressure also affects the density of the air. To obtain the corrected density factor:

$$\frac{P_1}{P_2} = \frac{d_1}{d_2}$$

$$\frac{407 \text{ inches wg}}{385.6 \text{ inches wg}} = \frac{0.74}{d_2}$$

$$d_2 = 0.70$$

To determine the corrected VP_i:

$$v = \frac{Q}{A}$$

$$v = \frac{20,710}{5.585}$$

$$v = 3708 \text{ fpm}$$

Then to obtain VP_i

$$v = 1096.2 \sqrt{VP_i/\rho} \quad (2.3.1)$$

where $\rho = 0.075 \times d = 0.075 \, (0.74)$

$VP_i = 0.64$ inches wg

8. Duct discharge losses

    The loss in the discharge section must be determined. Since the static pressure losses in the discharge section will be low, it will not be necessary to correct for pressure differences. The air volume and density will be as calculated before correction: i.e., $Q = 19,620$ and $d = 0.74$.

    Loss in discharge (use 34 inch diameter duct)

    0.44 inches wg/100 ft. x 40 ft x 0.74 = 0.13 inches wg

9. Select fan and rating

    $$SP_f = SP_o - SP_i - VP_i \quad (2.10.7)$$
    $$= 0.13 - (-21.42) - 0.61$$
    $$= 20.94 \text{ inches wg}$$

    Correcting for density since fan rating tables assume standard conditions:

    $$Fan_{SP} = \frac{20.94}{d} = \frac{20.94}{0.74} = 28.20 \text{ inches wg}$$

    Using the fan rating table below for the values:

    SP = 28.30 inches wg
    Q = 20,710 cfm

Table 2.15.1

CFM Volume	22" SP RPM	BHP	24" SP RPM	BHP	26" SP RPM	BHP	28" SP RPM	BHP	30" SP RPM	BHP	32" SP RPM	BHP
16,000	1130	74.6	1220	82.0	1305	91.5	1380	100	1450	108	1510	115
18,500	1180	81.8	1270	89.2	1355	98.7	1430	107	1500	115	1560	122
21,000	1228	88.8	1318	96.2	1403	106	1478	114	1548	122	1608	129
23,500	1274	95.6	1364	103	1449	113	1524	121	1594	129	1654	136
26,000	1318	102	1408	110	1493	119	1568	128	1638	136	1698	142
28,500	1360	109	1510	117	1535	126	1610	135	1680	142	1740	148
31,000	1400	115	1550	123	1575	133	1650	141	1720	148	1780	154
33,500	1438	121	1588	129	1613	139	1688	147	1758	154	1818	160

Interpolating between the values:

Q = 18,500 cfm and 21,000 cfm
SP = 28 inches wg and 30 inches wg

the following characteristics are obtained:

RPM = 1482
BHP = 114

Summary

When the air is other than standard, it is necessary to make corrections for the fact that the air has a different density, since the operation of a ventilation system is affected by this change. In general, as the air becomes less dense, the effect of losses as a result of turbulence and friction also becomes less. This in turn affects the size and operating characteristics of the air mover. Normally the correction is necessary for air if the temperature is greater than 100°F, if the altitude varies beyond 1000 ft from sea level, or if the moisture content of the air is greater than 0.02 pounds of water per pound of dry air.

16. Thermal Ventilation Effects

Quite often an industrial process involves significant amounts of heat. Such processes require that the designer consider the effect of the addition of heat to the air surrounding the process when designing a ventilation system to control process contaminants. Special techniques have been developed to handle this problem.

General Principles of Air Motion About a Hot Process

As air is heated, its molecules become more active, and the volume of air increases if unconstrained by an enclosure. As the volume of the air increases, its density is reduced. Thus, the air rises as a result of this reduced density; and colder air moves into the low pressure area vacated by the heated air. This creates an air movement about the hot process. The movement of the heated air is upward, while that of the cold air is inward to the hot process. For the purpose of this discussion, this air movement will be designated as the draft pressure. A difference in pressure between a heated column of air and the surrounding air causes air motion.

A number of formulas have been derived from theoretical consideration of the motion of air about a hot process. These formulas will be presented below. No attempt has been made to derive the relationships involved from the theory. For the interested reader, such a discussion can be found in the book, Plant and Process Ventilation, W. Hemeon, Chapter 8.

Draft Pressure

$$(2.16.1) \quad P = \frac{dH(T_c - T_o)}{5.2 \, T_c}$$

where

P = draft pressure, inches wg
H = height of heated column in ft
T_c = absolute temperature of heated air, °R
T_o = absolute temperature of surrounding air, °R
ρ = density of air at 0°F, lb/ft^3

Velocity of Air in a Heated Column

$$(2.16.2) \quad v = 480 \sqrt{H(T_c - T_o)/T_c}$$

where
> v = the velocity of heated air in feet per minute.
> Other variables are as described above.

To determine Q or the rate of flow, one would normally use the formula $Q = v \times A$, where A is the cross-sectional area of the column of air. However, the heated column does not have a constant temperature since mixing between the heated column and the surrounding air occurs as the column of air rises. Thus, a formula for Q must be developed that considers mixing.

Figure 2.16.1

Rate of air flow.

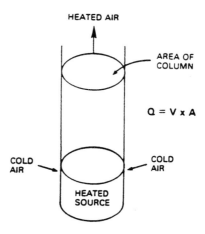

Formula for Rate of Flow of Hot-Air Column

(2.16.3) $Q = 29 \ [H_t A^2 h]^{1/3}$

where
> Q = the air flow rate at the upper limits of a hot body i
> cfm
> H_t = the heat transfer rate by convection in BTU/min
> A = the cross-sectional area of air stream, ft^2
> h = the height of a column receiving heat or the height o
> the body giving off heat, ft

In the above case, the object giving off heat has a height or vertical dimension. Where a horizontal surface is involved, some questions arise as t the value of h, or the height of the object. Some experimental data suggest that the value for h for horizontal surface is the diameter of the horizontal surface. In some special cases, the value of h is considered to be equal to to allow for calculations. The value of A or the stream area in the formula is taken to be the area of the horizontal surface.

Figure 2.16.2

Effect of mixing.

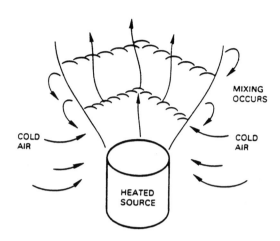

The heat loss that is of interest in ventilation of hot processes is the convectional heat loss (H_t). The total heat loss of the object involves losses occurring by convection, conduction, and radiation. However, the loss that is transferred to the air by convection is by far the most significant when considering the control of contaminants.

Convectional Heat Loss Formula

$$(2.16.4) \quad H_t = \frac{h_c A(T_b - T_o)}{60}$$

where

H_t = the heat loss of a hot body to surrounding air by convection, BTU/min

h_c = the convection coefficient

A = the surface area emitting heat, ft^2

T_b = the temperature of the hot surface, °F

T_o = the temperature of the surrounding air, °F

Note that degrees Fahrenheit are used in the formula, since the absolute temperature values will cancel when the difference in temperature is considered. A heat loss coefficient is used in the formula. This heat loss coefficient has been determined experimentally for various configurations of objects. Some typical heat loss coefficients are presented in the accompanying table.

Table 2.16.1

Heat loss coefficients (h_c)
for loss by convection.

Configuration	Heat loss by natural convection
Vertical Plate Over 2 ft High	$0.3(\Delta t)^{1/4}$
Vertical Plate Less than 2 ft High (X = height in feet)	$0.28(\Delta t/X)^{1/4}$
Horizontal Plates Facing Upward	$0.38(\Delta t)^{1/4}$
Horizontal Plates Facing Downward	$0.2(\Delta t)^{1/4}$
Single Horizontal Cylinders (where X' is diameter in inches)	$0.42(\Delta t/X')^{1/4}$
Vertical Cylinders Over 2 ft High	$0.4(\Delta t/X')^{1/4}$
Vertical Cylinders Less Than 2 ft High where	$f \times 0.4(\Delta t/X')^{1/4}$

Height (ft)	f
0.1	3.5
0.2	2.5
0.3	2.0
0.4	1.7
0.5	1.5
1.0	1.1

Plant and Process Ventilation, 2d Edition. W. Hemeon,
Industrial Press, Inc., New York, 1963.

Control of Contaminants from Processes--The Low Canopy Hood

When placed above a cold process, the low canopy hood (vertical distance
from source less than or equal to 3 feet) acts like a booth. The face
velocity is determined at the perimeter of the open space between the hood and
the source. A difference in velocity exists between the rim of the hood and
point near the source of contaminant. In general, this difference in velocity
is corrected by assuming that the area is 40 percent larger than that of the
actual area.

When a low canopy hood is placed above a hot process, a different
situation exists. The low canopy hood acts as a receiving hood above a hot

process. The air that has become heated rises from the hot process into the hood itself. As a result, the exhaust rate of the canopy hood should be equal to the rate at which the contaminated air is entering the hood. The rate of flow into the hood is assumed to be the same as that generated at the surface of the body since the hood is relatively close to the source and any correction for this difference would result in only a small change in the rate of flow.

Figure 2.16.3

Low canopy hood.

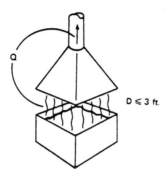

Assuming a dry heat source, determine the convectional heat transfer and rate of flow involved. From the heat transfer equation given previously,

$$H_t = \frac{g_c A(T_b - T_o)}{60} \qquad (2.16.4)$$

the appropriate convection coefficient for the configuration of the process involved can be inserted. In this case, assume that the source was an upward facing plane. From the table of heat loss coefficients, the formula for a horizontal plane facing upward is given as

$$h_c = 0.38(T_b - T_o)^{1/4}$$

Substituting in the heat transfer formula gives

$$H_t = \frac{0.38}{60} A(T_b - T_o)^{5/4}$$

where
H_t = the heat transfer by convection from a horizontal plane, BTU/min

A = the area of the source body since it is assumed that very little mixing will occur between the source body and a low canopy hood, ft^2

T_c = the temperature of the body surface, °F

T_o = the temperature of the surrounding air, °F

Substituting in the original rate of flow formula gives

$$Q = 29 \ [H_t A^2 h]^{1/3} \qquad (2.16.3)$$

or

$$Q = 5.4A \ [h(T_b - T_o)^{5/4}]^{1/3}$$

If a different source configuration is present, then the Q formula will be different. Also, the area of the source body is the actual area that is giving off heat to surrounding air. This is in contrast to the cross-sectional area of the air stream that is rising. For a low canopy hood, it is assumed that the cross-sectional area does not increase over the distance involved.

If the heated source involves steam from a tank of hot water, then the heat transfer formula becomes

$$H_t = 1000 \ GA$$
where
   G = the pounds of steam evaporated per minute per square foot

This relationship can be substituted in the rate of flow formula to obtain the following relationship:

$$(2.16.5) \qquad Q = 290A \ [G \ h]^{1/3}$$

The low canopy hood should be designed in such a manner that dimensions of the hood face are the same as the dimensions of the source or hot process. Since the hood is placed relatively close to the source (within 3 feet), little mixing with surrounding air occurs, and the column of air rising from the hot process remains at approximately the same cross-sectional area as the hot process.

In some cases, a low canopy hood may already be present that is larger than the source from which the heated air is rising. In this case, it is necessary that a correction in the rate of flow from the hood be made in order to accommodate the surrounding air that enters the hood in addition to that rising in the column. This correction is made by increasing Q to create a face velocity at the perimeter of the hood. If the correction is not made, it is likely that contaminated hot air will spill out from the hood and enter the workroom atmosphere. The formula for correcting the rate of flow in this case is given as:

$$(2.16.6) \qquad Q' = Q + vA$$

where

   Q' = the new rate of flow to capture the contaminated air and additional surrounding air entering the hood, cfm

Q = the calculated flow from the hot surface, cfm

v = the face velocity in ft/min to overcome any possible spillage of contaminated air from the hood

A = the area of the face, ft^2

Figure 2.16.4

Large hood--small source.

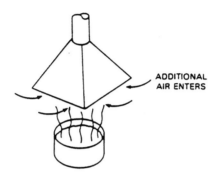

ADDITIONAL
AIR ENTERS

Examples

1. A hot furnace that is 3 ft by 3 ft by 3 ft (l, w, h) has a surface temperature of 1100°F and emits toxic fumes. A 3 ft by 3 ft low canopy hood is to be used to control the fumes. At what rate should air be exhausted from the hood?

Solution

The convection heat transfer rate (H_t) is calculated from the convection coefficient (h_c) for a vertical plate.

$$h_c = 0.3(T_b - T_o)^{1/4}$$
$$h_c = 0.3(1100 - 70)^{1/4}$$
$$h_c = 1.7$$

Using the heat transfer formula

$$(2.16.4) \quad H_t = \frac{h_c A(T_b - T_o)}{60}$$

and substituting in the appropriate values as follows:
$$h_c = 1.7$$

$$A = 45 \text{ ft}^2 \ (5 \text{ surfaces} \times 9 \text{ ft}^2/\text{surface})$$
$$T_b = 1100$$
$$T_o = 70$$

we obtain

$$H_t = 1313 \text{ BTU/min}$$

Substituting this value into the rate of flow formula gives

$$Q = 29 \ [1313 \times 9^2 \times 3]^{1/3} \qquad (2.16.4)$$

$$Q = 1982 \text{ cfm}$$

2. Assume in the above problem the area of the hood face is 6 ft by 6 ft. What exhaust rate should be specified?

Solution

Since a larger hood is being used, the exhaust rate must be corrected. The correction is calculated from the formula:

$$Q' = Q + vA \qquad (2.16.6)$$

If v = 100 feet per minute, to prevent contaminant from escaping the hood face
$$Q' = 2181 + 100(36 - 9)$$
$$Q' = 4881 \text{ cfm}$$

3. If a hot tank of boiling water (8 ft by 3 ft) evaporates at 15 pounds per square foot per hour, at what rate should a low canopy hood exhaust to remove the steam?

Solution

For a steam process
$$Q = 290A \ [G \ h]^{1/3} \qquad (2.16.5)$$

$$G = \frac{15}{60} \text{ or } 1/4 \text{ lbs/ft}^2/\text{min}$$

and assume h = 1 since the heat generated is only at the surface of the tank, then

$$Q = 290 \times 24 \ [1/4 \times 1]^{1/3}$$

$$Q = 4405 \text{ cfm}$$

Control of Contaminants from Hot Processes--High Canopy Hood

A high canopy hood is defined as any hood located more than 3 feet above process. These hoods have certain problems and are not normally recommended for installation above a hot process. As the heated air rises, the air stream widens because of mixing of the heated air column with the surrounding cooler air. In addition, if the air must travel very far from the process to the hood, it is subject to cross drafts. These cross drafts can divert the rising column of air away from the hood, thus allowing contaminants to enter the workroom atmosphere.

If a high canopy hood is to be used to exhaust contaminated air rising from a hot process, certain precautions must be taken. First, the flow rate at the hood must be significantly greater because of the larger volume of air that is entering the hood as a result of mixing. In addition, the effect of cross drafts must be controlled. This can be done in some cases by inserting baffles that separate the column of air from the surrounding workroom atmosphere. This, in effect, creates a chimney in which the hot air rises and acts like a low canopy hood if the baffles can be brought down close to the process.

Figure 2.16.5

High canopy hood.

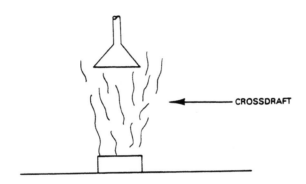

CROSSDRAFT

Enclosures for Hot Processes

In some cases, the hot process may be enclosed in an air-tight chamber. In such cases, the heated air develops a positive static pressure within the enclosure. This positive pressure can cause the hot toxic air to escape into the lower pressure atmosphere if any openings or leaks are present within the chamber. This effect can cause contamination to enter the workroom atmosphere and must be controlled. Since it is very difficult to construct a completely air-tight enclosure, the possibility of escape of contaminated air is a real problem and must be faced.

In order to prevent contaminated air from escaping, an adequate face velocity must be supplied in the areas where leaks can occur. This is accomplished by creating a negative static pressure within the enclosure. This negative pressure must be equal to or greater than the draft pressure caused by the heated air. If this is done, then the air will enter the enclosure from the outside through any leaks rather than escaping into the workroom atmosphere.

Natural Ventilation in Buildings

If the indoor air temperature is different from the outdoor air temperature, a flow of air will be created. Normally, the air within the building is warmer than that outside the building. In this case, the hot air will leave the work area at openings in the upper levels of the building. Cold outside air will enter at ground level to replace the exiting hot air. The difference in height between the inlet and outlet affects the flow. In order for such a flow to occur, there must be a continuous source of heat in the building.

Figure 2.16.6

Natural draft.

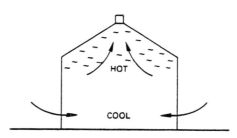

A formula for determining the natural ventilation rate based on thermal effects is given as follows:

(2.16.7) $Q = 9.4A \sqrt{h(T_i - T_o)}$
    where

Q = the rate of flow of air for natural ventilation, cfm
h = the difference in height between inlet and outlet areas, ft
A = the area of the inlet or outlet, assuming that each is the same, ft^2
T_i = the indoor temperature, °F
T_o = the outdoor temperature, °F

Example. An industrial building has an average inside temperature of 75°F while the outside temperature is 40°F. If three roof louvers (4 ft by 6 ft each) exist at the roof level of 20 ft and equivalent openings are present at ground level, calculate the effect of natural thermal ventilation.

Solution

Using the formula presented above:

$Q = 9.4A \sqrt{h(T_i - T_o)}$ (2.16.7)

$Q = 9.4 \times 72 \times \sqrt{20 \times 35}$

$Q = 17,906$ cfm

Summary

The following table summarizes the important formulas presented in this chapter.

REFERENCE	RELATIONSHIP	FORMULA
2.16.1	Draft pressure caused by heated column of rising air	$P = \dfrac{dH(T_c - T_o)}{5.2T_c}$
2.16.2	Velocity of a heated column of air	$v = 480 \sqrt{H(T_c - T_o)/T_c}$
2.16.3	Rate of flow for a heated column Of air	$Q = 29 \, [H_t A^2 h]^{1/3}$
2.16.4	Convectional heat loss of a body surrounding air	$H_t = \dfrac{h_c A(T_b - T_o)}{60}$
2.16.5	Rate of flow from heated source involving steam	$Q = 290A \, [G \, h]^{1/3}$
2.16.6	Correction of Q for a large canopy hood	$Q' = Q + vA$
2.16.7	Natural ventilation rate	$Q = 9.4A \sqrt{h(T_i - T_o)}$

17. Testing Procedures in the Plant

The installation of a ventilation system in the plant does not complete the responsibility of the industrial hygiene engineer. To assure adequate control of contaminants, the industrial hygiene engineer must develop a testing procedure that can be used to assure that the ventilation system is operating within the design parameters. Testing of ventilation systems can be carried out to accomplish a number of purposes.

Reasons for Ventilation System Tests

One reason the industrial hygiene engineer may wish to test a ventilation system is to determine if the system is in compliance with regulations of local, state, or Federal government and represents good industrial hygiene practice. Where state guidelines do not exist, good practice guidelines are usually available. An operating system should be periodically tested to assure that regulations and guidelines are being met and that the worker is being provided adequate protection.

Before placing a ventilation system on-line, it is necessary to check out the newly designed and installed ventilation system to determine if the system is operating as it was designed. Design and installation errors can and often do occur. The check-out provides the data to pinpoint where these errors have occurred and allows for correction before the system is put into actual operation. The industrial hygiene engineer should not depend upon worker complaints to determine if the design criteria have been met.

In obtaining measurements of a newly installed system, an additional benefit is obtained. The data that are gathered during the test provide checkpoint values that can be used as bench marks for future measurements. Differences obtained in future tests can then be used to indicate the possibility that a problem has arisen in the operation of the ventilation system.

Another reason for testing a ventilation system is to determine if the capacity exists for addition to the system. In many cases it is less costly to add on to an existing system than it is to provide a new local exhaust system. However, the system must have the capacity for such an addition. If an addition to the system is made that exceeds its capacity, not only will the new addition fail to provide adequate protection to the worker, but the existing sections of the ventilation system will also be inadequate.

Data obtained from measurements of a well-designed and well-operated system can be valuable to the industrial hygiene engineer. This data can be used to provide bench marks for similar designs that may be used in the future. The effects of minor modification to a well-designed ventilation system can be determined when this design is reused in another section of the plant.

When a blast-gate design has been installed, it is obvious that tests will be required to determine the setting of the blast gates to obtain proper operation. Such a system cannot be place in operation without a complete testing procedure. Once the blast gates have been set on such a system, it is desirable that they be locked in place so that tampering with their settings cannot occur. The movement of one blast gate within such a system can produce an undesirable result throughout the entire system.

A ventilation system that has been operating continuously over a period of time should also be checked by the industrial hygiene engineer. Such a check indicates where it may be necessary to perform maintenance to return the operation of the system to its design level. Variations from initial values in the measurements indicate that some type of problem is present in the operation of the system.

Another reason for making ventilation measurements within the plant is to determine if adequate make-up air is being supplied to the system. A poorly operating system may not be the result of the design itself but of the inadequacy of make-up air. Later in this chapter, a method will be discussed for determining the presence of an inadequate make-up air supply system.

One final reason for testing ventilation systems, which has already been mentioned in the chapter on recirculation of exhaust air, is to determine if a lower ventilation rate can be used. This lower ventilation rate can result in a smaller power requirement to operate the system and reduces the operating cost of the ventilation system. If less air is ventilated, then less tempered air is required to be supplied to the operation.

Types of Ventilation System Tests

There are basically three types of tests that can be conducted for a ventilation system: a test that estimates the effectiveness of the system, a test that determines parameters of operation for the total system, and special tests conducted to determine the operation of components of the system. Often the situation will dictate which type of test should be conducted by the industrial hygiene engineer. The determining factor as to the type of test that should be conducted is the information that is desired from the test.

Often only a quick estimate is required concerning the operation of a ventilation system. Does it seem to be operating to remove the potential health hazard from the workplace? It is not necessary that all facets of a ventilation system be checked out to determine whether such operation is present. One or two measurements may be sufficient to determine the adequacy of the ventilation being provided.

On the other hand, it may be necessary to check out the design of an existing system or to determine checkpoint values or bench marks for a system. In this case, it is necessary that a complete test procedure be developed to determine values at all critical points within the ventilation system. Such a test may be necessary to determine the location of a problem that was indicated during an internal checkout of the ventilation system.

Further, the industrial hygiene engineer may wish to conduct tests to determine the operation of certain components of the system. For example, it may be desirable to determine if the make-up air supply is adequate for the operation of the system. Other special tests might include determining if a particular hood is providing adequate capture velocity at the point of operation, if the appropriate transport velocity for particulate matter within the ducts is being maintained, or if any cleaner and/or fan is operating to specification.

The Location and Purpose of Ventilation System Tests

There are two basic types of ventilation systems, the local exhaust system and the general dilution ventilation system. Each of these systems requires that different procedures be used for system tests.

Within a local exhaust ventilation system, tests can be conducted in the ducts. Such tests determine the transport velocity, the rate of flow (Q) at which air is moving through the system, the static pressure at various points through the system, and fan and/or air cleaner pressure drops.

The entry to the system or the hood is a critical area. Certain tests can be conducted to determine if the hood is operating as designed. For example, the face velocity of the air being captured by the hood can be determined. The static pressure of the hood can indicate the volume of air being moved through the hood. In addition, the capture velocity at the source or point of operation can be determined for a given hood.

Other tests can be conducted to determine the effect of cross drafts on the operation of a ventilation system, the quantity of contaminant escaping the system, and the contaminant generation at the source.

In terms of a general ventilation system, the make-up supply velocity and rate can be determined using testing procedures. In addition, the exhaust volume can be estimated from tests. It may be necessary to determine the extent of contaminant buildup in certain dead spots within a system serviced by a general ventilation system.

Testing Local Exhaust Systems

Determining the Static Pressure of the System. The most common type of instrument used to determine static pressure within a ventilation system is the U-tube manometer. Measurement of static pressure with a U-tube manometer is obtained by determining the difference in the levels of liquid in the legs of the manometer. Generally the fluid used in a U-tube manometer is water, although manometer oil can be used where increased sensitivity is desired. A U-tube manometer is illustrated in Figure 2.17.1.

To obtain increased sensitivity in the measurement of static pressure, the inclined manometer may be used. (Figure 2.17.2.) The <u>inclined manometer</u> operates on the same principle as the U-tube manometer but is constructed in such a way that one leg is inclined to produce a ratio of 10:1 between the vertical leg and the inclined leg. This results in a greater sensitivity and accuracy of measurement. Special manometers are made that produce a 20:1

Figure 2.17.1

U-tube manometer.

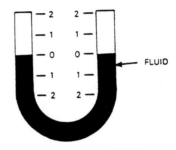

MEASURES STATIC PRESSURE

ratio for even greater sensitivity. However, this type of manometer is not usually used in the field, since the manometer oil levels so slowly that it is possible to introduce an error in reading the level before it reaches equilibrium. The inclined manometer is generally filled with manometer oil at 0.826 specific gravity. Special inclined-vertical manometers are also available that are designed to obtain a greater sensitivity in the lower range. In these manometers, the first inch of pressure differential is on an inclined scale (10:1), and the higher pressures are on a vertical scale. The inclined-vertical manometer is smaller than the standard 10:1 inclined manometer and, as a result, has some advantages for field use.

Static pressure measurements within a ventilation system should be taken at points where the air flow is as nearly parallel to the wall of the duct as possible. Measurements should be made at a point downstream of any obstructions and away from any turbulence that might be caused by the obstructions. Static pressure measurements at the hood should be made one diameter from a tapered hood and three diameters away from a plain or flanged hood. The difference in distance between the two types of hoods is a result of smoother air flow that is obtained through a tapered hood than is obtained through a plain or flanged hood.

Figure 2.17.2

Inclined manometer.

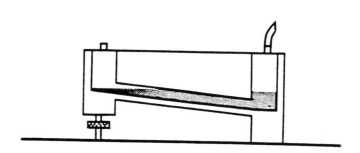

A great deal of information can be acquired concerning the operation of a ventilation system through the measurement of static pressure. For example, pressure drops or resistance through various sections of the ventilation system--such as the hood, a given duct section, an air cleaner, or fan--can give information concerning the operation of that section of the system. In the case of an air cleaner, if the manufacturer's specifications indicate a 3-inch drop between inlet and outlet, any measurement significantly different from this value indicates that a problem may be present.

It is possible to estimate the flow of air through a hood using only static pressure measurements. In this case, four orthogonal (90°) measurements are taken 3 diameters downstream. Using the following equation and substituting in the average static pressure obtained by the four measurements, a quick estimate of Q can be obtained.

$$Q = 4005C_eA \sqrt{SP_h} \qquad (2.7.7)$$
where

A = the area of the duct, ft^2
C_e = the coefficient of entry for the particular hood configuration
SP_h = static pressure at the hood, inches wg

In many cases where field measurements are taken, the Magnehelic® gauge, which is an aneroid gauge, is used in place of the manometer. The Magnehelic® gauge is easy to read and has a quicker response than the manometer. In addition, it is portable and readings can be taken without care in mounting the instrument. For this reason, it is preferred by some individuals. However, the Magnehelic® gauge does require calibration, and it is subject to mechanical failures.

Determining Velocity Pressure--The Pitot Tube. The pitot tube can be used to measure velocity pressure. This measurement is expressed in inches water gauge (inches wg). The device consists of two concentric tubes, the center tube measuring the total pressure while the outer tube measures static pressure. The center tube is connected to a tap at the bottom of the pitot tube, and the outer tube is connected to a tap halfway up the vertical leg.

Velocity pressure can be measured by attaching a manometer to the pitot tube such that one leg is connected to the bottom tap, and the second leg is attached to the upper tap. This arrangement provides an analog to the familiar Bernoulli's theorem, TP = SP + VP.

The standard pitot tube has a stem diameter of 0.312 inches (5/16 inches) and requires a minimum duct drill hole of 3/8 inches for insertion. Smaller sized pitot tubes that use the same geometric proportions are available for ducts smaller than 10 inches in diameter. The 1/8-inch pitot tube requiring a 3/16-inch diameter hole in the duct is of this type.

A special type of pitot tube, Type S, has been developed for use in very dusty areas. The Type S pitot tube has larger static pressure and total pressure holes that greatly reduce the tendency of these holes to plug in a dusty atmosphere. This pitot tube gives higher readings than the standard tube and requires a correction factor. The Type S tube requires calibration initially while the standard pitot tube does not.

As mentioned above, the pitot tube can be used to measure velocity pressure directly in ducts. Velocity is not constant within a duct. Because of obstructions and because of the frictional drag that occurs at the side walls, the velocity contour is not vertical. Therefore, it is necessary to obtain measurements throughout the contour to obtain an estimate of the velocity through the system. The point of stable air flow in a duct system is 7.5 diameters or more downstream from any major disturbance. Any measurements of velocity pressure using a pitot tube should be taken at this minimum distance from any obstruction.

In order to obtain a value for the velocity in a duct, it is necessary that a pitot traverse be conducted. The procedure for conducting a _pitot traverse_ is to divide the duct into cross sections of small equal areas. Two series of orthogonal measurements are then taken at the centers of the equal areas. The velocity pressures obtained are then converted into velocities using the equation

$$v = 4005 \sqrt{VP}$$

after correcting for any nonstandard condition. The velocities are then averaged, and this average velocity is used as the average velocity within the duct.

Tables are available that can be used to determine the traverse points for various sizes of duct. The number of points increases with the duct size. Commonly, the tables are for 6, 10, and 20 point traverses of round ducts. Where rectangular ducts are present, a different set of traverse points is used. Normally, the traverse points for rectangular ducts are not more than 6 inches apart.

Often it is necessary to obtain a quick estimate of the velocity pressure, and time does not allow for a pitot traverse. The velocity can be estimated by obtaining a centerline measurement of velocity. The average velocity within the duct is then said to be

$$v = 0.9 v_{cm}$$

Figure 2.17.3

Pitot tube.

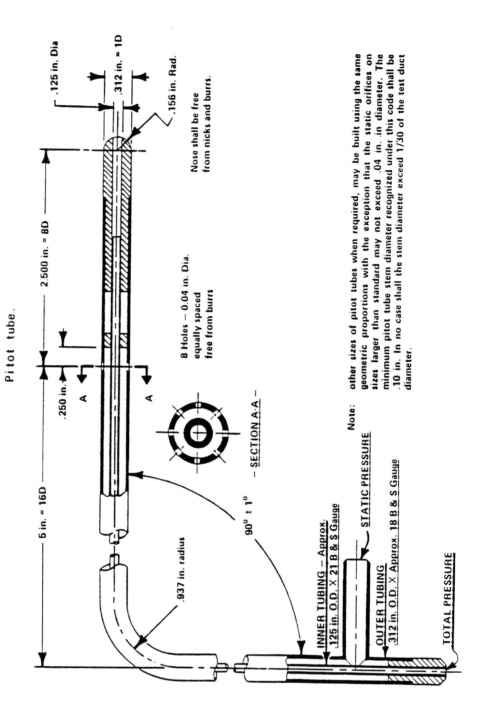

.125 in. Dia

.312 in. = 1D

.156 in. Rad.

Nose shall be free
from nicks and burrs.

2.500 in. = 8D

8 Holes — 0.04 in. Dia.
equally spaced
free from burrs

.250 in.

A

A

– SECTION A-A –

5 in. = 16D

.937 in. radius

90° ± 1°

INNER TUBING – Approx.
.125 in. O.D. X 21 B & S Gauge

STATIC PRESSURE

OUTER TUBING
.312 in. O.D. X Approx. 18 B & S Gauge

TOTAL PRESSURE

Note: other sizes of pitot tubes when required, may be built using the same geometric proportions with the exception that the static orifices on sizes larger than standard may not exceed .04 in. in diameter. The minimum pitot tube stem diameter recognized under this code shall be .10 in. In no case shall the stem diameter exceed 1/30 of the test duct diameter.

Figure 2.17.4

Pitot tube detail.*

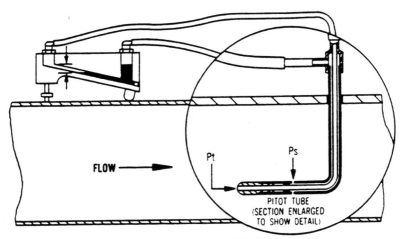

PITOT TUBE SENSES TOTAL AND STATIC PRESSURES.
MANOMETER MEASURES VELOCITY PRESSURE —
(DIFFERENCE BETWEEN TOTAL AND STATIC PRESSURES).

Figure 2.17.5

Traverse points.*

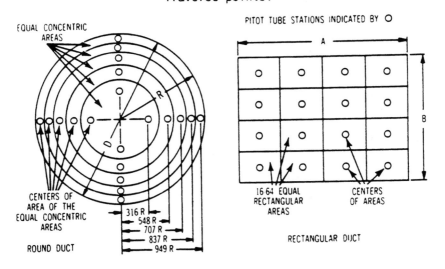

One problem with the pitot tube is that it is not effective in obtaining velocity pressure at low velocities. The accuracy of the pitot tube has been estimated to be ±6% at 800 feet per minute and ±15% at 600 feet per minute. Thus, some other method must be used to measure velocity pressure at these lower ranges. However, this is not generally a problem in exhaust ventilation systems because of the normally high velocity that is required to transport particulate matter through the system.

Determining Velocity Pressure—Other Instruments. The pitot tube is limited in its application to obtaining velocity pressure within ducts where the velocity is less than 600-800 feet per minute. It is sometimes necessary that velocity measurements be obtained where the duct velocity is below this critical range or where the velocity being measured is not within the duct but is at the face of the hood or within the workroom space. In these cases, other types of equipment must be used.

One type of equipment that can be used in these cases is the swinging vane anemometer. The Alnor velometer is of this type. The velocity is measured by a mechanical device that operates on a principle similar to the pitot tube. The velocity pressure is exerted on a vane traveling in a circular tunnel. This causes a pointer to indicate the velocity obtained directly on a gauge. The swinging vane anemometer generally measures velocity pressure on five different scales. These scales are shown in Table 2.17.1.

Table 2.17.1

Scales for velocity measurement
using an Alnor velometer.

30-300	fpm
0-1250	fpm
0-2500	fpm
0-5000	fpm
0-10,000	fpm

In addition, there are two scales on the Alnor velometer for measurement of static pressure. The first scale measures from 0 to 1 inches wg, while the second scale measures from 0 to 10 inches wg.

Three velocity probes are available for the Alnor velometer. The first is a low velocity probe that is contained within the instrument itself. This probe measures in the range of 30 to 300 feet per minute. However, such a probe cannot be used in the duct since it is not generally possible to insert the instrument into the duct without creating a disturbance that would affect the measurement being obtained. A pitot probe is available for measurements from 100 feet per minute to 10,000 feet per minute. The pitot probe is used for in-duct measurements. A diffuser probe is also included that can be used to determine velocity at supply and exhaust openings. The diffuser probe can measure in the range from 100 to 5000 feet per minute.

Two static pressure probes are also included with the Alnor velometer, the first for measuring in the lower range of 0 to 1 inches wg and the second for measuring in the upper range of 0 to 10 inches wg.

The advantages of the Alnor velometer include the fact that it is a direct reading device. Also, the velometer measures over a wide range of velocities. It can be used both inside and outside the ducts, and it is small enough to be easily portable. Since the velometer measures in the range below the pitot tube, it is useful for making measurements in heating and air-conditioning ducts which normally operate in the lower range.

However, there are certain disadvantages to the Alnor velometer. Because it is a mechanical device, it requires frequent calibration. Also, since the scale range is short and the pointer sensitive, readings are often rough. For in-duct measurements, the pitot probe requires a larger opening (1/2 inch) and the holes in the pitot probe, and thus the velometer, are not such as to allow measurement in a heavy dust atmosphere.

The velometer is most often used for measuring velocities of 50 feet per minute or greater at the hood, booth, or slot openings of a local exhaust system; for measuring duct velocity between 300 and 800 feet per minute; and, because of the probe size, only when the duct is large. The velometer can also be used for measuring velocity at supply diffusers and grilles.

The second type of instrument that is often used for measuring velocity is the heated thermocouple anemometer. This equipment operates based on a hot/cold thermocouple junction where one wire is heated. As the air passes across the probe, it cools the heated wire. The temperature change is sensed and causes a reduction in the millivolt output to the meter. The meter is scaled to read the velocity in feet per minute. Two scales are commonly included on such an instrument, from 10 to 300 feet per minute and 100 to 2000 feet per minute.

The advantages of the thermoanemometer include the fact that it can measure at low velocities, and its probe size is smaller than the velometer. It is a direct-reading instrument and is small; thus, it is easily carried to the point where measurement is desired.

On the negative side, this type of equipment is not recommended for use in dusty, corrosive, or combustible atmospheres. The probe sensor is fragile and care must be taken when it is being used. In addition, since the equipment is battery operated, the battery can lose power quickly and should be checked often.

The thermoanemometer is used for measuring low velocities. Often these measurements are at openings to the system. Its use is limited to areas where the air temperature ranges from 20°F to 150°F and where the air is relatively clean. It is preferred over the velometer for determining duct velocity below 800 feet per minute since the probe is smaller.

A third type of equipment that can be used to measure air velocity is the rotating vane anemometer. In this equipment, a rotating vane propeller is attached to a gear train. The gear is attached to a dial that reads linear feet of air passing through the vane. In order to obtain measurement of velocity, it is necessary to take a timing of the measurement so that the velocity in feet per minute can be obtained. Generally, the measurement range of this instrument is between 200 and 2000 feet per minute.

The rotating vane anemometer is accurate and can be used for measuring relatively low velocities. However, because of its size, it cannot be used for in-duct measurements. As with the thermoanemometer, it cannot be used in corrosive, dusty, or high-temperature air. The equipment must be calibrated frequently, and a method for measuring time must be provided.

The rotating vane anemometer is used most often in large supply and exhaust openings. Special designs are available to measure velocities as low as 25 feet per minute.

One other type of instrument is available for measuring air velocity--the heated wire anemometer. The principle of operation of the heated wire anemometer is similar to the thermoanemometer. Since the resistance of wire varies with temperature, as a stream of air passes over a heated wire, the varying resistance is indicated on the dial. This equipment measures velocities from 10 to 8000 feet per minute.

The heated wire anemometer can be used for low velocity measurement. It is a fairly accurate instrument that requires a relatively small probe (3/8 inch). However, as with the thermoanemometer, it is a fragile instrument and requires frequent calibration. In addition, it cannot be used in dusty, corrosive, or combustible atmospheres.

Testing Dilution or Make-Up Air Systems

To obtain measurements of the air flow in a dilution ventilation system, a measurement at the exhaust fan does not provide adequate data. The procedure that is recommended is that all openings be closed and any supply systems shut off. With the exhaust system operating, one door or area is opened. The air coming in at this area is measured using multiple traverse points. The opening should provide an average velocity of approximately 500 feet per minute to obtain accurate measurements. Either the velometer, thermoanemometer, or rotating vane anemometer can be used for these measurements. A relatively calm day should be chosen, since the effect of wind entering at the opening can introduce errors in the measurement.

After the measurements have been taken, the volume can be calculated by determining the area opened and the average velocity that is obtained. A correction factor should be applied for any cracks that may allow air to enter the closed-off area. Using the formula, $Q = vA$, the rate of flow can be determined.

In a similar way, the adequacy of make-up air for a local exhaust ventilation system can be determined. All exhaust fans and hoods are turned on and operating. All supply air and make-up air systems are also operating.

Figure 2.17.6

Application of velometer.

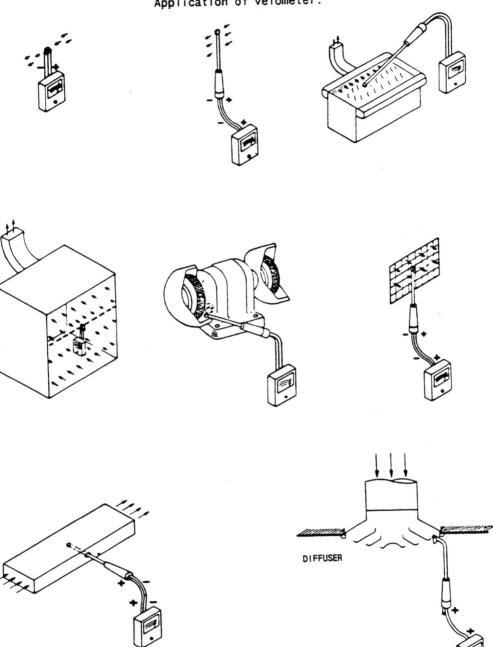

DIFFUSER

All openings are closed except one. This open area is then traversed to determine the velocity of air entering the workroom. The volume of air entering can be calculated after correcting for any incidental air entering through cracks. The rate of flow of air entering through the opening being measured then indicates the deficiency that is present in the supply system.

In some cases, it may be desirable to obtain measurements of the velocity at the supply and exhaust grilles of a system. Often these openings are not clear and grilles or louvers partially block the opening. The free opening is the percentage of gross opening not blocked and should be estimated in these cases. Measurements made by holding the probe against the grille will not give accurate results. The manufacturer supplies a correction factor tha can be used.

The general procedure for obtaining such measurements is to determine the traverse point at the opening being measured and to use a velometer with a probe if the area is small or the velocity is above 300 feet per minute. The probe is held flush with the grille, and at each point a reading is obtained. The readings are then averaged, and the correction factor supplied by the manufacturer is applied to the results. The rate of flow can then be calculated based upon the free area or gross area, depending upon the manufacturer's specifications. In the case where the manufacturer's correction factor is not available, measurements should be taken one inch awa from the grille. The same procedure is used; however, the gross area is used for calculation of the rate of flow.

Where it is desirable to obtain a measurement at a diffuser, a velometer with a diffuser probe attachment can be used. The manufacturer generally specifies the positions where such measurements should be made. Four measurements should be taken, each one 90° from the other. These readings are then averaged, and any correction factor specified by the manufacturer is applied.

Other Methods Available for Testing Ventilation Systems

One method that can be used to obtain a quick check on the operation of a ventilation system is the smoke tube. Some smoke tubes contain titanium tetrachloride. Air is blown through the tube with a squeeze bulb, and a visible smoke is produced.

The smoke tube can be used to indicate the direction of air flow within an area or near an exhaust opening. It can be used to indicate leaks in ducts, booths, or enclosures. The velocity in a duct or a long tunnel can be estimated if the time for passage of the smoke from one point to a second point is taken. By holding the smoke tube near a hood, the capture efficiency of the hood can be observed. If the smoke appears to dissipate or be blown away from the hood, this will indicate the presence of cross drafts that affect the hood's ability to capture contaminants.

The smoke tube is a low-cost visual indicator. It is easy to use and can provide a quick estimate of the adequate operation of a ventilation system.

However, this is only an estimate and does not take the place of more accurate measurements where needed. The smoke tube is not applicable for velocities above 150 feet per minute because of the effects of such rapid air flow in the dissipation of the smoke. In addition, the smoke tube is not effective in hot, dry air, since it depends on the moisture in the air to produce the smoke.

Smoke candles, which are tubes containing combustible materials that produce smoke when burned, can also be used. These operate on the same principle as the smoke tube.

One method that should not be overlooked when conducting tests of ventilation systems is the use of the powers of observation. Certain signs should be considered. Any smoke, fume, or particulate matter that is observed around the operation or escaping from the duct indicates a problem. If an odor is present within the workroom environment, it is likely that the system is not operating properly. Hoods, ducts, and fans can be inspected to determine if clogging, corrosion, or damage has occurred that will affect their operation.

Determining Where Problems Exist

When checking out a ventilation system for the presence of problems, certain key factors indicate the possibility of particular problems in the system. In the case of low system air flow, the following points should be checked:

1. Check fan for direction of rotation since incorrect installation will deliver only about 30 percent of the required air.
2. Check the fan rpm to see if it meets specifications.
3. Check the fan condition for clogging or corrosion.
4. Check the duct for clogging. This is often indicated by a high hood static pressure and a low flow. Cleanouts within the duct should also be checked to see if accumulations are present.
5. Check for closed dampers.
6. Check for tampering of blast-gate settings.
7. Check the air cleaners for clogging.
8. Check all outlets for clogging.
9. Check for poor design of duct and branches.
10. Check for inadequate make-up air supply.

In some cases, the proper flow is being obtained, but poor contaminant control exists. In these cases, the following should be checked:

1. Presence of cross drafts that cause the contaminant to escape from control by the system.
2. Process air movement which results in contaminant escape.
3. The point of operation too far from the hood capture range.
4. Changes in the hood after installation that result in a less efficient operation.

Summary

It is often necessary to perform tests of the operation of ventilation systems. Such tests provide information concerning the actual operation of the system. The results can be compared to the design specifications to indicate the presence of any problems.

Measurement of static pressure can be obtained by using the U-tube manometer, inclined manometer, or the Magnehelic® gauge. Velocity pressure measurements can be obtained through the use of the pitot tube, velometer, and various types of thermoanemometers. The pitot tube is accurate for measurements above 800 fpm while the velometer or thermoanemometer may be used for lower velocities. The pitot tube is limited to in-duct measurements while the other instruments can be used at diffusers, inlets, doors, etc. When velocity pressure reading is desired, it is necessary to perform a traverse since the velocity pressure profile is not constant throughout the duct.

18. Environmental Air Pollution

<u>Beyond the Plant</u>

Often the tendency is to assume that once the contaminant has been removed from the plant, the responsibilities of the industrial hygiene engineer are complete. In the past, the practice has been to discharge contaminants in the air outside the plant and depend upon natural dilution to remove the hazard. However, this situation can create problems. Natural dilution does not always exist. During periods of weather inversions, contaminants can build up to a point where a hazard or nuisance to the surrounding area is created. The industrial hygiene engineer should consider the effects of pollution to the surrounding area and should determine the extent of pollution that occurs. Controls should be developed to minimize the potential hazard that can result from environmental air pollution.

Air pollution is not limited to that which is produced by industrial processes. There are certain natural types of air pollution which have existed since the beginning of time. Dust that is picked up and moved from area to area is an example. The dust bowl that occurred during the mid-thirties was an extreme case of such natural air pollution. Other sources of natural air pollution include smoke resulting from naturally caused fires and pollen that floats through the air, raising havoc among certain people. Chemical reactions that occur in nature also produce contaminants which pollute the atmosphere. However, for the most part, these natural sources of air pollution are beyond the control of man. Also, since they have existed from the beginning of time, certain defense mechanisms have been built up within man to protect against this type of pollution.

On the other hand, man-made pollution is a relatively new phenomenon. The great majority of pollution that exists in the atmosphere today has probably come into being only since the beginning of the industrial revolution. Man-made pollutants include the exhaust from automobiles and emissions from fuel and energy production. Heat production at local plants as well as homes also pollutes the atmosphere. Industrial processes and open burning can be a major source of hazardous pollutants.

The Effects of Air Pollution. The presence of air pollution can result in many harmful effects. Among the most important of these effects are:

1. Health effects--This area has become the subject of much controversy. Statements have been made that cancer is related to industrial pollutants. The accuracy of such statements may be subject to question; however, there are documented cases where acute

air pollution has resulted in excessive deaths. Certain chronic
effects have been studied. These studies seem to indicate that a
cause/effect relationship between air pollution and health does
exist. Further studies are being conducted, and it is likely that
this subject will remain a controversial one for the foreseeable
future.

2.   Community relations--Excessive air pollution can be harmful to
     community relations for the industries involved. The workers may
     react to the dangers that threaten their families' health if they
     live in the immediate area. Community groups may form to put
     pressures on the industry to reduce the amount of pollution present.
     In addition, the public relations image obtained by the plant
     involved may be harmed, resulting in a negative effect on sales and
     profits.

3.   Property damage--One needs only to drive around a heavily
     industrialized area to see indications of the property damage that
     can occur as a result of air pollution. The economic effects of this
     damage are hard to determine. Equipment may operate over a shorter
     life because of corrosion caused by pollution. Buildings must be
     cleaned more often, and the exterior surfaces may be subject to
     excessive aging.

4.   Economic climate of the community--Excessive air pollution can affect
     the economic climate of the community. New businesses are less
     likely to move into a dirty area because of the difficulty in finding
     workers willing to live in the vicinity of the plant.

5.   Plant life--Botanists have done studies on the effects of air
     pollution on various types of plant life. Direct cause and effect
     relationships have been discovered for certain types of pollution.

6.   Animal life--As in the case of health factors affecting humans,
     certain acute pollution problems have been shown to exist in
     animals. Currently, the controversy surrounding PCB's and Kepone
     indicate the possibility of long-range chronic effects of pollution
     on animals, not to mention the potential second-level effects on
     man. As a part of the natural food chain, pollutants that affect
     plant life are often carried over to animals and thus to humans. The
     chronic effects of this type of transfer are not well known or
     understood.

Determining the Extent of Air Pollution--Measuring the Ambient Air

There are two methods that are available to determine the extent of air
pollution. The first of these methods is the measuring of the ambient air.
Such measurement involves determining the extent and dispersion of pollution
in the surrounding area. Pollution is affected by the weather patterns and
topography present. In addition, any synergistic effects between two
pollutants from different industrial plants can also be considered by this
method. Measuring the ambient air is somewhat akin to measuring the

contaminant within the workplace. Though it does not give specific information related to the pollutants from a particular source, it does present information concerning the potential hazards that may be present in the atmosphere.

The sampling train that is used in measuring the ambient air includes the following items:

1.   Collector for contaminants.
2.   Air mover or vacuum source.
3.   Airflow measuring device.
4.   Sample probe or collection device.
5.   Equipment to measure other factors in the environment, such as heat, humidity, and pressure.

The type of collection device that is used in the sampling train depends on the type of pollutant that is present. The basic types of pollutants are gases and vapors or particulate matter. Collection devices for gases and vapors are generally of two types. Either a grab sample (without concentration of contaminant) is taken, or a continuous sample with concentration of contaminant is taken. For grab samples, an evacuated container or a liquid displacement method is used. Continuous collection with concentration involves either absorption in liquids (both chemical and physical absorption), adsorption on solids such as activated charcoal, or condensation or freeze-out methods.

Collection devices in the sampling train for particulate matter involve sedimentation, inertial separation, electrostatic precipitation, thermal precipitation, filtration, or the use of photometers. It is beyond the scope of this discussion to go into the various advantages and disadvantages of each of these methods. The reader is referred to The Air Pollution Manual, Part I, Evaluation, published by the American Industrial Hygiene Association for further study and references on this subject. In general, the methods are similar to the methods for cleaning air previously discussed.

Certain observations of the smoke plume can also give some estimate of the amount of air pollution that is present. The Ringelmann chart has been used in the past for such observations. In addition, observers can be trained to estimate the pollution due to particulate matter by observing the smoke plume.

The second major component of a sample train is the air mover. The purpose of the air mover is to create a flow of air through the collector. Two major types of air movers are used--the pump and the ejector.

There are various types of pumps that are used in such sample trains. The piston-and-diaphragm pump is commonly used. In addition, pumps may be powered by a motor or by a hand crank. When small grab samples are desired, the system is often powered by a squeeze bulb. Ejectors that work on the venturi principle are often used in an area where the atmosphere is explosive.

Some method must be present in the sampling train to meter the amount of air that is being drawn into the collector. To determine the concentration of contaminant, it is necessary that the amount of sample air is known. A number

of measuring devices are available, including the dry gas meter, the wet tes
meter, and the cycloid type meter. These methods measure the quantity of ai
being delivered. The rate of flow can be measured by the use of head meters
including the venturi, flow nozzle, and orifice types. Rate of flow can also
be measured by laminar flow meters and rotameters.

In any case, each of the above methods requires a calibration to assure
that the proper metering occurs. The spirometer is a primary standard again:
which all meters are calibrated. Secondary standards of calibration are ofte
used. This method involves calibration of a meter against a primary
standard. This meter, which is generally more accurate, is then used to
calibrate a second type of meter.

Other equipment necessary for the sampling train includes the sampling
probe which must be inert to contaminants and resist clogging by particulate
matter. It is also necessary that an accurate method for measuring the
temperature, humidity, pressure, and time be provided. Valves to regulate
flow rate should also be present in the sampling train.

Among the factors that should be considered when taking a sample are the
following:

1.   How long to sample.
2.   How much to sample.
3.   Where to sample.
4.   The methods to be used to obtain the sample.
5.   The methods of sample analysis.
6.   The storage of the sample.
7.   The handling of the sample.
8.   The influence of variables such as weather, topography, and other
     factors on the representativeness of the sample.

Determining the Extent of Pollution--Measuring at the Source

A second method to determine the extent of pollution is to measure the
pollution that is resulting from a single source. This provides information
concerning the pollutants that are leaving the plant. From this information,
a determination can be made as to whether the methods of control used within
the plant are adequate.

When it is decided that measurements at the source should take place, the
industrial hygiene engineer must consider all sources of pollutants that may
escape from the plant. These pollutants may result from industrial processes
or may be the result of service equipment such as boiler equipment. All
outlets to the atmosphere and vents from exhaust system or stacks must be
monitored to determine the total extent of the pollution that is entering the
atmosphere from the source.

The procedure for obtaining measurements of pollutants at the source
involves, first, an identification of the pollutant. Is the pollutant a gas,
vapor, or particulate matter? What is the chemical composition of the
pollutant? Do any chemical reactions occur during exhaust that must be

considered? It may be necessary that a qualitative analysis of the emission be taken to determine the type of pollutants that are being exhausted.

The industrial hygiene engineer should determine <u>where the sample is to be taken</u>. It can be taken in the exhaust system prior to the fan, or it may be taken in the stack or at the vents. The location chosen depends on the particular situation involved. In some cases, it may be difficult to take measurements within the stack, while in other cases these measurements may yield a combined pollutant resulting from a chemical reaction that is unknown if measurements are taken in each of the individual exhaust ducts.

The next step is to <u>determine the velocity of the air</u> traveling through the duct or in the stack. In order to ascertain this, a traverse of the duct or stack is necessary. A pitot tube or anemometer can be used for this traverse, depending upon the velocity and temperature of the air within the duct. Using the average velocity obtained and a measurement of the diameter of the outlet, the industrial hygiene engineer can determine the rate of flow at which the pollutant is entering the surrounding atmosphere.

A determination should be made of the <u>pressure, gas, temperature, and moisture content</u> that is present in the emission. These factors will affect the rate of flow if significantly different from nonstandard conditions.

As in the case of sampling ambient air, it is necessary to develop a sampling train to <u>collect and measure the sample</u> from the source. If particulate matter is involved, it is desirable to determine the expected particle size since, unless special care is taken, agglomeration as well as particle breakup can occur during the collection process. Filtration is commonly used to collect particulate contaminants within the stack. A cyclone dust separator may also be used prior to the filter to remove large particles. Other methods that may be used include impingement and electrostatic precipitation. If a gas or vapor is present, the collection can be through either adsorption or absorption equipment as in measuring ambient air. Air movers and metering devices are also required when sampling from the source. Movers are much like the pumps and ejectors that are used in sampling ambient air, and the air metering methods are also the same. However, it is necessary that the velocity of the sampling train match that of the duct or stack (isokinetic conditions). This is often accomplished by using a static balanced tube or probe or by adjusting the sampling rate and nozzle size to match the velocity in the duct or stack. If these precautions are not taken and the duct or stack velocity differs significantly from that of the sampling train, then either too much or too little air will be sampled.

After the collection of the sample, a <u>measurement and analysis</u> must be made to determine the quantity and chemical composition of the materials gathered. These results can be compared to regulated standards and/or desired results to determine if the proper control is being exercised.

Other observations can be made concerning the plume appearance, the presence of water droplets in gas, the presence of deposits in the stack, and the nature of these droplets. In addition, the production schedule for the process producing the contaminants should be considered. Some production facilities operate on a cyclic basis while others are continuous. Obviously,

the timing of the sample must coincide with the production schedule.   Sampli
during the worst possible conditions will provide a measure of safety in ter
of errors made and pollutants emitted to the atmosphere.

Control of Environmental Air Pollution

This subject has been discussed in much detail in the previous chapter
concerning air-cleaning devices.   However, it is useful to review the genera
methods that are available.   The basic types of air cleaners are--

Cleaners for Particulate Matter

        Mechanical collectors
            Settling chambers
            Cyclones
            Impingers
            Dynamic precipitators
        Filtration
            Deep-bed filters
            Fabric filters (bag houses)
            High-efficiency panel filters
        Wet collectors
            Cyclone scrubbers
            Chamber scrubbers
            Self-induced spray scrubbers
            Wet impingement scrubbers
            Venturi scrubbers
            Mechanical scrubbers
        Electrostatic precipitators

Cleaners for Gases and Vapors

        Adsorbers
        Absorbers (generally equivalent to scrubbers)
        Incinerators
        Catalytic combustion

Weather Considerations for Pollution Control

As has been stated many times, weather is something we all discuss but ca
do very little about.   This is also true in the case of air pollution.
Weather factors cannot be changed.   However, it is desirable to consider
weather in terms of where to locate a plant or process as well as to determin
the location and size of any particular stack or vent.   Weather conditions
will also help to determine the vector of travel as well as the dispersion of
pollutants that are emitted from the plant.

The first factor to consider when looking at weather patterns is the
wind.   Generally, an area has a prevailing wind: that is, a wind that blows
from a particular direction the greatest percentage of the time.   The speed a

which this wind travels as well as the variability of speed are important considerations in determining the dispersion of pollution. In addition to the wind, one must consider the effects of topography and the height of the pointof emission on the pollution generated. If the topography is relatively rough, then a turbulence can be expected that results in a high variability of wind direction, thus making it difficult to predict the path of the contaminant flow.

A second factor to consider when looking at the weather is the temperature lapse rate. The <u>temperature lapse rate</u> is defined as the rate of decrease of temperature with height. Given certain meteorological conditions, a warm blanket of air can be trapped close to the earth by a cold air blanket above; this phenomenon is called an inversion. When this situation occurs, pollutants that are introduced into the atmosphere tend to stay close to the ground and do not disperse widely, causing difficulties because of their concentration. It is during these periods of inversion that major air pollution problems have occurred.

Precipitation cleans the air, much like water sprayed in a spray-tower air cleaner. As precipitation falls, it removes particles from the air and may absorb gases or vapors in the air. These contaminants are then washed to the ground.

The actual temperature range that is experienced within an area can be of importance in air pollution problems. The range of temperature from morning to evening provides a rough index concerning the stability of the air layers. In addition, when the temperature ranges to very cold, a significant pollution effect may be expected from the operation of heating systems.

Humidity is a factor that must also be considered. If the air is too dry, the result is a loading of dust through natural causes. If the air becomes too humid, the resulting fog can hold an inversion longer by preventing the sun from heating the lower air and making it rise. This traps pollutants that can attach themselves easily to water vapors in the air.

In the same manner, cloud cover affects the temperature lapse rate and results in a higher possibility of inversion. In any case, even though there is nothing we can do about the weather, it is important that we understand those factors that can affect the rate of pollution present in a given area.

Summary

The installation of a ventilation system to remove contaminants from the workplace area does not complete the responsibility of the industrial hygiene engineer. It is necessary to assure that the contaminants are not dumped outside the plant where harmful effects to the general population and environment will result. In order to prevent such a situation from arising, an air cleaner can be attached to the ventilation system to remove contaminants before they enter the atmosphere.

In order to determine if air pollution is present, two general methods of sampling can be employed. The industrial hygiene engineer may sample the ambient air in the community. This provides information concerning the concentration of contaminants to which various segments of the population a exposed. On the other hand, sampling of the exhaust stack can be performed which will indicate the extent of contaminants being introduced at a single source. Both methods involve essentially the same equipment but provide different information.

19. References

Alden, John L. and John M. Kane. Design of Industrial Exhaust Systems, 4th edition. New York: Industrial Press, Inc., 1970.

American Conference of Governmental Industrial Hygienists. Air Sampling Instruments for Evaluation of Atmospheric Contaminants, 4th edition. Cincinnati: American Conference of Governmental Industrial Hygienists, 1972.

American Conference of Governmental Industrial Hygienists, Committee on Industrial Ventilation. Industrial Ventilation: A Manual of Recommended Practice, 13th edition. Lansing: American Conference of Governmental Industrial Hygienists, 1974.

American Industrial Hygiene Association. Heating and Cooling for Man in Industry. Akron: American Industrial Hygiene Association, 1970.

Caplan, Knowlton J., ed. Air Pollution Manual Part II--Control Equipment. Akron: American Industrial Hygiene Association, 1968.

Giever, Paul M., ed. Air Pollution Manual Part I--Evaluation. 2d. edition. Akron: American Industrial Hygiene Association, 1972.

Hagopian, John H. and E. Karl Bastress. Engineering Control Research Recommendations. United States Department of Health, Education, and Welfare, Public Health Service, Center for Disease Control, National Institute for Occupational Safety and Health, Cincinnati: U. S. Government Printing Office, 1976.

Hagopian, John H. and E. Karl Bastress. Recommended Industrial Ventilation Guidelines. United States Department of Health, Education, and Welfare, Public Health Service, Center for Disease Control, National Institute for Occupational Safety and Health. Cincinnati: U. S. Government Printing Office, 1976.

Hanna, George. Principles of Ventilation. Unpublished. Cincinnati: National Institute for Occupational Safety and Health.

Hemeon, W. C. L. Plant and Process Ventilation, 2d. edition. New York: Industrial Press, Inc., 1963.

Hewitt, Paul G. Conceptual Physics . . . A New Introduction to Your Environment, 2d. edition. Boston: Little Brown and Company, 1974.

Horvath, Steven M. and Roger C. Jensen, eds. Standards for Occupational Exposures to Hot Environments. Proceedings of Symposium, February 27-28, 1973. U. S. Department of Health, Education, and Welfare, Public Health Service, Center for Disease Control, National Institute for Occupational Safety and Health, Cincinnati: U. S. Government Printing Office, 1976.

Jorgensen, Robert. Fan Engineering, 7th edition. New York: Buffalo Forge Co., 1970.

___. Recirculation of Exhaust Air--Proceedings of Seminar. U. S. Department of Health, Education, and Welfare, Public Health Service, Center for Disease Control, National Institute for Occupational Safety and Health, Cincinnati: U. S. Government Printing Office, 1976.

Schaum, Daniel. College Physics, 6th edition. New York: McGraw-Hill Book Company, 1961.

___. Basic Course -- Particulate Contaminants, Unpublished. Cincinnati: National Institute for Occupational Safety and Health, 1972.

___. Gas and Vapor Sampling Course Manual, Unpublished. Cincinnati: National Institute for Occupational Safety and Health.

___. Lectures on Sampling for Gases and Vapors, Unpublished. Cincinnati: National Institute for Occupational Safety and Health.

___. The Industrial Environment: Its Evaluation and Control. Washington: U. S. Government Printing Office, 1973.

Section 3

Thermal Stress

1. Heat Exchange and Its Effects on Man

<u>Heat Exchange</u>

Heat is a form of energy, while cold is the absence of heat or the absenc of this energy. Quite often there exists a confusion between the terms "heat and "temperature." <u>Heat</u> itself is a measure of the energy in terms of quantity. <u>Temperature</u> on the other hand, is a measure of the intensity of th heat or the hotness of an object.

A review of two examples will help to clarify the difference between heat and temperature. Consider a large block of iron and a small block of iron that are being heated with the same amount of energy. If the source of energy is removed after a given amount of time, the temperature of the smaller block will be higher than that of the larger block. The same amount of heat has been transferred to the blocks of iron, but the temperature readings differ. On the other hand, suppose a small quantity of water and a large quantity of water are both brought to the boiling point. The temperature of both quantities of water will be the same; i.e., 100°C or 212°F. However, it will take a longer period of time to bring the large quantity of water to the boiling point; thus, the amount of heat required will be greater. In this case, the temperature of each body of water is the same, but the amount of heat required to raise the body to this temperature is different.

Temperature is measured in terms of degrees. This measurement may be in degrees Fahrenheit, degrees Celsius, degrees Kelvin, or degrees Rankine. Conversion from one temperature scale to another can be accomplished using the following formulas:

$$(3.1.1) \quad °F = 9/5°C + 32$$
$$(3.1.2) \quad °C = 5/9(°F - 32)$$
$$(3.1.3) \quad °K = °C + 273$$
$$(3.1.4) \quad °R = °F + 460$$

Note: The actual values for the constants in (3.1.3) and (3.1.4) are 273.16 and 459.69, respectively. However, the rounded values are accurate enough for most work.

The measurement of heat energy is in terms of either calories or British Thermal Units (BTU). The <u>calorie</u> is defined as the quantity of heat necessary to raise the temperature of 1 gram of water 1°C. Since there is some variance between quantities of heat required depending on the beginning and ending temperature, the calorie is based on a standard temperature of 16.5°C to 17.5°C. The <u>BTU</u> is the quantity of heat necessary to raise the temperature of 1 pound of water 1°F.

Not all materials require the same amount of heat to raise their temperature one degree Celsius or Fahrenheit. The concept of specific heat has been conceived to handle this fact. The <u>specific heat</u> of a material is the quantity of heat that is necessary to raise 1 gram or 1 pound of the substance 1°C or 1°F. Again, this figure is based on a standard of 16.5°C to 17.5°C. The heat capacity is related to the specific heat in that it is the quantity of heat necessary to raise the temperature of a given material 1°. <u>Heat capacity</u> is stated as the amount of heat necessary to raise a unit mass of a substance 1 degree (°C or °F resulting in calories or BTU's).

As heat is added or removed from a substance, there is a point when the substance will undergo a change in phase. That is, the substance, if a solid, will become a liquid or, if a liquid, will become either a solid or a gas. For example, as heat is added to water, it reaches a point called the boiling point where the water begins to change its phase to a vapor. On the other hand, as heat is removed from water, it reaches a point where it freezes and becomes a solid. The change of phase does not occur instantaneously. A quantity of heat is required to cause this change in phase. As this phase change is occurring, the temperature does not vary, and the heat appears to be lost in the substance. Two concepts have been introduced to quantify this occurrence. The <u>heat of vaporization</u> is the quantity of heat that is required to vaporize one unit mass of a liquid without changing its temperature. The <u>heat of fusion</u> is the quantity of heat necessary to melt one unit mass of a solid without changing its temperature. The concept of <u>enthalpy</u> or stored energy is somewhat similar to that of heat absorbed during a change of phase.

Figure 3.1.1

Change of phase.

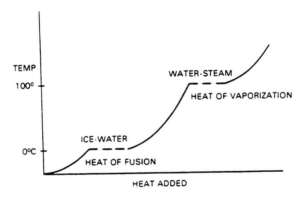

Since heat is energy, a hot body has more energy than a cold body, given the same mass and material for both bodies. The flow of energy is from the highest to the lowest level. Thus, a hot body gives off heat or energy to a colder body. A process in which heat is given off is termed an exothermic process. The converse, or a process in which heat is absorbed, is called an endothermic process.

Methods of Heat Exchange. There are three basic methods for the transfer or exchange of heat between materials. The first method of exchange is by conduction. In conduction heat passes from one part of the body to another. If two bodies are in direct contact, the heat will pass from one body directly to the other as if the two bodies were one single body. Conduction takes place only if a difference in temperature exists between the two bodies or parts of a single body. The conduction of heat is different for different materials. Metals usually conduct heat well; solids are generally better conductors of heat than liquids; and gases are the poorest conductors. For the most part, conduction is of little importance when considering problems involving hot environments and heat stress situations since the worker must be in contact with the surface for conduction to take place.

The second method of heat transfer is convection. Convection is a process where the transfer of heat occurs as a result of the movement of a fluid past a source of heat. The rate of convection is affected by the characteristics of the fluid that is moving past the source of heat, the surface of the heat source, the position of the source surface, the velocity of the fluid, and the relative temperature of the source and fluid. In most situations, the fluid is air; and the heat is transferred to the surrounding environment by induced air current movement. Convection itself causes the movement of the fluid. As the air is heated, it expands and becomes lighter. The lighter air rises away from the hot source, and colder air flows in to replace the heated air. The heated air mixes with the environment to cause a general increase in temperature. If the air and source are the same temperature, no movement will be induced. The transfer of heat can be increased by increasing the flow in the fluid using mechanical means. Convection is of major significance as a method of heat transfer in a hot environment. Thus, the industrial hygiene engineer must be very concerned with convective heat transfer.

The third method of heat transfer is radiation. Radiation differs from convection and conduction in that no fluid or solid need be present for the heat to be transferred from one object to another. The heat energy is transferred from a hot body to its surroundings in the form of electromagnetic waves or infrared radiation. An example of radiant heat is the thermal energy that is transferred to the earth from the sun. Generally, the wavelength of radiant heat is not visible; however, as an object becomes hotter, the wave length shortens and enters the visible spectrum. When an object is termed "red hot," this means that it is hot enough to emanate radiation in the red spectrum which is approximately 700°C. The color of light from the hot object indicates its approximate temperature. Thus, white hot is an extremely high temperature (approximately 1200°C).

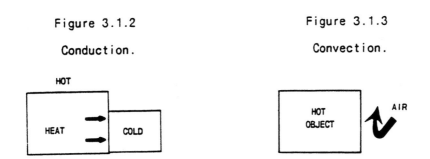

Figure 3.1.2

Conduction.

Figure 3.1.3

Convection.

Figure 3.1.4

Radiation.

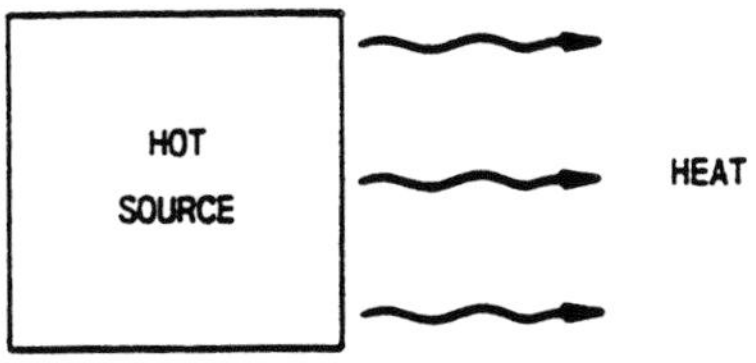

Radiant heat may be either reflected or absorbed. Highly polished surfaces, such as aluminum, are generally good reflectors. On the other hand, black bodies are good absorbers. A common example of this phenomenon can be seen by the fact that dirty snow, which is darker, melts faster than clean, white snow which reflects more of the radiant energy.

The rate of heat exchange by radiation depends on a number of factors. The difference in absolute temperature of the surfaces of the body and its surroundings affects the rate of heat exchange by radiation. If a body and its surroundings are the same temperature, then no radiant heat energy will be transferred from the body to its surroundings. A second factor is the relative emissivity of the body and its surroundings. Emissivity is the ratio of the energy radiated by a given surface and that which would be radiated by a perfect black body at the same surface temperature. This leads to a general statement of Kirchoff's law of radiation. This law states essentially that a body is as effective as a radiator as it is as an absorber. Thus, a poor absorber is likewise a poor radiator; a good absorber is a good radiator; and a poor absorber is a good reflector. This information is of significant value when determining control methods for radiant heat stress.

Sources of Heat

Two major sources of heat that are of concern are the environment itself and metabolic heat generated by the workers within the environment. In order to provide adequate control of heat within the workplace, it is necessary to identify the heat sources.

Often the climate and solar radiation generate significant amounts of heat within a workplace. Workers who are required to perform their job functions out of doors in hot climates are subjected to heat and humidity present in the air as well as solar radiation. These factors are also present within plant structures themselves. Hot outside air entering a hot plant will provide no relief from the heat within the plant. Also, solar radiation absorbed by the plant roof can add an additional heat load within the industrial building.

In many cases, the industrial process adds significant heat to the workers' environment. The air temperature may be increased as convectional currents pass by hot processes. Radiation emanating from high-temperature processes can provide an additional heat load. Steam that is used in many processes adds not only heat but also humidity to the air. Mechanical and electrical equipment can generate large quantities of heat in their normal operation. Finally, normal plant facilities, such as illumination and steam distribution piping, can also be a significant factor in increasing the overall heat load in the environment.

A second source of heat that is of concern is <u>metabolic heat</u>. Heat is a normal by-product of the body's activity. As the cells work to perform their functions, heat is generated. This heat is generally termed <u>basal heat</u>. If the individual is involved in physical work, additional heat is generated as by-product of the muscular activity. The basal heat and work heat must be dissipated into the atmosphere, or they can present a hazard to the worker. If the environmental conditions in the workplace do not provide appropriate relief to the worker for this metabolic
and work heat, an accumulation of heat will occur in the worker's body. Such an accumulation of heat can result in various physiological reactions that can be harmful to the worker's health. The resulting heat-induced illnesses will be further discussed later in this chapter.

Physiological Responses to Extreme Temperatures

The hypothalamus, located in the base of the brain, is the regulatory center that controls the response of the human system to heat. The hypothalamus acts to attempt to maintain a thermal balance within the body. This balance is maintained with a deep body or core temperature of approximately 37°C (98.6°F). The skin temperature normally varies between 33°C and 34°C (91.4°-93.2°F), but it may be near the core temperature or be 10° lower than the core temperature if the individual is exposed to extreme temperature ranges. The oral temperature that is familiar to all ranges from 36°C to 37°C (97° to 98.6°F).

As the body begins to build up heat, the hypothalamus initiates certain physiological reactions. The heart rate increases, and the blood vessels dilate to increase circulation in the body. This increased blood flow carries heat away from the inner core of the body to the skin surface where heat is dissipated into the surrounding environment. Increased respiratory activity also occurs. In this manner, exhaled air carries heat away from the body. Along with this increased circulation and respiration, the body begins to sweat. The heat of vaporization, that is, the heat necessary to cause a liquid to vaporize, requires a significant expenditure of heat energy. As the body sweats and the sweat is evaporated into the atmosphere, the vaporization requires significant amounts of heat. In this manner, heat generated within the body is dissipated without raising the body temperature.

On the other hand, the absence of heat, or cold, can also present a problem. In general, man's tolerance to cold is less than his tolerance to heat. Clothing makes up for this lack of tolerance and allows working in temperatures that are far below that which a nude human would be able to tolerate. The general physiological response that occurs when a human is exposed to extreme cold is shivering. This shivering creates muscle activity and results in the generation of heat. Shivering is the method that the body uses to generate heat to maintain its core temperature in equilibrium. When the body is exposed to cold, the blood vessels contract to restrict the flow of blood to the surface, thus conserving heat within the core of the body. Humans will also attempt to remain active during exposure to cold, though they may not be aware of it, thus generating additional heat to maintain thermal equilibrium. The lethal lower core temperature for the human body is 26°C (78°F).

Stress and Strain

Stress is the acting force on the body. Thermal stress is either the presence of excess heat or the absence of sufficient heat. Stress may be thought of as the cause of a given human response.

Strain, on the other hand, is the result of stress. Strain may be thought of as the cost or consequence in the human body of a given stress being placed upon it. When the response of the human system is abnormal, this is a result of some strain that has been experienced. Strain can be measured in terms of the physiological response, in terms of heart rate, respiratory rate, etc.; or it may be indicated from the disorders that arise.

Indicators of Thermal Strain

As was discussed above, the objective of the physiological response of the human system is to maintain the core temperature in equilibrium. If the core temperature drops below 26°C or rises above 41°C (106°F), damage and potential death will occur. In particular, as the temperature rises above 41°C, the regulating ability of the hypothalamus is depressed. Thus, the body's ability to regulate its temperature is depressed, resulting in a vicious cycle in which the core temperature continues to rise. Only external action, such as an alcohol bath or immersion in cold water, will prevent death to such an exposed individual.

Figure 3.1.5

Stress vs. strain.

STRESS

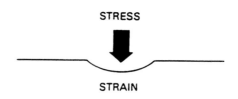

STRAIN

A chain of events is initiated when the human system is exposed to heat stress. The first response of the body is for the regulatory functions to begin to work. If these functions can work properly, and if excessive heat stress is not present, the body will attain thermal equilibrium. On the other hand, if the heat stress is such that the regulatory functions cannot control the buildup of heat, the result is a heat disorder.

There are generally four categories of heat disorders that are of interest. The first disorder that is recognized by many medical personnel is termed heat syncope. Because of excessive pooling of the blood in the extremities resulting from the body's attempt to dissipate heat by increased circulatory activity and dilation of the blood vessels, the brain does not receive an adequate supply of oxygen. The result is that the exposed individual loses consciousness. This reaction is similar to heat exhaustion except that it is likely to occur much more quickly without any accompanying physical exertion on the part of the worker. Heat syncope is directly related to the circulatory response of the affected individuals.

A second disorder is heat exhaustion. As the worker performs physical tasks in the hot environment, profuse sweating occurs, and the circulatory and respiratory activity is increased. If the worker sustains the physical activity for an extended time period, the body will become dehydrated and/or the circulatory system will become overworked. Then the worker will experience fatigue, nausea, headache, and giddiness. The skin will be moist and clammy, indicating that sweating is still present, but the circulatory system may cause a pooling of blood that leads to fainting. The skin may appear either pale or flushed.

The third disorder that may occur is heat cramps. Heat cramps are a result of profuse sweating that dissipates body salt along with the loss of fluids. The general sign of such a disorder is a painful muscle cramp spasm. Heat cramps are generally caused by sweating and hard work without adequate fluid and salt replacement.

Finally, the most severe heat disorder is heat stroke. Heat stroke is a failure of the body's thermal regulatory system. Unless controlled immediately, heat stroke can result in an increased body temperature beyond which cell damage occurs. Death is likely unless external action is taken to control the rising temperature. Heat stroke is evidenced by hot, dry, red

skin, rapid pulse, and an absence of sweating. Figure 3.1.6 illustrates the
progression of the human physiological response to heat stress.

In terms of treatment, heat cramps are generally easily prevented by
providing adequate salt for the worker. This may be either in the form of
salt tablets or in a one-tenth percent (0.1%) salt and water solution that the
worker should ingest frequently. For heat syncope, the worker can be
acclimatized (to be discussed later in this chapter) or encouraged to remain
somewhat active to stimulate return circulation to the heart. If a worker is
suffering from heat exhaustion, it is adequate to remove the worker from the
source of heat and provide fluid and salt replacement along with adequate rest
to allow the body to recover. Provision of salt should be done with care,
since an excess of salt can be harmful to individuals suffering from
cardiovascular disorders.

Heat stroke requires immediate positive action. The worker should be
removed from the heat and action taken to cool the body, either through cold
compresses, immersion in cold water, or an alcohol bath. Fluids should be
replaced as soon as possible, since one of the initial causes of heat stroke
is the dehydration of the body.

Figure 3.1.6

Effects of heat stress.

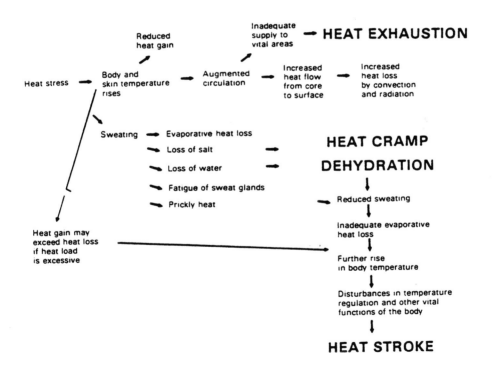

Factors in Heat Stress

For a given temperature, the thermal stress that is placed on an individual varies. There are a number of factors, both environmental and individual, that cause this variance.

The environmental factors that affect stress are the movement of air, the moisture content of the air, and the radiant heat load. Air movement is important in reducing heat stress. As the air moves past the worker, it carries away vapor from the evaporated sweat on the worker's skin, thus cooling the body. Without such air movement, the body would become insulated by the surface sweat, and sufficient cooling could not take place.

The moisture content of the air, or humidity, is also important. If the vapor pressure in the environment is high, then sweat does not evaporate. As a result, the cooling that normally occurs during the evaporation of sweat does not take place, and heat builds up in the body.

The radiant heat load is in addition to that which results from convection and metabolic heat. This heat load can be high enough to produce an excessive thermal stress on the individual even in cases where adequate air movement is present to allow for evaporative cooling.

The thermal stress that occurs in workers varies between given workers as a result of certain individual factors. The surface to weight ratio for a worker is of importance since heat loss is a function of area, and heat production is a function of weight. Because of this, obese or stocky individuals are affected by heat more than slender individuals, since they produce a greater amount of heat and have a proportionally smaller area in which the heat can be dissipated.

Age is another factor that can affect the physiological response to heat stress. Workers in the range of 40 to 65 years of age are not so tolerant of heat as are younger workers. This may be somewhat as a result of the fact that young workers have a better respiratory and circulatory response system.

Workers who have a history of cardiovascular disease are especially subjected to strain resulting from heat stress. This is a result of the reduced capacity of the cardiovascular system to react to dissipate heat from the body.

The physical fitness of the worker is also important. Through improved conditioning, the individual develops an increased cardiovascular response and, in addition, an increased efficiency of muscle use. This increased muscular efficiency results in lower heat generation when performing a particular task.

The alcoholic habits of the worker will also affect his tolerance to heat. Alcohol dehydrates the body, and as a result, dehydration can occur more quickly when the worker is subjected to heat stress.

Acclimatization. Experiments have shown that individuals respond to heat stress with strain at the first exposure. If these individuals are exposed regularly to heat stress, the amount of strain is reduced. After one to two weeks of exposure to above normal temperatures, no strain is present. These experiments have led to the practice of acclimatizing workers. During acclimatization, the worker is gradually exposed to longer periods of heat stress until the possibility of heat strain is minimized. In general, acclimatized workers exhibit an increased sweat rate (thus, more efficient cooling) with a lower salt loss than those workers who are not acclimatized.

However, acclimatization is lost quickly. In fact. experiments have shown that there is some loss of acclimatization after a weekend away from work. After two weeks away from work, this loss is substantial. Therefore, in order for acclimatization to be effective in reducing heat strain, it must be reinforced regularly.

On the other hand, humans do not generally become acclimatized to cold temperatures. There is no significant differences between the tolerance to cold of Eskimos in Alaska and that of native southern Americans.

Other Effects of Heat Stress. Aside from the physiological effects of heat stress, there are other effects that may result. Psychologically, the individual exposed to heat stress becomes edgy and develops a lassitude toward accomplishing a given task. The performance efficiency of these individuals is lowered, resulting in a potential for increased accidents.

Excessive heat stress can also have an effect on the morale of the worker. As a result, difficulties in handling workers in heat stress areas may be significantly greater than those experienced with workers performing under normal temperature conditions. Also, the performance of individuals exposed to heat stress may be decreased not only as a response to heat but also as a response to the lowered morale of the worker.

Summary

Often within the industrial environment the worker is subjected to extreme temperatures. If these temperatures are above normal, the worker can be subjected to developing illnesses such as heat cramps, heat syncope, heat exhaustion, and heat stroke. In these cases, the thermal load is such that the body's thermal regulatory functions cannot act to dissipate the heat buildup rapidly enough.

Strain resulting from a given thermal stress differs between individuals. Important factors, such as the physical build, age, condition, and alcoholic habits of the worker act to cause these differences.

Repeated exposure to thermal stress can acclimatize the worker. The acclimatization helps to lower the strain experienced for a given thermal stress.

2. Thermal Measurement

Introduction

It is not simple to determine the thermal stress to which the worker is subjected. Obviously the temperature of the work environment is significant. However, temperature alone does not determine thermal stress. The presence of water vapor in the air (humidity) must also be considered, since humidity is a determining factor in the rate of sweat evaporation. Also, air movement in the workroom environment must be considered. Without adequate air movement, evaporated sweat cannot be carried away from the worker, and the vapor pressure around the worker increases, thus reducing the evaporative cooling that can occur. In addition, the industrial hygiene engineer must determine if a radiant heat load is present, since radiant heat can be a major factor in the thermal stress present in an environment. Also to be considered are the problems associated with the metabolic heat generated by the workers' activities and the individual differences of the workers in response to heat stress. It is obvious, then, that a simple measurement of the temperature of the ambient air in the environment is not sufficient to determine thermal stress.

The temperature reading with which we are all familiar is taken using a dry-bulb thermometer. It is obvious from the discussion above that the dry-bulb thermometer alone is not adequate for determining the level of thermal stress. Consideration must be given to the presence of water vapor, air movement, radiant heat, and worker activity in order to determine the total thermal stress present in the environment. The instrumentation should always be located so that the readings obtained are representative of the environmental conditions to which the workers are exposed. The sensors should be located at chest height of the worker, and due consideration should be given to the location of radiation sources and the direction of air movement.

Measurement of Air Temperature

Air temperature may be measured by a variety of instruments, each of which may have advantages under certain circumstances. Mercury (or alcohol)-in-glass thermometers, the usual common glass thermometer, is often used for determining air temperature. Because of its very common nature, sometimes the simplest of precautions are neglected.

Thermometers may be in error by several degrees. Each thermometer should be calibrated over its range in a suitable medium (usually a temperature-controlled oil bath) against a known standard, e.g., National Bureau of Standards--certified, thermometer. Only thermometers with the graduations marked on the stem should be used. Those with scale markings on a mounting board can be off by 10 degrees; further the stem can shift relative to the mounting board. It seems superfluous to specify that the range of the thermometer should be selected to cover the anticipated environment where the mercury will not break the capillary glass tube; this is not an unusual occurrence in practice.

Sometimes the liquid column in a thermometer will separate. Before readings are taken, the continuity of the column should be checked. Separated columns may be rejoined by shaking, or by heating in hot water (never a flame!). When measurements are taken, it is important that the dry-bulb thermometer be sheltered from any source of radiant heat since the measurement that is desired is that of the ambient air. For example, in outdoor measurements, an unshielded dry-bulb thermometer may be several degrees higher than a shielded dry-bulb thermometer.

The second method that can be used to measure the temperature of the ambient air is a thermoelectric thermometer. The operation of this device is based on the fact that when two dissimilar metals are joined, and the temperature of the junction is changed, a small voltage is generated. Two junctions in a circuit, with one held at a known temperature ("reference junction") form the basic elements of a thermocouple. The current flowing in the circuit resulting from the voltage (electromotive force) generated may be measured directly by a galvanometer, or the electromotive force may be balanced by a known source potentiometrically. The latter technique is preferred, as the length of the thermocouple (hence its resistance) becomes of no consequence when the current flowing becomes zero. Each thermocouple used with a current measuring device must be calibrated individually. Figure 3.2.1 shows a schematic arrangement of the components in a thermocouple system. Instruments of this type must be calibrated to assure accuracy in measurement.

Figure 3.2.1

Thermocouple.

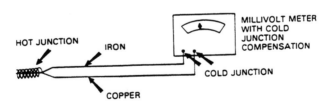

A thermocouple has certain advantages over a mercury-in-glass thermometer:

1. Provides a method for obtaining the surface temperature of an object where the bulb of a thermometer would not be appropriate, e.g., skin surface.

2. Thermojunctions may be placed at the measurement site and read remotely over long distances, if desired.

3.   Simultaneous readings from several locations may be read at one place using one potentiometer with a rotary selector switch in the circuit.

4.   Adaptable for use when continuous monitoring and recording are necessary.

5.   Equilibrium time with changing temperatures is virtually instantaneous, whereas mercury-in-glass thermometers may require several minutes to reach a steady state.

Another method that can be used to measure the ambient air temperature is the thermistor. Thermistors are semiconductors which exhibit substantial change in resistance in response to a small change in temperature. As the resistance of the thermistor itself is measured in thousands of ohms, the resistance imposed by lead wires up to 25 meters or so is immaterial, permitting remote readings as with thermocouples. Readout equipment is battery-powered, relatively light, and portable which is convenient for field studies. The advantages of thermistors are:

1.   Simple to use with minimum training.

2.   Less bulky and complicated to use than thermocouples.

3.   Requires no reference junction.

4.   Output signal may be recorded.

5.   Variety of probes available for special applications.

Thermistor probes, though they are called "interchangeable," require individual calibration before use. Calibration of thermistor beads will shift somewhat with age, requiring annual or biennial recalibration. The advantages of the thermistor thermometer make it the instrument of choice for field use when mercury-in-glass thermometers are inappropriate.

Measurement of Radiant Heat

The standard method for measuring radiant heat is the black globe thermometer (Vernon Globe). A black globe thermometer is constructed of a 6-inch diameter thin-copper sphere that is painted matte black. A hole is drilled in the sphere into which a rubber stopper can be placed. A mercury-in-glass thermometer, having a range of 30° to 220°F with 1°F graduations and accurate to ± 1°F is inserted through a rubber stopper in a hole in the top of the shell and the thermometer bulb is located at the center of the globe. Where it is desirable for quicker readings, a thermocouple or thermistor can be used in place of the mercury-in-glass thermometer.

The black globe acts to absorb the radiant heat that is being emitted from a source. The thermometer inside the globe reaches equilibrium after a period of time, generally between twenty and thirty minutes.

Figure 3.2.2

Globe thermometer.

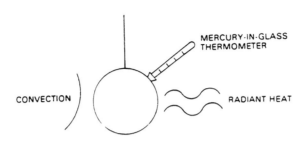

The globe itself is subject to convective air temperatures on its outer surface. The convection acts to reduce some of the heat that is absorbed by the globe. Thus, it is not the actual radiant energy that is being measured but some lesser amount of energy. The energy being measured is generally termed the "mean radiant temperature." The mean radiant temperature can be calculated after equilibrium has been reached between the convective heat loss on the outside of the globe and the radiant heat gain inside the globe. The mean radiant temperature is calculated as follows:

$$(3.2.1) \quad T_w = [(T_g + 460)^4 + (0.103 \times 10^9 v^{0.5})(T_g - T_a)]^{0.25} - 460$$

where

T_w = the mean radiant temperature °F
T_g = the measured globe temperature at equilibrium in °F
v = velocity of the air in ft/min
T_a = temperature of the air from a dry bulb reading in °F

Notice that the formula above takes into account both the measured globe temperature and the dry-bulb temperature. In this way, the formula accounts for heat energy lost by convection around the globe.

Measurement of Air Velocity

As noted previously, heat transfer by convection and by evaporation are functions of movement of the ambient air. While the units associated with air motion--distance per unit time--suggest movement of the mass of air past a point, turbulent air with little net mass movement will be as effective in heat transfer as linear movement.

Directional instruments, useful in ventilation engineering or meteorology, are usually not applicable for assessment of heat stress. On the other hand, instruments which depend upon a rate of cooling of a heated element provide readings meaningful in terms of "cooling power" of the moving air, and are thus the instruments of choice.

One useful instrument of this type is a thermoanemometer. There are several variations of this available. One measures air motion by the rate of cooling of a heated thermocouple at the tip of the probe. One thermojunction is heated by a constant current supplied to a heater wire; the other junction is located in the air stream. The air speed governs the rate of heat removal from the heated thermocouple, which in turn determines its millivolt output. The scale is calibrated directly in feet per minute. The low mass of the thermocouple permits almost instantaneous response of the instrument. Batteries supply the power to the unit, thus making it portable and self-contained. The heater supports and the thermocouple restricts airflow somewhat; in order to obtain the maximum reading, the probe should be slightly rotated.

Another version of the thermoanemometer has two matched thermometers which are mounted about 5 cm apart in the environment. One of the thermometer bulbs is wrapped with a fine resistance wire. Current from a battery passing through the wire heats the bulb. The second thermometer is bare. The temperature differential between the heated and the unheated thermometers depends on the current through the wire (adjustable), and the air speed. The voltage is set between 2 to 6 volts, depending on the range of air speed encountered. At high air speeds, greater heat input is required to obtain sufficient differential between the thermometers for reliable readings. Knowing this temperature differential and the voltage, the operator may find the air speed from the calibration curves supplied with each instrument. Achieving equilibrium requires 2 to 5 minutes. On the one hand, this provides an integrating effect in turbulent air, but on the other hand makes determination of air speed at many locations tedious. Its design, however, assures relatively non-directional response.

The Anemotherm, which is similar in operation to the first thermoanemometer mentioned, uses a heated resistance wire instead of a heated thermocouple circuit as one leg of the wheatstone bridge. The Anemotherm can be used to measure temperature and static pressure also.

The Kata thermometer was developed to determine the cooling power of air as a measure of efficiency of ventilation in factories, mines, etc. It is essentially an alcohol-filled thermometer with an outsized bulb. The bulb is heated in warm water until the column rises into the upper reservoir and is then wiped dry. The instrument is suspended in the air stream (it may be hand held, provided the body of the operator does not interfere with the flow of air); the fall of the column from the upper to the lower mark etched on the stem is timed with a stopwatch. The cooling time of the Kata is a function of air speed and air temperature; the air speed is determined from nomograms accompanying the instrument.

Measurement of Humidity

The amount of water vapor in the air (humidity) controls the rate of evaporation of water from skin surface and from other moist tissues, e.g., lungs, respiratory passages, conjunctiva of the eyes, etc. Water, like other liquids, will tend to saturate the surrounding space with vapor. In an enclosed vessel, the amount of water vapor per unit volume in the space above

Figure 3.2.3

Kata thermometer.

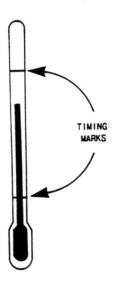

TIMING
MARKS

the water is dependent only on the temperature of the system (assuming
constant pressure). In accordance with Dalton's law of partial pressures,
presence or absence of other species of gases in the space will have no effect
on the amount of water vapor present. If all other gases are evacuated, the
pressure developed is termed the true vapor pressure (or saturation pressure)
of the liquid at the existing temperature. If the temperature is raised,
saturation vapor pressure will increase. When the vapor pressure equals total
atmospheric pressure, boiling occurs. In an open vessel where ambient air
currents carry away the water vapor, continuous evaporation takes place.

"Relative humidity" (RH) is defined as the amount of moisture in the air
compared with the amount that the air could contain at saturation at the same
temperature. It is usually expressed as a percentage. Thus, the amount of
moisture in the air at 50% RH will vary depending on the air temperature.
Since it is the amount of water vapor in the air ("absolute humidity") which
influences evaporation, the relative humidity cannot be used directly to
compute evaporative loss.

As an example, water vapor in air saturated at 0°C exerts a vapor pressure
of about 5 mm Hg. This condition might prevail on a winter's day with
freezing drizzle. When this air is inhaled into the lungs, it passes over
mucous membranes coated with liquid water at 37°C, corresponding to a vapor
pressure of about 45 mm Hg. With this gradient of 40 mm Hg, evaporation
occurs, quickly saturating the air, now warmed to 37°C. Thus air at 100% RH
enters at 0°C, and air at 100% RH leaves at 37°C, yet evaporation has
occurred, and the moisture content differs greatly from inhaled to exhaled

air. On exhalation, the air cools and the new moisture burden condenses out, creating a visible cloud.

Given the relative humidity and the temperature, the water vapor pressure may be determined. In fact, any two properties (temperature, total heat content, dew point, relative humidity, etc.) completely define the thermodynamic state of the air-water vapor mixture. The psychrometric chart is a convenient graphical representation of the mathematical interrelationships of these parameters.

The Psychrometric Chart. The wet-bulb thermometer does not directly measure the presence of humidity in the air. To determine this, it is necessary that a psychrometric chart be used. The psychrometric chart is designed to give the relationship between the temperature of the air as measured on dry and wet bulb thermometers, the relative humidity, the vapor pressure, and the dew point. The dew point is the temperature at which the air becomes saturated without a gain or loss in moisture. The psychrometric chart is constructed assuming standard barometric pressure. Conversion to nonstandard conditions must be made as required.

Multiple charts are generally available to simplify reading at various temperature levels. Not all psychrometric charts are constructed providing exactly the same information. However, the similarities are such that it is fairly easy to transfer from one type of chart to another.

The basic information on a psychrometric chart is presented in Figure 3.2.4. Dry-bulb temperature in degrees Fahrenheit is presented on the abscissa, while grains of water or vapor pressure in millimeters mercury is presented on the ordinate. The wet-bulb temperature can be found by consulting the left-hand margin of the graph section.

As was mentioned previously, you only need two properties to enter the chart and obtain the remaining properties. Generally speaking, however, the two most frequently used properties are the wet-bulb temperature and the dry-bulb temperature. These readings are found on the chart, as well as the additional data concerning the relative humidity, vapor pressure, and dew point. At saturation, the dry-bulb, wet-bulb, and dew-point temperatures are equal.

An example is presented here to illustrate the use of the psychrometric chart. Assume a wet-bulb temperature reading of 75°F and a dry-bulb reading of 100°F are obtained. The psychrometric chart in Figure 3.2.4 shows the intersection of the vertical line from 100°F and the diagonal from a wet-bulb temperature of 75°F. At this point, a relative humidity of 30% exists with a dew point of 62.5°F. The vapor pressure exerted by the water vapor in the air in this situation is 15 mm Hg, which corresponds to approximately 90 grains of water per pound of dry air. Other types of psychrometric charts list additional information, such as enthalpy at saturation and pounds of water per pound of dry air.

Equipment for Measuring Humidity. A sling psychrometer is one of the most popular instruments used for measuring humidity. This instrument consists of

Figure 3.2.4

Psychrometric chart.

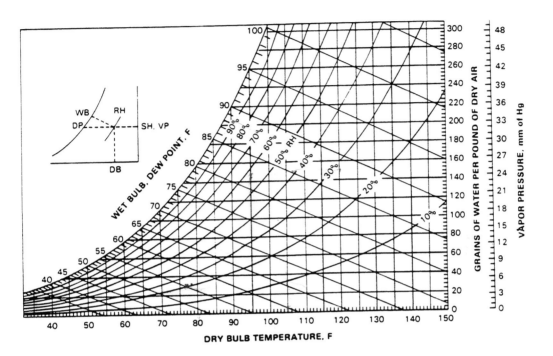

two mercury-in-glass thermometers clamped in a frame which is fastened to a
swivel handle. A cotton wick shielded from radiation and dipped in distilled
water covers one thermometer; the other is bare. The terms "wet-bulb" and
"dry-bulb" temperatures originated from this type of instrument. When it is
rapidly whirled (so that the velocity of air past the thermometers is between
15 and 16 feet per minute) water evaporates from the wick, cooling the bulb.
The rate of evaporation from the wick is a function of the vapor-pressure
gradient, determining in turn the depression of the wet-bulb thermometer
reading below the dry bulb. The vapor pressure can be read directly from the
psychrometric chart or tables.

     To ensure that correct readings are obtained, a few simple precautions
should be observed when using the sling psychrometer. Usually one minute of
swinging adequately cools the wet bulb to its lowest reading. It is advisable
to check the reading, and then swing again for a few seconds. Repeat this
procedure if the temperature continues to fall. You need to achieve the
minimum wet-bulb temperature. Make sure there are no obstructions in the path
of the swinging thermometers. The useful life of the wick can be extended by
using distilled water only. Remember, thermal radiation can cause rather
large errors in both dry- and wet-bulb temperatures taken with a sling
psychrometer.

There are also several types of aspirated psychrometers available, battery-powered for field use, as well as conventional laboratory instruments. These accomplish the same end as the sling psychrometer; air motion across the thermometer bulbs is created mechanically rather than whirling by hand.

Another device used for measuring humidity in the atmosphere is the hair hygrometer. Human hair absorbs and desorbs moisture with changes in atmospheric humidity. The length of hair under tension changes in turn with its moisture content. This motion is transmitted through a system of levers to a pointer indicating the relative humidity. Filled with a pen, the pointer records the relative humidity on a revolving drum.

Figure 3.2.5

Wet bulb thermometer.

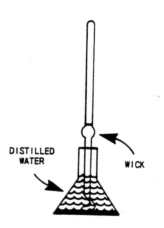

DISTILLED
WATER   WICK

Summary

As has been discussed in this chapter, a measurement of dry-bulb temperature alone is not sufficient to determine the level of heat stress. Other important factors are air movement, the absolute humidity of the air, and the radiant heat load in the environment. These factors can be measured using the equipment discussed in the chapter. One other important factor in determining the thermal stress is individual differences of the workers. Methods for measuring such individual differences do not exist at the present time. Only experience and past history can be used to estimate their effects.

Measurement alone does not determine the level at which a thermal stress will exert a strain on the human body. The measurements obtained must be converted in some manner to a stress level that indicates the point at which a physiological strain will be encountered for most individuals. Various attempts have been made to develop such a method. These attempts will be discussed in the next chapter.

3. Thermal Stress Indices

<u>Introduction</u>

Excessive thermal stress can result in a physiological and psychological strain on the exposed worker. The amount of thermal stress that is present in a work environment is a function of certain environmental measures, such as the temperature of the air, the humidity of the air, the radiant heat load, and the air movement present. These measures have been discussed in the previous chapter.

In addition, stress is a function of certain physiological conditions involving the worker. The amount of acclimatization to which the worker has been exposed affects the stress to which a specific worker is being subjected. The worker's metabolic rate and work rate are also important. In addition, the body surface area-to-weight ratio, as previously discussed, can affect the worker's stress level.

Other important factors have been discussed previously: the worker's clothing, the worker's age, sex, and physical condition. It has been shown that older workers are more subject to strain resulting from thermal stress than younger workers. The worker's sex is also a factor since experiments have shown that tolerance to heat is higher among males than females. The worker's general health and physical condition are also factors that affect the stress that is placed on an individual worker. Since each worker represents a different mixture of the various factors, there are individual variations in the ability to withstand heat stress. This alone presents some difficulties when attempting to determine how much heat will be hazardous to a given group of workers.

On the other hand, the physiological strain that results from thermal stress is a function of the circulatory capacity of the individual, his capacity for sweating, and tolerance to elevated body temperature. In addition, the exposure time is an important factor in determining the strain that is felt by an individual. The human body can withstand high temperatures for short periods of time without causing harmful effects to the health of the exposed individual.

In order to determine the amount of thermal stress above which workers should not be exposed, it is necessary to develop a method that relates stress to strain. That is, it is necessary to state in some manner strain as a function of the stress variables:

$$\text{Strain} = f(\text{Stress})$$

Attempts have been made to develop such a thermal stress index for this relationship. Although many indices have been developed, none are entirely satisfactory. In developing criteria for a thermal stress index, it is important that the following factors be considered:

1.   The index that is developed should be quantitative and yield scalar values relating to stress and strain.

2.   The index should be calculated from available data concerning the conditions that are present in the environment.

3.   The index should be tested and proved applicable through use.

4.   All important factors should be included in the index.

5.   The method should be simple to use and not lead to rigorous calculation or difficult measurements.

6.   All factors included should be related to physiological strain in a weighted manner.

7.   The method should be applicable and feasible for determining regulatory limits or threshold limit values for exposure to heat stress.

In the following discussion, various heat stress indices will be presented. None of the indices totally meets the criteria outlined above. In some cases the calculations and measurements are difficult to obtain. In other cases not all factors are included. However, the indices are the best that are available and are the tools that the industrial hygiene engineer has available to determine if thermal stress is present in the work environment.

The ultimate test of validity of an environmental heat stress index is its ability to provide a number which can be used to accurately predict how people will respond to environmental conditions being measured. Numerous investigators have conducted studies relating human response to various environmental heat levels. Unfortunately the investigators have used several different indices to describe the levels to which the subjects were exposed.

Effective Temperature

The Effective Temperature (ET) is a widely used index that is related to the comfort that is felt in a given atmosphere by individuals subjected to this environment. The Effective Temperature was developed by the American Society of Heating, Refrigeration, and Air-Conditioning Engineers (ASHRAE) in 1923 and was revised in 1950.

The Effective Temperature combines into a single value the temperature of the environment, the humidity of the air, and the air movement. The Effective Temperature scale was developed from empirical data gathered from individuals who indicated the thermal sensation they felt upon entering a given atmosphere. The individuals involved in responding to the environment were either sedentary or normally clothed or stripped to the waist performing light work. The Effective Temperature scale has been used extensively in the field of comfort ventilation and air-conditioning work.

The relationship of Effective Temperature to the wet bulb temperature, the dry bulb temperature, and the air velocity has been plotted for both sedentary individuals and those performing light work. Figure 3.3.1 illustrated the relationship between Effective Temperature and the factors listed for individuals performing light work.

Figure 3.3.1

Effective temperature.

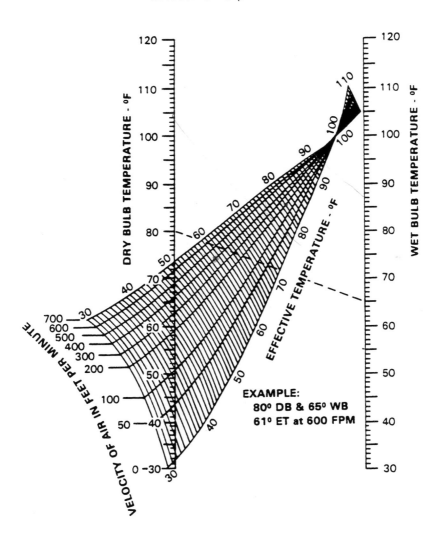

As an example of how to use the graph, consider a dry-bulb temperature of 80°F and a wet-bulb temperature of 65°F in an atmosphere in which the air is moving at 100 feet per minute. Drawing a line between the dry-bulb temperature and the wet-bulb temperature on the vertical graphs, one can determine the point at which this line intersects with the diagonal lines indicating air velocity. Reading diagonally down the Effective Temperature scale, a value of 68.5°F is obtained. These values indicate the degree of warmth felt by individuals in an environment with the conditions listed.

Somewhat akin to the Effective Temperature is the ASHRAE comfort chart (Figure 3.3.2). This index presents the subjective feeling of warmth of an individual after being in an environment for three hours. It is based upon

Figure 3.3.2

Comfort chart for still air.

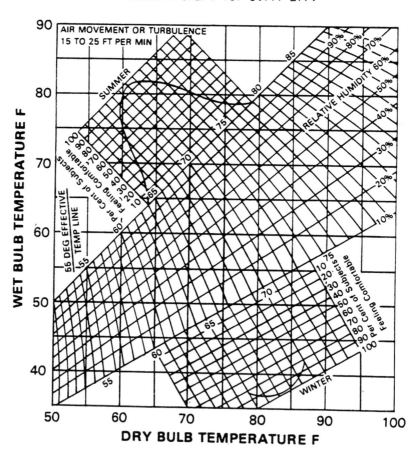

esponses from sedentary individuals wearing light clothing in both summer and winter. This index is quite often used for comfort ventilation determinations.

The Effective Temperature has certain problems when one considers its use as a measure of thermal stress. In the first place, the Effective Temperature requires a radiation correction. The accuracy of this correction has been questioned. In addition, the Effective Temperature does not consider varying work rates and the resulting varying metabolic heat-generation rates. Experience has shown that the Effective Temperature exaggerates stress in hot, dry conditions at air velocities of 100-300 fpm. On the other hand, the Effective Temperature underestimates stress at low air movement with hot, wet conditions. As a result, the Effective Temperature has not proved of significant value in determining the level of heat stress present in a work environment.

Heat-Stress Index

The Heat-Stress Index (HSI) was developed by Belding and Hatch in 1965. The Heat-Stress Index considers the radiant heat load, convective heat load, and metabolic heat generated by the worker. The heat stress relationship is stated below.

(3.3.1) $E_{req} = M \pm R \pm C$

where

E_{req} = the required sweat-evaporation rate to dissipate the heat load in BTU/hr
M = the metabolic heat produced in BTU/hr
R = the radiant heat load in BTU/hr
C = the convective heat load in BTU/hr

Using this relationship, a Heat-Stress Index is developed. The strain relationship is stated as

(3.3.2) $HSI = \dfrac{E_{req}}{E_{max}} \times 100$

where

HSI = the Heat-Stress Index
E_{max} = the maximum evaporative heat loss in BTU/hr

From the relationship for the Heat-Stress Index stated above, it can been seen that if the ratio $E_{req}/E_{max} = 1$, the environment will not provide relief from heat stress.

E_{max}, or the maximum evaporative cooling that is possible in the environment, can be determined by making measurements of environmental conditions such as the air velocity and vapor pressure. On the other hand, under hot, dry conditions E_{max} is confined to man's ability to sweat which is never more than 2400 BTU's per hour or one liter per hour.

Formulas have been empirically developed for calculating the variables in the heat stress relationship. These formulas are presented below.

Radiant Heat Load

$$(3.3.3)\quad R = 17.5\ (T_w - 95)$$

Convective Heat Load

$$(3.3.4)\quad C = 0.756v^{0.6}(T_a - 95)$$

Maximum Evaporative Capacity

$$(3.3.5)\quad E_{max} = 2.8v^{0.6}(42 - PW_a)$$

where
T_w = the mean radiant temperature °F
T_a = the dry-bulb temperature of the ambient air °F
v = the air velocity ft/min
PW_a = the vapor pressure of water in the air measured in mm Hg

In order to evaluate the various levels of the Heat-Stress Index, Beldin and Hatch also presented an interpretation of these levels to the physiological implications of an 8-hour exposure to various levels of the Heat-Stress Index. A summary of the Belding Hatch information is presented Table 3.3.1.

Table 3.3.1

Heat-Stress Index implications of 8-hour exposure.

-20 to -10	Mild cold strain. Frequently exists in heat recovery are
0	No thermal strain.
+10 to +30	Mild to moderate heat strain. Subtle to substantial decrements in performance may be expected where intellectual forms of work are performed. In heavy work, little decrement is to be expected unless worker is physically fit.
+40 to +60	Severe heat strain, involving threat to health unless men are physically fit. Acclimatization required. Not suitable for those with cardiovascular or respiratory impairment. Also not suitable where sustained mental effort required.
+70 to +90	Very severe heat strain. Personnel should be selected by (1) medical examination and (2) trial on the job after acclimatization. Slight indisposition may render worker unfit for this exposure.
+100	The maximum strain tolerated by fit, acclimatized young me

Though the Heat-Stress Index considers all the environmental factors and the work rate, it is not totally satisfactory as an index for determining the heat stress on an individual worker. The Heat-Stress Index requires that a measurement of the air velocity in the workplace be made. In actual practice, such measurements are difficult to obtain with accuracy since workers move around and the turbulence of the workplace atmosphere is such that differing velocities exist in different areas. In addition, the procedure is relatively complicated and requires that the metabolic rate of the worker be estimated. This estimate can be determined using tables of the metabolic rate for given types of activities.

In 1966, McKarns and Brief developed nomographs that can be used to estimate the Heat-Stress Index. These nomographs give an allowable exposure time. The allowable exposure time (AET) is defined as the time necessary to raise the body temperature 2°F. The formula from which this allowable exposure time is developed is as follows:

$$(3.3.6) \quad AET = \frac{250 \times 60}{E_{req} - E_{max}}$$

In addition, the minimum recovery time (MRT) from exposure to heat stress can be calculated using the formula

$$(3.3.7) \quad MRT = \frac{250 \times 60}{E_{req} - E_{max}}$$

In order to illustrate the McKarns and Brief nomograph, consider the following example and the accompanying charts:

Given

T_g = 120°F
T_a = 100°F
T_{wb} = 78°F
v = 40 feet per minute
M = 1500 BTU's per hour

Procedure

Step 1.   Determine the convective heat load (C). Connect Column I or air velocity with Column II or air temperature. Read convection or C in BTU's per hour in Column III. C then has a value of 35 BTUh. Since the air temperature is above 95°, this is a positive value. Below 95°, the left-hand side of the Column II is read and indicates a negative value.

Step 2.   Determine the maximum evaporative cooling (E_{max}). The dew-point temperature must be calculated from a psychrometric chart. Given the values stated, the dew-point temperature determined is 68°F. Connecting the air velocity with the dew-point temperature in Column IV, the intersection of Column V for E_{max} is read. The E_{max} value obtained is 610 BTUh.

Figure 3.3.3

Heat stress nomograph.

Chart 1

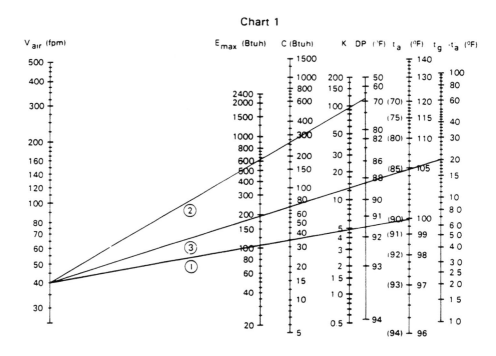

Step 3.   Determine the constant value, K. Connecting Column I or
air velocity with the temperature difference between the
globe thermometer and the ambient air in Column VI and
reading Column VII for the constant value K, the value
obtained for K = 13.

Step 4.   Determine the mean radiant temperature. Locate the value
for K in Column VII of the second chart. Connect this
value with the globe thermometer reading in Column VIII.
Read IX for the mean radiant temperature. In this case,
T_w = 135°F.

Step 5.   Determine the radiant heat load (R). Following the
diagonal line upward from 140° to Column X, a radiant heat
load of approximately 700 BTUh is obtained.

Step 6.   Determine the sum of the radiant heat load and the
metabolic heat load. An estimate of the metabolic heat
rate must be made. Assume in this case that the metabolic
heat rate is estimated to be 1800 BTUh. Connecting Column

Figure 3.3.3 (continued)

Chart 2

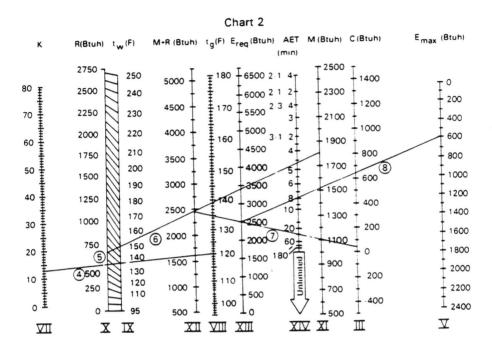

X for R and Column XI for the metabolic heat load and reading Column XII for M + R, a value of approximately 2400 BTUh is obtained for M + R.

Step 7.   Determine the required evaporative rate (E_{req}). Using the value obtained in Chart 1 for C, or 35 BTUh, connect Column XII for the value of M + R to Column III on Chart 2 for C = 35 BTUh. Read Column XIII for E_{req}. The value obtained is approximately 2500 BTUh.

Step 8.   Determine the allowable exposure time (AET). The allowable exposure time is calculated by connecting the value for E_{req} in Column XIII with the value obtained in Chart 1, Column V, for E_{max} on Column V of Chart 2. Reading Column XIV for the allowable exposure time, the value obtained is approximately 8 minutes.

The minimum recovery time can then be calculated using the formula previously stated. The values of E_{max} and E_{req} in calculating MRT are based upon that which the worker would experience in the rest area.

The Predicted Four-Hour Sweat Rate

The Predicted Four-Hour Sweat Rate, commonly denoted as P_4SR, is based upon the sweat loss in liters for various environments. A graph is used to calculate the four-hour sweat rate. Using the graph, determine the value for P_4SR in the following example. The example is based upon sedentary individuals.

$$T_{wb} = 80°F$$
$$T_g = 95°F$$
$$v = 50 \text{ feet per minute}$$
$$M = 150 \text{ K calories per meter}^2 \text{ per hour}$$

To obtain the P_4SR, follow the line intersecting the T_{wb} to the velocity line. This point is then connected to the T_g, and the intersection of the connecting line with the P_4SR for the appropriate velocity yields the resulting P_4SR. In the example, $T_{wb} = 80°F$, and the intersection of the T_{wb} and $v = 50$ ft/min is connected to a value of $T_g = 95°F$. The connecting line intersects the P_4SR line for $v = 50$ ft/min ($v = 10 - 70$ ft/min) at .6 liters. If the workers are involved in a work activity in which a metabolic rate is estimated, the small chart in the upper left-hand quadrant is used, and a correction for T_{wb} is made for the appropriate estimated metabolic rate.

The P_4SR index is based upon young men working in shorts and, as such, has limitations when applied in the industrial environment. The index also requires an estimate of the metabolic rate and a measurement of air velocity.

The Wet-Bulb Globe Temperature Index

The wet-bulb globe temperature index, commonly designated as WBGT, is based upon a measurement of the globe thermometer reading, a dry-bulb thermometer reading, and a natural wet-bulb thermometer reading. The natural wet-bulb thermometer (T_{nwb}) reading is obtained using no artificial air movement with only evaporation in the ambient air occurring.

Two formulas have been developed, one for outdoor use and the other for indoor use. The formula for indoor use does not involve a dry bulb reading. These formulas are presented below:

Outdoor Use
(3.3.8) $WBGT = 0.7T_{nwb} + 0.2T_g + 0.1T_a$
(3.3.9) $WBGT = 0.7T_{nwb} + 0.3T_g$

The WBGT formula is easy and simple to use. It is the basis for the ACGIH guide for a heat stress TLV. It is also the basis for the NIOSH recommended standard.

Although the WBGT is easy and simple to use, it does not in itself include a factor for the rate in which the individual is working. In addition, it is not possible to determine an allowable exposure time directly from the WBGT. However, in the following section discussing the ACGIH TLV guideline, certain steps have been taken to eliminate these difficulties.

Figure 3.3.4

Predicted four hour sweat rate.

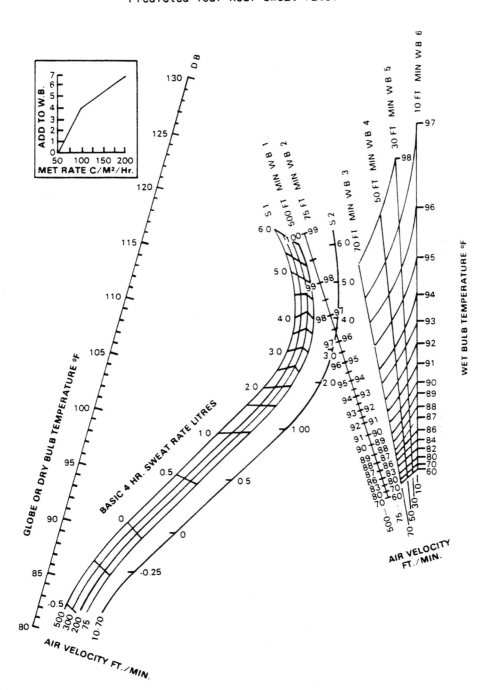

Whenever a worker is exposed to different heat loads for various time periods during his work schedule, a time-weighted WBGT must be used. A formula for calculation of this time-weighted WBGT is presented below.

$$(3.3.10) \quad WBGT_{avg.} = \frac{WBGT_1(t_1) + WBGT_2(t_2) + \ldots WBGT_n(t_n)}{t_1 + t_2 + \ldots t_n}$$

The ACGIH Guide for Assessing Heat Stress

The ACGIH has developed a guide for determining heat stress and has set forth a TLV based upon the work rate of the worker exposed to this heat stre
The basis for measurement of this index is the WBGT temperature. The procedure required for such a measurement is as follows:

A. Dry- and wet-bulb thermometer in the range of -50°C to +50°C with a accuracy of ±0.5°C.
B. The dry bulb is to be shielded from the sun when outdoor measuremer are being made.
C. Allow 1/2 hour for the wet bulb to reach equilibrium.
D. The wick should be entirely wetted 1/2 hour before reading.
E. The globe is to be a 15-centimeter (6 inches) diameter hollow coppe sphere painted matte black.
F. the globe thermometer range should be -5°C to 100°C with an accurac of ±0.5°C.
G. Allow 25 minutes for the globe thermometer to reach equilibrium.

Table 3.3.2 sets forth the criteria for determining the work load of the exposed worker. This table can be used to estimate the metabolic rate of th worker. Another method that is much more time consuming is to measure the worker while he is performing the job.

Sample Calculation: Using a heavy hand tool on an assembly line

A.	Walking Along	2.0 kcal/min
B.	Intermediate value between heavy work with two arms and light work with the body	3.0 kcal/min
		5.0 kcal/min
C.	Add for basal metabolism	1.0 kcal/min
	Total	6.0 kcal/min

Adapted from Lehmann, G. E., A. Muller and H. Spitzer: Der Kalorienbeda bei gewerblicher Arbeit. Arbeitsphysiol. 14:166, 1950.

A permissible heat exposure threshold limit value has been presented bas on the amount of time the worker is involved in continuous work and the leve of work that the worker is performing. This TLV is presented in Table 3.3.3 The TLV is applicable only for acclimatized workers and assumes that the workers are wearing light summer clothing. If the rest area is maintained a a temperature below 24°C WBGT, then the amount of rest that is required may reduced by 25%.

Table 3.3.2

Assessment of work load.
Average values of metabolic rate during different activities.

A. Body Position and Movement	kcal/min
Sitting	0.3
Standing	0.6
Walking	2.0-3.0
Walking up hill	add 0.8 per meter (yard rise)

B. Type of work	Average kcal/min	Range kcal/min
Hand work		0.2 - 1.2
light	0.4	
heavy	0.9	
Work with one arm		0.7 - 2.5
light	1.0	
heavy	1.8	
Work with both arms		1.0 - 3.5
light	1.5	
heavy	2.5	
Work with body		2.5 - 15.0
light	3.5	
moderate	5.0	
heavy	7.0	
very heavy	9.0	

Light hand work: writing, hand knitting
Heavy hand work: typewriting
Heavy work with one arm: hammering in nails (shoemaker, upholsterer)
Light work with two arms: filing metal, planing wood, raking a garden
Moderate work with the body: cleaning a floor, beating a carpet
Heavy work with the body: railroad track laying, digging, barking trees

Table 3.3.3

Permissible heat exposure Threshold Limit Values.
(Values given are in °C WBGT.)

Work-Rest Regimen	Work Load		
	Light	Moderate	Heavy
Continuous Work	30.0	26.7	25.0
75% Work-- 25% Rest, Each hour	30.6	28.0	25.9
50% Work-- 40% Rest, Each hour	31.4	29.4	27.9
25% Work-- 75% Rest, Each hour	32.2	31.1	30.0

The Wind-Chill Index

Many workers are exposed to extremely cold temperatures. In general, the strain produced in the worker by the stress of the cold environment is based on many factors. Little work has been done in this area. However, a wind-chill index has been developed that indicates where danger areas may be present.

Since convection causes heat loss and helps to reduce thermal stress, it stands to reason that, as the wind increases additional heat is lost from the body. Thus, when the temperature is cold, this additional heat loss can present a problem to the workers. A wind-chill index has been developed that equalizes the temperature and wind factors for these two conditions. Table 3.3.4 illustrates values for the wind-chill index.

Summary

Significant work has been done to develop a relationship between thermal stress and physiological strain. Among the indices that have been developed are the Effective Temperature, the Heat-Stress Index, the P_4SR, and the WBGT. None of these indices are perfect and at best provide only an estimate of the relationship between thermal stress and physiological strain. However until such time as a better method is developed, the industrial hygiene engineer has the indices that have been developed to evaluate thermal stress in the industrial environment.

Table 3.3.4

Equivalent temperatures (°F) on exposed flesh
at varying wind velocities.[1]

Wind Velocity, mph								
0	1	2	3	5	10	15	20	25
23	47.5	53.5	57	60	65	67	68	69.5
-11	20	34.5	39	44.5	52	55	57	59
-27	0	11	18.5	28	38	42.5	45	47
-38	-23.5	-9	0	11	25	30.5	34	36
-40*	-40*	-40	-16.5	-5	11	18	23	25
		-40*	-40	-19	-2	6	11	14
			-40*	-35	-15	-6	0	3
				-40	-29	-18	-12	-8
				-40*	-40	-30	-23	-18
					-40*	-40	-35	-30
						-40*	-40*	-40*

*Less than value indicated

[1]Adapted from Consolazio, Johnson, and Pecora, Physiologic
Measurements of Metabolic Functions in Man, McGraw-Hill Book Company,
New York, 1963.

4. Methods for Controlling Thermal Exposures

Introduction

In the preceding chapters, the discussion centered about the fact that man at work in an industrial environment can be exposed to thermal stress. The industrial process generates heat by convection and radiation, while the worker in the environment generates body heat as a result of metabolism and general physical activity. The industrial hygiene engineer must develop methods to control the exposure to thermal stress in order to protect the worker from physical strain. There are three general methods that are available to accomplish this task. These methods are:

1. Administrative controls
2. Modifying the thermal environment
3. Personal protective equipment

Before undertaking a method for controlling thermal stress, it is important to determine the type of thermal stress that is present in the environment. Since the methods of control differ for radiant heat and convective heat, it is important to determine the relative heat load from each of these sources. In addition, it is important to identify the source of heat and measure its intensity. As discussed in the previous chapter, in most cases, the WBGT method is the simplest method for such measurement while the HSI method takes into account the total heat load on the worker. The industrial hygiene engineer should consider the work rate at which the worker accomplishes his tasks. This work rate will determine the metabolic heat generated by the worker. Incidental environmental heat such as that resulting from the operation of equipment in the area, lighting, the general climatic conditions, and heat and steam distribution lines should be considered.

After the industrial hygiene engineer has identified the source of heat, measured its intensity, and determined the type of heat stress to which the worker is being exposed, the work of developing controls can begin. The remainder of this chapter will discuss the various methods of control that are available to control thermal stress. It is unlikely that any single method will be totally satisfactory. In most cases, it may be necessary to combine various approaches to control the thermal environment of the worker.

General Administrative Methods for Reducing Heat Stress

Decreasing the Work Required. One obvious method that can be used to control the exposure to heat stress is to decrease the amount of work required on the part of the workers exposed to the heat. As the physical activity of the worker lessens, the metabolic rate is lower and the possibility of heat strain developing is thus lessened. Quite often this approach does not result in a significant reduction in heat stress as is evident from the discussion related to the Heat Stress Index. However, in many situations where a marginal exposure exists, this reduction may be sufficient to eliminate the possibility of heat strain occurring.

In order to determine if the physical activity of the worker can be decreased, it is necessary to observe the jobs being performed. During this observation, the amount and type of physical activity of the workers can be noted. Analysis can then be made to determine if these activities can be modified in some manner to reduce the physical exertion of the worker. Can a particular tool be modified to reduce the amount of muscular activity? Can the total procedure be automated in a manner that allows the worker to be removed from the source? Can various procedures be implemented that decrease the worker's activity?

Modifying the Worker's Exposure to Heat Stress. In addition to decreasing the work required. it may be possible to determine methods for modifying the exposure of the worker. One general method available is to provide relief to the workers on a regular schedule. By providing rest areas where the worker can escape the heat and cool down, the possibility of heat strain developing is significantly lessened. Such rest areas should preferably be air conditioned at or below 75°F (24°C). These rest areas should be located near the workplace to facilitate their regular use. A rest area located at some distance from the workplace is not likely to be used by the worker because of time lost going to and from the area.

Another method for modifying the exposure is to schedule the performance of hot jobs. Where possible, hot jobs should be scheduled in the cooler part of the day. Thus, the environmental heat load will be lessened. If such scheduling is not possible, it is wise to balance the work load throughout the day. It is better to have the worker intersperse hard, physical tasks with tasks of a less physical nature than to attempt to do all the difficult physical tasks at once.

A supply of cool water (50°F to 60°F) at or near the workplace is important in reducing the possibility of heat dehydration, resulting in heat stroke. The supply of water should be in close proximity to the workplace to encourage its use. By placing a 0.1% salt solution in the drinking water, the possibility of the worker developing heat cramps is significantly lessened. This method is preferred to the use of salt tablets since it assures that salt replacement occurs when the fluid is ingested.

Screening of Workers. Since it is known that certain individual characteristics of workers make these workers more susceptible to heat strain resulting from stress, it is important that a screening procedure be developed. Such screening can occur prior to employment or placement in a hot area. Such things as illness, particularly that involving the cardiovascular system, and general physical condition are important.

After the workers have been placed in a hot job, it is desirable that periodic examinations of the exposed workers be scheduled. The purpose of the examination is to determine if the worker's physical condition has changed in such a manner that exposure to heat stress will be harmful.

Education and Training of Workers. Before a worker is placed in a heat stress environment, education and training should be provided to assure that the employee is aware of the thermal hazards involved in the job. This training should include such items as:

1. The effects of acclimatization.
2. Need for liquid replacement.
3. Need for salt replacement.
4. Recognition of the symptoms and treatment of heat disorders.
5. The effects of alcohol, lack of sleep, illness, etc., on heat tolerance.
6. The appropriate clothing to wear on the job.
7. The need for rest away from the workplace.

By participating in such training and education, the worker can become more aware of the dangers involved in exposure to thermal stress. In this way the worker will act to police his own activities in such a manner to reduce the possibility of strain occurring.

Acclimatization of Workers. Whenever a worker is being placed in a hot environment for the first time, it is important that an acclimatization procedure be used. Data from experimental studies indicate that a properly designed acclimatization program will reduce the possibility of strain developing in workers exposed to heat stress. Generally, a two-week program of acclimatization is required. During this period, the worker is progressively exposed to the hot environment and physiological adjustments occur in the body to reduce the strain experienced. The NIOSH recommendations for a standard for work in hot environments suggest that the unacclimatized employee be acclimatized over a period of six days, with 50% of the anticipated total work load and time exposure on the first day. Each day following the first day, a 10% increase in exposure is scheduled, building up to a 100% total exposure on the sixth day. In addition, the recommended standard recognizes the fact that acclimatized employees tend to lose the effects of acclimatization after a layoff. The recommended standard states that after nine or more consecutive days leave, the employees should undergo a four-day acclimatization period with daily increments of 20%, beginning with a 50% exposure on the first day. In addition, if the employee has been away from work four days or more because of illness, the same four-day reacclimatization period should be instituted. (Criteria for a Recommended Standard . . . Occupational Exposure to Hot Environments. USDHEW, HSMHA, NIOSH, U. S. Government Printing Office, HSM-72-102-69. Washington, DC, 1972.

Other Administrative Controls. Other administrative controls that can be used to reduce the exposure to thermal stress include the monitoring of the hot workplace to determine the level of thermal stress present. This is basically an identification task that determines where further controls are necessary. However, before a control can be instituted, it is necessary to determine where such a control is required.

Table 3.4.l

Summary of administrative controls
for control of heat exposure.

Decrease the Work Required
Modify the Worker's Exposure
  • rest
  • scheduling
Screen Workers
Education and Training
Acclimatization
Record-keeping

An additional method for helping to identify where heat exposure exists is to keep historical records of heat illnesses as they occur. These records can point out workers who have a low tolerance to heat exposure. Also, these records can point out areas of extreme thermal stress that can then be the subject of further investigation and control efforts.

Modifying the Thermal Environment for Radiant Heat

One of the major sources of heat stress in the industrial environment is radiant heat. The reduction of the radiant heat load in a work area can make a significant contribution to the control of thermal exposures. There are three general methods that are available to reduce the radiant heat load. These methods are:

1. Lower the radiation level.
2. Shield or isolate the worker.
3. Provide the worker with protective clothing.

Lower the Radiant Heat Level. The surface of a hot body often radiates significant amounts of heat. If the surface can be treated with a material of low emissivity, the amount of radiant heat can be significantly reduced. In order to accomplish this, the surface can be painted with a reflective or shiny paint, preferably an aluminum-type paint. In addition to reducing the radiant heat level exterior to a hot source, this approach conserves the heat inside the body where the process requires this heat.

A second method for reducing the radiant heat load is to insulate the radiant source. A thermally conductive material can be placed on the outside of a hot body that will in turn reduce the radiant heat load and cause it to be converted to heat that can be carried away by convection. An alternate method of insulating the outside of the radiant source is to provide a water jacket through which water is circulated. The water absorbs the heat energy and carries it away before entry to the workroom environment.

Shielding for Control of Radiant Heat. One of the most effective ways to reduce the level of radiant heat to which the worker is exposed is to use shielding. By applying shielding between the worker and the source, infrared radiation is intercepted. Since radiant heat travels in a straight line, it is important that the shield be located between the worker and the source and extend in such a manner that the entire worker is protected from any straight line infrared radiation.

There are basically three types of shielding methods available. These are reflective shielding, absorbing shielding, and heat-exchange shielding. Examples of reflective shielding include aluminum sheet, aluminum foil, aluminum paint on the surface of another metal, special reflective glass, wire or chain mesh, or flexible material. Depending upon the application, one type of material will have an advantage over the other. For example, aluminum foil is relatively inexpensive but does not hold up well over time and is easily torn. Reflective glass, wire, or chain mesh provides the operator with the ability to observe the process while limiting the exposure to radiant heat. However, neither material is as effective in reflecting radiant heat as aluminum sheeting.

Figure 3.4.1

Shielding.

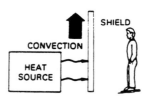

The shield should be located with space between the shield and the source of heat. This space will act as a chimney that will carry away heat that is reflected back towards the source. Otherwise, the possibility of overheating of the structure of the source is possible. Whatever surface is used must be kept clean in order that it acts effectively as a reflector. A thin film of dirt can substantially reduce the reflective ability of aluminum sheeting.

A second method of shielding is to place an absorbing surface between the worker and the source of infrared radiation. A flat, black surface will absorb the infrared radiation. The radiant heat is then converted to convective heat by air passing over the surface. However, in these situations, some reradiation occurs, and this method is not as satisfactory as using reflective shielding.

The absorptive shield may be combined with a water-cooled jacket. Water is circulated inside the shield and carries away the heat buildup in the shield. This approach, though effective, tends to be relatively expensive for installation as compared to reflective shielding.

Personal Protective Equipment. In certain situations it is desirable that the worker enter a hot environment with a high radiant heat load to perform maintenance functions. In these situations the fixed shield is not feasible. It is necessary to provide protection to the worker from the radiant heat load during exposure. Personal protective clothing provides a solution to this type of situation. Though this clothing is somewhat restrictive to motion and does not breathe, thus prohibiting evaporative cooling, it does provide the worker with a short protection against the radiant heat load.

Where it is necessary that longer exposures occur or where additional convective heat loss is required, refrigerated suits can be used. Generally the refrigeration involves either water cooling, compressed air passing through a vortex and thus expanding, or refrigerated air. Though these units are very restrictive to activity, they are useful for emergency entry into extremely hot areas.

In situations where only one portion of the worker's body is exposed to radiant heat, experiments have shown that partial protection using reflective clothing can be effective. Such items as aprons, gloves, hats, and face shields can be used where the worker must be exposed to radiant heat for short periods of time. However, again these methods do not replace the more long-term controls such as shielding.

Modifying the Thermal Environment for Convective Heat

Where the worker is exposed to convective heat stress, the industrial hygiene engineer should consider the methods of substitution and isolation as possible controls. An investigation should be made to determine if it is possible that the process can be changed to eliminate the heat requirements. Can another process be substituted that generates less heat? Can the worker be isolated from the heat source and thus protected? An example of isolation is the provision of a separate air-conditioned control room for the workers. Another method is to isolate the hot processes in an area away from other activities, thus centralizing the source of heat in an area where control can be implemented.

One other method for controlling convective heat is to determine if the heat itself can be removed from the work area. This can be accomplished by insulating the source of heat as was discussed in the section on radiant heat. In addition, vents and local exhaust hoods can carry away significant portions of the convective heat generated.

General Dilution Ventilation. In many situations involving convective heat loads, general dilution ventilation can be used to reduce the thermal stress encountered. Recirculation of air from man-cooling fans can increase the convective heat loss of the workers. However, it should be remembered that such a recirculation of ambient air does not reduce the temperature. Thus, if the temperature is above 95°F, recirculation will only increase the heat gain of the workers rather than accomplishing the desired result of reducing this heat gain.

Where the general heat load of a work area is high, thermal draft may assist in providing protection to the workers. Since hot air rises and escapes through ventilators in the roof or is drawn out by fans, effective cooling can be accomplished by supplying air at the outside temperature. Again, this air must be of significantly lower temperature in order to be effective in lessening the heat load. This air supply can be distributed throughout the entire work zone. Where spot cooling is required in specific hot areas, the supply then can be directed to these areas.

Removing Heat from the Air

In certain situations, the outside air is not sufficiently cool to provide relief from the hot environment. Thus, it is necessary to cool the outside supply air. This can be done either through evaporative cooling or through refrigeration of the air.

Evaporative cooling involves passing the air through a water spray. As the water evaporates into the air from the spray, heat is removed from the air because of the required BTU's necessary to accomplish this evaporation. The air thus becomes cooler as it is supplied to the worker. A totally efficient unit will reduce the dry-bulb temperature of the air to that of the incoming wet-bulb temperature. To further increase the cooling capacity of the evaporative cooler, water below the wet-bulb temperature can be utilized in the spray system.

The second method available is to refrigerate the air. Direct expansion refrigeration units can be used to supply a general area or for spot cooling of a local enclosure or area. When a large industrial area must be cooled, this method tends to be expensive for installation and operation.

Protection from Climatic Conditions. The climatic conditions of the plant location can add an additional heat load to the interior environment. Radiation from the sun as well as hot and humid air in the environment can materially increase the potential for heat stress. Reflective glass can be placed in the windows that will reduce the radiation level passing through into the work environment. Water sprays can be placed on the roof that remove heat during evaporation. In addition, adequate insulation in the walls and below the roof can result in savings when the interior plant requires that cool air be supplied.

Modifying the Environment for Moisture

In some cases it is necessary to change the water vapor pressure in the air. A reduction in humidity allows for evaporative cooling in the worker's body to take place. On the other hand, an increase in humidity may be necessary to reduce the potential for static electricity buildup. In an explosive atmosphere, such static electricity buildup can result in the existence of a potential hazard.

The moisture content in the air can be increased by applying steam jet humidifiers and air washers to the incoming air. In these cases, a water vapor is introduced to the incoming air that increases the vapor content of the plant atmosphere.

Lowering the moisture content can be accomplished in a number of ways. Direct expansion refrigeration results in a lowering of moisture content since the air is cooled and reaches its dew point. In addition to cooling the air, the water vapor contained in the air condenses, thus lowering the humidity.

Chilled water can be sprayed into the incoming air. By lowering the temperature of the air, water vapor within the air condenses. A second method for introducing chilled water is through coils. As the air passes over the chilled water coils, it is cooled, thus lowering the dew-point temperature and causing water vapor to condense.

Absorption of water vapor as the air is passed through certain solids and liquids can result in lowering the humidity. Certain problems exist when using solid absorption materials since, once the solids have absorbed the water vapor, the process cannot be reversed. Liquids can be heated to release the water vapor, and thus recycling of the liquid can occur. In general the liquids are sprayed through the incoming air, gathered, heated, and then cooled and recycled back to the incoming air. One problem with such a system, however, is that there is a slight increase in the temperature of the air as a result of the dehumidification process.

Solid adsorption is another method for removing moisture from the air. Solids such as silica gel are often used as an adsorption medium. Heating of the adsorption material regenerates its adsorption properties. As in the case with absorption, heat is generated during the adsorption process, thus raising the heat of the incoming air. In many cases it is advantageous to include a refrigeration of the air prior to the adsorption process. This not only maintains the air at a comfortable incoming temperature but also removes some of the moisture prior to the adsorption process.

Modifying the Environment for Cold

During the winter months in cold climates, it is necessary to add heat to the air within an industrial facility. Heating the air can be accomplished through general heating of the make-up air or, in cases where general heating is not feasible, through the use of local heating with unit heaters and radiation panels. A further discussion of this topic is beyond the scope of this book. The interested reader is referred to the ASHRAE Engineers Guide and Data Book or the AIHA publication, "Heating and Cooling for Man in Industry."

Personal Protective Clothing. Workers are often subjected to extreme cold temperatures when working out of doors or in refrigerated areas. General heating cannot provide protection in these cases. Thus, the best approach is to provide personal protective clothing for the workers.

In general, individuals do not become acclimatized to cold. In fact, man's tolerance to cold is somewhat less than one might expect. Particularly dangerous is the exposure of the extremities and respiratory passages. Thus there is a need to protect the worker from exposure to extreme cold that can result in frostbite and even death if the exposure lasts over a long period of time.

Where heavy work is required, there is an additional problem of evaporation of sweat. The body can become overheated as the sweat collects on the skin and cannot evaporate. During rest periods after heavy activity, the sweat that is collected evaporates and exposes the body to excessive cooling. Therefore, it is important that the worker dress for the activity in which he is involved. Air that is held between layers of clothing provides additional insulation against heat loss and, as a result, multi-layered clothing is preferable. The outer layer should be wind resistant to protect the worker against convective heat loss. Layers should be such that they can be removed during heavy work periods and added during rest periods or periods of lighter physical activity. Protection of the hands and feet can be accomplished by using mittens and insulated boots. Mittens are preferred over gloves since they provide better protection of the hands. Boots should be waterproof leather as opposed to rubber since the leather will breathe and allow for evaporation of moisture on the feet.

Summary

When controlling the work environment for thermal stress, the industrial hygiene engineer must consider both radiation and convection heat loads. The general control methods available include decreasing the work load, modifying the exposure, screening the workers, education and training of the workers, acclimatization, monitoring the workplace, and maintenance of historical records of heat illness. For control of radiant heat, action can be taken to lower the radiation level by insulation or surface treatment, by placing shields between the source and the worker, and by providing personal protective equipment to the worker. For control of convective heat, the process may be modified, the source can be isolated from the work area, local exhaust can be used to remove the heat, general dilution can be used, or the workroom can be air conditioned. The industrial hygiene engineer must also take action to control exposure to high humidity and cold.

5. References

American Conference of Governmental Industrial Hygienists. <u>Threshold Limit Value for Chemical Substances and Physical Agents in the Workroom Environment with Intended Changes for 1976</u>. Cincinnati: American Conference of Governmental Industrial Hygienists, 1976.

____. Committee on Industrial Ventilation. <u>Industrial Ventilation: A Manual of Recommended Practice</u>, 13th ed. Lansing: American Conference of Governmental Industrial Hygienists, 1974.

American Industrial Hygiene Association. <u>Heating and Cooling for Man in Industry</u>. Akron: American Industrial Hygiene Association, 1974.

Baumeister, Theodore, ed. <u>Marks Standard Handbook for Mechanical Engineers</u>, 7th ed. New York: McGraw-Hill Book Company, 1967.

Giever, Paul M., ed. <u>Air Pollution Manual Part I--Evaluation</u>, 2d ed. Akron: American Industrial Hygiene Association, 1972.

Hewitt, Paul G. <u>Conceptual Physics . . . A New Introduction to Your Environment</u>, 2d ed. Boston: Little, Brown & Co., 1974.

Horvath, Steven M. and Roger C. Jensen, eds. <u>Standards for Occupational Exposures to Hot Environments</u>. Proceedings of Symposium, February 27-28, 1973. U. S. Department of Health, Education, and Welfare, Public Health Service, Center for Disease Control, National Institute for Occupational Safety and Health. Cincinnati: U. S. Government Printing Office, 1976.

International Labor Office. <u>Encyclopaedia of Occupational Safety and Health</u>, 2 vols. New York: McGraw-Hill Book Company, 1971.

Jensen, Roger C. and Hems, Donald A., <u>Relationships Between Several Prominent Heat Stress Indices</u>, DHEW (NIOSH) Publication No. 77-109, Cincinnati, Ohio: NIOSH, Division of Biomedical and Behavioral Science, October, 1976.

McElroy, Frank E., ed. <u>Accident Prevention Manual for Industrial Operations</u>, 7th ed. Chicago: National Safety Council, 1975.

Mutchler, John E., Delno Malzahn, Janet L. Vecchio and Robert D. Soule. <u>An Improved Method for Monitoring Heat Stress Levels in the Workplace</u>. U. S. Department of Health, Education, and Welfare, Public Health Service, Center for Disease Control, National Institute for Occupational Safety and Health. Cincinnati: U. S. Government Printing Office, 1975.

Olishifski, Julian B. and Frank McElroy, eds. <u>Fundamentals of Industrial Hygiene</u>. Chicago: National Safety Council, 1971.

Patty, Frank A. <u>Industrial Hygiene and Toxicology</u>, 2d ed., 2 vols., New York: Interscience Publishers, Inc., 1958.

Schaum, Daniel. College Physics, 6th ed. New York: McGraw-Hill Book Company
     1961.

___. Theory and Problems of College Chemistry, 5th ed.
     New York: McGraw-Hill Book Company, 1966.

U. S. Department of Health, Education, and Welfare, Public Health Service,
     National Institute for Occupational Safety and Health. The Industrial
     Environment: Its Evaluation and Control. Washington: U. S. Government
     Printing Office, 1973.

Section 4

Sound

1. Physics of Sound

Introduction

This chapter discusses the definition of sound, sound waves, sound power, sound pressure, and sound intensity. The concepts presented in this chapter are the basis for solving industrial noise control problems.

What is Sound?

What is sound? What is noise? Are the two different? Yes, sound is different from noise. Noise is frequently defined as any unwanted sound. The question of whether sound is wanted or not depends not only on the individual but also on the circumstances. What is considered noise (unwanted sound) is therefore subjective. The definition of noise is a functional definition, not a physical definition.

What is sound? Very simply, sound is something that can be heard. Machines make sounds, pianos make sounds, people make sounds, and tuning forks make sounds. Sound is nothing more than an oscillation in atmospheric pressure (a traveling vibratory movement of molecules) within an elastic medium (material) of any phase (gas, liquid or solid). This is a complex definition, containing many, perhaps unfamiliar, terms.

An Example of Sound

Suppose a vibratory machine surface is in an air medium. As the surface vibrates, a sound is heard. What is happening that causes the sound, and why can a sound be heard? As the surface of the machine vibrates in one direction acting as a sound source, the air molecules adjacent to the machine become compressed. This area of compression is an area of increased atmospheric pressure. This area of high pressure acts to push immediately surrounding air molecules at lower pressure. As the surface moves in the opposite direction, the air molecules adjacent to the surface create a low pressure area, an area of rarefaction. So as the machine surface vibrates, it creates alternating areas of compression and rarefaction of the adjacent air molecules. These molecules in turn affect molecules that are adjacent to them. These alternating areas of compression and rarefaction are nothing more than fluctuations in atmospheric pressure. This disturbance in air molecules travels through the air and reaches the listener's ears. As the disturbance reaches the ears, components of the ears begin to vibrate. This mechanical vibration in the ears is eventually changed to electrical energy and is transmitted to the brain, and thus the listener hears the sound.

The areas of compression and rarefaction are illustrated in Figure 4.1.1, with the sound source being a tuning fork.

Figure 4.1.1

Areas of compression and rarefaction.

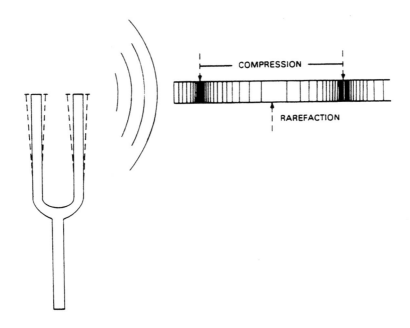

Sound Wave

As the areas of compression and rarefaction travel in a medium, a sound wave is produced. A sound wave (in an air medium) is the pattern of fluctuation (alternating areas of compression and rarefaction) in the air pressure over a specific distance or time. That is, a sound wave is the pattern of changes in air pressure. This pattern can be graphed as shown in Figure 4.1.2.

In Figure 4.1.2, the vertical axis represents air pressure. The horizontal axis represents either distance or time. By combining Figure 4.1.1 and Figure 4.1.2, it is obvious that there is a correspondence between the wave and the areas of compression and rarefaction of the movement of air molecules. This resulting figure would be as shown in Figure 4.1.3.

The air molecules do not move along the path of the sound wave; rather, the air molecules stay in one place and oscillate around their central location, just as the vibrating source does.

Figure 4.1.2

Pattern of sound--a sound wave.

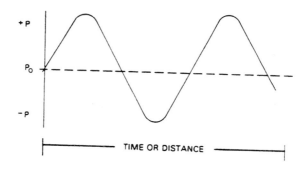

Figure 4.1.3

Areas of compression and rarefaction
and a sound wave.

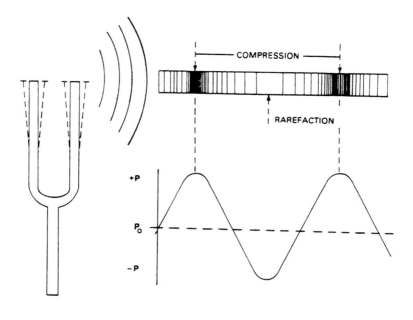

Velocity of Sound

The speed or velocity at which sound travels through a medium is dependent upon (a) the density of the medium (density equals mass divided by volume), and (b) the elasticity of the medium (i.e., the ability of a material to change size and/or shape when subjected to an external force). Mathematically, the relationship between density, elasticity, and velocity is given as

$$C^2 = \frac{\text{elasticity}}{\text{density}}$$

where C denotes velocity.

The above expression is the general expression for the velocity of sound in a medium. In a gas (such as air), the expression can be written as

$$C^2 = \frac{\gamma P_o}{\rho}$$

where C denotes velocity, γ denotes specific heat ratio, ρ denotes density (mass divided by volume), and P denotes atmospheric pressure. Under normal conditions, air at 68°F and $\gamma = 1.41$, it can be shown that the velocity of sound in air is equal to 1127 feet per second or 344 meters per second.

The velocity of sound will be affected by the temperature of the medium. In air the velocity of sound will change about one foot per second for each increase in one degree Fahrenheit (or about two feet per second for each increase in one degree Celsius).

Frequency of Sound

Another important characteristic in describing sound in addition to its velocity is frequency. Frequency refers to the rate at which complete cycles of high and low pressure regions are produced by the sound source. Frequency is usually measured in cycles per second or Hertz (Hz) and is the number of times maximum sound pressure occurs in one second. The ear can hear frequencies between 20 and 20,000 cycles per second.

Period (T) refers to the time it takes for one complete cycle or vibration. It is equal to the reciprocal of frequency.

$$T = \frac{1}{f}$$

where T denotes period and f denotes frequency.

Wavelength

Another interesting characteristic of a sound wave is wavelength. At a given velocity (C), how far would a wave travel in one period (T)? To answer this recall from basic physics that

$$velocity = \frac{distance}{time}$$

where distance refers to how far a wave can travel, and time is represented by the period; that is, the time required for one cycle of pressure change.
Substituting these in the equation gives

$$C = \frac{\lambda}{T}$$

where λ denotes the wavelength and T denotes the period.

Substituting 1/f for the period and solving for wavelength results in the following equation:

$$\lambda = \frac{C}{f}$$

Using the above equation, what is the wavelength of a 1000 Hz wave being propagated through air at 68°F? Recall that the velocity of air under normal conditions is 1127 feet per second.

The answer is as follows:

$$\lambda = \frac{1127 \ ft/sec}{1000 \ cycles/sec}$$

$$\lambda = 1.127 \ ft/cycle$$

This represents the distance a wave would travel in one period (one cycle).

What is the wavelength of a 1000 Hz wave in air at 90°F? Recall that velocity increased one foot per second for each degree Fahrenheit. Therefore, the velocity of sound at 90°F would be 1149 ft/sec.

The answer is as follows

$$\lambda = \frac{1149 \ ft/sec}{1000 \ cycles/sec}$$

$$= 1.149 \ ft/cycle$$

A wavelength can be graphically represented as shown in Figure 4.1.4.

Figure 4.1.4

Representation of a wavelength.

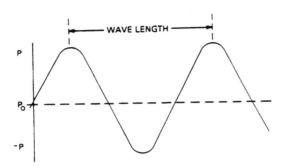

One can further visualize a wavelength by using a spring or a slinky toy. Stretch the spring vertically and then suddenly push down on the top coil and continue to repeat this motion. You will see groupings of compressed coils traveling down the spring. Between these compressed coil groupings will be groupings whose coils are expanded farther apart than usual. Of course, the coils do not move down; they stay in one average position and oscillate about it--the same as the air molecules. The groupings of spring elements move in the wave motion. This motion of the groupings of elements travels with a definite speed. If you change the rate of the up-and-down motion of your hand holding the top of the spring, you will change the frequency of groupings; but the speed of the groupings will stay the same; i.e., the grouping will still travel through the spring at the same speed (the sounds of all frequencies travel at the same speed in the same media). By changing the frequency, you will change the spacing between the groupings. This spacing is the wavelength. The wave speed in the spring remains constant while the wavelength changes. Increasing the frequency decreases the wavelength--the distance between the groupings. Decreasing the frequency increases the wavelength. The same situation occurs with sound in air.

The wave motion in air involves particles (molecules) that vibrate because of the sound energy present. The number of complete cycles per second executed by these molecules is called the frequency of the wave. In the spring analogy, the frequency could be changed, but the speed of sound would not change. This is because speed in a given medium remains constant.

Summary

So far, sound has been defined as an oscillation in pressure within an elastic medium of any phase that evokes an auditory sensation. It has been said that the velocity of sound is dependent upon the density and elasticity

of the medium, where the velocity of sound in normal air is 1127 ft per
second. The temperature of the air will affect the velocity of sound (an
increase in velocity of one foot per second for each increase in degrees
Fahrenheit). Frequency has been discussed and defined as the rate at which
complete cycles of high and low pressure regions are produced by the sound
source. The period has been defined as the time required for one cycle of
pressure change. Thus, the period is equal to the reciprocal of frequency.
Wavelength is the distance a wave will travel in one period (one cycle).

It is now time to discuss three important terms that are the basics for
understanding the physics of sound: sound pressure, sound power, and sound
intensity. Equations to represent these characteristics of sound will be
developed, and the relationship between these expressions will be discussed.
A conceptual understanding of these terms is important.

Sound Pressure

In the previous discussion, sound was defined as an oscillation in
atmospheric pressure within an elastic medium of any phase. Sound pressure is
defined as the difference between atmospheric pressure and the actual pressure
during rarefaction and compression. One can see that sound pressure is
unrelated to frequency or wavelength. Sounds in the same medium and with the
same frequency may generate different sound pressure. Consider a tuning
fork. The fork may be hit lightly and produce a faint sound or may be hit
firmly and produce a loud sound. Both sounds will have exactly the same
frequency and wavelength since the tines (the forks) will vibrate back and
forth the same number of times in a second. The harder the fork is struck,
however, the greater the distance the tine travels during each cycle. This
increased distance traveled by the tines will cause greater pressure
fluctuations above and below atmospheric pressure. This situation is
graphically illustrated by Figure 4.1.5.

Figure 4.1.5 illustrates that the harder the tines are struck, the greater
the height of the sound wave above atmospheric pressure. It should be noted
that the wavelengths are exactly the same. There is a difference between the
wave produced by lightly striking the tines and the wave produced by striking
the tines a little harder. This difference is the difference in sound
pressure. The harder the tines are struck, the greater the fluctuations in
atmospheric pressure.

Atmospheric pressure--force per unit area--is usually measured in bars
(14.7 pounds per square inch). However, a fluctuation of only 0.1% of
atmospheric pressure represents an intolerably loud sound. Since fluctuations
in pressure that generate sound are extremely small compared to a bar, it is
convenient to use a much smaller unit, the microbar. This unit is abbreviated
"μbar" and is equal to one-millionth of a bar. (μbar equals atmospheric
pressure times 10^{-6}.) Sound pressure can also be expressed in dynes per
square centimeter or newtons per square meter. (One dyne equals
10^{-5} newtons). Normal pressure exerted by the atmosphere is approximately
1,000,000 dynes per square centimeter.

Figure 4.1.5

Wave having same wavelength
but diffferent sound pressure.

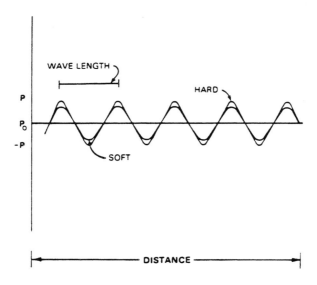

The faintest sound that can be detected by the ear is produced by pressure variations of approximately 0.0002 dynes/cm^2 (or 0.0002 newtons/m^2). Discomfort occurs around 20 newtons/m^2, and the threshold of pain is around 200 newtons/m^2. The sounds heard in offices are around one dyne per square centimeter.

The sound pressure generated by a sound source is dependent upon the location of the hearer. The farther away the hearer is from the sound source, the smaller the variations in sound pressure from atmospheric pressure. Because of this, sound pressure is not a good way to evaluate the sound generated by the sound source.

Sound pressure changes over time and is not constant. Since sound pressure is not constant, it is difficult to come up with a single number to describe sound pressure. What has been done is to integrate sound pressure over time. However, most measuring devices do not do this; they use a simpler method, the root mean square (RMS) method. This method amounts to measuring sound pressure at certain places, squaring the sound pressures at those places, summing the sound pressures squared, and dividing by the number of measures taken, and then taking the square root of the average. This method works for pure tone or steady state noise. The time interval over which a single periodic sound pressure pattern must be measured is equal to an integral number of periods of that sound pattern, or the interval must be long compared to a period. There must be more than ten peaks per second for noise to be considered steady state for measurement purposes.

There are two types of measuring instruments: instruments to measure
sound pressure in RMS and instruments to measure peak pressures. Maximum peak
pressure is normally used when peak pressure is repeated no more than two per
second. Peak pressure instruments are used when the noise or sound is not
steady state noise or sound.

Sound Power

Sound was described as the movement of air molecules adjacent to a
vibratory surface. A tuning fork is the simplest sound generating unit. When
it is struck, it begins to vibrate at a definite frequency. Its vibrations
transmit energy (where energy is defined as force times distance) to the
atmosphere (creating waves having alternating points of maximum and minimum
pressure). The amount of energy in the sound is a function of the amount of
energy imparted to the tuning fork when it is struck. Every sound source,
such as a tuning fork, has a sound power it generates. From basic physics
recall that

$$\text{Power} = \frac{\text{energy}}{\text{time}}$$

Sound power can best be defined, then, as the total sound energy radiated by a
sound source per unit time.

Energy is usually measured in foot-pounds. A weight of one pound lifted
one foot off the ground requires the expenditure of one foot-pound of energy.
If it took one second to lift the one pound weight, the power involved would
be one foot-pound per second. Power can also be expressed in horsepower,
where 550 foot-pounds per second equals one horsepower. In the metric system,
power is measured in joules per second, where one joule per second is equal to
one watt. A watt is equivalent to about three-quarters of a foot-pound per
second.

Table 4.1.1. shows the sound powers radiated by familiar sound sources in
watts. (Note: A kilowatt is 1000 watts; a microwatt is one-millionth of a
watt.)

Power is also expressed in dyne-centimeters (or newton-meters) per
second. One watt equals one joule per second, which equals 10^7 dyne-
centimeters per second (one joule equals 10,000,000 dyne-centimeters), or one
joule equals one newton-meter (i.e., one joule of energy is expended when one
newton of force is exerted over one meter; if it takes one second, then the
power involved is one newton-meter per second).

The sound power generated by a machine (sound source) is not measured but
calculated from measurements made under controlled laboratory conditions.
Manufacturers usually provide the sound power created or generated by their
equipment. The industrial hygiene engineer is not responsible for calculating
sound power.

Table 4.1.1

Approximate power radiated by some familiar sound sources.

Watts	Prefix Notation	Exponential Notation	Sound Source
10,000,000.	10 megawatts	10^7	
1,000,000.	1 megawatt	10^6	
100,000.	100 kilowatts	10^5	Future turbo-jet (est.)
10,000.	10 kilowatts	10^4	Turbo-jet engine, after-burner
			Turbo-jet engine, take-off
1,000.	1 kilowatt	10^3	2-engine airliner, take-off
100.	100 watts	10^2	Large wood planer
			2-engine airliner, cruising
10.	10 watts	10^1	Chipping hammer, large castings
1.	1 watt	10^0	Chipping hammer, small castings
0.1	100 milliwatts	10^{-1}	Circular saw, ripping plank
0.01	10 milliwatts	10^{-2}	Voice, shouting
0.001	1 milliwatt	10^{-3}	Auto on highway
0.000,1	100 microwatts	10^{-4}	Typewriter
0.000,01	10 microwatts	10^{-5}	Voice, conversational level
0.000,001	1 microwatt	10^{-6}	
0.000,000,1	100 millimicrowatts	10^{-7}	Telephone dial
0.000,000,01	10 millimicrowatts	10^{-8}	Voice whisper
0.000,000,001	1 millimicrowatt	10^{-9}	Pencil writing on paper
0.000,000,000,1	100 micromicrowatts	10^{-10}	
0.000,000,000,01	10 micromicrowatts	10^{-11}	Normal breathing
0.000,000,000,001	1 micromicrowatt	10^{-12}	Man's wrist watch
0.000,000,000,000,1	0.1 micromicrowatt	10^{-13}	

Remember that sound power is the total sound energy radiated per unit time by the sound source. It is the energy per unit time radiated by the sound source that causes the fluctuations in atmospheric pressure. Therefore, sound power rather than sound pressure is usually used to describe the sound source. However, it should be noted that conceptually sound pressure and sound power are related. At a given distance from a sound source, the increases in sound power will result in increases in sound pressure.

Sound Intensity

Sound power per unit area is called the sound intensity. If sound power is distributed over an area in such a way that one watt of power falls on each square foot of area, the sound intensity is one watt per square foot. Sound power is an indication of the concentration of power. Thus, when a certain sound power is distributed over a large area, the sound intensity will be much smaller than when the same sound power is concentrated in a smaller area.

Sound intensity is affected by the observer's distance away from the sound source. If a sound source is a point source and that point source radiates a given sound power, the definition of sound intensity makes it clear that the farther away an observer is from that point source, the larger the area in which the sound power is concentrated. Thus, the intensity would become smaller as the observer travels farther from the point source.

When pebbles are dropped into a still pond at a constant rate, the crests of the waves radiated outward are in ever-increasing circles. If it were possible to drop a series of pebbles with proper timing, a pattern similar to that shown in Figure 4.1.6 would be observed. Here the width of the black

Figure 4.1.6

Conceptualization of sound intensity.

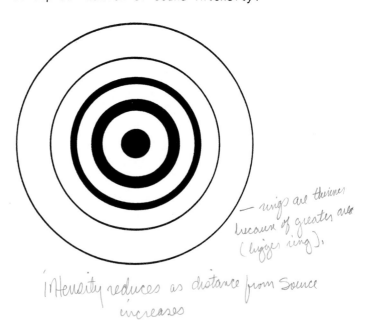

— rings are thinner because of greater area (bigger ring).

Intensity reduces as distance from Source increases

rings is intended to indicate the height of the wave. Note that the width of the rings decreases as the diameter increases. Naturally, this is a picture of the surface of the body at only one instant. Since the waves are traveling outward, each ring will expand rapidly until it takes the place of the next larger ring shown in the diagram. This process will continue over and over again so that the picture will always appear to be changing, yet is always the same.

Sound waves radiating from a tuning fork or any other sound source can also be represented by the rings shown in the diagram. Of course, since the sound wave travels in all directions, there will be a pattern similar to this in a vertical plane or in any other plane chosen. Therefore, instead of a set of expanding circular rings there is a set of expanding spherical shells.

In the case of the sound wave, the thickness of the shells corresponds to the intensity of the sound, the concentration of sound power. And, as can be seen, the intensity becomes less as the observer gets farther away from the sound source; i.e., as the diameter of the rings increases, the intensity decreases.

If sound intensity is defined as the sound power per unit area, then the relationship between sound intensity and sound power can be expressed as

$$\text{Sound intensity} = \frac{\text{sound power}}{4\pi r^2}$$

where $4\pi r^2$ represents the surface area of a sphere (r denotes the radius).

If the sound power of a machine is given as 12.5664 foot-pounds per second and an observer is 1.0 feet from the sound source, then the sound intensity at that distance can be computed as

$$\text{Sound intensity} = \frac{12.5664 \text{ ft-pounds/sec}}{4(3.1416)(1.00\text{ft})^2}$$
$$= 1 \text{ foot-pound/sec-ft}^2$$

This means that a sound source of 12.5664 foot-pounds per second will produce a sound intensity of 1 foot pound per square foot at the surface of a hypothetical sphere 1.0 feet from the sound source. This relationship between sound intensity and sound power only holds true in a free-field condition, a condition where the sound is permitted to radiate without bouncing off walls, ceilings, or floors.

The relationship between sound power and sound intensity is often referred to as the inverse square law. From the above expression, it can be noted that if sound power remains constant, the intensity must vary inversely with the square of r, the distance from the source (since π and 4 are always constant).

Assume a sound source that radiates a sound power of 1   watt (one millionth of a watt or one millionth of a joule per second). Further, assume that the hearer moves away from this sound source a distance of 1 centimeter, then 2 centimeters, then 4 centimeters. Notice that the distances are doubled. Using the formula above, the sound intensity at each of these distances can be computed. At 1 centimeter, the sound intensity would be 0.08 watts per square centimeter; at 2 centimeters, the sound intensity would be 0.02 watts per square centimeter, and at 4 centimeters, the sound intensit would be 0.005 watts per square centimeter. Note that as the distance double from the source, the intensity drops by one quarter, or the sound intensity i equal to the inverse of the square of the distance. This relationship is extremely important. It will be used when the solution to noise control problems is discussed.

Sound intensity can also be expressed in terms of sound pressure. Sound intensity is defined as

$$\text{Sound intensity} = \frac{\text{sound power}}{\text{area}} \qquad (4.1.1)$$

Recall that sound power can be expressed as energy per unit time.

$$\text{Sound power} = \frac{\text{energy}}{\text{time}} \qquad (4.1.2)$$

Substituting expression (4.1.2) in expression (4.2.1) above results in

$$\text{Sound intensity} = \frac{\text{energy}}{\text{area x time}} \qquad (4.1.3)$$

From basic physics, recall that

$$\text{Energy} = \text{force x distance} \qquad (4.1.4)$$

Substituting expression (4.1.4) in expression (4.1.3) results in

$$\text{Sound intensity} = \frac{\text{force x distance to move particle}}{\text{area x time to move particle}} \qquad (4.1.5)$$

Recalling from basic physics that

$$\text{Pressure} = \frac{\text{force}}{\text{area}} \qquad (4.1.6)$$

and

$$\text{Velocity} = \frac{\text{distance to move particle}}{\text{time to move particle}} \qquad (4.1.7)$$

Then expression 4.1.5 can be written as

$$\text{Sound intensity} = \text{sound pressure x velocity of the particle} \qquad (4.1.8)$$

The particle velocity in the material of propagation is found from basic impulsive momentum changes.

$$\text{Impulsive force = change in momentum} \tag{4.1.9}$$

and

$$\text{Force x time = mass x change in particle velocity} \tag{4.1.10}$$

where

$$\text{Mass = density x volume} \tag{4.1.11}$$

Substituting (4.1.11) in (4.1.10) results in

$$\text{Force x time = density x volume x change in particle velocity} \tag{4.1.12}$$

Rearranging (4.1.12) gives

$$\text{Velocity of particle} = \frac{\text{force x time}}{\text{density x volume}} \tag{4.1.13}$$

$$= \frac{\text{force x time}}{\text{density x area x distance}}$$

$$= \frac{\text{pressure}}{\text{density x velocity in medium}}$$

Substituting this in expression (4.1.8), results in

$$\text{Sound intensity} = \frac{\text{sound pressure x sound pressure}}{\text{density x velocity in medium}}$$

or

$$I = \frac{p^2}{\rho C} \tag{4.1.14}$$

where I denotes sound intensity, P denotes pressure, ρ denotes density of the medium, and C denotes velocity of sound in a medium.

Expression (4.1.14) denotes sound intensity at an instant in time as the impulsive force acts. The total mean sound intensity over time is the integration of

$$I = (1/T \int_{o}^{T} p^2 \; x \; dt)/ \; \rho C$$

By definition, the integral is equivalent to the square of the root mean square (RMS), or

$$I = \frac{P^2_{RMS}}{\rho C}$$

Under normal atmospheric conditions, where I is in μwatts per square feet and P is in μbars, Cox (p. 626, Industrial Hygiene and Toxicology, Volume I) reports the relationship to be

$$I = (1.52P)^2$$

Sound intensity is not steady but varies in a pulsating fashion. With each vibration of the sound source, a pulse of energy is carried from the sound source. One way to measure intensity is to look at the maximum intensity. For a pure tone--such as that resulting from a tuning fork--maximum intensity will be a constant at each compression. For more complicated sounds, this will not be true. The average intensity of a pure sound is equal to one-half the maximum intensity. For more complicated sounds, the average intensity is more meaningful than the maximum intensity. Sound intensity can be averaged. This information will be used later.

Relationship Between Sound Power and Sound Pressure

In the last section, it was shown how sound intensity is related to sound power (by definition).

$$I = \frac{W}{4\pi r^2} \tag{4.1.1}$$

where I denotes sound intensity, W denotes sound power, r denotes radius of a hypothetical sphere around the sound source. Note: r must be measured in the system being used (either in cm or feet).

In addition, it was shown how sound intensity is related to sound pressure

$$I = \frac{p^2}{C} \tag{4.1.2}$$

where I denotes sound intensity, P denotes sound pressure (in μbars), denotes density of the medium, and C denotes velocity of sound in the medium.

It is often convenient to express a relationship between sound power and sound pressure. To arrive at this relationship, substitute expression (4.1.2) in expression (4.1.1) and solve for P (sound pressure).

$$\frac{p^2}{\rho C} = \frac{W}{4\pi r^2}$$

$$p^2 = \frac{W\rho C}{4\pi r^2}$$

therefore

$$P = [W\rho C/4\pi r^2]^{1/2} \qquad\qquad (4.1.3)$$

If W is given in watts, r in feet, and P in newtons per square meters with standard conditions, equation (4.1.3) can be written as (see The Industrial Environment: Its Evaluation and Control, p. 302).

$$P = [3.5W \times 10^2/r^2]^{1/2} \qquad\qquad (4.1.4)$$

The relationship between sound pressure and sound power is very important. It will be used in subsequent chapters.

Given the expression above, predict the sound pressure that would be produced at a distance of 100 feet from a pneumatic chipping hammer. The manufacturer states that the hammer has an acoustic power of 1.0 watts.

Solution

$$W = 1.00 \text{ watts}$$

$$r = 100 \text{ feet}$$

$$P = [3.5 \times 1.0 \text{ watt} \times 10^2/(100 \text{ ft})^2]^{1/2}$$

$$P = 0.187 \text{ N/m}^2 \text{ (newtons per square meter)}$$

Expression (4.1.4) is only appropriate in a free-field condition. A free-field condition means that the sound created by the sound source is free to travel in all directions; for example, a sound source suspended in the middle of a large room has a free field. The sound would radiate towards the walls, floor, and ceiling without meeting any obstacles or bouncing back. Although a free-field condition is not the normal condition in industrial noise problems, it is the basis for understanding the physics of sound.

Summary

For convenience, the important aspects of this chapter are summarized below.

1.   Sound is defined as an oscillation in pressure (a traveling vibratory movement of molecules) within an elastic medium (material) of any phase (gas, liquid, or solid) which evokes an auditory sensation.

2.   Noise is subjectively defined as unwanted sound.

3. When a vibratory surface moves back and forth, areas of compression and rarefaction of the adjacent air molecules are created.

4. A sound wave is the pattern of fluctuations in air pressure over distance or time.

5. Velocity of sound depends upon the elasticity and density of the medium.

6. Velocity is given by the following equation:

$$c^2 = \frac{\text{elasticity}}{\text{density}}$$

In air (a gas), the expression can be rewritten as

$$c^2 = \frac{\gamma P_0}{\rho}$$

where γ denotes specific heat ratio and ρ denotes density of the medium.

7. Velocity of sound in normal air is 1127 feet per second, or 344 meters per second.

8. Velocity is affected by temperature. Velocity increases 1 foot per second for each increase in degree Fahrenheit.

9. Frequency (f) is the rate at which complete cycles of high and low pressure regions are produced by the sound source. Frequency is measured in cycles per second or Hertz (Hz).

10. Wavelength is the distance traveled by a wave in one period.

11. A period (T) is the time required for one cycle of pressure change: i.e., $T = 1/f$.

12. The relationship between velocity and wavelength and frequency is given as

$$\lambda = \frac{c}{f}$$

13. Sound pressure is defined as the difference between atmospheric pressure and actual pressure during rarefaction.

14. Sound pressure is not related to frequency. A low frequency sound can have a large sound pressure, and a high frequency sound can have a low pressure.

15. Sound pressure (P) is measured in fractions of bars, usually bars, which is one-millionth of bar. Sound pressure can also be expressed in dynes per square centimeter or newtons per square centimeter.

16. Sound pressure can be measured in root mean squares (RMS) or peak pressures.

17. Sound power (W) is the total sound energy radiated per unit time by a sound source. Sound power is not related to the distance the hearer is away from the sound source as sound pressure is. Sound pressure can be expressed in foot-pounds per second, horsepower, or joules per second (watts).

18. Sound intensity (I) is defined as the sound power per unit area. Sound intensity can be expressed as foot-pounds per second per square foot, watts per square foot, or watts per square centimeter.

19. Sound intensity and sound pressure are related by the inverse square law, which is given by the following equation:

$$W = I4\pi r^2$$

20. Sound intensity and sound pressure are related by the following equation under normal atmospheric conditions (see Industrial Hygiene and Toxicology, Volume I, p. 626).

$$I = (1.52P)^2$$

where I is in μwatts per square foot and P is in μbars.

21. Given that sound intensity is related to sound power and sound pressure, it can be shown that there is a relationship between sound power and sound pressure. This relationship is expressed as

$$P = [W\rho C/4\pi r^2]^{1/2}$$

under normal atmospheric conditions where W is given in watts, C in feet per second, r in feet, and ρ in newtons per square meters. The expression can be written as (see The Industrial Environment: Its Evaluation and Control, p. 302).

$$P = [3.5W \times 10^2/r^2]^{1/2}$$

22. Free-field is defined as a situation where a sound is free to radiate in all directions. The equations developed in this chapter assume a free-field.

2. Physics of Sound

Introduction

The concepts of sound, sound power, sound pressure, and sound intensity were discussed in the last chapter. Further, the relationships between sound power, sound pressure, and sound intensity were conceptually and arithmetically presented. During the presentation of these topics, only pure tones were discussed.

In this chapter, complex sound is examined; and the concepts of sound-pressure level, sound-power level, and sound-intensity level are discussed. By the end of this chapter, the student should be able to convert sound pressure, sound power, and sound intensity into sound-pressure levels, sound-power levels, and sound-intensity levels. In addition, the student should be able to add and subtract decibels (sound pressure, power, and intensity levels).

This chapter also expresses the relationship between sound-pressure level and sound-power level. This relationship is used in subsequent chapters as the basis for making corrections in conditions other than in the free-field.

Complex Sound

The last chapter discussed only pure tones or very simple sounds. However, most industrial sound is not simple. It is complex. Figure 4.2.1 shows complex sound.

This complex sound can be broken up into pure tones or very simple sounds. (See Figure 4.2.2.) The top of Figure 4.2.2 shows the pattern of complex sound. The bottom of the figure shows that the complex sound can be broken down into three simple pure tones; one having a frequency of 100 Hz (cycles per second, CPS), one having a frequency of 200 Hz or CPS, and one having a frequency of 300 Hz or CPS. The combination of these three simple sounds generates the complex sound at the top of the figure. Most sounds, such as musical sounds, are composed of a superposing of many frequencies. The lowest frequency in the complex sound is the fundamental. The fundamental determines the pitch of the sound (or musical note). (Note: The pitch of a sound corresponds to its frequency—low pitch sounds are low frequency sounds; high pitch sounds are high frequency sounds.)

Figure 4.2.1

Illustration of complex sound.

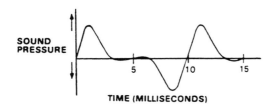

Figure 4.2.2

Analysis of complex sound.

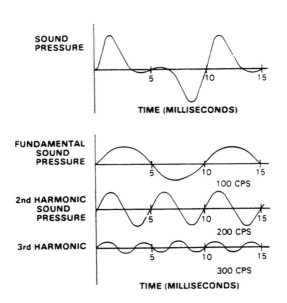

    The higher frequencies making up the complex sound are <u>overtones</u> or
<u>harmonics</u>. It is these overtones that give sound its quality. The tones of
the same pitch (frequency) that have different qualities either will have
different overtones, or the relative intensities of the overtones will be
different. This is why the same tones from a clarinet and a piano sound
different. The frequencies of the overtones are not haphazard but are whole
multiples of the lowest frequency, the fundamental. If the frequency of one
sound cannot be related simply to the frequency of another sound, the

combination of the two sounds will be discordant (i.e., the sounds will be
unharmonically related).

Notice in Figure 4.2.2 that the peak pressure variation caused by the
combination of tones is only slightly greater than the peak pressure variation
caused by the fundamental alone. If sound is expressed in terms of sound
intensity, the sum of the average intensities of the components is equal to
the average intensity of the combination. The sound in Figure 4.2.3 is the
same sound as in Figure 4.2.2 except it is plotted by intensity and time
rather than by pressure and time. The top left part of Figure 4.2.3 shows the
complex sound for 10 milliseconds. The average intensity of that complex
sound is given by the bar labeled "OA" (overall average). The bottom left
part of Figure 4.2.3 shows the intensities of the fundamental and overtones
for the same 10 milliseconds. The bottom right part of the figure shows the
average intensities of the fundamental and the two overtones. The top right
part of Figure 4.2.3 shows that the sum of the average intensities of the
fundamental and overtones equals the average intensity of the complex sound.
From the components, it is easy to determine the shape of the complex sound.
However, it is more difficult to determine the components of the complex sound.

Figure 4.2.3

Sound intensity and complex sound.

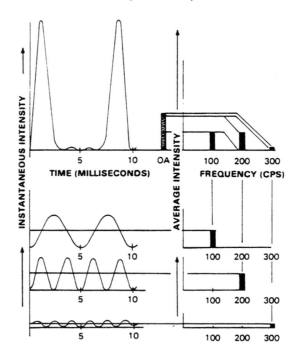

In 1822 the French mathematician, Joseph Fourier, discovered a mathematical regularity to the components of a sound wave motion. He found that even the most complex sound could be broken down into simple sine waves (pure tones). The mathematical operation for doing this is <u>Fourier analysis</u>. The mathematics involved will not be explained in this text. Given complex sound, it is possible to break it into its components; that is, it is possible to plot the components as sound pressure or intensity as time passes.

In many situations, it is more important to know the frequency of sound than to know the exact behavior as time passes (the plot of intensity over time). Therefore, an alternate method of describing sound, <u>frequency analysis</u>, is often used. The right side of Figure 4.2.4 shows a frequency analysis for three sounds; the left side shows the pattern of sound intensity as time passes. Again, notice that the overall average intensity (OA) is equal to the sum of the average intensities making up the sound. The right side of Figure 4.2.4 is meaningful in that it shows the average sound intensity of the components making up the total or complex sound. The left side is meaningful only if the fundamental and overtones are also shown.

Figure 4.2.4

Frequency analysis.

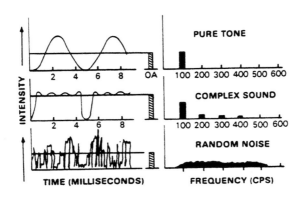

Frequency Bands

Since many sounds encountered in the industrial setting are complex sounds or even random sounds as shown in the bottom of Figure 4.2.4, it becomes impractical to measure the intensity of each component at each frequency in a frequency analysis. It is much easier to measure the total sound intensity in each of a set of frequency bands. A frequency band is nothing more than a range of frequencies.

Three frequency bands are typically used: the octave band, the half octave band, and the third octave band.

In the octave band, audible frequencies are divided into eight or more equal segments where each segment represents a band. (See Figure 4.2.5.) The word "octave" is used here because it means the upper limit of the frequency band is twice the lower limit.

$$F_2 = 2F_1$$

where F_2 denotes the upper limit of the band and F_1 demotes the lower limit of the band.

The center frequency of an octave band is equal to the geometric mean; that is

$$F_m = \sqrt{F_1 F_2}$$

where F_m denotes the center frequency, F_1 represents the lower limit or lower frequency, and F_2 represents the upper limit of the band or the upper frequency.

Two octave bands have been reported in the literature. (See Figure 4.2.5)

Figure 4.2.5

Octave bands.

Center Frequency (In Hz or CPS)	31.5	63	125	250	500	1000	2000	4000	8000
Center Frequency (In Hz or CPS)	53		106	212	425	850	1700	3400	6800

In the half-octave band, the band width narrows so that references to the frequency can be more specific. In the half-octave band, the upper frequency of the band is equal to the square root of 2 times the lower frequency of the band, or

$$F_2 = \sqrt{2F_1} \qquad \sqrt{2} * F_1$$

where F_2 denotes the upper limit of the band, and F_1 denotes the lower limit of the band. Again, the geometric mean is the center frequency.

The third-octave band is still a narrower band width. It is given by the following relationship:

$$F_2 = \sqrt[3]{2F_1} \qquad \sqrt[3]{2} \cdot F_1$$

where F_2 denotes the upper frequency, and F_1 denotes the lower frequency. The center frequency is also computed as the geometric mean.

Rather than looking at the average intensity of each of the components at each frequency, it is more realistic and more practical to look at the average intensity of each component at the octave bands, either the full-octave band, the half-octave band, or the third-octave band. The band that is selected depends upon the specificity desired (that is, how narrow the bands should be). The average sound intensity in any frequency band is equal to the sum of the average intensities of the components within the frequency limits of that band. By the same rule, the overall intensity or the average intensity must be equal to the sum of the average intensities of each of the frequency bands. That is, nothing is lost by using bands rather than a single specific frequency since intensity is a quantity that can be averaged.

Decibels

    In the last section, frequency and sound intensity were plotted. An example of this using frequency bands is given in Figure 4.2.6. The vertical

Figure 4.2.6

Sound intensity plotted by frequency.

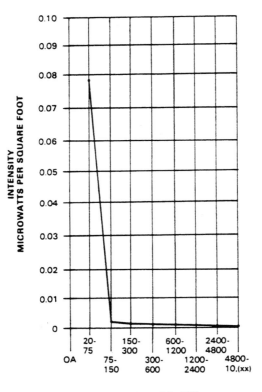

OCTAVE BANDS (CPS)

axis gives sound intensity in μwatts per square foot. The horizontal axis gives the frequency limits of the band in which the intensity is measured. (Note: The first and last bands are not exact octave bands for convenience i. presentation.)

It can be noted from Figure 4.2.6 that the sound intensities in all but the lowest frequency bands are too small to plot accurately. The noises in the higher octave bands, however, are very important in determining the overall intensity of the sound in a room. Therefore, plotting sound intensity by frequency is inadequate, because it overemphasizes the large components of sound and makes other components almost too small to notice. What is needed is a scheme that expands the differences at small intensities (the bottom par of the vertical axis) and contracts the differences at large intensities (the top part of the vertical axis). The human ear responds to a very broad range of sound intensities. Sound intensity as computed in the last chapter may result in very small intensities--so small that the differences when plotted are hardly noticeable. What is needed, then, to represent sound intensity is a scale that avoids small numbers. The scale used to avoid small numbers is the decibel scale.

When sound intensity is changed to the decibel scale and plotted against frequency bands, the differences in the smaller intensities become noticeable. (See Figure 4.2.7.) On the right hand side of the figure, the vertical axis represents sound intensity converted to the decibel scale, while the horizontal axis remains the frequency bands.

A decibel is the log of a ratio. The ratio of concern is the measured quantity over a reference quantity. Usually the reference quantity is the threshold of hearing. For example, when referring to intensity, the concern is with the ratio of the measured intensity to the reference intensity which is usually given as 10^{-12} watts per square meter. (In air, this reference corresponds closely to the reference pressure, 0.00002 newtons per square meter.) Thus, the ratio becomes

$$\frac{I}{I_{ref}} = \frac{I \text{ watts/meter}^2}{10^{-12} \text{ watts/meter}^2}$$

where I denotes the measured intensity and I_{ref} denotes the reference intensity (10^{-12} watts per square meter).

If the log of this ratio is taken, the result is

$$Log \frac{I}{I_{ref}}$$

This log of a ratio, does not give the decibel scale. A bel is a dimensionless unit related to the ratio of two quantities. A decibel is equal to ten bels. To express the ratio in terms of decibels, take 10 times the log of the ratio, which is written as

$$10 \text{ Log } \frac{I}{I_{ref}}$$

where I denotes the measured intensity and I_{ref} denotes the reference intensity, 10^{-12} watts per square meter.

By expanding the above expression, it can be seen that intensity expressed in decibels is given as

$$10 \text{ Log } \frac{I}{I_{ref}} = 10 \text{ Log } I + 10 \text{ Log } I_{ref}$$
$$= 10 \text{ Log } I - 10 \text{ Log } 10^{-12}$$
$$= 10 \text{ Log } I + 120$$

where I denotes the measured sound intensity.

When sound intensity is expressed in the decibel scale, it is known as the sound-intensity level.

Figure 4.2.7

Decibel scale by frequency.

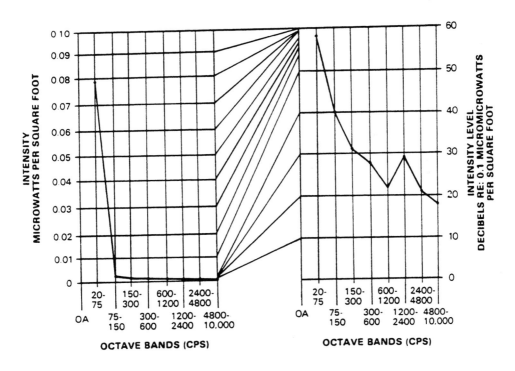

Reprinted from Industrial Hygiene and Toxicology, 1958, Vol. I, 2nd ed., Patty, F.A. (ed.), by permission of John Wiley & Sons, Inc., copyright © 1958.

Although this discussion has been concerned with intensity, it is convenient also to transform sound power and sound pressure into decibel units.

The range of sound pressures encountered is extremely wide. The minimum sound pressure detected by the ear is 0.00002 newtons per square meter. Sound pressures of 200 newtons per square meter represent the threshold of discomfort. Sound pressures of more than 10^6 newtons per square meter cannot be scaled linearly with practical instruments because the scale might be many miles in length in order to obtain the desired accuracy at various pressure levels. In order to cover this wide range of sound pressures, it is convenient to use the decibel scale; i.e., to convert sound pressure into a sound pressure level. The reference quantity used in 0.00002 newtons per square meter, 0.00002   bars, or 0.00002 dynes per square centimeter.

$$\text{Sound Pressure Level} = 10 \ \text{Log} \ (P/P_{ref})^2$$

$$ref = 0.00002 \ N/m^2$$

or

$$\text{Sound Pressure Level} = 20 \ \text{Log} \ P + 94$$

$$ref = 0.00002 \ N/m^2$$

The ratio for sound pressure is squared because sound pressure is usually measured as a root mean square.

Table 4.2.1 shows the relationship between sound pressure level in N/m^2 (ref = 0.00002 N/m^2) and sound pressure in N/m^2. This table illustrates the advantage of using the decibel scale rather than the wide range of direct pressure measurements.

Sound power can also be converted to sound-power level. The reference quantity is given as 10^{-12} watts. Thus

$$\text{Sound-Power Level} = 10 \ \text{Log} \ \frac{W}{W_{ref}} \quad , \ ref = 10^{-12} \ watts$$

$$= 10 \ \text{Log} \ W + 120$$

Table 4.2.2 shows the relationship between sound power and sound-power level.

Given the following sound intensity, sound pressure, and sound power, convert them to sound-pressure level, sound-power level, and sound-intensity level.

What is the sound-intensity level (SIL) if the sound intensity is 0.08 watts per square meter? (Use $I_{ref} = 10^{-12} watts/M^2$.)

$$\begin{aligned}
SIL &= 10 \ \text{Log} \ I + 120 \\
&= 10 \ \text{Log} \ 0.08 + 120 \\
&= 10(0.9 - 2.0) + 120 \\
&= 109 \ \text{decibels}
\end{aligned}$$

Table 4.2.1

Sound pressure level and sound pressure.

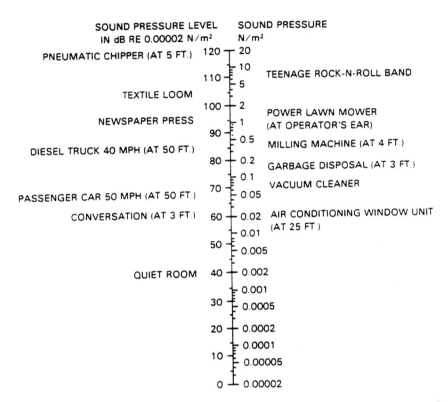

What is the sound-pressure level (SPL) if the sound pressure is 20 N/m²? (Use 0.00002 N/m² as the reference.)

$$SPL = 20 \text{ Log } P + 94$$
$$= 20(1.301) + 94$$
$$= 26.02 + 94$$
$$= 120 \text{ decibels}$$

What is the sound-power level (SWL) if the sound power is 4.0 watts? (Ref = 10^{-12} watts.)

$$SWL = 10 \text{ Log } 4 + 120$$
$$= 126 \text{ decibels}$$

Assume a sound source has the sound power of 1 watt, and sound intensity at 1, 2, and 4 meters is of concern. Recall from the inverse square law that the relationship between sound power and sound intensity is given as

$$I = \frac{W}{4\pi r^2}$$

where I denotes sound intensity, W denotes sound power and r denotes the radius (distance from the sound source).

Table 4.2.2

Sound-power level and sound power.

SOUND POWER LEVEL. dB RE 10^{-12} WATT		SOUND POWER IN WATTS
	170	100,000
TURBOJET ENGINE	160	10,000
	150	1000
	140	100
	130	10
COMPRESSOR	120	1
	110	10^{-1}
	100	10^{-2}
	90	10^{-3}
	80	10^{-4}
CONVERSATION	70	10^{-5}
	60	10^{-6}
	50	10^{-7}
	40	10^{-8}
	30	10^{-9}
	20	10^{-10}
	10	10^{-11}
	0	10^{-12}

With the above information, find the sound-intensity levels at distances 1, 2, and 4 meters.

Hint: Convert or calculate the intensity at distance 1, 2, and 4 meters, and then change the sound intensities to sound-intensity levels, using 10^{-12} watts per square meter. Doing this, it will be noted that the sound-intensity levels are 109 decibels at 1 meter, 103 decibels at 2 meters, and 98 decibels at 4 meters. Notice that a change of six decibels occurs for every doubling of distance. That is, as the distance doubles, the sound-intensity levels decrease by six decibels.

If the sound-intensity level at a given distance is known, then the sound-intensity level at some other distance can be computed using the following expression:

$$SIL_{(r)} = SIL_{(1)} - 20 \, Log \, 10(r/r_1)$$

where $SIL_{(r)}$ denotes the sound-intensity level at distance r, $SIL_{(1)}$ denotes the known sound-intensity level at distance r_1, and r and r_1 denote the distances corresponding to the two sound-intensity levels.

For example, if the sound-intensity level at $r_1 = 1$ is 109 dB, then the sound-intensity level at $r = 2$ can be computed as follows:

$$SIL_{(r=2)} = SIL_{(r=1)} - 20 \text{ Log } 10(r/r_1)$$

$$= 109 \text{ dB} - 20 \text{ Log } 10(2/1)$$

$$= 109 \text{ dB} - 20 \text{ Log } 10(2)$$

$$= 109 \text{ dB} - 6.0 \text{ dB}$$

$$= 103 \text{ dB}$$

Adding and Subtracting Decibels

Although converting sound pressure, sound power, and sound intensity to the decibel scale is useful for graphic representation, converting them to the decibel scale also has its disadvantages. Decibels cannot be directly added and subtracted. Converting sound pressure, power, and intensity to decibels (the log of ratios) changes the nature of the numbers of involved. This presents a problem. Recall that when sound intensity was plotted against frequency it was noted that the overall average intensity was equal to the sum of the average intensities of each of the component frequencies. When dealing with sound-intensity levels, they cannot be directly added to find the overall average sound-intensity level.

Suppose for a complex sound composed of a fundamental and one overtone that the fundamental has an average sound-intensity level of 50 dB and the overtone has an average sound-intensity level of 55 dB. (Note: dB is a shorthand notation for decibel.) It is not possible to simply add the 50 dB and 55 dB to find the overall average sound-intensity level of the complex sound because they are logs. To add decibels (sound-intensity levels, sound-power levels, or sound-pressure levels), the following equation is used:

$$L_c = 10 \text{ Log } (10^{L_1/10} + 10^{L_2/10}) \qquad (4.2.1)$$

where L_c denotes combined level, L_1 denotes level 1, and L_2 denotes level 2

or

$$L_c = L_1 + 10 \text{ Log } [10^{(L_2 - L_1)/10} + 1] \qquad (4.2.2)$$

where L_c denotes combined level, L_1 denotes the lowest level, and L_2 denotes the highest level.

Expression (4.2.2) can now be used to find the overall average sound intensity level of two sounds, one at 50 dB and one at 55 dB. Substituting these values in the expression results in the following:

$$L_c = 50 + 10 \text{ Log } [10^{(55 - 50)/10} + 1]$$
$$L_c = 40 + 10 \text{ Log } (4.16)$$
$$= 50 + 6.19$$
$$= 56.2 \text{ dB}$$

When there are only two quantities to be added, this method is simple. If there are more than two quantities, the formula becomes unmanageable because two levels must be added to get a combined level; this must be added to the third to get a new combined level, and so on. However, a table is available for adding and subtracting decibels (Table 4.2.3). Use of the table is very simple. Find the difference between level 1 and level 2, and use the table to determine how much to add to the higher level.

Example

For the following sound-intensity levels at each of the following octave bands, find the overall sound-intensity level.

Center Frequency	SIL (dB)
31.5	85
63	88
125	94
250	94
500	95
1000	100
2000	97
4000	90
8000	88

Solution

Rearrange the sound intensity levels from the lowest to the highest and add them together, using Table 4.2.3. The result is as follows:

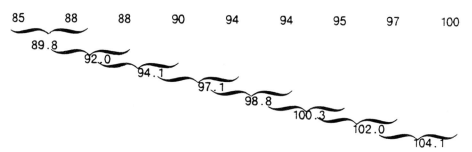

The Relationship Between Sound-Power Level and Sound-Pressure Level

Recall from the last chapter that the relationship between sound power and sound pressure was given as:

$$P = [3.5W \times 10^2/r^2]^{1/2}$$

Table 4.2.3

Adding and subtracting decibels.

Numerical Difference Between L_1 and L_2	Amount to be Added to the Higher of L_1 and L_2
0.0 to .1	3.0
.2 to .3	2.9
.4 to .5	2.8
.6 to .7	2.7
.8 to .9	2.6
1.0 to 1.2	2.5
1.3 to 1.4	2.4
1.5 to 1.6	2.3
1.7 to 1.9	2.2
2.0 to 2.1	2.1
2.2 to 2.4	2.0
2.5 to 2.7	1.9
2.8 to 3.0	1.8
3.1 to 3.3	1.7
3.4 to 3.6	1.6
3.7 to 4.0	1.5
4.1 to 4.3	1.4
4.4 to 4.7	1.3
4.8 to 5.1	1.2
5.2 to 5.6	1.1
5.7 to 6.1	1.0
6.2 to 6.6	.9
6.7 to 7.2	.8
7.3 to 7.9	.7
8.0 to 8.6	.6
8.7 to 9.6	.5
9.7 to 10.7	.4
10.8 to 12.2	.3
12.3 to 14.5	.2
14.6 to 19.3	.1
19.4 to ∞	0.0

Step 1: Determine the difference between the two levels to be added (L_1 and L_2).

Step 2: Find the number (L_3) corresponding to this difference in the table.

Step 3: Add the number (L_3) to the highest of L_1 and L_2 to obtain the resultant level. $L_R = (L_1$ or $L_2) + L_3$

Source: The Industrial Environment: Its Evaluation and Control.

Note that this relationship is between sound power and sound pressure, not sound-power level and sound-pressure level. The relationship between sound-power level and sound-pressure level is given as follows: (See The Industrial Environment: Its Evaluation and Control, p. 307)

$$L_p \quad SPL = SWL - 20 \text{ Log } r - 0.5 \text{ dB} \qquad (4.2.3)$$

or

$$L_w \quad SWL = SPL + 20 \text{ Log } r + 0.5 \text{ dB}$$

where SWL denotes sound-power level in decibels (reference 10^{-12} watts), SPL denotes sound-pressure level in decibels (reference 0.00002 newtons per square meter), and r is in feet. If r is measured in meters, replace the constant 0.5 with 11.
This relationship is true only in the free-field condition in normal atmosphere.

Example. Predict the sound-pressure level that will be produced in a free-field at a distance of 10 feet in front of a machine. (Assume an omnidirectional noise source--a free-field.) The source has a sound power of 0.1 watts. (Note: To convert sound power to sound-power level, use 10^{-12} watts as the reference.)

Solution. Substituting the given values in the expression results in the following:

$$L_p \quad SPL = SWL - 20 \text{ Log } r - 0.5 \text{ dB}$$

$$L_p \quad SPL = 10 \text{ Log } \frac{W}{10^{-12} \text{ watts}} - 20 \text{ Log } 100 \text{ feet} - 0.5 \text{ dB}$$

$$L_p \quad SPL = 10(\text{Log } 0.1 - \text{Log } 10^{-12} \text{ watts}) - 20 \text{ Log } 10^2 - 0.5 \text{ dB}$$

$$L_p \quad SPL = 10 (-1 + 12) - 40 \text{ dB} - 0.5 \text{ dB}$$

$$L_p \quad SPL = 69.5 \text{ dB (SPL reference 0.00002 N/m}^2)$$

Correction for Atmospheric Conditions

Expression (4.2.3) given in the last section is true only under normal atmospheric conditions. If conditions are nonstandard, correction for these nonstandard conditions can be made using the following expression:

$$L_p \quad SPL = SWL - 20 \text{ Log } r - 0.5 \text{dB} + T$$

where T denotes the correction factor.

The correction factor can be obtained from the Figure 4.2.8. This correction factor takes into consideration the velocity of sound under different temperatures and pressures.

Figure 4.2.8

Computation of correction factor.

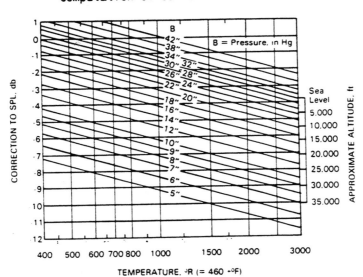

Correction for the Directivity of a Sound Source

The relationship between sound-pressure level and sound-power level can be modified for the directivity of the sound source. In the last sentence, the expression given is appropriate only in a free-field condition. However, sometimes the sound source is directional rather than nondirectional; that is, the sound source spreads in only one direction. This directivity factor (Q) of the sound source will disrupt the relationship between sound-pressure level and sound-power level.

The directivity factor is defined as the measure of the degree to which a sound is concentrated in a certain direction rather than radiated evenly in a full spherical pattern. There are several patterns that are possible. The first pattern is a nondirectional point source pattern (free-field condition). It is related to the area of a sphere, $4\pi r^2$. In this pattern, Q would be equal to 1.

Figure 4.2.9

Directivity factor, Q = 1.

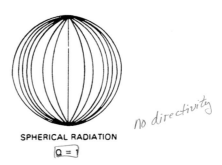

no directivity

SPHERICAL RADIATION

Q = 1

The second possible pattern is a half spherical radiation where the source is in the field but on the ground. Here Q would be equal to 2. (See Figure 4.2.10.)

Figure 4.2.10

Directivity factor, Q = 2.

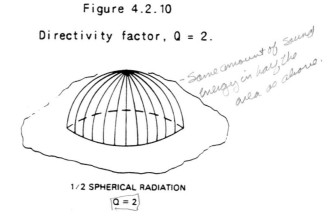

- Some amount of sound energy in half the area as above.

1/2 SPHERICAL RADIATION

Q = 2

The third directional pattern would be the sound source on a floor next to the wall. In this case, Q would be equal to 4. The sound-radiation area has been reduced by a factor of 4; that is, $4\pi r^2$ divided by 4.

The fourth radiation pattern is a source next to two walls sitting on the floor. In this case, Q would be equal to 8.

The relationship between sound-pressure level and sound-power level can be modified for this directivity factor as follows: (See The Industrial Environment: Its Evaluation and Control, p. 307.)

SPL = SWL - 20 Log r - 0.5 dB + 10 Log Q + T

Figure 4.2.11

Directivity factor, Q = 4.

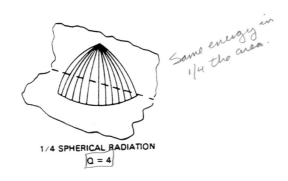

Same energy in 1/4 the area.

1/4 SPHERICAL RADIATION
Q = 4

Figure 4.2.12

Directivity factor, Q = 8.

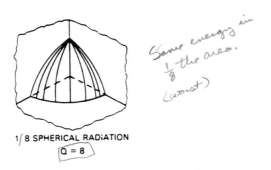

Same energy in 1/8 the area.
(worst)

1/8 SPHERICAL RADiATION
Q = 8

Example. Using the above expression, predict the sound-pressure level that will be produced at a distance of 3 feet directly in front of a machine. The machine has a directivity factor of 5 (this factor is provided by the machine manufacturer). The noise source has a sound power of 0.1 watts. In solving the problem, assume normal atmospheric conditions; i.e., T = 0.

Solution. Using the above expression, the solution is as follows. Use 10^{-12} watts as the reference.

Given: Q - 5, r = 3 ft, W = 0.1 watts
         SPL = SWL - 20 Log r - 0.5 dB + 10 log Q + T dB

$$SPL = 10 \ Log[0.1 \ watt/10^{-12} \ watt] - 20 \ Log \ 3 \ ft - 0.5 \ dB +$$

$$10 \ Log \ 5$$

$$SPL = 106.95 \ dB \ (reference \ 0.00002 \ N/m^2)$$

Summary

The following principles were discussed in this chapter.

1. Complex sound can be broken down into simple sound components--a fundamental and the component harmonics.

2. Harmonics give sound its quality.

3. The plot of sound intensities or sound pressure by frequency (frequency analysis) is meaningful and useful. At times it is more meaningful than the pattern of sound intensity or pressure as time passes.

4. Rather than measuring sound pressure (or computing sound intensity) at every frequency, frequency bands are used. There are three common bands that are used: full-octave band, half-octave band, and one-third octave band. The narrowest band is the one-third octave band. Sound intensity or sound pressure is usually plotted against the center of the band being used.

5. The sound intensity in any frequency band is equal to the sum of the intensities of the components within the frequency limits of that band. The overall average intensity of a complex sound is equal to the sum of the intensities in each of the frequencies.

6. A sound intensity expressed in decibels is a sound-intensity level (SIL). Sound-intensity level is computed as follows:

$$SIL = 10 \ Log \ I + 120$$

    where I denotes sound intensity, and the reference quantity is 10^{-12} watts per square meter.

7. A sound pressure expressed in decibels is a sound-pressure level (SPL). Sound-pressure level is computed as follows:

$$SPL = 20 \ Log \ P + 94$$

    where P denotes sound pressure and the reference quantity is given as 0.00002 newtons per square meter.

8. A sound power expressed in decibels is a sound-power level (SWL). Sound-power level is computed as follows:

$$SWL = 10 \ Log \ W + 120$$

where W denotes sound power and the reference quantity is given as 10^{-12} watts.

9. The decibel scale is used because the range of sound audible by the human ear is wide. If scaled linearly, the scale might be many miles long.

10. Decibels cannot be directly added or subtracted. To add decibels, the following expression is used.

$$L_c = L_1 + 10 \text{ Log } [10^{(L_2 - L_1)/10} + 1]$$

where L_c denotes the combined level, L_1 denotes the lowest level, and L_2 denotes the highest level.

If several levels are being added, tables are available to eliminate many calculations.

11. The relationship between sound-pressure level and sound-power level is given by

$$SPL = SWL - 20 \text{ Log } r - 0.5 \text{ dB}$$

where r is distance in feet and SPL (ref: 0.00002 N/m^2) and SWL (reference 10^{-12} watts) denote sound-pressure level and sound-power level respectively.

This expression assumes a nondirectional sound source and normal atmospheric conditions.

12. The relationship between sound-pressure level and sound-power level can be modified for nonstandard atmospheric conditions.

$$SPL = SWL - 20 \text{ Log } r - 0.5 \text{ dB} + T$$

where T denotes the correction factor, obtained from a correction table.

13. The relationship between sound-pressure level and sound-power level can be modified for the directivity of the sound source.

$$SPL = SWL - 20 \text{ Log } r - 0.5 \text{ dB} + T + 10 \text{ Log } Q$$

where Q denotes the directivity factor of the sound source.

Q is usually supplied by the manufacturer. When Q = 1, there is spherical radiation in all directions from the sound source. When Q = 2, the sound radiated is in a hemispherical pattern; when Q = 4, there is quarter-sphere radiation; and when Q = 8, there is one-eighth spherical radiation.

3. Physics of Sound

Introduction

In the last chapter, the relationship between sound-pressure level and sound-power level was discussed. The relationship was given as:

$$SPL = SWL - 20 \text{ Log } r - 0.5 \text{ dB} + T + 10 \text{ Log } Q$$

where SPL denotes sound-pressure level (reference: $0.00002N/m^2$), SWL denotes sound-power level (reference: 10^{-12} watts), r denotes distance from the sound source in feet, T denotes the correction for atmospheric conditions in dB, and Q denotes the directivity factor of the sound source.

This chapter discusses sound in a room. The relationship between sound-pressure level and sound-power level will be modified to account for the behavior of sound in a room. Also discussed in this chapter is how sound travels from one room to another. This will include the concepts of transmission loss and noise reduction.

Sound in a Room

Sound in a free-field, a condition where sound from a sound source is free to radiate in all directions, was presented in the last chapter. Sound in a free-field can be graphically represented by Figures 4.3.1 and 4.3.2.

Figure 4.3.1

Sound in a free field.

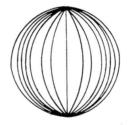

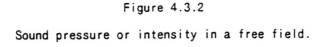

Figure 4.3.2

Sound pressure or intensity in a free field.

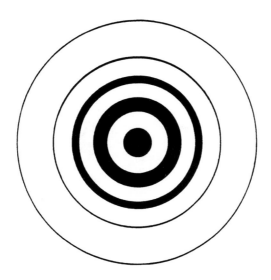

But what would happen if walls were put around the sound source? By putting the sound source in a room, what is going to happen when the sound reaches a wall? Naturally, the sound will be reflected off the walls--the sound will generate a reflected wave off the wall. (See Figure 4.3.3.) Actually, there would be multiple reflections; the sound waves will bounce off the walls repeatedly. (See Figure 4.3.4.)

From Figure 4.3.4, it can be seen that there are three fields of sound. There is sound that is in the near field--the field near the sound source. There is a field that acts like the inverse-square field in a free-field condition--the field that is some distance away from the sound source. In the inverse-square field, the sound of the sound source predominates, rather than the sound bouncing off the walls. And there is the sound field near the walls. This is the reverberant sound field where sound is reflected off the walls, and the reflected sound predominates rather than the sound from the sound source.

In Figure 4.3.4, sound intensity is used to show the three fields. However, sound pressure could have been used since sound intensity and sound pressure are related.

When the sound source is in a room, the sound pressure (or sound-pressure level) in the near field cannot be predicted. However, in the inverse-square field, the sound-pressure level or the sound-intensity level can be predicted if the sound-power level is known:

Figure 4.3.3

Sound in a room.

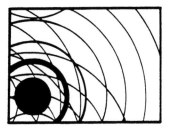

Figure 4.3.4

Multiple reflections.

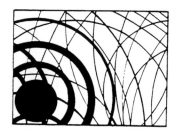

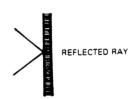

REFLECTED RAY

$$\text{Sound intensity} = \frac{\text{Sound power}}{4\pi r^2}$$

where r denotes the distance from the sound source.

The sound pressure predicted is dependent upon the distance from the sound source. In the reverberant field, as can be seen from Figure 4.3.4, the sound pressure (and sound intensity) will eventually become constant near the walls and may have nothing to do with the distance and direction of the sound source; i.e., the sound pressure in the reverberant field will be independent of distance from the sound source. A method for predicting the sound pressure in the reverberant field is presented later in this chapter.

An important concept when considering sound in a room is the critical distance. The critical distance is the distance at which the noise level (sound pressure or intensity) changes from inverse-square-law behavior to reverberant field behavior. An expression for computing the critical distance will be given later in this chapter. There is a way of determining precisely the location where the inverse-square law no longer holds, and the reverberant field behavior of sound becomes the important sound. One can roughly estimate the critical distance by ear. This can be done by focusing your attention on a predominately identifiable noise source. Walk away from the source machine until the level appears relatively constant to your ears. Then walk rapidly toward the source, stopping when you are first aware of the increase in level. Repeat this procedure until you have localized the point at which the

direct sound begins to predominate, at the critical distance position.   Then
measure from there to the sound; this gives the critical distance.

Absorption

What factors will affect sound in the reverberant field? An obvious
answer is the composition of the walls in the room. If the walls of the room
are constructed of a hard material, the sound will reflect. On the other
hand, if the walls of the room are constructed of a soft surface, sound will
be absorbed rather than reflected. A soft surface is a surface that is made
of porous material. This porous material has interconnecting air spaces that
allow the sound to be absorbed. As the sound enters these interconnected air
spaces, the sound energy is transformed into heat energy. (At normal sound
intensities, this heat buildup is insignificant.) Thus, as the wall becomes
more absorbent, there is less reflected sound; thus, there is less reverberant
sound in the reverberant sound field.

The ability of a surface to absorb sound is given by the absorption
coefficient, usually denoted by alpha (α). A surface that has an absorption
coefficient equal to 1 is a perfectly absorbing medium, such as open space.
Open space will not reflect any sound at all. A hard surface, such as marble,
has an absorption coefficient equal to 0; that is, no sound is absorbed at
all, and it is reflected back into the room.

The absorption coefficient of a given material is not the same for all
frequencies. Given materials, such as marble, wood, plaster, etc., all have
absorption coefficients; but these coefficients are different for different
frequencies. There are tables available that give the absorption coefficient
of a given material at a given frequency. Figure 4.3.5 shows the absorption
coefficients of various materials at various frequencies.

Most walls in industrial settings are not composed of just one material.
For example, brick walls may have glass windows. Thus, what is needed is a
system to compute the average absorption coefficient of a wall that is made of
different kinds of materials. If a wall is made of glass and brick, what is
the absorption coefficient of this wall? Before this question can be
answered, the frequency of concern must be known since the absorption
characteristics of the wall are dependent upon the frequency of the sound.
Also, the area of the wall that is made of brick and the area of the wall that
is made of glass must be known. Once this information is given, the average
absorption coefficient of the wall can be computed using the following
expression:

$$\alpha_{avg} = \frac{\sum\limits_{i=1}^{n} S_i \alpha_i}{\sum\limits_{i=1}^{n} S_i}$$

where α_{avg} denotes the average absorption coefficient of the wall constructed of combined materials; S_i denotes the surface area of the ith building material; and α_i denotes the absorption coefficient of the ith building material. (α_i would be obtained from a figure or table, such as Figure 4.3.5, given a specific frequency.)

Figure 4.3.5

Absorption coefficient.

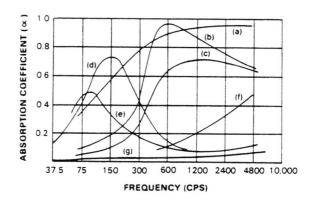

The absorption coefficient of various materials (a reverberant sound field is assumed): (a) 4-inch glass wool blanket (6 lb/ft³ density), against wall--no facing; (b) average for perforated acoustic tiles cemented directly to a hard backing and 1 inch thick; (c) average for perforated acoustic tiles cemented to a hard backing and 1/2-inch thick; (d) 1-inch mineral wool blanket (Aerocor--2 lb/ft³) covered by perforated facing (12 percent open area) and separated from hard backing by 1-inch air space; (e) 3/8-inch plywood panel with 4-inch air space, one cross brace, and 2 inches of mineral wool at wall; (f) heavy carpet on concrete. (g) unpainted brick wall.

For example, a room is 8 feet high, 10 feet wide, and 12 feet long. The ceiling is composed of acoustical tile that has an absorption coefficient of 0.95 at the frequency of concern; the floor is carpeted and has an absorption coefficient of 0.37 at the frequency of concern; and the walls are all made o brick which has an absorption coefficient of 0.03 at the frequency of concern. What is the average absorption coefficient of the room?

$$\alpha_{avg} = \frac{\sum\limits_{i=1}^{n} S_i \alpha_i}{\sum\limits_{i=1}^{n} S_i}$$

$$= \frac{(10 \times 12)0.95 + (10 \times 12)0.37 + 2(10 \times 8)0.03 + 2(12 \times 8)0.03}{2(10 \times 12) + 2(10 \times 8) + 2(12 \times 8)}$$

$$= \frac{168.96}{592}$$ — total surface area of room.

$$= 0.285$$

But 0.285 what? What units are attached to the absorption coefficient? The absorption coefficient is commonly expressed in <u>sabins</u>. One sabin is equivalent to one square foot of a perfectly absorbent surface. The closer the absorption coefficient is to 1, the more absorbent that surface is. The closer the absorption coefficient is to 0, the harder the surface is, and more of the sound will be reflected.

Room Constant

Along with the absorption coefficient of the surfaces, the room constant is also of concern. The room constant is a measure of the ability of a room to absorb sound. The room constant, R, is a value based on the summation of all areas and is given by the following expression:

$$R = \frac{\alpha_{avg} \sum\limits_{i=1}^{n} S_i}{1 - \alpha_{avg}} \quad \text{or} \quad R = \frac{\sum\limits_{i=1}^{n} S_i \alpha_i}{1 - \alpha_{avg}}$$

where R denotes the room constant, α_{avg} denotes the average absorption coefficient of a room, and α_i denotes the absorption coefficient of the ith surface.

Given this expression, what is the room constant of a room that has the following characteristics? 8 feet by 12 feet by 10 feet; the ceiling has an absorption coefficient of 0.95 sabins; the floor has an absorption coefficient of 0.37 sabins; and the walls are brick and have an absorption coefficient of 0.03 sabins. To find the room constant, first the absorption coefficient of the room must be computed using the following expression:

$$\alpha = \frac{\sum\limits_{i=1}^{n} S_i ft^2 \alpha_i sabins}{\sum S_i ft^2}$$

$$= \frac{168.96 \text{ ft}^2 \text{ sabins}}{592 \text{ ft}^2}$$

$$= 0.285 \text{ sabins}$$

Given the average absorption coefficient of the room, the room constant can be computed:

$$R = \frac{\alpha_{avg} \sum_{i=1}^{n} S_i}{1 - \alpha_{avg}}$$

$$= \frac{(0.285 \text{ sabins}) (592 \text{ ft}^2)}{1 - 0.285 \text{ sabins}}$$

Note that the room constant would be in units of ft^2.

$$= 235.97 \text{ ft}^2$$

Factors Affecting the Reverberant Field. From the last two sections, it should be clear that sound pressure in the reverberant field depends upon the room dimensions, the number and type of objects in the room, the placement of the objects in the room, and the absorption characteristics of the room and the objects in the room. In the reverberant fields where a high percentage of reflected sound is present, the sound-pressure levels may be essentially independent of direction and distance to the sound source.

Room Constant and Sound Pressure

The room constant will affect the sound-pressure level in various parts of the room. If the walls were perfectly absorbent and no sound were reflected, the sound-pressure level could be computed as follows:

$$SPL_{(r)} = SPL_{(1)} - 20 \text{ Log } (r/r_1)$$

Where $SPL_{(r)}$ denotes the sound-pressure level at distance r, $SPL_{(1)}$ denotes a known sound-pressure level at some distance r_1, and r and r_1 denote the distances corresponding to $SPL_{(r)}$ and $SPL_{(1)}$ respectively.

If the sound-pressure level is known at a certain position, then the sound-pressure level can be calculated at any other position in the room. Where the walls are perfectly absorbent, sound is going to behave as it would in a free-field condition. Where the walls are less than perfectly absorbent and the sound is reflected off the walls, the sound-pressure levels in various parts of the room will not follow the relationship given in the above expression. Given the room constant, however, the relative sound-pressure level in the reverberant field can be calculated. Calculations from rooms having various absorption coefficients, α_{avg}, are shown in Figure 4.3.6.

[Note: α_{avg} is a function of the room constant: $\alpha_{avg} = R/(\Sigma S + R)$.]

Figure 4.3.6

Relative sound pressure level.

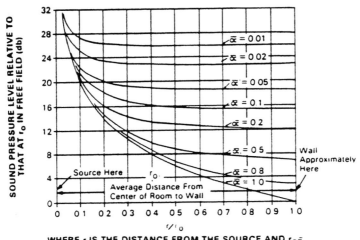

WHERE r IS THE DISTANCE FROM THE SOURCE AND $r_0 = $
$$\sqrt{\text{TOTAL SURFACE AREA OF ROOM}/4\pi}$$

The horizontal axis is the distance, r, from the source to some desired point divided by r_0, the radius of a sphere whose surface area is the same as that of the room; i.e.,

$$r_0 = \sqrt{\text{surface area}/4\pi}$$

For example, if the room is 8 feet by 12 feet x 10 feet, then r_0 can be computed as

$$r_0 = \sqrt{\text{surface area}/4\pi}$$

$$= \sqrt{2(10ft \times 8ft) + 2(8ft \times 12ft) + 2(10ft \times 12ft)/4(3.1416)}$$

$$= \sqrt{592/12.56}$$

$$= 6.865 \ ft$$

r_0 represents the average distance from the center of the room to the walls.

The vertical axis shows the increase in sound-pressure level that exists at any point in the room over the sound-pressure level that would exist at r_0 with the source radiating into the free space; e.g., perfectly absorbing walls. For example, if $\alpha_{avg} = 0.2$ and the room has the following dimensions, 8 ft by 12 ft by 10 ft, then at a distance of 3.865 feet from the source, the sound-pressure level would be 14 dB higher than the sound-pressure level that would exist at 6.865 feet with the sound source radiating into a free space.

From Figure 4.3.6, it can be seen that in an acoustically treated room (with less than perfectly absorbing walls) as the distance from the sound source increases, the sound-pressure level will decrease for a while; but a point will be reached where there is little or no decrease. Specifically, a point will be reached where the sound-pressure level will level off. The sound-pressure level will not continue to decrease because of the reverberan buildup near the walls. The curves in Figure 4.3.6 are appropriate only whe the observer and the sound source are at least one-half wavelength away from the walls. Thus, if the room is small or the frequency low, there will be positions in the room where Figure 4.3.6 will give incorrect results.

Given that the room constant affects the relative sound-pressure level a various distances from the sound source, it is obvious that the room constan also affects the relationship between the sound-power level and the sound-pressure level. The room constant affects the relationship between the sound-pressure level and the sound-power level in the following manner. (See: Industrial Noise Manual.)

$$SPL = SWL + 10 \, Log \, [(Q/4\pi r^2) + (4/R)] + 10.5 + T$$

Assume a chipping hammer that radiates one watt of power in the center o a room. The directivity factor of the machine is 1; that is $Q = 1$. The average distance from the wall to the sound source is 6.87 feet, and the roor constant is 229.39 ft^2. There is no correction for atmospheric temperature or pressure; i.e., $T = 0$. What is the sound-pressure level at the wall?

First, the sound-power level must be computed since the problem states only sound power and not sound-power level. Recall from the last chapter tha the sound-power level can be computed using the following expression:

$$SWL = Log \, W + 120 \, (reference: \, 10^{-12} \, watts)$$

Substituting the sound power in this expression results in

$$SWL = Log \, 1 + 120$$

$$= 120 \, dB \, (reference: \, 10^{-12} \, watts)$$

Now the sound-power level can be substituted in the expression that shows the relationship between sound-power level and sound-pressure level. This result in the following:

$$SPL = SWL + 10 \, Log \, [(Q/4\pi r^2) + (4/R)] + 10.5 + T$$

$$= 120 \, dB + 10 \, Log \, [(1/(4 \times 3.14 \times 6.87)) + (4/229.39)] + 10.5 +$$

$$= 113.316 \, dB \, (reference: \, 0.00002 \, N/m^2)$$

Thus, it can be seen that the sound-pressure level at the wall would be 6.68 dB less than the sound-power level (or 113.316 dB). Note that this sound-pressure level takes into consideration the reverberant field because the expression used considered the room constant (R).

Rather than using the above expression to compute the sound pressure relative to the sound-power level, the relative sound pressure can be found by using published curves. (See Figure 4.3.7.) The figure is used by entering the curves at the horizontal axis at the desired distance, r; following the diagonal lines to a given Q; then up to the appropriate room-constant curve and across to reveal the sound-pressure level relative to the sound-power level (SPL - SWL). In the example given above, enter the curves at r = 6.87 feet; follow the diagonal line to Q = 1; then move up to a room constant of 229.39 feet^2 and across to read the sound-pressure level relative to sound-power level (about 7 dB); i.e., the sound-pressure level would be about 7 dB less than the sound-power level.

Figure 4.3.7

Sound-pressure level in a room
relative to sound-power level.

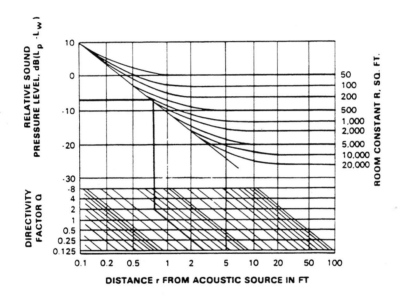

Critical Distance

In previous sections of this chapter, it was noted that there are three sound fields in a room; the near field, the inverse-square-law field, and the reverberant field. It was also noted that in the inverse-square-law field the relationship between sound-power level and sound-pressure level is given as

$$SPL = SWL - 20 \, Log \, r + 10 \, Log \, Q - 0.5dB + T \quad (4.3.1)$$

where r is given in feet, SPL reference: 0.00002 N/m^2, and SWL reference: 10^{-12} watts.

In the reverberant field, the relationship between sound-pressure level and sound-power level can be expressed as

$$SPL = SWL + 10 \ Log \ [(Q/4\pi r^2) + (4/R)] + 10.5 + T \qquad (4.3.2)$$

where r is given in feet, SPL reference: 0.00002 N/m^2, SWL reference: 10^{-12} watts, and R is given in square feet.

Pictorially, the three fields can be represented as in Figure 4.3.8.

Figure 4.3.8

Sound field in a room.

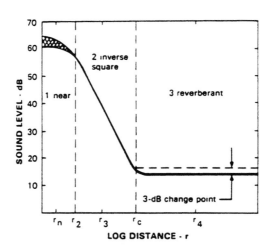

LOG DISTANCE · r

Of particular importance is the critical distance, r_c. The critical distance is the point at which the sound behavior changes from inverse-square-law behavior to reverberant field behavior. The junction between regions 2 and 3 in Figure 4.3.8 is the critical distance.

From expression (2) in this section, it is seen that the inverse-square-law and reverberant fields are equal. (See: Industrial Noise Control Manual, p. 59.)

$$\frac{Q}{4\pi r_c^2} = \frac{4}{R}$$

where r_c, denotes the critical distance in feet, Q denotes the directivity factor, and R denotes the room constant in square feet.

Solving the above identify for r_c results in

$$r_c = \sqrt{QR/16\pi} \qquad (4.3.3)$$

It is often convenient to use expression (4.3.3) in terms of α_{avg}, the average room coefficient. This can be done by recalling.

$$R = \Sigma S\alpha_{avg}/(1-\alpha_{avg}) \qquad\qquad (4.3.4)$$

Substituting expression (4.3.4) in expression (4.3.3) results in

$$r_c = \sqrt{[Q(\Sigma\alpha_{avg})/(1-\alpha_{avg})]/16\pi}$$

$$r_c = \sqrt{(Q\Sigma S\alpha_{avg})/16\pi(1-\alpha_{avg})}$$

$$r_c = 0.14 \sqrt{(Q\Sigma S\alpha_{avg})/(1-\alpha)_{avg}}$$

If a room is 8 ft x 10 ft x 12 ft and has an average absorption coefficient of 0.28 sabins and a sound source with a Q factor of 1, where does the inverse-square-law field end and the reverberant field begin? (In other words, calculate r_c.)

$$r_c = 0.14 \sqrt{1 \, [2(8 \times 10 + 2(10 \times 12) + 2(8 \times 12)] \, 0.28/(1 - 0.28)}$$

$$= 0.14 \sqrt{592(0.28)/0.72}$$

$$= 0.14 \sqrt{165.78/0.72}$$

$$= 2.12 \text{ feet}$$

The critical distance is important because most workers are between the sound source and the critical distance point. The critical distance is also important because it can be shown that making the room more absorbent will not significantly affect the sound-pressure level at the critical distance. The problem below illustrates this point. In the problem, the sound-pressure level will be calculated in three locations; somewhere in the inverse-square-law field, at the critical distance, and somewhere in the reverberant field. Then the room will be made more absorbent to see how the sound pressure is affected in these three locations. For purposes of simplicity, the problem will be concerned only with sound having a frequency of 500 Hz.

Problem. The room is 8 feet high, 12 feet wide, and 10 feet long. The ceiling has an absorption coefficient of 0.95 sabins at 500 Hz; the floor has an absorption coefficient of 0.37 sabins at 500 Hz; and the walls have an absorption coefficient of 0.03 sabins at 500 Hz (brick). The sound source is a compressor for which the manufacturer reports a sound power of 110 dB (reference: 10^{-12} watts) and a directivity factor of 2.0. Assume normal atmospheric conditions; i.e., T = 0.

Solution. First, compute the critical distance, the point where the inverse square law ends and the reverberant field begins. Recall

$$r_c = \sqrt{QR/16\pi}$$

where

$$R = \Sigma S_i \alpha_i / (1 - \alpha_{avg})$$

and where

$$\alpha_{avg} = \Sigma S_i \alpha_i / \Sigma S_i$$

then

$$\alpha_{avg} = \frac{(12 \text{ ft} \times 10 \text{ ft}) \, 0.95 \text{ sabins} + (12 \text{ ft} \times 10 \text{ ft}) \, 0.37 \text{ sabins} + 2(12 \text{ ft} \times 8 \text{ ft}) \, 0.03 \text{ sabins} + 2(10 \text{ ft} \times 8 \text{ ft}) \, 0.03 \text{ sabins}}{2(12 \text{ ft} \times 10 \text{ ft}) + 2(12 \text{ ft} \times 8 \text{ ft}) + 2(10 \text{ ft} \times 8 \text{ ft})}$$

$$= \frac{114 \text{ ft}^2\text{sabins} + 44.4 \text{ ft}^2\text{sabins} + 5.76 \text{ ft}^2\text{sabins} + 4.8 \text{ ft}^2\text{sabins}}{592 \text{ ft}^2}$$

$$= \frac{168.96 \text{ ft}^2\text{sabins}}{592 \text{ ft}^2}$$

$$= 0.285 \text{ sabins}$$

and

$$R = \Sigma S_i \alpha_i / (1 - \alpha_{avg})$$

$$= \frac{168.96 \text{ ft}^2 \text{ sabins}}{1 - 0.285 \text{ sabins}}$$

$$= 236.307 \text{ ft}^2 \text{ sabins or } 236 \text{ ft}^2$$

and then

$$r_c = \sqrt{QR/16\pi}$$

$$= [2(236 \text{ ft}^2)/16\pi]^{1/2}$$

$$r_c = 3.06 \text{ ft}$$

Now compute the sound-pressure level at the critical distance.

$$SPL = SWL + 10 \text{ Log } [(Q/4\pi r^2) + (4/R)] + 10.5 + T$$

$$= 110 \text{ dB} + 10 \text{ Log } [2/4\pi(3.06 \text{ ft})^2] + [4/236 \text{ ft}^2] + 10.5 + 0$$

$$= 110 \text{ dB} + (-14.692) + 10.5$$

$$= 105.808 \text{ dB (reference: } 0.00002 \text{ N/m}^2)$$

Now compute the sound-pressure level somewhere in the inverse-square-law field, 0.7 feet.

$$SPL = SWL + 10 \; Log \; [(Q/4\pi r^2) + (4/R)] + 10.5 + T$$

$$= 110 \; dB + 10 \; Log \; [(2/4\pi(0.7 \; ft)^2) + 4/236 \; ft^2] + 10.5 + 0$$

$$= 110 \; dB + (-4.663) + 10.5$$

$$= 115.837 \; dB \; (reference: \; 0.00002 \; N/m^2)$$

Now compute the sound-pressure level near the wall in the reverberant field at 7 feet.

$$SPL = SWL + 10 \; Log \; [(Q/4\pi r^2) + (4/R)] + 10.5 + T$$

$$= 110 \; dB + 10 \; Log \; [(2/4\pi(7 \; ft)^2) + 4/236 \; ft^2] + 10.5 + 0$$

$$= 110 \; dB + (-16.947) + 10.5$$

$$= 103.553 \; dB \; (reference: \; 0.00002 \; N/m^2)$$

In the given room, then, the sound-pressure levels are 115.837 dB in the inverse-square-law field, 105.818 dB at the critical distance, and 103.553 dB near the wall.

Now change the characteristics of the room to see what happens to sound pressure levels in these three locations. Let the ceiling absorption coefficient remain at 0.95 sabins; let the floor absorption coefficient remain at 0.37 sabins; but change the walls from brick (absorption coefficient 0.03 sabins) to a material that has an absorption coefficient of 0.10 sabins. Then

$$\alpha_{avg} = \Sigma S_i \alpha_i / \Sigma S_i$$

$$= \frac{(12 \; ft \; x \; 10 \; ft) \; 0.95 \; sabins + (12 \; ft \; x \; 10 \; ft) \; 0.37 \; sabins + 2(12 \; ft \; x \; 8 \; ft) \; 0.10 \; sabins + 2(10 \; ft \; x \; 8 \; ft) \; 0.10 \; sabins}{592 \; ft^2}$$

$$= \frac{193.6 \; ft^2 \; sabins}{592 \; ft^2}$$

$$\alpha = 0.327 \; sabins$$

and

$$R = \Sigma S_i \alpha_i / 1 - \alpha_{avg}$$

$$= \frac{193.6 \; ft^2 \; sabins}{1 - 0.327 \; sabins}$$

$$= 287.667 \; ft^2$$

At 0.7 ft in the inverse-square-law field (same distance as used above) the sound-pressure level in the more absorbent room would be

$$SPL = SWL + 10 \text{ Log } [(Q/4\pi r^2) + (4/R)] + 10.5 + T$$

$$= 110 \text{ dB} + 10 \text{ Log } [(2/4\pi(0.7 \text{ ft})^2) + (4/287.667 \text{ ft}^2)] + 10.5 + 0$$

$$= 110 \text{ dB} + (-4.702) + 10.5$$

$$= 115.798 \text{ dB (reference: } 0.00002 \text{ N/m}^2)$$

Recall that the sound-pressure level in the less absorbent room was 115.837 dB, a difference of only 0.039 dB.

At the critical distance (3.06 ft) the sound-pressure level in the more absorbent room would be

$$SPL = SWL + 10 \text{ Log } [(Q/4\pi r^2) + (4/R)] + 10.5 + T$$

$$= 110 \text{ dB} + 10 \text{ Log } [(2/4\pi(3.06 \text{ ft})^2) + (4/287.667 \text{ ft}^2)] + 10.5 + T$$

$$= 110 \text{ dB} + (-15.100) + 10.5$$

$$= 105.399 \text{ dB (reference: } 0.00002 \text{ N/m}^2)$$

compared to 105.808 dB in the less absorbent room, a difference of 0.409 dB.

Near the wall (7 feet) the sound-pressure level in the more absorbent room would be

$$SPL = SWL + 10 \text{ Log } [(Q/4\pi r^2) + (4/R)] + 10.5 + T$$

$$= 110 \text{ dB} + 10 \text{ Log } [(2/4\pi(7 \text{ ft})^2) + (4/287.667 \text{ ft}^2)] + 10.5 + 0$$

$$= 110 \text{ dB} + (-17.657) + 10.5$$

$$= 102.847 \text{ dB (reference: } 0.00002 \text{ N/m}^2)$$

compared to 103.553 dB in the less absorbent room, this is a difference of 0.71 dB.

It can be seen from this example that making the room more absorbent will not affect the sound-pressure level in the inverse-square region or at the critical distance. The benefits of making the room more absorbent appear in the reverberant field. Making the walls more absorbent will not help the worker who is in the inverse-square-law region or at the critical distance; it will help only when in the reverberant field.

Sound in an Adjoining Room

So far, sound in only a single room has been discussed. This section deals with how sound travels from room to room. The situation would be something like that shown in Figure 4.3.9. In this figure, the sound source is in the larger room. The problem is to find the sound pressure level in the adjacent, smaller room (room B). The problem of concern is how sound travels through the wall that joins the secondary room (room B) and the primary room (room A).

Figure 4.3.9

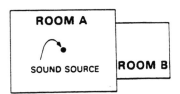

How does sound travel through a wall? If the wall is made of a highly absorbent material, a great deal of sound will go through the wall as depicted by Figure 4.3.10.

Figure 4.3.10

Sound travelling through a sound-absorbing wall.

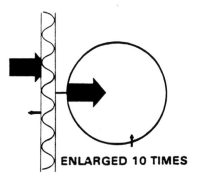

If the wall or partition is solid, less sound goes through; and much more sound is deflected as depicted by Figure 4.3.11.

Figure 4.3.11

Sound travelling through a solid wall.

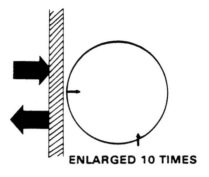

ENLARGED 10 TIMES

If a combination wall is built, a wall with highly absorbing material on one side and a hard or solid material on the other, little sound is reflected, and little sound goes through the wall as shown by Figure 4.3.12.

Figure 4.3.12

Sound travelling through a combination wall.

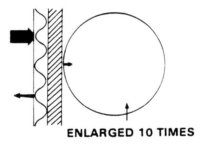

ENLARGED 10 TIMES

The amount of sound that is lost in the transmission through the wall depends upon the mass of the wall. Theoretically, the sound pressure on the source side of the wall or partition causes the partition to move in and out--vibrate. This motion causes a new sound wave on the opposite side of the partition. The movement of the partition or wall is dependent upon the mass of the material. A brick wall moves much less than a wood wall.

The transmission loss can be defined as the difference in the sound-pressure level on the source side compared to the sound-pressure level on the opposite side of the wall; i.e., the transmission loss of a wall may be defined in terms of sound-pressure level reduction afforded by the wall. However, mathematically, the transmission loss (TL) is expressed as

$$TL = 10 \, Log_{10}(Energy \ transmitted/ \ Energy \ of \ incident)$$

Transmission loss is difficult to measure. Only a few laboratories in the United States are qualified to make the standard measures (ASTM E90-61T). However, there are tables available that give the transmission loss of standard materials. (See Table 4.3.1.) Note from the tables that the transmission loss is not the same for a given material at all frequencies. The transmission loss is dependent upon the frequency of concern.

Transmission Loss of Combined Materials

Most walls are not made of a single material. For example, walls are made of brick and glass, plaster and glass, plaster and wood, etc. When a wall is constructed of more than one material, the materials that make up the walls have different transmission losses. The transmission loss of a wall composed of a combination of materials can be computed as

$$TL_{combined} = 10 \, Log \sum_{i=1}^{n} S_i - 10 \, Log \, (\Sigma S \, 10^{TL_i/10})$$

where TL_i denotes the transmission loss of the ith material composing the wall.

Problem. A wall is 8 ft high and 12 ft wide and is made of 6-inch hollow concrete block (cinder aggregate) with no surface treatment. In the center of the wall is a 1/4 inch thick glass window, 20 inches x 40 inches. What is the transmission loss of the wall? Assume the frequency of concern is 512 Hz.

Solution. From Table 4.3.1, the 6-inch hollow concrete block has a transmission loss of 45 dB, and the glass has a transmission loss of 31 dB. Thus, the combined transmission loss would be

$$TL_{combined} = 10 \, Log \sum_{i=1}^{n} S_i - 10 \, Log \, (\Sigma S \, 10^{TL_i/10})$$

where

$$\sum_{i=1}^{n} S_i = 8 \ ft \ x \ 12 \ ft$$

$$= 96 \ ft^2$$

and the surface area of the concrete block is

$$S_{block} = 16 \ ft^2 - (3.33 \ ft \ x \ 1.67 \ ft)$$

Table 4.3.1

Sound transmission loss of general building material and structures.

Item	Material or Structure	Weight Lbs/Ft²	Loss in Decibels at Indicated Frequencies, Hz								
			128	192	256	384	512	768	1024	2048	4096
A	**Doors**										
1	Heavy wooden door, approx. 2-1/2" thick, special hardware, rubber gasket & sides, drop felt on bottom	12.5	23	26	26	28	29	30	26	33	33
2	Approx. same as above (No. 1)		30	30	30	29	24	25	26	37	36
3a	Wooden door, 2-5/8" thick, 3' x 7' with double frame construction, frames insulated with hair felt, surface formed of 1/4" hardwood panels, door hung in split frame with felt insert & mounted in 12" brick wall. Two tubular gaskets gave a double seal around both sides & top of door, two drop felts at bottom	6.8	29	33	33	32	36	34	34	41	40
4a	Same as panel A-3, except door edges plastered to frame on both sides		32	38	38	35	39	38	42	49	53
5a	Door, steel clad (well sealed to door casing and threshold)		42	47	51	48	48	45	46	48	45
6a	Door, flush hollow core (well sealed to door casing and threshold)		14	21	27	24	25	25	26	29	31
7	Door, oak, solid 1-3/4", with cracks as ordinarily hung		12		15		20		22	16	
8a	Door, 3" x 30" x 84" wooden door, special soundproof construction, sponge rubber gasket around sides and top, approx. 1/2" square cross section, chamfered on hinge side; and a sponge rubber drop closure at bottom of door	7	31	27	32	30	33	31	29	37	41
B	**Glass**										
1a	Glass, 1/8" double strength, 40" x 20"		15		26		27		31	33	29
2a	Glass, 1/4" plate, 40" x 20"		25		33		31		34	34	32
	Walls - Homogeneous										
1	Single sheet of .025" aluminum, 40" x 21-1/2" (Approx. 22 ga)	0.35			18		13		18	23	25[b]
2	Single sheet of .03" galvanized iron, 40" x 21-1/2" (Approx. 22 ga)	1.2			25		20		29	35	32
3	Single sheet of lead 1/8" thick	8.2			31.0		27.2		37.5	43.8	32.6[b]
4	Single sheet of lead 1/16" thick	3.9			31.8		33.2		32.0	32.1	32.5[b]
5	PF fiberglas, 6 lb./ft.³ density, 1" thick	0.5	5	5	5	5	5	4.5	4.5	4	3.5
6	PF fiberglas, 6 lb./ft.³ density, 2" thick	1.0	8	8	8	8	7.5	7.5	7	7	6.5
7	PF fiberglas, 6 lb./ft.³ density, 3" thick	1.5	10	10	10	10	10	10	10	10	10
8	PF fiberglas, 6 lb./ft.³ density, 4" thick	2.0	12	12	12.25	12.5	12.5	12.5	12.5	13	13
	Glass brick partition, 3-3/4" x 4-7/8" x 8" thick		30.2	36.2	34.7	39.4	40.5	45.1	48.6	49.0	43.4
10	Concrete, reinforced, 4"		37	33	36	44	45	50	52	60	67
11	Concrete, reinforced, 8"		42	38	41	49	50	55	57	65	72
12	Cinder block, 4" solid	24.4	22	25	29	31	31	32	34	40	41
13	Cinder block, 6" solid	40.2	17	22	24	35	40	45.5	51.5	58.5	62.5

[a]Results obtained at 125, 175, 250, 350, 500, 700, 1000, 2000, 4000 cps

Table 4.5.1 (Continued)

Item	Material or Structure	Weight Lbs/Ft²	Loss in Decibels at Indicated Frequencies, Hz								
			128	192	256	384	512	768	1024	2048	4096
D	**Walls - Nonhomogeneous**										
1	2 x 4 studs, 1/2" insulating board on both sides (16" ctrs)	3.8	15.9	19.0	21.9	32.4	28.1	33.3	37.9	49.7	51.8
2	2 x 4 studs, 3/4" insulating board on both sides (16" ctrs)	4.3	20.7	17.8	21.4	26.6	20.7	32.1	37.6	49.3	52.7
3	2 x 4 studs, 3/8" Gypsum board lath & 1/2" gypsum plaster on both sides (16" ctrs)	15.0	33.4	23.9	24.5	30.2	28.3	37.7	35.5	41.7	58.8
4	2 x 4 studs, 1/2" insulating board lath & 1/2" gypsum plaster on both sides (16" ctrs)	12.6	28.3	27.3	30.9	37.8	40.7	44.4	46.3	46.7	65.6
5	2 x 4 studs, 1/2" dense wood fiberboard both sides (16" ctrs) joints at studs	3.8	16	19	22	32	28	33	38	50	52
6	2 x 4 studs, 2 sets staggered (16" cts with studs of one set 8" on ctrs and projecting 2" on ctrs from other set) 1/2" wood fiberboard both sides, joints filled	4.9		34[c]						59	60[c]
7	Concrete block - 4" hollow, no surface treatment) Cinder Aggregate		27	29	30	35	28	42	42	46	48
8	Concrete block - 4" hollow, one coat resin - emulsion paint)		30	33	32	36	37	45	45	55	53
9	Concrete block - 4" hollow, one coat cement base paint)		37	40	34	45	41	49	50	56	55
10	Concrete block - 6" hollow, no surface treatment)		28	34	36	41	45	48	54	52	47
11	Concrete block - 6" hollow, one coat cement base paint)		18	24	28	44	37	39	51	42	40
12	Concrete block - 8" hollow, one coat cement base paint)		30	36	40	36	46	48	40	50	41
13	Concrete block - 8" hollow, filled with vermiculite insulators)		20	29	33	31	38	38	51	45	47
14	Concrete block - 4" hollow, no surface treatment) Expanded Shale		21	26	28	34	35	38	41	44	43
15	Concrete block - 4" hollow, one coat resin-emulsion paint)		26	30	32	35	37	42	43	46	44
16	Concrete block - 4" hollow, two coats resin-emulsion paint)		24	31	33	38	38	42	44	47	44
17	Concrete block - 6" hollow, one coat cement-base paint) Aggregate		23	30	35	42	42	43	44	48	43
18	Concrete block - 6" hollow, two coats cement-base paint)		34	38	40	36	45	47	49	51	46
19	Concrete block - 6" hollow, no surface treatment)		22	27	32	41	40	43	46	45	43
20	Concrete block - 4" hollow, no surface treatment) Dense Aggregate		30	36	39	41	43	44	47	54	50
21	Concrete block - 4" hollow, one coat cement base paint on face)		30	36	39	41	43	44	47	54	49
22	Concrete block - 6" hollow, one coat cement base paint on face)		37	46	50	50	50	53	56	56	46
23	Concrete block - 6" hollow, one coat resin-emulsion paint)		37	50	54	52	53	55	57	56	46
24	Concrete block - 8" hollow, no surface treatment) each face		40	47	53	54	54	56	58	56	50
25	Concrete block - 8" hollow, two coats resin-emulsion paint each) face		38	50	54	54	55	58	60	38	49
26	Fluted steel, 18 gauge, stiffened at edges by 2 x 4" wood strips, joints sealed	4.4	30	20	20	21	22	17	30	28	31
27	Fluted steel, 18 gauge, 1-1/2" mineral wool - flat steel sheet, 18 gauge panel stiffened by 2 x 8" wood beam, joints caulked	7.8	36	30	25	36	37	42	46	44	44
28	Corrugated asbestos - bolted to 2 x 8" stiffening beam, braced at top and bottom by asphalt strips, joints sealed	7.0	33	29	31	34	33	33	33	42	39
29	Same as No. 29 except backed by 1-3/16" uncorrugated board, composed of 15/16" organic matl. covered both sides by 1/8" asbestos fiberboard, joints closed by 1 x 1" furring, joints sealed	10.4	40	36	33	38	40	43	46	45	42
30	Tile, hollow - 4 x 8 x 16" - surface untreated	15.5	8	8	5	7	9	12	14	18	17
31	Tile, hollow - 4 x 8 x 16" - one surface plastered	20.4	31	27	27	36	35	33	36	40	47

[c] Results obtained at 165 & 3100 cps instead of 192 & 4096 cps

Reprinted with permission by American Industrial Hygiene Association.

$$= 95 \text{ ft}^2 - 5.561 \text{ ft}^2$$

$$= 90.439 \text{ ft}^2$$

and the surface area of the glass is

$$S_{glass} = (3.33 \text{ ft} \times 1.67 \text{ ft})$$

$$= 5.561 \text{ ft}^2$$

and the combined transmission loss would be

$$TL_{combined} = 10 \text{ Log} \sum_{i=1}^{n} S_i - 10 \text{ Log} (\Sigma S\ 10^{TL_i/10})$$

$$= 10 \text{ Log } 96 \text{ ft}^2 - 10 \text{ Log } [90.439 \text{ ft}^2 \times 10^{-45 \text{ dB}/1C}] +$$

$$5.561 \text{ ft}^2 \times 10^{-31 \text{ dB}/10}$$

$$= 19.823 - (-21.38)$$

$$= 41.203 \text{ dB}$$

Possible leaks are of concern when a wall is composed of different kinds of materials. A tiny portion of the wall or partition constructed of a material of low transmission loss tends to nullify the effect of the remainder of the wall. Consider the transmission loss of a 6-inch concrete wall 10 feet high and 8 feet wide. This structure would have a transmission loss of 45 dB in the mid frequencies (512 Hz). But suppose that a mason did not realize the importance of small cracks in a noise-control structure and carelessly left an opening of just one-eighth of an inch wide along the top of the wall. The area of this small crack would then be 0.083 square feet while the area of the block would be 79.917 square feet. The combined transmission loss of the concrete wall with the one-eighth inch crack at the top will only have an effective transmission loss of 29.679 dB; this is substantially less than would be expected for the concrete wall (45 dB). One must always be alert for similar situations in construction for the purpose of noise control. Leaks around doors are extremely hard to eliminate unless great care is exercised. Poorly fitted panels and joints are also frequently sources of trouble. The point is that leaks are going to reduce the transmission loss. These leaks will cause more noise to go into the adjoining room.

Transmission loss is the amount of sound lost as it passes through a wall. The higher the transmission loss, the more sound that is lost.

Secondary Room

In the last section, transmission loss was discussed. When sound travels through a wall, the wall begins to vibrate and creates sound on the opposite side of the wall. If the adjoining room is small, the energy--the sound energy that gets through the wall--will bounce off the walls in the smaller room. This reverberant sound must also be considered if the sound-pressure level in the adjoining room is to be computed. Thus, if it is desired to compute the sound-pressure level in the secondary room as a result of the sound source in the primary room, it is necessary to consider the reverberant field in the secondary room.

The amount of reverberant sound in the secondary room depends upon the absorption coefficients of the walls, floor, and ceiling (the room constant) in the secondary room. This characteristic of the secondary room is taken into consideration in the computation of the noise reduction. Noise reduction is defined as the difference in the sound-pressure level from the source side of the wall to the opposite side of the wall when there is going to be reverberant buildup in the smaller room. The general formula for noise reduction (NR) is given as follows:

$$NR = TL - 10 \, Log_{10} \, [(1/4) + (S_W/R)]$$

where NR denotes the noise reduction--the difference in sound-pressure levels on the opposite sides of the walls; TL denotes the transmission loss through the partition or wall; S_W indicates the surface area of the wall between the two rooms; and R denotes the room constant in the secondary room.

Problem.   Assume the following layout:

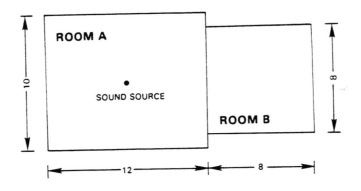

Both Rooms A and B are 8 feet high. In room A, let α_{avg} = 0.285 sabins and let R = 237 ft^2. In room B, let the walls, ceiling, and floor all have an absorption coefficient of 0.07 sabins. Further, let the transmission loss of the adjoining wall (8 ft by 8 ft) be 45 dB. What is the noise reduction of the wall, considering the reverberant buildup in the smaller room?

Solution.   The noise reduction can be computed from

$$NR = TL - 10 \, Log_{10} \, [(1/4) + (S_W/R)]$$

where $S_w = 64$ ft^2 and the room constant in the smaller room is given as

$$R = \alpha \Sigma S_i / (1 - \alpha_{avg})$$

where

$$\alpha = \Sigma S_i \alpha_i / \Sigma S_i$$

$$= \frac{6(8 \text{ ft} \times 8 \text{ ft})0.08 \text{ sabins}}{6(8 \times 8)}$$

$$= 0.08 \text{ sabins}$$

and thus

$$R = \frac{30.720 \text{ ft}^2 \text{ sabins}}{1 \text{ sabin} - 0.08 \text{ sabins}}$$

$$= 33.391 \text{ ft}^2$$

Thus

$$NR = TL - 10 \text{ Log}_{10} [(1/4) + (S_w/R)]$$

$$= 45 \text{ dB} - 10 \text{ Log} [(1/4) + (64 \text{ ft}^2/33.391 \text{ ft}^2)]$$

$$= 45 \text{ dB} - 3.358 \text{ dB}$$

$$= 41.642 \text{ dB}$$

Notice that the noise reduction is smaller than the transmission loss because the smaller room has a log average absorption coefficient, causing an excessive buildup of reverberant sound.

Given the noise reduction, the sound-pressure level in the smaller room can be computed if the sound-pressure level at the adjoining wall in the larger room is known. That is,

$$SPL_{in \text{ smaller room}} = SPL_{at \text{ wall of larger room}} - NR$$

For example, if the larger room has an $R = 237$ ft^2 and a sound source with a sound power level of 120 dB and $Q = 2$, then the sound-pressure level at the wall in the larger room (an average of 6.86 feet from the center of the room) would be

$$SPL = SWL + 10 \text{ Log} [(Q/4\pi r^2) + (4/R)] + 10.5$$

$$= 120 \text{ dB} + 10 \text{ Log} [(2/4\pi(6.86 \text{ ft})^2) + (4/237 \text{ ft}^2)] + 10.5$$

$$= 120 \text{ dB} + (-16.934) + 10.5$$

$$= 113.566 \text{ dB} \text{ (reference: } 0.00002 \text{ N/m}^2)$$

and sound pressure level in the adjoining room would be calculated as

$$SPL_{in\ smaller\ room} = SPL_{at\ wall\ in\ larger\ room} - NR$$

$$= 113.566\ dB - 41.642\ dB$$

$$= 71.924\ dB\ (reference:\ 0.00002\ N/m^2)$$

Summary

The following principles were discussed in this chapter:

1. Sound in a room will be reflected off the walls making sound behave differently than in the free-field condition.

2. There are three fields of sound in a room: the near field (sound near and around the source), the field that follows the inverse-square law, and the reverberant field (sound near the walls of the room). The predominant sound in the inverse-square-law field is the sound generated by the source. The predominant sound in the reverberant field is sound bouncing (reflecting) off the walls.

3. The sound-pressure level in the inverse-square-law field is affected by the direction and distance from the sound source. The sound-pressure level in the reverberant field will become constant and is not affected by the distance from the sound source.

4. The sound-pressure level in the reverberant field is affected by the absorption ability of the walls, ceiling, and floor. A more absorbent material reflects less sound back into the room. A less absorbent material reflects more sound back into the room.

5. The absorption coefficient (α) indicates the absorption ability of the material. A material that has an absorption coefficient of 1 ($\alpha = 1$) is a perfectly absorbing material (such as open air). A very hard surface, such as marble, has an absorption coefficient equal to 0 ($\alpha = 0$). In this case no sound is absorbed; it is all reflected back into the room.

6. The absorption coefficient of a material is not the same value at all frequencies.

7. The average absorption coefficient of a room is computed by

$$\alpha_{avg} = \frac{\sum\limits_{i=1}^{n} S_i \alpha_i}{\sum\limits_{i=1}^{n} S_i}$$

where S_i denotes the surface area composed of the ith material and α_i denotes the absorption characteristics of the ith material. α is measured in sabin units.

8. The room constant (R) is a measure of the ability of a room to absorb sound. It is a function of the average absorption coefficient.

$$R = \frac{\alpha_{avg} \sum\limits_{i=1}^{n} S_i}{1 - \alpha_{avg}}$$

R is in square feet units.

9. The average absorption coefficient (and therefore the room constant) affects the sound-pressure level in various parts of the room. If the average absorption coefficient equals 1 (a free-field condition), then

$$SPL_{(r)} = SPL_{(1)} - 20 \; Log \; (r/r_1)$$

where $SPL_{(r)}$ denotes the sound-pressure level at distance r; $SPL_{(1)}$ denotes a known sound pressure at some distance r_1; and r and r_1 denote the distances in feet corresponding to $SPL_{(r)}$ and $SPL_{(1)}$. This relationship will not hold, however, if the materials composing the walls, floor, and ceiling are less than perfectly absorbent. There are tables to predict the sound-pressure level in various parts of the room if the walls, ceiling, and floor are composed of materials with less than perfectly absorbing characteristics.

10. The room constant (R) also affects the relationship between sound-power level and sound-pressure level.

$$SPL = SWL + 10 \; Log \; [(Q/4\pi r^2) + (4/R)] + 10.5 + T$$

where SPL denotes sound-pressure level (reference: 0.00002 N/m^2), SWL denotes sound-power level (reference: 10^{-12} watts), Q denotes the directivity factor, r denotes distance from the sound source in feet, R denotes the room constant in square feet, and T denotes the correction for nonstandard atmospheric conditions.

11. The critical distance (r_c) is the point where the inverse square law field ends and the reverberant field begins.

$$r_c = \sqrt{QR/16\pi}$$

where Q is the directivity factor and R is the room constant. Alternatively, r_c can be expressed as

$$r_c = \sqrt{(Q\Sigma S\alpha_{avg})/16\pi(1-\alpha_{avg})}$$

where S denotes the surface area in feet of the material and α_{avg} denotes the average absorption coefficient.

12. The critical distance is important because most workers are within the critical distance zone. Further, it can be shown that making the floor, ceiling, and walls more absorbent does not significantly affect the sound-pressure level at the critical distance. However, making the room more absorbent will reduce the sound-pressure level near the walls.

13. Sound will travel from one room to another. Theoretically, the sound-pressure level on the source side of a wall will cause the wall to vibrate. This motion causes a new sound wave on the opposite side of the wall.

14. The transmission loss (TL) of a wall can be defined in terms of the sound-pressure level reduction afforded by the wall. Mathematically,

$$TL = 10 \, Log \, (Energy \, transmitted \, / \, Energy \, of \, incident)$$

Transmission loss of materials is usually published in table form.

15. If an adjoining wall is composed of various material, the combined transmission loss can be computed as follows:

$$TL_{combined} = 10 \, Log \, \sum_{i=1}^{n} S_i - 10 \, Log \, (\Sigma S \, 10^{TL_i/10})$$

where S_i denotes the surface area (in square feet) of the ith material composing the wall and TL_i denotes the transmission loss of the ith material composing the wall.

16. If there are leaks in the adjoining wall (air spaces around windows, doors, etc.), the effective transmission loss is considerably reduced.

17. If the room adjoining the sound source room is small, then the sound transmitted from the adjoining wall will cause a reverberant buildup in the small room, thus possibly increasing the sound-pressure level in the smaller room.

18. Noise reduction is defined as the difference in the sound-pressure level from the source side of the wall to the opposite side of the wall. When there is going to be reverberant buildup in the smaller room, the noise reduction is computed as follows:

$$NR = TL - 10 \, Log_{10} \, [(1/4) + (S_w/R)]$$

where TL denotes the transmission loss of the adjoining wall, S_w denotes the surface area of the adjoining wall in square feet, and R denotes the room constant of the adjoining room.

19. The amount of noise reduction is related to the room constant (and thus to the average absorption coefficient) of the adjoining room. If the adjoining room has a small average absorption coefficient, the noise reduction achieved will be 5 to 6 dB less than transmission loss. The noise reduction will be less than the transmission loss due to the extreme

buildup in the adjoining room. If the average room absorption coefficient is average, the noise reduction achieved will be 1 to 2 dB greater than the transmission loss. If the adjoining room has a very high average absorption coefficient, the noise reduction achieved will be about 5 dB greater than the transmission loss because the sound transmitted will be absorbed by the wall, ceiling, and floors of the adjoining room.

20. The sound-pressure level in the adjoining room can be computed as follows:

a.   Compute the average distance the wall is from the source in the sound source room using

$$r_{\text{average to wall}} = \sqrt{\Sigma S/4\pi}$$

where S denotes the surface area in the source room.

b.   Compute the average absorption coefficient in the source room.

$$\alpha_{\text{avg}} = \frac{\sum\limits_{i=1}^{n} S_i \alpha_i}{\sum\limits_{i=1}^{n} S_i}$$

where S_i denotes the surface area of the ith building material and α_i denotes the absorption coefficient of the ith building material.

c.   Compute the room constant of the source room.

$$R = \frac{\alpha_{\text{avg}} \sum\limits_{i=1}^{n} S_i}{1 - \alpha_{\text{avg}}}$$

d.   Compute the sound-pressure level at the wall in the source room using

$$SPL = SWL + 10 \, Log \, [(Q/4\pi r^2) + (4/R)] + 10.5 + T$$

where r becomes the average distance to the wall (step a) and R becomes the room constant of the source room (step c).

e.   Compute the transmission loss of the material forming the adjacent wall (if wall is composed of many materials, using the following formula):

$$TL_c = 10 \, Log \, \Sigma S_i - 10 \, Log \, (\Sigma S_i \, 10^{-TL_i/10})$$

f.   Compute the surface area of the adjoining wall (S_w).

g. Compute the average absorption coefficient in the adjoining room.

$$\alpha_{avg} = \frac{\sum\limits_{i=1}^{n} S_i \alpha_i}{\sum\limits_{i=1}^{n} S_i}$$

and then compute the room constant in the adjoining room.

$$R = \frac{\alpha_{avg} \sum\limits_{i=1}^{n} S_i}{1 - \alpha_{avg}}$$

h. Compute the noise reduction of the wall by

$$NR = TL - 10 \, Log_{10} \, [(1/4) + (S_w/R)]$$

where TL is the transmission loss computed in step e, S_w is the surface area of the adjoining wall (step f), and R denotes the room constant in the adjoining room (step g).

i. Compute the sound pressure level in the adjoining room by

SPL adjoining room = SPL at wall in source room - NR

where SPL (at wall in source room) is given by step d and NR is given by step h.

4. The Ear and the Effects of Sound

Introduction

The title of this chapter may be somewhat misleading. Rather than discussing the anatomy and physiology of the ear (refer to Chapter 24, The Industrial Environment: Its Evaluation and Control, for a discussion of the ear), this chapter discusses effects of noise on the ear. If the effects of sound on the ear are known, then it is possible to establish suitable criteri for the acceptable level of noise. Then if the existing noise level is measured, the difference between this level and the acceptable level is the noise reduction that is necessary.

First, this chapter discusses the threshold of hearing and hearing loss. Then it discusses some of the possible causes of such hearing losses. The chapter closes by discussing such other characteristics of sound as loudness, perceived noise level, annoyance of noise, and speech interference.

The Threshold of Hearing

A sound is at the threshold of hearing when it is just intense enough to evoke a response from the listener. Since a listener's threshold may vary slightly from moment to moment, the average of a response to a number of trials is usually obtained. To describe a threshold completely, one must report the nature of the sound, the physical measurements made to specify the sound, and, in addition, the exact nature of the response or series of responses required of the listener. Many different sounds have been used in measuring the threshold of hearing, including pure tones, speech, and noise. For instance, the pure tone may be presented at any frequency in the audible range, may be interrupted or steady, and may have a gradual or abrupt beginning. The speech material may be sentences, words, or syllables. Noise may be presented with a vast variety of spectra and band widths. Only thresholds obtained with the same kinds of sounds can be expected to be the same.

Many experiments have made measurements of the threshold of hearing of various listeners. When young persons with good hearing are tested, a curve representing the threshold of hearing can be obtained. See Figure 4.4.1. Here sound pressure level is plotted against frequency.

From Figure 4.4.1, it can be seen that certain frequencies are perceived at lower intensities (sound-pressure levels) than other frequencies. From 16 Hz to about 1000 Hz, it takes progressively lower sound-pressure levels (less

Figure 4.4.1

Auditory sensitivity curve.

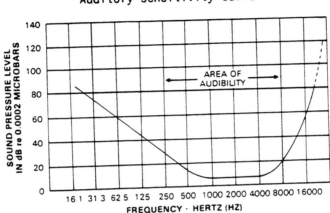

Reprinted with permission by American Industrial Hygiene Association.

intensity) for a tone to be audible. From 1000 Hz to 4000 Hz, the ear's
response is relatively constant. From 4000 Hz to higher frequencies, this
trend reverses and a greater sound-pressure level (intensity) is required to
make the sound audible. (Note: In Figure 4.4.1, the sound-pressure level
reference is 0.00002 microbars.)

The curve in Figure 4.4.1 is deceiving, however. "Normal hearing" is the
"threshold of hearing" found in young people with no evidence or history of
infection or other diseases of the ear. As with height and weight, hearing
thresholds are not all the same, but are distributed over a range of
sound-pressure levels of about 25 dB. The thresholds of these young people
are distributed throughout this range in a nonuniform manner, as are their
heights and weights. Many are near the center of the range, and only a few
are at the extremes. The line in Figure 4.4.1 represents the average of the
average. The variations or deviations about this average are not usually
depicted on such graphs; however they should be kept in mind.

For convenience in comparing thresholds of hearing sensitivity, a decibel
scale is used. The reference level for most hearing scales is set arbitrarily
at the most common (modal) threshold sound-pressure level (not the lowest
sound-pressure level) for a group of listeners with "normal hearing." This
modal value is often referred to as the "audiometric zero." The difference
between this arbitrary reference level and the sound-pressure level at a given
listener's threshold is called that individual's hearing loss. The use of the
word "loss" here may be somewhat misleading, because the smaller hearing
losses lie within ranges of normal hearing, the 25 dB range.

Another common cause of confusion is the existence of "negative hearing
losses." Since the reference level is the most common threshold for normal
listeners, there will be many whose threshold sound-pressure level is less
than the reference level. Thus listeners with "negative hearing losses"

should be expected when any group of normal listeners is tested under the appropriate conditions.

Because "hearing losses" is a term reserved for a particular use, it should not be applied to the amount of hearing lost by an individual between two audiometric examinations. Changes in an individual's hearing over two audiometric examinations are called threshold shifts. For example, a man has a 30 dB hearing loss as a result of a threshold shift of 20 dB. His original 10 dB "hearing loss" may have been quite normal for him, contrary to the misleading implication of the words "hearing loss."

Another consideration in measuring the range of hearing is the limit of sound intensity or sound pressure which the ear can tolerate. When the sound pressure level reaches 120 dB (reference 0.00002 microbars) in the normal ear, the listener describes the sound as "uncomfortable." With about another 10 dB, he reports a tickling; and around 130 to 140 dB, actual pain results. Interestingly enough, this tolerance threshold does not vary remarkably with frequency (although higher frequencies more often seem unpleasant than lower frequencies of equal intensity or pressure). Sustained exposure to sound of sufficient intensity or pressure can produce auditory damage even without noticeable pain or discomfort.

Hearing Loss and Age

The expected loss in hearing sensitivity with age has been determined by statistical analysis of hearing threshold measurements on many people. (See Figure 4.4.2.) It is clear from Figure 4.4.2 that, on the average, auditory sensitivity as a function of age is increasingly diminished as one goes from 1000 Hz to 6000 Hz. It is also clear that hearing at the lower frequencies (1000 to 2000 Hz) does not deteriorate until late in life. On the other hand, the higher frequencies--especially 4000 to 6000 Hz--show relatively early effects of age.

The shifts in hearing sensitivity as shown by the figure represent the effects of a combination of aging (presbycusis) and the normal stresses of nonoccupational noises of modern civilization.

Other Causes of Hearing Loss

Other causes of hearing loss include:
- exposure to loud noise
- congenital defects
- anatomical injuries
- diseases

The physiological effects of exposure to noise are discussed in Chapter 24, The Industrial Environment: Its Evaluation and Control. However, the following factors should be kept in mind:

1.   Low-frequency sounds tend to be less damaging than mid-frequency sounds.

Figure 4.4.2

Hearing level as a function of age.

N=2518

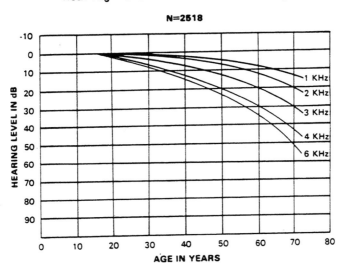

Reprinted with permission by American Industrial Hygiene Association.

2. Beyond certain levels, increased intensity and increased exposure
    time produce increased hearing loss.

3. Individuals show a differential susceptibility to noise-induced
    hearing loss.

4. Hearing loss due to noise is most pronounced in the region near 4000
    Hz but spreads over the frequency range as exposure time and level
    increase.

Other Effects of Noise

Although noise results in hearing loss, it can also result in other
effects. Noise can interfere with communication, thus causing accidents or
perhaps increasing errors in the performance of tasks. No adequate measures
of the annoyance level of noise have yet been devised (Handbook of Noise
Measurement, General Radio, p. 20). This is because there are psychological
difficulties in designing experiments that investigate annoyance. The extent
of annoyance depends greatly upon what a person is trying to do at the moment,
previous conditioning, and the character of the noise itself.

The annoyance level of a noise is sometimes assumed to be related directly
to the loudness level of the noise. In this section, then, loudness, loudness
level, and a procedure for calculating loudness level from physical
measurements (sound-pressure level) will be discussed, along with other
indices that are sometimes used to measure annoyance.

There are two measures of loudness, loudness level and loudness number (sometimes just called loudness). The loudness level is defined as the sound-pressure level of a narrow band noise (e.g., a pure tone) at 1000 Hz, frontally presented to a listener, that sounds to him equal in loudness to the noise (sound) being rated. When experimentally judging loudness level, a noise whose loudness level is to be determined would be frontally presented to a person. While switching back and forth between that noise and a reference noise, the listener would adjust the level of the latter until the two noises sound equally loud. The sound-pressure level (reference: 2×10^{-5} N/m^2) of the reference noise would then be measured at the position of the listener's head with the listener removed. This measured level would be called the <u>loudness level</u> of a given noise in phons. The results of these determinations (based on an average of many listeners) are usually given as equal loudness contours (see Figure 4.4.3).

Figure 4.4.3

Equal-loudness curves.

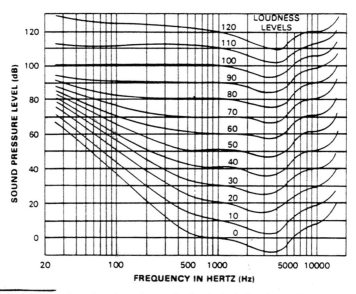

In Figure 4.4.3, the number of each curve is the sound-pressure level of a 1000 Hz tone used for the comparison of that curve (in phons). To use the curves for determining the equally loud levels at other frequencies, find the point on the curve corresponding to the desired frequency and read off the corresponding sound-pressure level as the ordinant. For example, the 60 dB contour line shows that a 72 dB level at 100 Hz is just as loud as a 60 dB, 1000 Hz tone. The figure also shows that a 60 dB, 100 Hz sound is equally as loud as a 40 dB, 1000 Hz tone. The loudness level can also be calculated rather than determined experimentally. When this is done, the result is called the <u>calculated loudness level</u>. Procedures for calculating the loudness level are given below.

Loudness differs from loudness level although they are related logarithmically. Loudness is a numerical designation that, for a given noise (sound) is proportional to the subjective magnitude of the "loudness" of that sound as judged by a normal listener. The unit of loudness is the <u>sone</u>. The loudness of a 1000 Hz tone with a sound-pressure level of 40 dB (reference: 0.00002 N/m^2) (a loudness level of 40 phons) is taken to be 1 sone. A tone that sounds twice as loud has a loudness of 2 sones. A doubling in loudness (in sones) is commonly taken to be equal to an increase of 10 phons. (Note: S. S. Stevens has shown that a majority of listeners would probably judge a doubling in loudness to correspond to an increase of 9 phons in loudness level.) However, to be consistent with the current American and international standards, it will be assumed that a change of 10 phons corresponds to a doubling or halving of loudness. The conversion of phons to sones and sones to phons will be given in the tables.

A number of people have found it useful to translate their noise measurements into such loudness terms. They can then say that the measured sound is about equal in loudness to another more familiar sound. To the lay person, this may be more meaningful than levels quoted in decibels.

When sound is divided by an analyzer into frequency bands covering the audible range, the loudness can be calculated by the following procedure:

1.   From Table 4.4.1, find the proper loudness index(s) for each band.

2.   Then use the following expression to determine the loudness in sones.

$$\text{Loudness}_{(\text{sones})} = 0.3 \sum_{i=1}^{n} S_1 + 0.7\, S_{max}$$

where S_{max} denotes the largest loudness index within the given frequency bands.

3.   Then convert the total loudness in sones to the loudness level in phons by using the relation shown in the right-hand columns of Table 4.4.1.

For example, suppose for the following frequency bands the following sound pressures are recorded:

Octave Frequency Band (Hz)	Sound Pressure Level (dB)
31.5	75
63	72
125	69
250	66
500	63
1000	60
2000	56
4000	54
8000	54

Table 4.4.1

Band level conversion to loudness index.

Band Level dB	31.5	63	125	250	500	1000	2000	4000	8000	Loudness Sones	Loudness Level Phons
20						.18	.30	.45	.61	.25	20
21						.22	.35	.50	.67	.27	21
22					.07	.26	.40	.55	.73	.29	22
23					.12	.30	.45	.61	.80	.31	23
24					.16	.35	.50	.67	.87	.33	24
25					.21	.40	.55	.73	.94	.35	25
26					.26	.45	.61	.80	1.02	.38	26
27					.31	.50	.67	.87	1.10	.41	27
28				.07	.37	.55	.73	.94	1.18	.44	28
29				.12	.43	.61	.80	1.02	1.27	.47	29
30				.16	.49	.67	.87	1.10	1.35	.50	30
31				.21	.55	.73	.94	1.18	1.44	.54	31
32				.26	.61	.80	1.02	1.27	1.54	.57	32
33				.31	.67	.87	1.10	1.35	1.64	.62	33
34			.07	.37	.73	.94	1.18	1.44	1.75	.66	34
35			.12	.43	.80	1.02	1.27	1.54	1.87	.71	35
36			.16	.49	.87	1.10	1.35	1.64	1.99	.76	36
37			.21	.55	.94	1.18	1.44	1.75	2.11	.81	37
38			.26	.62	1.02	1.27	1.54	1.87	2.24	.87	38
39			.31	.69	1.10	1.35	1.64	1.99	2.38	.93	39
40		.07	.37	.77	1.18	1.44	1.75	2.11	2.53	1.00	40
41		.12	.43	.85	1.27	1.54	1.87	2.24	2.68	1.07	41
42		.16	.49	.94	1.35	1.64	1.99	2.38	2.84	1.15	42
43		.21	.55	1.04	1.44	1.75	2.11	2.53	3.0	1.23	43
44		.26	.62	1.13	1.54	1.87	2.24	2.68	3.2	1.32	44
45		.31	.69	1.23	1.64	1.99	2.38	2.84	3.4	1.41	45
46	.07	.37	.77	1.33	1.75	2.11	2.53	3.0	3.6	1.52	46
47	.12	.43	.85	1.44	1.87	2.24	2.68	3.2	3.8	1.62	47
48	.16	.49	.94	1.56	1.99	2.38	2.84	3.4	4.1	1.74	48
49	.21	.55	1.04	1.69	2.11	2.53	3.0	3.6	4.3	1.87	49
50	.26	.62	1.13	1.82	2.24	2.68	3.2	3.8	4.6	2.00	50
51	.31	.69	1.23	1.96	2.38	2.84	3.4	4.1	4.9	2.14	51
52	.37	.77	1.33	2.11	2.53	3.0	3.6	4.3	5.2	2.30	52
53	.43	.85	1.44	2.24	2.68	3.2	3.8	4.6	5.5	2.46	53
54	.49	.94	1.56	2.38	2.84	3.4	4.1	4.9	5.8	2.64	54
55	.55	1.04	1.69	2.53	3.0	3.6	4.3	5.2	6.2	2.83	55
56	.62	1.13	1.82	2.68	3.2	3.8	4.6	5.5	6.6	3.03	56
57	.69	1.23	1.96	2.84	3.4	4.1	4.9	5.8	7.0	3.25	57
58	.77	1.33	2.11	3.0	3.6	4.3	5.2	6.2	7.4	3.48	58
59	.85	1.44	2.27	3.2	3.8	4.6	5.5	6.6	7.8	3.73	59
60	.94	1.56	2.44	3.4	4.1	4.9	5.8	7.0	8.3	4.00	60
61	1.04	1.69	2.62	3.6	4.3	5.2	6.2	7.4	8.8	4.29	61
62	1.13	1.82	2.81	3.8	4.6	5.5	6.6	7.8	9.3	4.59	62
63	1.23	1.96	3.0	4.1	4.9	5.8	7.0	8.3	9.9	4.92	63
64	1.33	2.11	3.2	4.3	5.2	6.2	7.4	8.8	10.5	5.28	64
65	1.44	2.27	3.5	4.6	5.5	6.6	7.8	9.3	11.1	5.66	65
66	1.56	2.44	3.7	4.9	5.8	7.0	8.3	9.9	11.8	6.06	66
67	1.69	2.62	4.0	5.2	6.2	7.4	8.8	10.5	12.6	6.50	67
68	1.82	2.81	4.3	5.5	6.6	7.8	9.3	11.1	13.5	6.96	68
69	1.96	3.0	4.7	5.8	7.0	8.3	9.9	11.8	14.4	7.46	69
70	2.11	3.2	5.0	6.2	7.4	8.8	10.5	12.6	15.3	8.00	70
71	2.27	3.5	5.4	6.6	7.8	9.3	11.1	13.5	16.4	8.6	71
72	2.44	3.7	5.8	7.0	8.3	9.9	11.8	14.4	17.5	9.2	72
73	2.62	4.0	6.2	7.4	8.8	10.5	12.6	15.3	18.7	9.8	73
74	2.81	4.3	6.6	7.8	9.3	11.1	13.5	16.4	20.0	10.6	74
75	3.0	4.7	7.0	8.3	9.9	11.8	14.4	17.5	21.4	11.3	75
76	3.2	5.0	7.4	8.8	10.5	12.6	15.3	18.7	23.0	12.1	76
77	3.5	5.4	7.8	9.3	11.1	13.5	16.4	20.0	24.7	13.0	77
78	3.7	5.8	8.3	9.9	11.8	14.4	17.5	21.4	26.5	13.9	78
79	4.0	6.2	8.8	10.5	12.6	15.3	18.7	23.0	28.5	14.9	79
80	4.3	6.7	9.3	11.1	13.5	16.4	20.0	24.7	30.5	16.0	80
81	4.7	7.2	9.9	11.8	14.4	17.5	21.4	26.5	32.9	17.1	81
82	5.0	7.7	10.5	12.6	15.3	18.7	23.0	28.5	35.3	18.4	82
83	5.4	8.2	11.1	13.5	16.4	20.0	24.7	30.5	38	19.7	83
84	5.8	8.8	11.8	14.4	17.5	21.4	26.5	32.9	41	21.1	84
85	6.2	9.4	12.6	15.3	18.7	23.0	28.5	35.3	44	22.6	85

Table 4.4.1 (Continued)

Band Level dB	Band Loudness Index									Loudness Sones	Loudness Level Phons
	31.5	63	125	250	500	1000	2000	4000	8000		
86	6.7	10.1	13.5	16.4	20.0	24.7	30.5	38	48	24.3	86
87	7.2	10.9	14.4	17.5	21.4	26.5	32.9	41	52	26.0	87
88	7.7	11.7	15.3	18.7	23.0	28.5	35.3	44	56	27.9	88
89	8.2	12.6	16.4	20.0	24.7	30.5	38	48	61	29.9	89
90	8.8	13.6	17.5	21.4	26.5	32.9	41	52	66	32.0	90
91	9.4	14.8	18.7	23.0	28.5	35.3	44	56	71	34.3	91
92	10.1	16.0	20.0	24.7	30.5	38	48	61	77	36.8	92
93	10.9	17.3	21.4	26.5	32.9	41	52	66	83	39.4	93
94	11.7	18.7	23.0	28.5	35.3	44	56	71	90	42.2	94
95	12.6	20.0	24.7	30.5	38	48	61	77	97	45.3	95
96	13.6	21.4	26.5	32.9	41	52	66	83	105	48.5	96
97	14.8	23.0	28.5	35.3	44	56	71	90	113	52.0	97
98	16.0	24.7	30.5	38	48	61	77	97	121	55.7	98
99	17.3	26.5	32.9	41	52	66	83	105	130	59.7	99
100	18.7	28.5	35.3	44	56	71	90	113	139	64.0	100
101	20.3	30.5	38	48	61	77	97	121	149	68.6	101
102	22.1	32.9	41	52	66	83	105	130	160	73.5	102
103	24.0	35.3	44	56	71	90	113	139	171	78.8	103
104	26.1	38	48	61	77	97	121	149	184	84.4	104
105	28.5	41	52	66	83	105	130	160	197	90.5	105
106	31.0	44	56	71	90	113	139	171	211	97	106
107	33.9	48	61	77	97	121	149	184	226	104	107
108	36.9	52	66	83	105	130	160	197	242	111	108
109	40.3	56	71	90	113	139	171	211	260	119	109
110	44	61	77	97	121	149	184	226	278	128	110
111	49	66	83	105	130	160	197	242	298	137	111
112	54	71	90	113	139	171	211	260	320	147	112
113	59	77	97	121	149	184	226	278	343	158	113
114	65	83	105	130	160	197	242	298	367	169	114
115	71	90	113	139	171	211	260	320		181	115
116	77	97	121	149	184	226	278	343		194	116
117	83	105	130	160	197	242	298	367		208	117
118	90	113	139	171	211	260	320			223	118
119	97	121	149	184	226	278	343			239	119
120	105	130	160	197	242	298	367			256	120
121	113	139	171	211	260	320				274	121
122	121	149	184	226	278	343				294	122
123	130	160	197	242	298	367				315	123
124	139	171	211	260	320					338	124
125	149	184	226	278	343					362	125

By permission of Gen Rad, Inc.

From Table 4.4.1, the loudness indices at each frequency band and sound pressure are 3.0, 3.7, 4.7, 4.9, 4.9, 4.9, 4.6, 4.9, and 5.8. Thus the loudness in sones is

$$\text{Loudness(sones)} = 0.3 \sum_{i=1}^{9} S_i + 0.7\, S_{max}$$

$$= 0.3(41.4) + 0.7(5.8)$$

$$= 12.42 + 4.06$$

$$= 16.48 \text{ sones (OB)}$$

and from the right-hand side of Table 4.4.1, 16.48 sones is approximately 80.44 phons (OD). The calculated loudness is labeled sones (OB) and the loudness level is labeled phons (OD) to denote they have been calculated from

octave band levels (0) and for a diffuse field (D). A similar calculation ca
be made for third-octave bands, and they are labeled (TD). (See Noise and
Vibration Control, p. 561 to 563.)

Another index that is important to consider is the Speech Interference
Level (PSIL). Because of the annoyance of interference with speech and also
because noise interferes with work where speech communication is necessary, a
noise rating based on the speech interference level is useful. The procedure
rates steady noise according to its ability to interfere with communication
between two people in an environment free of nearby reflecting surfaces that
might strengthen the talker's voices.

There are two speech interference levels that have been used; one related
to octave band filter sets with the "old" cutoff frequencies,[1] the other
with the new (preferred) band center frequencies.

The speech interference level with the old cutoff frequencies is the
arithmetic average of the sound-pressure levels in three octave bands;   600 t
1200, 1200 to 2400, and 2400 to 4800 Hz.

The speech interference level (with the preferred band center frequencies
is the arithmetic average of the sound-pressure levels in the three octave
bands with center frequencies of 500, 1000, and 2000 Hz. This is often calle
the three band preferred octave speech interference level.[2]

Given the following information, compute the three band preferred octave
speech interference level.

Octave Band Hz	Sound Pressure Level dB
31.5	78
63	75
125	78
250	82
500	81
1000	80
2000	80
4000	73
8000	65

---

[1] Below 75 to 75, 75 to 150, 150 to 300, 300 to 600, 600 to 1200, 1200 to
2400, 2400 to 4800, and 4800 to 9600.

[2] For a full discussion of why the arithmetic average is used, see Handbook
of Noise Measurement, General Radio, p. 36-37.

The three band preferred octave speech interference level is:

$$PSIL_{three\ octave\ band} = \frac{81\ dB + 80\ dB + 80\ dB}{3}$$

$$= \frac{241\ dB}{3}$$

$$= 80.33\ dB$$

Table 4.4.2 shows the speech interference levels (three octave band) in dB at which reliable communication is barely possible between two male voices at various distances and voice efforts with speaker and listener facing each other using unfamiliar words and numbers. The table assumes no nearby reflecting surfaces. For female voices, subtract 5 dB.

Table 4.4.2

Relationship of PSIL, voice effort, and distance.

Distance in Feet	Voice Effort			
	Normal	Raised	Very Loud	Shouting
0.5	74	80	86	92
1	68	74	80	86
2	62	68	74	80
4	56	62	68	74
6	52	58	64	70
12	46	52	58	64

For example, if the PSIL (three octave band) of an intruding noise were 80 dB, the average male would need to communicate in a "very loud" noise to make himself understood outdoors at a distance of 1 foot; he would need to "shout" at a PSIL of 80 dB if he wanted to be understood at a distance of 2 feet. The levels reflected in Table 4.4.3 reflect the background noise level.

Other indices for engineering and control include:

1.   Perceived Noise Level: Listeners are asked to compare noises on the basis of their acceptability or their "noisiness." The resulting judgments have been found to be similar to those for loudness.

2.   Perceived Level--Stevens' Mark VII: A procedure for calculating loudness that was developed by S. S. Stevens after considerable review of the available evidence on "loudness," annoyance, noisiness, acceptability, objectionability, etc. (See Handbook of Noise Measurement, General Radio, p. 28 to 33.)

Table 4.4.3

PSIL criteria indoors.

Type of Room	Maximum PSIL dB (Measured when room not in use)
Small Private Office	45
Conference Room for 20	35
Conference Room for 50	30
Movie Theater	35
Concert Hall (No Amplification)	25
Secretarial Office (Typing)	60
Home (Sleeping Area)	30
School Room	30

Source: Handbook of Noise Measurement.

3.   Noise Curves (NC) and PNC (Preference Noise Curves): A set of curve that give criteria of sound-pressure level in a set of frequency bands. Typically used to determine satisfactory background noise inside office buildings and in rooms and halls of various types.

4.   Noise and Number Index (NNI): An index based on the perceived nois levels for aircraft noise. (It takes into consideration the number of aircraft per day in the annoyance.)

5.   Noise Pollution Level: A procedure for rating community noise, whe the noise fluctuates between relatively quieter periods and noisier periods.

Sound (Noise) Level, dBA

In previous chapters it has been suggested that a frequency analysis of sound be done. That is, the sound-pressure level or sound-intensity level should be identified for each frequency band, as in Table 4.4.4.

Further, it has been suggested that the overall sound-pressure level can be obtained by properly adding the sound-pressure level dB in each frequency band. In the example in Table 4.4.4, the overall sound-pressure level is about 104 dB. This overall sound-pressure level corresponds to the value tha would be found by reading a sound level meter at a specific location with the frequency weighting set so that each frequency in the spectrum is weighted equally (a flat weighting system).

However, many noise regulations refer to an A-weighted sound-pressure level. An A-weighted sound-pressure level can be obtained for the data in Table 4.4.4 by adding the corrections given in Table 4.4.5 to the

Table 4.4.4

Frequency analysis.

Octave Band Center Frequency	Sound Pressure Level dB
31.5	85
63	88
125	94
250	94
500	95
1000	100
2000	97
4000	90
8000	88

sound-pressure levels given in dB in Table 4.4.4. (Table 4.4.6 shows the corrections being added to the values in Table 4.4.4 to get the dBA values.)

The overall sound-pressure level in dBA can now be obtained by properly adding the values in the last column of Table 4.4.6. The overall sound pressure in dBA would be about 103 dBA. This would be the value obtained if the A network were used on a sound level meter. Note: The sound-pressure level gives only one value; it is not capable of giving a value at each frequency band. (For this, an octave band analyzer would be needed.)

General purpose sound measuring instruments are normally equipped with three frequency weighting networks: A, B, and C. The frequency weightings are shown in Figure 4.4.4. Also shown is the flat response that weights all frequencies equally. These weightings are used because they approximate the ear's response characteristics at different sound levels and because they can be produced with a few electronic components.

The A-weighting approximates the ear's response for low-level sound, below 55 dB (reference: 0.00002 N/m^2). The B-weighting is intended to approximate the ear's response for levels between 55 and 85 dB, and the C-weighting corresponds to the ear's response level about 85 dB.

Although the sound level meter gives a single number, the distribution of noise can be approximated by comparing the levels measured with each weighting network. If

$$L_C - L_A = 0$$

i.e., sound level on C-weighting is equal to the sound level on the A-weighting, then it can be reasoned that most of the sound is at 1000 Hz

Table 4.4.5

A-frequency weighting adjustments.

f (Hz)	Corrections
25	-44.7
32	-39.4
40	-34.6
50	-30.2
63	-26.2
80	-22.5
100	-19.1
125	-16.1
160	-13.4
200	-10.9
250	-8.8
315	-6.6
400	-4.8
500	-3.2
630	-1.9
800	-0.8
1000	0.0
1250	+0.6
1600	+1.0
2000	+1.2
2500	+1.3
3150	+1.2
4000	+1.0
5000	+0.5
6300	-0.1
8000	-1.1
10000	-2.5
12500	-4.3
16000	-6.6
20000	-9.3

(because this is the only position on the spectrum where the weightings are similar).

If

$$L_C - L_A > 0$$

i.e, if the sound level on the C-weighting is greater than that on the A-weighting, then it can be reasoned that most of the sound is at low frequencies. And if

$$L_C - L_A < 0$$

Table 4.4.6

Corrections being added to values in Table 4.4.4.

Octave Band Center Frequency	Sound Pressure Level dB	Correction	Sound Pressure Level dBA
31.5	85	-39.2	45.8
63	88	-26.2	61.8
125	94	-16.1	77.9
250	94	- 8.6	85.4
500	95	- 3.2	91.8
1000	100	0	100.0
2000	97	+ 1.2	98.2
4000	90	+ 1.0	91.0
8000	88	- 1.1	86.9

Be ear hears these better than mic.

& because of tubal resonance.

Figure 4.4.4

Frequency characteristics for sound level meters.

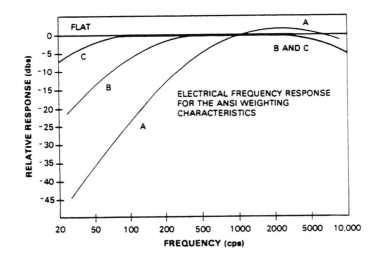

then it can be reasoned that most of the sound is above 1000 Hz. In most cases, particularly in engineering and control, the information provided by the A-B-C weightings is not adequate to describe the sound. Hence, frequency analysis is normally used. However, the A-B-C weighting can provide a quick, on-the-spot analysis of the noise.

The A-weighting scale, because it approximates the hearing sensitivity of the human, has become the common legal description for sound levels. It shows a good single approximation which correlates with such effects as loudness, speech interference, annoyance, and hearing loss.

Extra-Auditory Effects

It has been said that exposure to noise can cause hearing loss as well as interference with sound reception and job performance. Aside from hearing loss, noise may trigger changes in the cardiovascular, endocrine, neurological, and other body functions, all of which are suggestive of a general stress reaction. These physiological changes are usually produced by intense sound of sudden onset but can also occur under continued high levels. Whether continued, noise-induced reactions of this type can ultimately damage a person's physical and mental health is still uncertain.

Damage-Risk Criteria

How damage-risk criteria are established is beyond the scope of this text. The criteria now being used are designed to protect most workers from hearing losses which would impair their ability to hear and understand normal speech.

The Industrial Noise Manual, American Industrial Hygiene Association, has this to say about the criteria:

> On August 4, 1972, NIOSH submitted to the U.S. Department of Labor (DOL) a criteria package entitled "Occupational Exposure to Noise" in accordance with Section 20(a)(3) of the Occupational Safety and Health Act. This NIOSH publication included the permissible levels as found in the Walsh-Healy Standard. However, it proposed that permissible levels for new installations be dropped 5 dBA. Furthermore, their proposal recommended that these lower permissible levels become generally applicable following an extensive feasibility study.

This recommended standard is given in Table 4.4.7.

The recommended standard also specifies:

1. Exposure to impulse or impact noise should not exceed 140 dB peak sound pressure.

2. When the daily noise exposure is made up of two or more periods of noise exposure of different levels, their combined effect should be considered.

Table 4.4.7

Permissible noise exposures[1].

Duration Per Day, Hours	Sound Level dBA Slow Response	
	Existing	New
8	90	85
6	92	87
4	94	89
3	97	92
2	100	95
1.5	102	97
1	105	100
0.5	110	105
0.25 or less.	115	110

[1] When the daily noise exposure is composed of two or more periods of noise exposure of different levels, their combined effect should be considered rather than the individual effects of each. If the sum of the following fractions: C1/T1 + C2/T2... + Cn/Tn exceeds unity, then the mixed exposure should be considered to exceed the limit value. Cn indicates the total time of exposure at a specified noise level, and Tn indicates the total time of exposure permitted at that level.

If

$$C_1/T_1 + C_2/T_2 \ldots + C_n/T_n > 1$$

where C_n denotes the total time of exposure at a specified noise level and T_n denotes the total time of exposure permitted at that level, then the mixed exposure should be considered to exceed the limit value.

Summary

1.   The threshold of hearing is determined by testing young, healthy adults.

2.   Hearing loss is defined as the difference between an individual's threshold and the average threshold for young, healthy adults. Hearing loss should not be confused with threshold shifts.

3.   Most significant noise-induced hearing losses occur first in the frequency range of 400 Hz. With increased exposure, losses grow and broaden to involve other frequencies in the range of 500 to 3000 Hz.

4. Hearing loss occurs as age increases due to exposure to societal
    noises and age.

5. In addition to hearing loss, noise can interfere with speech and job
    performance. That is, noise can become an annoyance.

6. Noise exposure may also cause physical and psychological disorders;
    e.g., changes in the cardiovascular system, endocrine system, and
    neurological system.

7. There are many indices available to measure the effects of noise.

    a. Loudness (in sones)
    b. Loudness Level (in phons)
    c. Speech Interference Level; the arithmetic average of
        sound-pressure levels in the frequency bands centered around
        500, 1000, and 2000 Hz.
    d. Perceived Noise Level
    e. Perceived Level
    f. Preferred Noise Curves
    g. Noise Number and Index
    h. Noise Pollution Level
    i. A-Weighted Network on a sound level meter

8. Individuals find the following noise characteristics annoying.

    a. A loud noise is more annoying than a less loud noise.
    b. Noise varying in intensity and frequency is more annoying than
        continuous, steady-state noise.
    c. Nondirectional noise is more annoying than directional noise.
    d. Noise that appears to be moving is more annoying than noise that
        appears to be stationary.

5. Vibration

Introduction

This chapter discusses the characteristics of vibration, the theory of vibration, and the effects of vibration on man. In addition, it discusses the methods of controlling vibration; in particular, how to select isolators that isolate a disturbing force from a radiating surface.

Definition of Vibration

In general, vibration can be described as an oscillary motion in a system about an equilibrium position produced by a disturbing force. The three key words are motion, system, and disturbing force.

The motion may be flexorial, torsional, compressional, or more complex. There may be one or more modes of vibration at different frequencies for each type of motion. The disturbing force may be periodic or nonperiodic. Periodic disturbing forces are.produced mechanically by unbalanced, misaligned, loose, or eccentric parts of rotating machinery; for example, bad gears or bent shafts. Forces are also produced hydraulically and aerodynamically; for example, by pump propellers, centrifugal compressors, or fans. In either case, the frequency spectrum occurs at the basic rotational speed or some multiple of it. Nonperiodic forces are produced by sliding or rolling parts, turbulent fields, or jet discharges; for example, bad bearings or cavitation. The resulting frequency spectrum is determined by the interaction of the inherent properties of the system with the disturbing force. It is not necessarily related to the rotational speed for nonperiodic forces.

The system referred to in the definition of vibration may be gaseous, liquid, or solid. When the system is air (gaseous) and the motion involves vibration of air particles in the frequency range of 20,000 Hz, sound is produced. However, usually the word "vibration" is used to describe motions of the structures found in machinery, bridges, or battleships and is classed as solid-borne or mechanical vibration.

Periodic Vibration

Vibration is considered periodic if the oscillating motion of a particle around the position of equilibrium repeats itself exactly after some period of time. The simplest form of periodic vibration is called "pure harmonic motion" which can be represented by a sinusoidal curve as a function of time. Such a relationship is illustrated in Figure 4.5.1.

455

Figure 4.5.1

Periodic vibration.

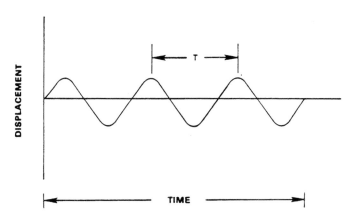

The motion of any particle can be characterized at any time by (1) displacement from equilibrium position, (2) the velocity or rate of change in displacement, or (3) acceleration, or the rate of change in velocity. For pure harmonic motion, the three characteristics of motion are related mathematically.

The instantaneous displacement of a particle from its reference position under the influence of harmonic motion can be described mathematically as follows:

$$s = S \sin(2\pi t/T)$$
$$= S \sin (2\pi f)$$
$$= S \sin \omega t$$

where s denotes instantaneous displacement, S denotes maximum displacement, t denotes time, T denotes period of vibration, f denotes frequency, and ω denotes angular frequency ($2\pi f$).

Of the possible vibration measurements (displacement, velocity, and acceleration), displacement is probably the easiest to understand. Displacement can be measured directly only if the rate of motion, i.e., frequency of vibration, is low enough.

In many practical problems, displacement is not the most important property of vibration. For example, experience has shown that velocity of a vibrating part is the best single criterion for use in preventive maintenance of rotating machinery.

Although peak-to-peak displacement measurements have been widely used for this purpose, it is necessary to establish the relationship between the limits for displacement and rotational speed for each machine. Since the velocity of a moving particle is a change in displacement with respect to time, velocity can be mathematically defined as

$$v = ds/dt$$

$$= \omega S \cos (\omega t)$$

$$= v_{max} \cos (\omega t)$$

$$= v_{max} \sin (\omega t + \pi/2)$$

where v denotes instantaneous velocity and v_{max} denotes maximum velocity.

In many cases of vibration, especially when mechanical failure is a consideration, actual forces set up in the vibrating parts are critical factors. Since the acceleration of a particle is proportional to these applied forces and since equal and opposite reaction forces result, particles in vibrating structures exert forces that are a function of the masses and acceleration of the vibrating parts on the total structure. Thus, acceleration measurements are another means by which the motion of vibrating particles can be characterized.

The instantaneous acceleration--the time rate of change of velocity of a particle in pure harmonic motion--can be described as follows:

$$a = dv/dt$$

$$= d^2s/dt^2$$

$$= -\omega^2 S \sin (\omega t)$$

$$= A \sin(\omega t + \pi)$$

where "a" denotes instantaneous acceleration and "A" denotes maximum acceleration.

The expressions given above have utilized peak values. This approach is quite useful in the consideration of pure harmonic vibration. However, in the situation of more complex vibration, peak values are not that useful. What needs to be known is the behavior of the vibration over its history. Peak values do not take into account the previous history of the vibration. One descriptive quality that does take history into account is the average absolute value.

$$S_{average} = 1/T \int_{o}^{T} |s| \, dt$$

Although the above expression does take the time history of the vibration into account (over one period), it has very limited practical usefulness. The root mean square value is much more useful.

$$S_{rms} = [1/T \int_o^T s^2 t dt]^{1/2}$$

For pure harmonic vibration, it can be shown that

$$S_{rms} = \pi/2 \sqrt{2}$$

Attempts have been made to introduce the concepts of displacement level, velocity level, and acceleration level. These are similar in concept to sound-pressure level, where displacement, velocity, and acceleration are expressed in decibels. Displacement level is defined as

$$\text{Displacement level} = 20 \, Log_{10}(d/d_o)$$

where d_o denotes the reference quantity usually given as 10^{-11} meters or 39.4×10^{-11} inches.

Velocity level is given as

$$\text{Velocity level} = 20 \, Log_{10}(v/v_o)$$

where v_o denotes the reference quantity usually given as 10^{-8} m/sec or 39.4×10^{-8} inches/sec.

The acceleration level is given as

$$\text{Acceleration level} = 20 \, Log_{10}(a/a_o)$$

where a_o denotes the reference quantity usually given as 10^{-5} m/sec^2 or 39.4×10^{-5} inches/sec^2.

When to Use What

Vibration can be examined by looking at displacement, velocity, or acceleration. Although displacement of the moving part is easiest to understand, in many practical problems displacement is not the most important property.

A vibrating part will radiate sound in much the same way as a common loudspeaker does. In general, velocities of the radiating part (which corresponds to the cone of the loudspeaker) and the air next to the part will be the same; and if the distance from the front of the part to the back is large compared with one-half of the wavelength of the sound in air, the actual sound pressure in air will be proportional to the velocity of the vibration. Furthermore, the sound energy radiated by the vibrating surface is the product of the velocity squared and the resistance components of the air load. Under these conditions, it is the velocity of the vibrating part and not its displacement that is of greater importance.

In the above paragraph, it was shown that in the case where the vibrating part is large compared to the wavelength of the sound that velocity was of importance. However, in most machines this relationship does not hold, since relatively small parts are vibrating at relatively low frequencies. This situation can be compared to a small loudspeaker without a baffle (cone). At low frequencies, the air may be pumped back and forth from one side of the cone to the other with high velocity but without building up much pressure or radiating much sound energy because of the very low air load. Under these conditions, an acceleration measurement provides a better measure of the amount of noise radiated than does the velocity measurement.

Acceleration measurement has been extensively used to analyze the situation where vibration is severe enough to cause mechanical failure. In mechanical failure, the actual forces set up in the vibrating parts are important factors. The acceleration of a given mass is proportional to the applied force, and the reacting force will be equal but in the opposite direction. Members of a vibrating structure, therefore, exert forces on the total structure that are a function of the masses and the accelerations of the vibrating parts. Thus, acceleration measurements are the important measure when actual mechanical failure due to vibration is considered.

In summary, for a given sinusoidal displacement, velocity is proportional to frequency; and acceleration is proportional to the square of the frequency. The higher-frequency components of a vibration are progressively more important in velocity and acceleration measurements than in displacement readings.

Resonance

An object when struck will vibrate at its own frequency. This frequency depends upon the elasticity and shape of the object. Resonance occurs when successive impulses are applied to a vibrating object in time with its natural frequency. When an elastic object is struck with the sound wave of the same natural frequency, the wave will set the object into resonance--motion. If there are two matching tuning forks and one is set into motion, the other one can be set into motion. When tuning forks are placed a specified distance apart, the first tuning fork, when put into motion, will cause the other tuning fork to vibrate since they both are at the same frequency. What happens is this: The areas of compression give the prongs of the fork a tiny push. Since these pushes correspond to the natural frequency of the fork, they will successively increase the amplitude (displacement) of the vibration.

The effects of resonance can be extremely disastrous. In 1940, the Tacoma Narrows Bridge was destroyed by wind generating a resonance.

During the discussion on how to select isolators to control vibration, the term and concept of resonance will be used.

Vibration Measurement

A wide variety of systems can be used to measure vibration; mechanical systems, electrical systems, and optical systems such as stroboscopic observation are examples. A stroboscopic system is discussed in <u>Handbook of Noise Measurement</u>, General Radio, page 224. The most common system used has three components: a vibration pickup, which transforms mechanical motion into an electrical signal; an amplifier, to enlarge the signal; and an analyzer, to measure the vibration in specific frequency ranges. Various types of each measuring device are available; e.g., pickups can measure displacement, velocity, or acceleration. The most common type of pickup is the accelerometer.

The problems involved in measuring vibration are determining what quantity to measure--displacement, velocity, or acceleration; determining the points at which the vibration pickup should be placed; determining how to fasten the pickup; and determining how to arrange the equipment in the field.

The quantities to be measured and some general rules of when to use what have already been discussed.

The correct pickup location is sometimes not obvious, and some exploration of the vibration position is required. Furthermore, the pickup must be correctly oriented, and this too sometimes requires exploration. The pickup must be oriented with respect to the direction of motion. In general, vibration instruments are most sensitive to vibrations in the direction perpendicular to the largest flat surface of the pickup.

The direction of maximum vibration at a point is often obvious from the vibrating structure; it is usually in the direction of least stiffness. However, this rule is sometimes misleading because of the many possible modes of vibration, some of which are perpendicular to the obvious direction of least stiffness. Such a mode can be strongly excited if close to the frequency of a component of the driving or disturbing force. Furthermore, the nature of the motion may favor one mode of vibration rather than another.

The measuring location is then related to the detection of the source of the disturbing force and to the identification of surfaces contributing significantly to airborne sound. Seemingly insignificant differences in location can result in significant differences in the observed reading. Usually readings are taken at more than one location and then compared. The comparison then helps to locate the significant sources. Rotating machinery provides a good example. Radial (perpendicular to the shaft), horizontal, and vertical readings on the bearing housing (as close as possible to the shaft) are compared to axial (parallel to the shaft) readings, based upon the knowledge that pickup response is directional.

Unbalance usually produces radial vibration at the basic rotational speed. Misalignment does the same, but is also associated with axial vibration at two or three times the basic speed. Looseness produces radial vibration at twice the basic rotational speed. Bad bearings produce high-pitched sounds unrelated to the basic speed. Gears, fans, impellers, etc., produce vibrations at tooth-on-blade passing frequencies, which equal rotational speed multiplied by the number of passes per rotation. More complex procedures can be used which are beyond the scope of this text. (See <u>Handbook of Noise Measurement</u>, General Radio, pages 207 to 215.)

Pickups can be fastened to the vibrating surface in a number of different ways. Pickups may be attached temporarily with magnets, putty, double-sided tape, and grease (jelly). Or, they may be attached permanently with bolts or epoxy cement. Permanent attachments may be necessary for maintenance tests. Care must be taken when fastening the pickup since the method of fastening may cause the vibrating surface to change its characteristics which would result in erroneous readings.

In some cases, for example, to make a quick check of vibration amplitude or to explore a vibration pattern, a hand-held pickup might be used. If the vibrating machine is massive and is vibrating with a significant amplitude, this technique can be useful for frequencies below about 1000 Hz. There are enough serious limitations to this technique, however, so that it should not generally be expected to yield accurate or highly reproducible results.

Other errors in measurement can be introduced by magnetic and electrical fields such as a ground loop-induced electrical hum. Thus, care must be taken to eliminate any mechanical vibration of the cables used in the field situation. Temperature can also affect vibration measurement, particularly measurement of very low frequency and amplitude.

The Effects of Vibration

Besides the disturbing force setting a surface into vibration and creating noise, vibration can cause other problems--problems that are not necessarily related to the noise produced by vibration.

The human body is an extremely complex physical and biological system. When looked upon as a mechanical system, it contains a number of linear and nonlinear systems, the mechanical properties of which differ from person to person. Biologically, and certainly physiologically, the system is by no means simple. On the basis of experimental studies, as well as documented reports of industrial experience, it is apparent that exposure of workers to vibration can result in profound effects on the human body mechanically, biologically, physiologically, and psychologically. Although not much is known about the effects of vibration on the human body, there is some literature available, mainly in European countries.

There are really two types of vibration effects on the human body, whole-body vibration, and segmental vibration. The human body is subjected to mechanical vibration just as any other system is. For example, when the body sits on a tractor seat, the body can vibrate just as the tractor seat does. This is called "whole-body vibration." "Segmental vibration" refers to the vibration of only parts of the body such as the hands using hand tools, the feet, etc. In segmental vibration, only the body part is free to vibrate while the rest of the body is firmly supported.

As a mechanical system, the body and even the body parts have their own natural frequencies. That is, the body and its parts will vibrate or be sent into resonance. Whole-body resonance occurs at 3 to 6 Hz and from 10 to 14 Hz. Body parts can also be sent into vibration. For example, the head and shoulders will vibrate at 20 to 30 Hz; the eyeballs will vibrate from 60 to 90 Hz; and the lower jaw and skull will vibrate at 100 to 200 Hz.

The effects of whole-body vibration are not completely understood. When the whole body vibrates, there is increased consumption of oxygen which affects the pulmonary system and cardiac output. In addition to pulmonary and circulatory changes, whole-body vibration can cause tendon reflexes. It can also impair the ability to regulate posture. In addition, there is some evidence to suggest that whole-body vibration can affect the electrical activity of the brain. It can also affect visual acuity and the ability to perform different types of motor activities.

The effects of segmental vibration are various. There are four types of disorders that can result from segmental vibration.

1.   Raynaud's phenomenon, sometimes called "white fingers."

2.   Neuritis and degenerative alterations, particularly in the ulnary and axillary nerves; that is, the loss of touch, the loss of sensitivity to heat, and even paralysis.

3.   Decalcification of the bones.

4.   Muscle atrophy (tenosynovitis).

Raynaud's Syndrome. Raynaud's syndrome affects about one-half of the workers exposed to segmental vibration. Sometimes this syndrome is called "dead fingers" or "white fingers." In Raynaud's syndrome the circulation of the hand becomes impaired; and when exposed to cold, the fingers become white and void of sensation as though mildly frosted. The condition usually disappears when the fingers are warmed for some time, but a few cases have been sufficiently disabling that some workers have been forced to seek other types of work. In some instances, both hands have been affected. The syndrome has been observed in a number of occupations including the use of fairly light vibrating tools such as air hammers for scraping and chipping metal surfaces, stone cutting, lumbering, and cleaning departments of foundries where workers have a good deal of overtime work. Most commonly the frequency implicated in Raynaud's syndrome is between 40 and 125 Hz. Exposure time of a few months can cause the symptoms to appear. When exposure ends, symptoms will improve; however, complete recovery is rare. There are no standards available concerning Raynaud's disease or symptoms, and most of the studies concerning the disease have been performed in European countries. Table 4.5.1 presents some of the evidence that has been found in these European countries for segmental and whole-body vibration. In recent years there has been an increase in studies concerning vibration.

Control of Vibration

Before control techniques are discussed, it should be pointed out that at the present time there are no generally accepted safe vibration levels for whole body or segmental vibration. Some standards do exist, but these are based on studies that produce variable results. Consequently, no reliable

Table 4.5.1

European countries in which clinical evidence
of overexposure to workers to vibration has been reported.

Industry	Vibration Type	Common Vibration Sources
Agriculture	Whole body	Tractor operation
Boiler making	Segmental	Pneumatic tools
Construction	Whole body Segmental	Heavy equipment vehicles, pneumatic drills, jackhammers, etc.
Diamond cutting	Segmental	Vibrating hand tools
Forestry	Whole body Segmental	Tractor operation. chain saws
Foundries	Segmental	Vibrating cleavers
Furniture manufacture	Segmental	Pneumatic chisels
Iron and steel	Segmental	Vibrating hand tools
Lumber	Segmental	Chain saws
Machine tools	Segmental	Vibrating hand tools
Mining	Whole body Segmental	Vehicle operators rock drills
Riveting	Segmental	Hand tools
Rubber	Segmental	Pneumatic stripping tools
Sheet metal	Segmental	Stamping equipment
Shipyards	Segmental	Pneumatic hand tools
Stone dressing	Segmental	Pneumatic hand tools
Textile	Segmental	Sewing machines, looms
Transportation (operators and passengers)	Whole body	Vehicle operation

Source: The Industrial Environment: Its Evaluation and Control

standards have been constructed. In addition, most authors point out that the available standards should be used with caution in the industrial setting, mainly because the standards that have been developed are for short-term exposures and, therefore, do not reflect the typical industrial setting. Also, because these standards were developed using physically fit individuals (pilots), they do not necessarily represent the typical industrial population.

Vibration can be controlled in the following ways:

1. By reducing the mechanical disturbance (driving force) causing the vibration.

2. By isolating the disturbing force from the radiating surface.

3. By reducing the response of the radiating surface.

In order to discuss how to reduce the mechanical driving force, it should be understood that there are different kinds of forces: rotational force, impact force, and sliding force. Rotational forces can be controlled by:

1. Balancing;
2. Alignment;
3. Reducing clearances;
4. Replacing worn parts;
5. Proper lubrication;
6. Reducing the speed of the machine.

Impact forces can be reduced by:

1. Having a smaller force over a longer period of time;
2. Using helical instead of spur gears;
3. Putting fiber gears between metal gears;
4. Cushioning applications to control impact of parts falling against chutes.

Sliding forces can be controlled by proper lubrication and reduction of friction.

Another way of controlling vibration is to isolate the driving force from the vibrating surface. For example, if a vibratory object like an unbalanced machine is set on an ordinary wood table, the vibration will radiate to the table when the machine is started; and the table will begin to vibrate. The vibration being transmitted from the machine to the table can be reduced by somehow isolating the machine from the table. Isolators such as rubber washers can be put under the machine. The rubber washers will stop the machine from transmitting force to the table and, thus, stop the table from vibrating.

Installation and selection of isolators can be a difficult job because improper application of isolators can make the problem worse and may further increase the force being transmitted to the vibratory surface. Further, isolation is a difficult job because vibration can exist in six modes. For example, there are three linear modes: horizontal, vertical, and transverse. The other three are known as rotational modes, and they appear as rocking actions around the center of gravity of the load that vibrates back and forth around the x, y, and z axis.

When developing an isolation system, there are several things that must be known--the natural frequency of the system and the frequency of the driving force. In the linear modes, the natural frequency can be computed using the following:

$$f_n \doteq (1/2\pi)\sqrt{Kg/W}$$

where

      f_n denotes natural frequency (Hz)
      K denotes stiffness of the isolator (lbs/in)
      g denotes acceleration in gravity, 386 inches (32.2 x 12) per
         $second^2$
      W denotes weight of the system per mount (lbs)

An alternate method, the static deflection method, could be

$$f_n = 3.13 \times \sqrt{1/S_{st}}$$

where
      f_n denotes natural frequency (Hz)
      S_{st} denotes static deflection of the mount (inches), usually
         provided by the manufacturer of the isolator

For rotational modes, the following equation can be used:

$$f_n = (1/2\Pi) \sqrt{Kr/i} = 0.167 \sqrt{Kr/i}$$

where
      f_n denotes the natural frequency (Hz)
      Kr denotes the rotational stiffness of the mount (in-lb/radian
         of angular displacement about a given axis)
      i denotes mass moment of inertia of supporting load about a given
         axis through the center of gravity ($pounds/inches^2$)

The natural frequency can change if any of the following factors change: weight of the system, stiffness of the mount, moment of inertia, and rotational motion of the mount. These changes will change the static deflection and, therefore, the natural frequency. In most cases, changing the stiffness of the mount is the easiest way to alter the rotational frequency.

The second thing item must be known in order to design a good isolation system is the frequency of the driving force. If there are many frequencies involved, the lowest frequency of the system must be used.

Transmissibility is also a factor of concern when designing an isolation system. Transmissibility is a term used to express the efficiency of the isolation system. It is a ratio of forces. For example: If an unbalanced motor was running at a speed of 180 rpm and was producing 100 pounds of centrifugal force and it was desired to limit the force to 2 pounds on the foundation that the machine was set in, the transmissibility would be 0.02 or 2/100.

The reduction of structural-borne noise by vibration isolation can also be expressed in terms of transmissibility. On a decibel scale, it is defined as

Noise Reduction (NR in dB) = 20 Log T

$$= 20 \text{ Log } \frac{\text{Exciting force}}{\text{Transmitted force}}$$

Figure 4.5.2 is an illustration of transmissibility curves. The left-hand side of the figure indicates that if a noise were at 30 dB and it was desired to reduce it to 25 dB, the transmissibility of the system would have to be 0.6.

Figure 4.5.2

Transmissibility curves.

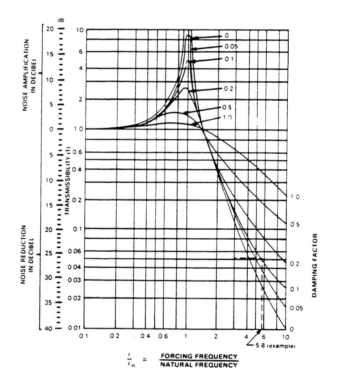

The figure not only shows the relationship between transmissibility and the decibel scales but also gives transmissibility curves over various ratios of forcing frequency to natural frequency. On the horizontal axis is the ratio of forcing frequency to the natural frequency, and on the vertical axis is the transmissibility. Since low transmissibilities are essential for effective vibration isolation, it is only necessary to examine the transmissibility curves to find the desirable frequency ratio (forcing frequency to natural frequency) which must be attained to make the system effective. Notice from the curves that a reduction in noise in decibels occurs when the transmissibility is less than 1. If the transmissibility is greater than 1, there is an amplification in the noise. Other facts can be observed from the curves.

1. When the forcing frequency equals the natural frequency of the mounted system, the transmissibility becomes much greater than 1.0, and no isolation is attained. Instead, an amplification of the existing force or motion occurs (resonance).

2. It is not until the forcing frequency is 1.4 or more times the natural frequency of the mounted system that any isolation is achieved.

3. To achieve a transmissibility of 0.1, which means 90% isolation efficiency, the frequency ratio must be at least 3.3.

The above paragraphs suggest a step-by-step procedure for selecting a vibration isolator. These steps are:

1. Determine the lowest forcing frequency in the machine to be isolated.

2. Establish permissible transmissibility or desirable noise reduction level.

3. Using Figure 4.5.2, determine the required natural frequency.

4. Determine the necessary deflection to obtain the natural frequency required. Also consider the effect of the environmental conditions, such as creep, wear, resistance to corrosion, ozone, oil, or other detrimental agents.

5. Determine the weight of each mounting point on the machine to be isolated.

6. From the load deflection data supplied by the manufacturer of the vibration isolators, determine the size required.

A 200-pound machine is transmitting vibration at 40 Hz into a support structure with the force of 100 pounds. It is desired to limit the force to 5 pounds, by the use of an isolator. This would require a transmissibility of 0.05 (5/100). The machine is exposed to grease; hence, an isolator made of neoprene is desired. The dampening factor of the isolator is 0.1 according to the vendor. Following the 0.1 curve on Figure 4.5.2 to the transmissibility of 0.05, the ratio of the forcing frequency to natural frequency is found to be as follows:

$$f/f_n = 5.8$$

Thus,

$$f_n = 40 \text{ Hz}/5.8 = 6.9 \text{ Hz}$$

From this information it can be seen that the static deflection of about 0.21 inches is required for the isolator. That is, the natural frequency of 6.9 Hz can be substituted in the following expression (assume load deflection curve is linear):

$$f_n = 3.13 \times 1/\sqrt{S_{st}}$$

Assuming equal distribution of load on the four points of support, the load per mount becomes 50 pounds, so that the stiffness of the isolator must be 50 lbs/0.21 inches, or 238 pounds per inch. From the information in the vendor's catalog, it is now possible to select the proper isolator.

Here is another example. If the vibration of a 200-pound machine is causing the supporting structure to radiate a 60-decibel noise, and it is desired to reduce the noise to 34 dB--a reduction of 26 decibels--the same procedure is used. First, follow the 0.1 curve on Figure 4.5.2 to the noise reduction of 26 dB, and the solution is obtained.

There are many types of isolators. Felt compositions called elastomers are effective at frequencies of about 30 Hz. There are spring elastomers which are not affected by oil or other contaminants. The type of isolator selected depends upon the particular problem to be solved.

The third method of control is reducing the response of the vibrating surface. This method would be particularly useful when the vibrating force is equal to the natural frequency of the vibrating surface, and resonance results. There are three methods of reducing the response of the vibrating surface: stiffening, increasing mass, and dampening. It should be noted that any of these methods would change the natural frequency of the system.

Usually large, flat surfaces will vibrate, and adding stiffeners will reduce the vibration. Along with the stiffening of a material, the shape of the vibrating surface can be changed. For example, the panel can be dished or curved so that the vibration is cut down. Also, the size of the radiating surface can be changed. A smaller surface will tend to radiate less sound.

The second method of reducing the response of the vibrating surface is through increasing the mass of the material or vibrating surface. Increased mass makes the material heavier and more resistant to vibration.However, when increasing the mass of a material, one must be careful of the resonant frequency of the new material.

The third method of reducing the response of the vibrating surface is through dampening. Dampening refers to restraining noise achieved by reducing the contact of the vibrating surface with the air. This contact can be reduced by the addition of an absorbing material to the vibrating surface. This absorbing material will transfer the vibration energy into heat energy, and less energy will be put into the air. Dampening materials include dampening felt, elastomers, tars, and any kind of masking material. Optimizing dampening treatment is usually a complicated procedure. In addition, it can be extremely expensive. Thus, it is suggested than a technical expert should be consulted when considering dampening.

Summary

The following are key items from this chapter.

1. Vibration can be periodic or nonperiodic.

2. Vibration can be measured by examining displacement, velocity, and acceleration. The quantity used depends upon the vibration and the vibrating source.

3. Vibration measurements involve:

    a. determining what quantity to measure.
    b. determining the location to measure.
    c. determining how to fasten the vibration measuring instrument.

4. Vibration measurements are usually taken in several locations; e.g., perpendicular to shaft or housing.

5. Vibration measurement instruments include:

    a. pickups
    b. amplifiers
    c. analyzers

6. Other vibration measurement techniques include stroboscopic examination.

7. Vibration not only causes airborne noise but also causes whole-body and segmental vibration effects. These effects can cause physiological and psychological problems.

8. No reliable criteria exist for determining the vibration effects in an industrial setting.

9. Vibration can be controlled by:

    a. reducing the mechanical driving force
    b. isolating the vibration driving force from the radiating surface
    c. reducing the radiation of the vibrating surface

10. Obtaining vibration measurements and controlling vibration depends to a large extent on experience.

6. Noise Control

Introduction

Noise control techniques discussed in this chapter include new plant planning, controlling noise in existing facilities (including the building of enclosures, barriers, and shields), and personal protective equipment.

There are no standard solutions to noise control problems; each one is unique and requires a unique solution. However, many case studies have been published to assist in evaluating certain techniques in certain situations. Before attacking a noise control problem, review the literature (e.g., case studies) to determine how effective your proposed noise solution will be.

Does Noise Control Pay?

Noise control can be complicated as well as time consuming. It may involve the interruption of production and, as such, may be expensive. Noise control must be viewed as a long-term investment in the employee's hearing, improvement in communications (reduction in speech interference), and perhaps improved performance. It may be difficult to observe the benefits of solving noise control problems.

The following course of action should be viewed as a preliminary procedure to solving noise control problems.

1. Measure noise levels in dB(A) using a sound level meter.

2. Measure employee exposure time.

3. Compare the results of the above steps with the standards.

4. Set priorities for solving the problems. (For example; if there are three noise sources, one at 90 dBA, one at 95 dBA, and one at 101 dBA, and the 90 dBA source were completely removed, the overall level would still be 102 dBA. If the 90 dBA and 95 dBA sources were removed completely, the level would be 101 dBA. If the 101 dBA source were removed only, the average would be 96 dBA. Thus, it is best to work on the noisiest source first.)

5. Analyze the top priority problems. This may include octave band analysis and comparison to the standards, or it may involve more in-depth measurement techniques.

6. Institute the control techniques. The effects of control techniques are usually very difficult to predict. This unpredictability is due to the complexity of noise sources, the varying environmental conditions that might be found in industrial settings, and the limitations due to maintenance and operational requirements.

7. Remeasure to estimate the degree of effect attained by the noise control technique that was instituted. Since it is difficult to predict the results of a noise control technique, after the noise control technique is instituted, remeasurements should be made to determine exactly how much noise reduction was achieved.

Basics of Noise Control

If noise is viewed as originating from a source, traveling along a path to the ear, and finally being received by the ear, then a fundamental approach to solving noise control problems has been established. Noise can be controlled at its source; it can be controlled along the path to the ear; and it can be controlled at the receiver--the ear. Usually when noise is controlled at the source, the control is most effective. Controlling noise at the source is also less expensive. The least desirable location to control noise is at the receiver or the ear. As a matter of fact, controlling noise at the ear can be viewed as only a temporary solution to the problem.

Plant Planning

When designing a new facility, the industrial hygiene engineer is in a good position to control potential noise problems. In order to design a less noisy new plant (and perhaps new processes), the noise characteristic of each machine and process must be known. It is essential to know what machine and process are going to be used as well as their locations in relation to the walls and the workers.

One thing involved with the designing of a new plant is the determination of the noise specifications for the machines and process to be purchased. These specifications should require that the manufacturer provide certain noise data. An example of how to structure a noise specification is given in the Industrial Noise Manual, American Industrial Hygiene Association, pp. 71-73. When purchasing new equipment, it is a good practice to avoid future noise problems by building the noise control solution into the machine itself. Most built-in noise control solutions should not significantly increase the cost of the machine.

A Simple Example of a New Plant Noise Prediction

Only experience with noise and noise control techniques will help the industrial hygiene engineer when designing a new plant. However, one problem often confronted is to predict the noise level of a machine in a new environment.

Problem.   A vendor's machine produces a maximum sound-pressure level of 140 dB at 1000 Hz when the worker is 3 feet away, Q = 4, and R = 2000 square feet.   You are considering purchasing the machine from the manufacturer but using it under these conditions: r = 10, Q = 2, and R = 2000 square feet. Will the new machine meet the criteria of 90 dB at 1000 Hz under your new plant conditions?   (Notice that the sound-power level of the machine is not specified, but it will be the same under the vendor's conditions as under you conditions.)

Solution.   First, determine the sound-power level radiated by the machine using

$$SWL = SPL - 10 \text{ Log } [(Q/4\pi r^2) + (4/R)] - 10.5 \text{ dB}$$

Under the manufacturer's conditions where r = 3 ft, Q = 4, R = 2000 sq. ft, and SPL = 140 dB

$$SWL = 140 \text{ dB} - 10 \text{ Log } [(4/4\pi(3 \text{ ft})^2)) + (4/2000 \text{ ft}^2)] - 10.5 \text{ dB}$$

$$= 140 \text{ dB} - 10 \text{ Log } [(1/3.14(9 \text{ ft}^2)) + (4/2000 \text{ ft}^2)] - 10.5 \text{ dB}$$

$$= 140 \text{ dB} - 10(-1.43) - 10.5 \text{ dB}$$

$$= 140 \text{ dB} + 3.8 \text{ dB}$$

$$= 143.8 \text{ dB}$$

Now compute the sound-pressure level under your conditions: r = 10 ft, Q = 2, R = 2000 ft^2, and SWL = 143.8 dB using

$$SPL = SWL + 10 \text{ Log } [(Q/4\pi r^2) + (4/R)] + 10.5 \text{ dB}$$

$$= 143.8 \text{ dB} + 10 \text{ Log } [(2/4\pi(10 \text{ ft})^2) + (4/2000 \text{ ft})] + 10.5 \text{ dB}$$

$$= 143.8 \text{ dB} - 24.45 \text{ dB} + 10.5 \text{ dB}$$

$$= 129.85 \text{ dB}$$

The sound-pressure level under your conditions will be 129.85 dB which is 39.85 dB greater than the desired 90 dB criteria.   Therefore, the machine will not meet your standards under your conditions.

New Plant Planning and Substitution of Equipment--Some General Rules

When designing a new plant, the following substitution rules should be kept in mind:

1.   Use welding instead of riveting.
2.   Use compression riveting instead of pneumatic riveting.
3.   Use mechanical forging instead of drop forging.

4.6.4

4. Use grinding instead of chipping.
5. Use electrical tools instead of pneumatic tools.
6. Use conveyors instead of chutes.
7. Use mechanical stripping from punch presses instead of air blast stripping.
8. Use hot instead of cold working metals.
9. Use belt drives instead of gear drives (screw drives instead of gears).
10. Use squirrel cage fans instead of axial fans.
11. Use a larger, slower speed fan instead of a small fan at higher speeds.
12. Use quieter material when and where possible.

Controlling Noise in an Existing Facility

The machines that are now in an existing plant are probably the most economical but not necessarily the most quiet. In those cases where the machines makes a lot of noise--so much noise that the criteria are not met--the noise will have to be controlled in the existing facility. The noise can be controlled at the source, along the path, or at the receiver.

Controlling Noise at the Source. This section considers noise originating from machines, noise originating from a driving force (vibration), and noise resulting from pressure-reducing valves.

One of the first techniques of controlling noise at the source is to substitute the equipment, process or material--substitute the existing source of noise for another, less noisy source. In substituting equipment, processes, and materials, the general rules discussed under new plant design in this chapter can be applied.

The second general method of controlling noise in an existing facility (at the source) is to direct the sound away from the point of interest, usually the worker. Most machines are directional. This quality of machines can be used to advantage by turning the machine so that the noise is radiating in a direction away from the worker. Intake and exhaust noise can usually be controlled in this way. It should be pointed out that this technique is usually not beneficial in the reverberant field. In the reverberant field, usually no reduction will result if the direction of the sound is changed. However, in a room the machine can be directed to a highly absorbent material. This may result in some benefit.

The third general technique is to remove the machine to another room. This is often possible when access to the machine is not required.

Vibration can be controlled at the course by the following methods:

1. Reduction of the driving force by balancing, lubricating, aligning, and general maintenance. Noise due to impact forces can be partially controlled by using a smaller force over a longer period of time or by using resilient bumpers at the point of impact.

2.   Isolation of the driving force from the responding surface by the selection of isolators. This was discussed in Chapter 5.

3.   Reduction of the response of the vibrating surface by dampening, improving the support of the vibrating surface, increasing the stiffness of the vibrating surface, decreasing the size of the vibrating surface, and/or changing the shape of the vibrating surface. It should be pointed out that dampening can be a complicated, expensive procedure. A general rule when using dampening is to use the sandwich approach--use an outer plate the same gauge as the vibrating plate.

When the noise originates from the flow of air or gas, there are some general principles to follow.

1.   For fans and blowers, usually backward curved blades are quieter.

2.   Try to avoid the use of high-velocity fluid. Velocity of fluid or gas is not the usual noise source. The problem generally is the pressure-reducing valve (sonic velocity of valve) that controls the flow of gas or fluid.

The problem of high-velocity fluid can be controlled by using a muffler, a special pressure-reducing valve, or by external pipe coverings. A velocity of 10,000 feet per minute can be used without excessive noise. Therefore, velocities higher than those that are necessary should not be used. Where the pressure ratio of upstream to downstream is 1.9 or greater, excessive noise is produced by the valve. (There are special valves that are made to achieve a gradual pressure drop. These special valves will not be discussed in this text. In some cases the special valves cannot be used because they will become clogged with dirt or grit.)

In cases where a muffler or special valve is not used, the pipe can be covered. However, external pipe covering is usually the least economical solution since a great deal of pipe has to be covered to achieve the same noise reduction.

Usually the easiest solution is to use a muffler which can be purchased from a vendor. However, the industrial hygiene engineer should be familiar with the calculations necessary to select the correct muffler.

When the ratio of absolute pressure upstream of the pressure-reducing valve to downstream of the valve is 1.9 or greater, the port velocity in the valve will be sonic; and the sound-power level of the valve will vary directly with the quantity of gas flow. Figure 4.6.1 is a graph from which the approximate sound-power level of valves can be estimated. The sound-power level obtained from this graph applies to the octave bands contained at and above the cutoff frequency of the pipe or duct downstream from the valve. The cutoff frequency can be calculated by

$$f_{co} = \frac{c}{2D}$$

where f_{co} denotes the cutoff frequency (Hz), C denotes the velocity of sound in the gas under consideration (ft/sec), and D denotes the inside diameter of the downstream pipe in feet.

Figure 4.6.1

Sound-pressure level gives mass flow.

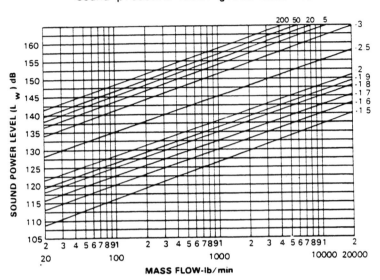

The velocity of sound, C, can be calculated as follows:

$$C = 1127 \sqrt{((t + 273)/300)(29/M)}$$

where C denotes velocity of sound (ft/sec), t denotes gas temperature in °C, and M denotes the molecular weight of the gas.

At and above the cutoff frequency, the sound power will drop approximately 6 dB for each octave band.

Assume the following situation where the gas is steam:

Upstream absolute pressure	= 165 psia
Downstream absolute pressure	= 30 psia
Gas temperature	= 185°C
Mass flow rate	= 3000 lbs/hour
Pipe downstream	= 4 inches diameter (inside)

To use the graph in Figure 4.6.1, the mass flow rate in lbs/minute needs to be calculated,

$$\text{Mass flow rate} = \frac{3000 \text{ lbs/hour}}{60 \text{ min/hour}}$$

$$= 50 \text{ lbs/min}$$

and the ratio of pressures also needs to be calculated

$$\frac{165 \text{ psia}}{30 \text{ psia}} = 5.5$$

Entering Figure 4.6.1 at 5.5 and 50 lbs/min, the sound power level is given as 141 dB.

The cutoff frequency can be computed as follows: first compute the velocity where M = 18 (molecular weight of steam).

$$C = 1127 \sqrt{((t + 273)/300)(29/M)}$$

$$= 1127 \sqrt{((185°C + 273)/300)(29/18)}$$

$$= 1770 \text{ ft/sec}$$

Then compute the cutoff frequency

$$f_{co} = \frac{C}{2D}$$

$$= \frac{1770}{2 \times 0.33}$$

$$= \frac{1770}{2(.33)}$$

$$= 2682 \text{ Hz}$$

Thus, the octave band spectrum is as follows:

Octave	Sound Power Level
63	105
125	111
250	117
500	123
1000	129
2000	135
4000	141
8000	141

he octave bands 63 Hz to 2000 Hz are computed by noting that there will be a
 dB drop for each band containing and below the cutoff frequency.

The octave band spectrum can be used to select an available commercial muf
ler or to specify the construction of a muffler.

In a previous paragraph it has been stated that if the pressure ratio
upstream to downstream ratio) is less than 1.9, sonic velocity will not be
reated. This situation describes a nonchoke valve, and the data given in
igure 4.6.1 are inappropriate. However, the graph can still be used if
orrected by the following factor:

$$K = 20 \, \text{Log} \left(\frac{0.9 \, (\text{absolute pressure downstream})}{\text{absolute pressure} - \text{absolute pressure}} \right)$$
$$\text{upstream} \qquad \text{downstream}$$

When this situation exists, follow the same procedure as before to compute
he octave band spectrum, then subtract K from each sound power level.

Mufflers. There are basically two types of mufflers, the dissipative
uffler and the nondissipative muffler. The dissipative muffler uses an
bsorption material in the lining. (See Figure 4.6.2.) This amounts
onothing more than having a pipe that is lined to dampen the noise. Usually
he straight-through type of pipe or muffler results in very little pressure
rop. Usually the diameter of the pipe is six inches or less. There is also
 center body type dissipative muffler, and it is illustrated in Figure 4.6.3.

There are procedures available for selecting the type and thickness of the
ining of mufflers. However, this is beyond the scope of this text. Mufflers
f these types are generally available commercially.

Nondissipative mufflers use the principle of resonance. The
ondissipative muffler reflects sound at particular frequencies back to the
ource of the sound. The design of this type of muffler is complicated and
ill not be discussed. However, Figure 4.6.4 is an illustration of a
ondissipative muffler.

Figure 4.6.2

Dissipative muffler--straight through type.

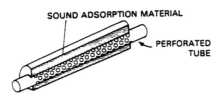

Figure 4.6.3

Dissipative muffler--centered body type.

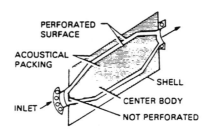

Figure 4.6.4

Nondissipative or reactive type.

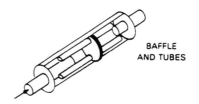

Controlling Noise Along Its Path

The last section discussed controlling noise at the source using mufflers substituting machinery, and changing the direction of the noise source. This section discusses controlling noise along its path. The techniques used to control noise along its path are shields and barriers, partial enclosures, total enclosures, and room absorption.

To understand these control techniques, it is essential to understand the physics of sound. Therefore, it is strongly suggested that you reread chapters 1, 2, and 3 so that you have a full understanding of the physics of sound before approaching these problems. Using enclosures, shields, or barriers involves nothing more than an understanding of how sound travels from one room to another. It involves concepts such as transmission loss and noise reduction.

In chapters 1 through 3, sound-pressure level in an adjoining room was computed when the sound-power level was given. This was done by computing the transmission loss of the wall and by computing the noise reduction that was achieved. Recall that the noise reduction calculations considered the reverberant buildup in the secondary room. To some degree, the problems that were discussed in the previous chapters were rather impractical and ones that would normally not occur.

Enclosures. Noise control by enclosure means building a room or wall between a sound source and the receiver. The concepts involved are essentially the same as computing the sound-pressure level in an adjoining room.

Suppose there is a room 30 feet by 30 feet and 10 feet high. The floor and ceiling are unpainted poured concrete with an absorption coefficient of 0.02 sabins, and the walls are constructed of unpainted brick (α = 0.09 sabins).

A machine that has a directivity factor of 2 (Q = 2) is in the middle of the room. At 4.0 feet from the sound source, the recorded sound-pressure readings are those recorded in line #1 of Table 4.6.1. The desired noise levels at 4.0 feet are indicated in line #2. From line #2, it is seen that the recorded sound-pressure levels are 1 dB at 500 Hz, and 8 dB at 1000 Hz, and 3 dB at 2000 Hz--higher than the desired criteria levels. To bring the sound-pressure levels to the desired criteria levels, it is decided to build an enclosure around the sound source. The sound enclosure is to be 3 feet by 3 feet by 3 feet and made of steel with an absorption coefficient of 0.02 sabins.

The problem is to compute the transmission loss of the steel enclosure. From the computed transmission loss, the thickness of the steel required can be determined. To be on the safe side, 5 dB are added to line #3 (noise reduction required) to allow for possible variations from the theoretical values. To compute the transmission loss required, it must be realized that putting an enclosure around the machine will cause reverberant buildup in the enclosure. This reverberant buildup will influence the amount of transmission loss required. To compute the reverberant buildup, compute the sound-pressure level at the wall of the enclosure before and after the wall is built. The difference between these two values will be the amount of buildup.

First, compute the sound-power level. (It will remain constant.) The analysis to follow will be confined to the 1000 Hz octave band to illustrate the procedure; the same calculations should be done, however, for the 500 Hz and 2000 Hz octave bands.

Recall that

$$SPL = SWL + 10 \text{ Log } [(Q/4\pi r^2) + (4/R)] + 10.5 \text{ dB}$$

such that

$$SWL = SPL - 10 \text{ Log } [(Q/4\pi r^2) + (4/R)] - 10.5 \text{ dB}$$

where SWL denotes sound-power level, SPL denotes sound-pressure level, Q denotes the directivity factor, r denotes the distance from the source in feet, and R denotes the room constant in square feet.

To use the above expression, let r = 4.0 feet (since SPL is known at this distance), let Q = 2 (specified by the manufacturer), let SPL = 93 dB (line #1, Table 4.6.1), and compute R as follows:

$$R_{1000} = \alpha_{avg} \Sigma S_i/(1 - \alpha_{avg})$$

Table 4.6.1

Summary data for problem.

Octave band (Hz)	63	125	250	500	1000	2000	4000	8000
SPL (at 4.0 ft) (dB)				82	84	87	86	93	88	80	81
Criteria (dB)				105	98	93	85	85	85	85	85
Required Noise Reduction (dB)							1	8	3		
Allowance for Safety (dB)							5	5	5		

where

$$\alpha_{avg\ 1000} = \Sigma S_i \alpha_i / \Sigma S_i$$

$$= \frac{(30\ ft\ \times\ 30\ ft)0.02\ sabins\ +\ (30\ ft\ \times\ 30\ ft)0.02\ sabins\ +\ 4(30\ ft\ \times\ 10\ ft)0.09\ sabins}{2(30\ ft\ \times\ 30\ ft)\ +\ 4(30\ ft\ \times\ 10\ ft)}$$

$$= \frac{144\ ft^2\ sabins}{3000\ ft^2}$$

$$= 0.048\ sabins$$

Thus

$$R_{1000} = \frac{0.048\ sabins\ \times\ 3000\ ft^2}{1\ sabin\ -\ 0.048\ sabins}$$

$$= 151.26\ ft^2$$

and

$$SWL = 93\ dB\ -\ 10\ Log[(2/4\pi(4.0\ ft)^2)\ +\ (4/151.26\ ft^2)]\ -\ 10.5\ dB$$

$$= 93\ dB\ -\ (-14.39\ dB)\ -\ 10.5\ dB$$

$$= 96.89\ dB$$

Given this sound-power level, the sound-pressure level at the wall of the enclosure (both before and after the enclosure is built) can be computed.

If the enclosure is to be 3 ft x 3 ft x 3 ft, then the average distance t the enclosure wall is calculated as

$$Average\ distance = \sqrt{S_i/4\pi}$$
to wall

$$= [6(3\ ft)^2/4\pi]^{1/2}$$

$$= 2.07\ ft$$

And the sound-pressure level at that distance without the enclosure being built is

$$SPL = SWL + 10 \ Log \ [(Q/4\pi r^2) + (4/R)] + 10.5 \ dB$$

$$= 96.89 \ dB + 10 \ Log \ [(2/4\pi(2.07 \ ft)^2) + (4/151.26 \ ft^2 + 10.5 \ dB$$

$$= 96.89 \ dB + (-11.97 \ dB) + 10.5 \ dB$$

$$= 95.42 \ dB$$

Now, after the enclosure is built, what will be the SPL at the wall of the enclosure? First, you need to compute the room constant of the proposed enclosure.

$$R_{1000} = \alpha_{avg} \ \Sigma S_i/(1 - \alpha_{avg})$$
where

$$\alpha_{avg} \ 1000 = \Sigma S_i \alpha_i / \Sigma S_i$$

$$= \frac{6(3 \ ft \ x \ 3 \ ft)0.02 \ sabins}{6(3 \ ft \ x \ 3 \ ft)}$$

$$= 0.02 \ sabins$$

Thus

$$R = \frac{0.02 \ sabins \ x \ 54 \ ft^2}{1 \ sabin \ - \ 0.02 \ sabins}$$

$$= 1.10 \ ft^2$$

And SPL at 2.07 feet when the enclosure is built is

$$SPL_{1000} = SWL + 10 \ Log \ [(Q/4\pi r^2) + (4/R)] + 10.5 \ dB$$

$$= 96.89 \ dB + 10 \ Log \ [(1/4\pi(2.07 \ ft)^2) + (4/1.10 \ ft^2 + 10.5 \ dB$$

$$= 96.89 \ dB + 5.63 \ dB + 10.5 \ dB$$

$$= 113.02 \ dB$$

Thus the reverberant buildup due to the enclosure is the difference between sound-pressure levels at 2.07 feet and after the enclosure is built or

$$Reverberant \ buildup = 113.02 \ dB \ - \ 95.42 \ dB$$
$$= 17.60 \ dB$$

Thus the transmission loss required would be the sum of the required noise reduction (8 dB), the safety factor (5 dB), and the reverberant buildup (17. dB) or

$$\text{Transmission loss} = 8 \text{ dB} + 5 \text{ dB} + 17.60 \text{ dB}$$
$$= 30.60 \text{ dB}$$

Given this transmission loss, the thickness of steel required can be determined from a table of transmission loss at 1000 Hz. The process should be repeated for 500 Hz and 2000 Hz octave bands to determine the transmissic losses at these frequencies.

Additional Notes About Total Enclosures. In the example in the last section, any other noise in the room after the enclosure was built was not considered. That is, any reverberant buildup that might be in the larger rc after the sound was transmitted through the enclosure wall was not considered. This is because the larger room was indeed larger, and reverberant buildup would be minimal. However, if the enclosure were to be built in a smaller room, the reverberation outside the enclosure would have be considered. This, however, is not the usual case; usually an enclosure i built in a large enough room so that the reverberant buildup in the larger room, after the enclosure is built, is insignificant.

Also not considered was putting an absorbent material inside the enclosure. Putting an absorbent material inside the enclosure would reduce the reverberant buildup within the enclosure. By reducing the reverberant buildup, the amount of transmission loss required from the enclosure would be reduced. If an absorbent material is put in the enclosure, a lighter enclosure material could be used because not so much transmission loss is required. The rule of thumb for putting an absorbing material inside an enclosure is as follows: If the enclosure is lined so that the average absorbent coefficient is 0.75 sabins or greater, for all practical purposes the transmission loss will equal the noise reduction required.

In the example above, the enclosure was made of steel with an absorption coefficient of 0.02 sabins. If the enclosure is lined with an absorption material equal to 0.90 sabins on five sides (everywhere but the floor), the average absorption coefficient would be equal to

$$\alpha_{\text{avg } 1000} = \frac{(3 \text{ ft} \times 3 \text{ ft})0.02 \text{ sabins} + 5(3 \text{ ft} \times 3 \text{ ft})0.90 \text{ sabins}}{6(3 \text{ ft} \times 3 \text{ ft})}$$

$$= 0.75 \text{ sabins}$$

and the sound-pressure level at the walls of the enclosure (2.07 feet from t sound source) would be

$$SPL = SWL + 10 \text{ Log } [(Q/4\pi r^2) + (4/R)] + 10.5 \text{ dB}$$

where r = 2.07 feet, Q = 2 (since the absorption material will maintain the directivity factor of the sound source), and R is computed as

$$R_{1000} = \alpha_{avg}\ \Sigma S_i / (1 - \alpha_{avg})$$

$$= \frac{0.75 \text{ sabins} \times 54 \text{ ft}^2}{1 \text{ sabin} - 0.75 \text{ sabins}}$$

$$= 162 \text{ ft}^2$$

such that

$$SPL = SWL + 10 \text{ Log } [(Q/4\pi r^2) + (4/R)] + 10.5 \text{ dB}$$

$$= 96.89 \text{ dB} + 10 \text{ Log } [(2/(2.07 \text{ ft})^2) + (4/162 \text{ ft}^2)] + 10.5 \text{ dB}$$

$$= 96.89 \text{ dB} + (-12.09 \text{ dB}) + 10.5 \text{ dB}$$

$$= 95.30 \text{ dB}$$

Thus the reverberant buildup would be the difference between the sound-pressure levels at 2.07 feet before and after the enclosure is built; or 95.30 dB - 95.42 dB or -0.12 dB. For all practical purposes, then, there will be no reverberant buildup, and the transmission loss would be equal to the noise reduction required plus the 5 dB safety factor or 13 dB.

Another factor not considered when the enclosure was built was the potential heat buildup in the enclosure. This can be a problem where the machine generates a great deal of heat, and the heat would be stored in the enclosure. Since noise is affected by temperature, the heat buildup can be a problem. This heat problem can be overcome by ventilating the enclosure properly.

Access to the machine within the enclosure also was not considered when the enclosure was built. Sometimes for maintenance and even for operation it is convenient to have an enclosure that has doors and windows. When an enclosure that has doors, windows, or access is built, the transmission loss must be computed carefully since a combined transmission loss will be involved because the enclosure will be built with more than one type of material. Also, if the doors and windows have leaks, the desired transmission loss will not be achieved.

Enclosures Inside a Noisy Work Area. In the last section, an enclosure was built around the noisy machine. However, there are times when an enclosure is built to keep the noise out of an area; for example, an office that is built in the center of a large, noisy room. In this instance, the office acts as an enclosure to keep the noise out.

A 10 foot by 10 foot by 8 foot office is to be built in the center of a 100 foot by 100 foot by 15 foot manufacturing area that has the noise levels shown in Table 4.6.2. Line 2 of the table indicates the noise levels that are desired in the office. The problem is to determine the required wall and ceiling transmission losses to meet the criteria, given these provisions:

1.   The only frequencies of concern are 250 and 500 Hz.

2.   The office ceiling must be acoustical tile with an absorption coefficient of 0.65 sabins at 500 Hz and an absorption coefficient 0.45 sabins at 250 Hz.

3.   The absorption coefficients of the floors and walls are to be 0.02 sabins at 500 Hz and 0.01 sabins at 250 Hz.

Table 4.6.2

Summary data for problem.

Octave band (Hz)		63	125	250	500	1000	2000	4000	8000
1. Existing Noise Level	(dB)	82	84	87	89	88	88	85	81
2. Criteria	(dB)	76	69	64	60	59	60	61	62
3. Line 1 - 2	(dB)	6	15	23	29	29	28	24	19
4. Allowance (Safety Factor)	(dB)	5	5	5	5	5	5	5	5
5. Required Noise Reduction	(dB)	11	20	28	34	34	33	29	24
6. Total TL Required (dB)				--	--				

The transmission loss required can be computed by rearranging the following expression:

$$NR = TL - 10 \, Log \, [(1/4) + (S_w/R)]$$

to

$$TL = NR + 10 \, Log \, [(1/4) + (S_w/R)]$$

where S_w denotes the surface area of the enclosure, NR denotes the required noise reduction, and R denotes the room constant.

S_w is computed as follows:

$$S_w = \sum_{i=1}^{n-1} S_i \text{ where } i = \text{floor area}$$

$$= (10 \text{ ft} \times 10 \text{ ft}) + 4(8 \text{ ft} \times 10 \text{ ft})$$

$$= 420 \text{ ft}^2$$

The floor area is not considered because the office is to be built on the existing floor.

R at 250 Hz is computed as follows:

$$R_{250} = \alpha_{avg} \Sigma S_i/(1 - \alpha_{avg})$$

where α_{avg} 250 Hz is computed as follows:

$$\alpha_{avg} \text{ 250 Hz} = \Sigma S_i \alpha_i / \Sigma S_i$$

$$= \frac{(10 \text{ ft} \times 10 \text{ ft})0.01 \text{ sabins} + (10 \text{ ft} \times 10 \text{ ft})0.45 \text{ sabins} + 4(8 \text{ ft} \times 10 \text{ ft})0.01 \text{ sabins}}{2(10 \text{ ft} \times 10 \text{ ft}) + 4(8 \text{ ft} \times 10 \text{ ft})}$$

$$= \frac{49.2 \text{ ft}^2}{520 \text{ ft}^2}$$

$$= 0.095 \text{ sabins}$$

and therefore

$$R_{250 \text{ Hz}} = \frac{0.095 \text{ sabins} \times 520 \text{ ft}^2}{1 \text{ sabin} - 0.095 \text{ sabins}}$$

$$= 54.59 \text{ ft}^2$$

Thus

$$TL_{250 \text{ Hz}} = NR_{250 \text{ Hz}} + 10 \text{ Log } [(1/4) + (S_w/R_{250 \text{ Hz}})]$$

$$= 28 \text{ dB} + 10 \text{ Log } [(1/4) + (420 \text{ ft}^2/54.59 \text{ ft}^2)]$$

$$= 28 \text{ dB} + 9.0 \text{ dB}$$

$$= 37 \text{ dB}$$

where $NR_{250 \text{ Hz}}$ (28 dB) comes from Table 4.6.2.

Following the same procedure at 500_{Hz} results in

$$\alpha_{avg} \text{ 500 Hz} = \Sigma S_i \alpha_i / \Sigma S_i$$

$$= \frac{(10 \text{ ft} \times 10 \text{ ft})0.02 \text{ sabins} + (10 \text{ ft} \times 10 \text{ ft})0.65 \text{ sabins} + 4(8 \text{ ft} \times 10 \text{ ft})0.02 \text{ sabins}}{2(10 \text{ ft} \times 10 \text{ ft}) + 4(8 \text{ ft} \times 10 \text{ ft})}$$

$$= \frac{73.4 \text{ ft}^2 \text{ sabins}}{520 \text{ ft}^2}$$

$$= 0.14 \text{ sabins}$$

and

$$R_{500 \text{ Hz}} = \alpha_{avg\ 500\ Hz} \Sigma S_i / (1 - \alpha_{avg\ 500\ Hz})$$

$$= \frac{0.14 \text{ sabins} \times 520 \text{ ft}^2}{1 \text{ sabin} - 0.14 \text{ sabins}}$$

$$= 84.6 \text{ ft}^2$$

Thus

$$TL_{500 \text{ Hz}} = NR_{500 \text{ Hz}} + 10 \text{ Log} [(1/4) + (S_w / R_{500 \text{ Hz}})]$$

$$= 34 \text{ dB} + 10 \text{ Log} [(1/4) + (420 \text{ ft}^2 / 84.6 \text{ ft}^2)]$$

$$= 34 \text{ dB} + 7.17 \text{ dB}$$

$$= 41.17 \text{ dB}$$

From a table of transmission loss for 37 dB at 250 Hz and 41.17 dB at 500 Hz, the building material can be determined.

Partial Enclosures. It is not always possible to build a total enclosure. Sometimes a partial enclosure is desired (for material flow or access to the machine). The more complete the partial enclosure, the greater the obtained noise reduction; that is, the closer the partial enclosure approaches a total enclosure, the more noise reduction that is achieved. Partial enclosures are useful in giving the worker some shadow effect from the noise. Partial enclosures usually will only reduce high frequency noise when the dimensions of the barrier are several times the wavelength. The shadow effect achieved by a partial enclosure depends upon the worker's distance and position from the opening of the partial enclosure, the absorption material that the room is made of, and the absorption material of the partial enclosure. There is a practical way to estimate the performance of a partial enclosure. The procedure consists of the following: The effect of the partial enclosure can be determined by estimating the percent of radiation pattern that is intercepted by the partial enclosure. For example, if 50% of the pattern is intercepted by the partial enclosure, the noise reduction achieved is about 3 dB. If 80% of the radiation pattern is intercepted, there is about a 7 dB drop; and if 90% of the radiation pattern is intercepted, there is about a 10 dB reduction. The maximum noise reduction achieved by a partial enclosure is about 15 to 20 dB.

The mathematics of building a partial enclosure will not be discussed here since they approximate those of building a total enclosure.

Shields and Barriers. A shield is a square piece of material usually of safety glass or clear plastic that is placed between the worker and the sound source. Shields are effective only if their smaller dimension is at least three times the wavelength contributing most of the noise. Shields are only effective against high frequency sounds. The maximum possible reduction due to shields is about 8 dB. Shields might be used where there is an air injection system in a punch press, in plasma guns, air guns, and in metal spray guns. Shields should be used carefully since the shield must allow access to the machine. Also, the shield must be carefully isolated from the machine or else the shield itself may become the vibrating surface and contribute to the sound.

Barriers are usually much larger than shields and usually are attached to the floor, placed between the machine and the worker. Barriers are effective only for medium and high frequencies. The problem is that sound escapes from around the sides of the barriers and from the top of the barriers. The amount of noise reduction achieved depends upon the height of the barrier, the wavelength of concern, and the angle of deflection. The angle of deflection is the angle in which the sound travels over the top of the barrier. (See Figure 4.6.5.)

Figure 4.6.5

Barriers and shields.

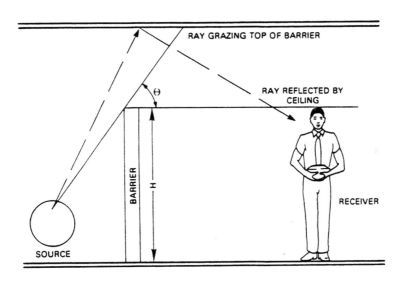

In general, the following rules should be used when designing barriers:

1.   The barrier should be as high as possible.

2.   The barrier should have a transmission loss compatible with the expected noise reduction.

3.   The barrier should have an absorption material on the source side.

4.   The barrier should be isolated from the noise that is transmitted
through the floor.

The amount of reduction achieved depends upon the height of the barrier,
the angle of deflection, and the wavelength of the sound source.   If a barrier
is 4 feet high and has an angle of deflection of 30° (θ = 30°), what is the
noise reduction achieved (i.e., the attenuation achieved at each octave band)?

The noise reductions achieved are given in graph form (Figure 4.6.6).   To
enter the graph (curve), H/λ must be computed, where H denotes height in
feet and λ denotes wavelength in feet.   Recall that

$$\lambda = C/f$$

where C denotes velocity of sound and f denotes frequency.

If the barrier is in standard air, C = 1127 ft/sec, such that at each of the
octave bands λ is given as

Octave Band	λ (ft)
63	17.89
125	9.02
250	4.51
500	2.25
1000	1.13
2000	0.56
4000	0.28
8000	0.14

and respectively H/λ is given as 0.22, 0.44, 0.89, 1.78, 3.54, 7.14, 14.29,
and 28.57.

From Figure 4.6.6, with θ = 30°, the noise reductions achieved at each
octave band are 7 dB, 9 dB, 11.5 dB, 14 dB, 17 dB, 20 dB, 22.5 dB, and 25 dB.

Controlling Noise Along Its Path Using Room Absorption.   Another way to
control noise along its path is by the use of room absorption.   The addition
of material to the walls of the room can cut down on the reverberant buildup.
When adding an absorption material to the surface of a room, it should be
recalled that the worker in the near field or the free field is not helped.
However, adding room absorption will cut down on the reverberant buildup; and
therefore, it is a useful technique for controlling noise along its path.

How much will adding room absorption material cut down on the noise?   The
noise reduction achieved by the absorption material can be computed as follows

$$NR = 10 \, Log \, (\alpha_{avg \, 2}/\alpha_{avg \, 1})$$

where
   NR denotes noise reduction

Figure 4.6.6

Noise reduction of barriers.

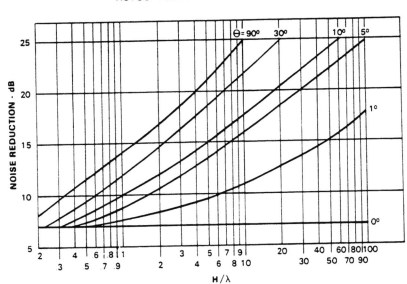

Reprinted with permission by American Industrial Hygiene Association.

α_{avg1} denotes the average room absorption coefficient
before the walls are treated

α_{avg2} denotes the average absorption coefficient after the
absorption material is used.

Consider the following information before absorption material is added to
the ceiling:

Room   30 x 60 x 10
Ceiling   Plaster (α = 0.02 sabins at 1000 Hz)
Floor   Concrete (α = 0.02 sabins at 1000 Hz)
Walls   Glazed tile (α = 0.01 sabins at 1000 Hz)
Steam Pipes   S = 180 square feet (α = 0.50 sabins at 1000 Hz,
                    magnesia covered)
Machinery   S = 180 square feet (α = 0.02 sabins at 1000 Hz)
People   4 people (4 sabins/person)

α_1 would be computed as follows:

Ceiling	(30 ft x 60 ft) 0.02 sabins	= 36
Floors	(30 ft x 60 ft) 0.02 sabins	= 36
Walls	2(30 ft x 10 ft) + 2(60 ft x 10 ft)0.01 sabins	= 18
Pipe	180 ft (0.50 sabins)	= 90
Machinery	180 ft (0.02 sabins)	= 4
People	4 people x 4 sabins	= 16

200 ft^2 sabins

If sound-absorbing material having an $\alpha = 0.80$ sabins is added to the ceiling, then the ceiling would be

$$(30 \text{ ft} \times 60 \text{ ft}) \ 0.80 \text{ sabins} = 1440 \text{ ft}^2 \text{ sabins}$$

and α_2 would be

$$1440 \text{ ft}^2 \text{ sabins} + 36 \text{ ft}^2 \text{ sabins} + 90 \text{ ft}^2 \text{ sabins} +$$
$$4 \text{ ft}^2 \text{ sabins} + 16 \text{ ft}^2 \text{ sabins} = 1586 \text{ ft}^2 \text{ sabins}$$

And the reduction achieved is given by

$$NR = 10 \ Log(\alpha_2/\alpha_1)$$

$$= 10 \ Log \ \frac{1586 \text{ ft}^2 \text{ sabins}}{200 \text{ ft}^2 \text{ sabins}}$$

$$= 8.99 \text{ dB (at 1000 Hz)}$$

The results might vary considerably for other frequencies; therefore, similar calculations should be repeated for all frequencies of interest.

Noise Control at the Receiver

Noise control at the receiver should be the last resort for controlling noise. Basically, there are two types of techniques--administrative controls and personal protective equipment.

Administrative controls consist of checking the criteria and designing administrative procedures to work around those criteria. For example:

1.   Workers at 90 dBA are not exposed to higher levels.

2.   Workers at higher levels should be removed from the noise after the indicated limits are reached; they should spend the balance of the day at levels lower than 85 dBA.
3.   Split shifts (work time should be divided between two or more operations).

4.   When less than full-time operation of a machine is required, time is split into partial-day instead of full-day operations.

5.   Exposure time is reduced by shift scheduling to reduce the number of exposed employees and the number requiring personal protective equipment.

Personal protective equipment can be used to control noise at the receiver. However, the Department of Labor guidelines indicate that personal protective equipment should be used only as an interim measure or procedure. The Department of Labor Bulletin 334 Guidelines gives the following:

1. Only approved ear protectors that have been tested in accordance with ANSI standards, S3.19, should be used.

2. Five dBA less than the stated attenuation of equipment should be allowed, because test data were obtained under ideal conditions that are not normal day-to-day operations.

3. Earmuffs and earplugs should be fitted and supplied through a properly trained person who can educate the workers in the use and maintenance of muffs and plugs.

4. Wax impregnated cotton and fine glass wool are acceptable, but cotton stuffed in the ears has very little value and is not acceptable.

Types of personal protective equipment include:

1. Earplugs (sized plugs, formable plugs, and individual molded plugs).

2. Earmuffs (including helmets).

The protection provided by earmuffs and earplugs varies by individual and by type of material. Understanding the advantages achieved by earplugs involves an understanding of how sound reaches the ears. Sound can reach the ears by passing through the bone and tissue of the ear and the protector itself. It can also enter the ear by causing vibration of the protector which will generate a sound in the ear. Sound can enter the ear through leaks in the protector, and sound can enter the ear by passing through leaks around the protector and the ear. There are ways to avoid leaks. The plugs can be made out of imperforated material; they can be made to fit well so that audible leaks around the protector will not occur; and they can be designed so that they do not vibrate.

Attenuation of earmuffs and earplugs is determined by strict standards which will not be discussed in this text.

It should be pointed out that wearing earplugs or earmuffs in a quiet environment interferes with speech and communication. However, wearing earplugs or earmuffs in noise levels about 90 dB will not interfere with speech or communication. In fact, communication might be increased.

7. References

American Industrial Hygiene Association. <u>Industrial Noise Manual</u>. Akron: American Industrial Hygiene Association, 1975.

Baumeister, Theodore, ed. <u>Mark's Standard Handbook for Electrical Engineers</u>. New York: McGraw-Hill Book Company, 1967.

Beranek, Leo L., ed. <u>Noise and Vibration Control</u>. New York: McGraw-Hill Book Company, 1971.

Hewitt, Paul G. <u>Conceptual Physics . . ., A New Introduction to Your Environment</u>. Boston: Little, Brown and Company, 1974.

Patty, Frank A. <u>Industrial Hygiene and Toxicology</u>, 2d. ed. New York: Interscience Publishers, Inc., 1958.

Peterson, Arnold P. G. and Ervin G. Gross, Jr. <u>Handbook of Noise Measurement</u> 7th ed. Concord, Massachusetts: General Radio, 1974.

Salmon, Vincent, James S. Mills, and Andrew C. Peterson. <u>Industrial Noise Control Manual</u>. HEW Publication No. (NIOSH) 75-183. Washington: U. S. Government Printing Office, 1975.

U. S. Department of Health, Education, and Welfare, Public Health Service, Center for Disease Control, National Institute for Occupational Safety and Health. <u>The Industrial Environment: Its Evaluation and Control</u>. Washington: U. S. Government Printing Office, 1973.

Section 5

Industrial Illumination

1. Light

Introduction

The purpose of industrial lighting is to provide an efficient and comfortable seeing of industrial tasks and to help provide a safe working environment. Adequate lighting is not for safety alone. Lighting adequate for seeing production and inspection tasks will be more than is needed for safety. Light is more for comfort and convenience than for safety.

It has been shown that adequate industrial lighting results in many benefits; for example:

1. Promotes reduced production and inspection mistakes.
2. Increases production.
3. Reduces accidents.
4. Improves morale.
5. Improves housekeeping.

What Is Light?

The nature of light is not easy to understand. The question, "What is light?" has been extremely elusive throughout the history of science.

Near the end of the seventeenth century, there were two theories to explain the nature of light; the particle or corpuscular theory and the wave theory. In the nineteenth century, the discovery of interference and diffraction--the bending of light as it passes through different media--made the wave theory of light the predominant theory; i.e., interference and diffraction could not be explained adequately by the particle or corpuscular theory.

In the late 1800's, light was thought to be electromagnetic waves, which at certain frequencies could be seen by the human eye. This conceptualization of light was primarily used to explain the propagation of light. To conceptualize the propagation of light, an understanding of electrical forces and fields and magnetic forces and fields is needed.

To illustrate electrical forces, the simple case of an electrical charge at rest will be discussed. Each atom has a positively charged core, the nucleus, which is surrounded by negatively charged electrons. The nucleus consists of a number of protons, each with a single unit of positive charge and one or more neutrons (except for hydrogen). A neutron is a neutral

particle. Normally, an atom is in a neutral or uncharged state because it
contains the same number of protons as electrons. If, for some reason, a
neutral atom loses one or more of its electrons, the atom will have a net
positive charge and is referred to as an "ion." A negative ion is an atom
which has gained one or more additional electrons. That is, an object which
has an excess of electrons is negatively charged; and an object which has a
deficiency of electrons is positively charged. Objects can be electrically
charged in many different ways.

It is known that objects with the same charge repel each other, while
objects with opposite charges attract each other. That is, some force exists
between charged objects. In 1784 Charles Augustine de Coulomb found that the
force of attraction or repulsion between two charged objects is inversely
proportional to the square of the distance separating them. Coulomb's law can
be stated as:

The force of attraction or repulsion between two point charges is
directly proportional to the product of the two charges and inversely
proportional to the square of the distance between them.
From Coulomb's law, the following may be written:

$$F \propto \frac{qq'}{r^2}$$

or

$$F = \frac{kqq'}{r^2}$$

where F denotes the magnitude of force; q and q' represent the magnitude of
two charges; r represents the distance between the charges; and k represents
Coulomb's constant, a proportionality constant that takes into account the
property of the medium separating the charged bodies. The units attached to
q, q', and k are of no concern for conceptual development. This relationship
can be graphically illustrated by Figure 5.1.1.

Electrically charged bodies then exhibit a force. The presence of an
electrically charged object alters the space around it. This alteration in
the surrounding space can be described by introducing the concept of fields.
An electrical field is said to exist in a region of space in which an electric
charge will experience an electrical force. The strength of the electrical
field at any point will be proportional to the force a given charge
experiences at any point; i.e., the strength of an electrical field can be
represented by the force per unit charge. The electrical field intensity, E,
is then defined at a point in terms of the force, F, experienced by an
arbitrary positive charge, +q, when it is placed at that point. Thus

$$E = \frac{F}{+q}$$

Figure 5.1.1

Illustration of Coulomb's law.

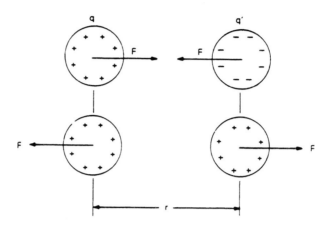

Since the electrical field intensity is defined in terms of a positive charge, its direction at any point would be the same as the electrostatic (at rest) force on a positive charge at that point.   (See Figure 5.1.2.)

Figure 5.1.2

Direction of electrical fields.

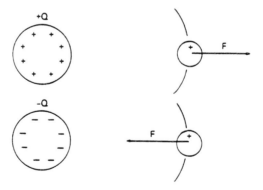

On this basis, the electrical field in the vicinity of a positive charge would be outward or away from the charge, while in the vicinity of a negative charge the direction of the field would be inward or toward the charge.   (See Figure 5.1.3.)

Figure 5.1.3

Direction of electrical fields.

ELECTRIC FIELD OF
NEGATIVE CHARGE

ELECTRIC FIELD OF
POSITIVE CHARGE

If an electrically charged particle is brought into the field created by another electrically charged particle, then

$$E = \frac{F}{q'} = \frac{kqq'/r^2}{q'} = \frac{kq}{r^2}$$

where E denotes the electrical field intensity, F denotes force, r denotes the distance between the two emitted charges, q and q' denote the magnitude of the charges, and k denotes Coulomb's constant.

Magnetic forces and fields are similar to electrical forces and fields. The magnetic law of forces states: Like magnetic poles repel each other while unlike magnetic poles attract each other. In the eighteenth century, de Coulomb discovered that (1) the force of attraction or repulsion between the poles of two magnets is inversely proportional to the square of the distance, r, between the poles; and (2) the force of attraction or repulsion between two poles is along a line joining the two poles and directly proportional to the product of the pole strengths, p_1 and p_2. These two statements may be combined to form a mathematical statement:

$$F = \frac{kp_1p_2}{r^2}$$

where F denotes the force between two poles of strength p_1 and p_2 which are separated by a distance, r. The value of the proportional constant, k, depends upon the units chosen and the medium surrounding the magnets.

Every magnet is surrounded by a space in which the magnetic effects are present. These regions are called "magnetic fields." The strength of the magnetic field at any point is referred to as the magnetic field intensity, H, and is defined in terms of the force exerted on a unit north pole; i.e. the magnetic field intensity, H, at any point is the magnetic force per unit north pole placed at that point:

$$H = \frac{F}{p}$$

where H denotes the magnetic field intensity, F denotes force, and p denotes the magnitude of the unit north pole.

A more useful expression for computing the magnetic field intensity is given by

$$H = \frac{F}{p'} = \frac{kpp'/r^2}{p'} = \frac{kp}{r^2}$$

where p' denotes a test pole placed distance r from the pole p, and the remaining symbols are defined as before.

Magnetism is believed to result from movements of electrons within the atoms of substances. That is, magnetism results from a change in motion. The magnetic polarity of two atoms stems primarily from the spin of electrons about their own axis and is due also to their orbital motions around the nucleus. (See Figure 5.1.4.) As can be seen, magnetism is closely related to electrical phenomena.

Figure 5.1.4

A charge in motion.

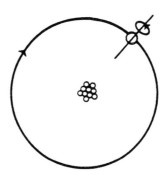

If compass needles were placed around an electrical current, a magnetic field would be produced. (Figure 5.1.5.) If a moving charged particle creates a magnetic field, will a moving magnetic field create an electrical field? The answer is "yes." (Figure 5.1.6) This figure consists of a wire with some loops in it and a regular bar magnet. If the magnet is moved up and down, the meter to the right will register an electrical current or electrical field. A magnetic field is created by the movement of a charged particle, and the movement of a magnetic field creates an electrical field.

The upper part of Figure 5.1.7 indicates that when a wire with no initial current is moved downward, the charges in the wire experience a deflecting force perpendicular to their motion. Since there is a conducting path made by the wire in this direction, the electrons follow it, thereby constituting a

Figure 5.1.5

A moving charge creates a magnetic field.

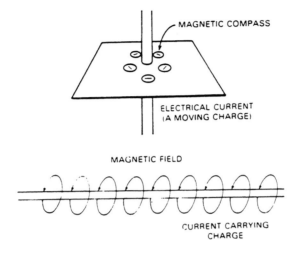

Figure 5.1.6.

A moving magnetic field creates
an electrical field.

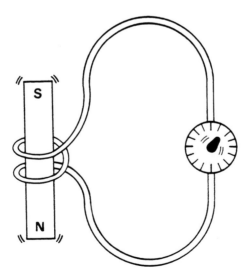

Figure 5.1.7

Moving charges experience a force that is
perpendicular to the magnetic field lines they traverse.

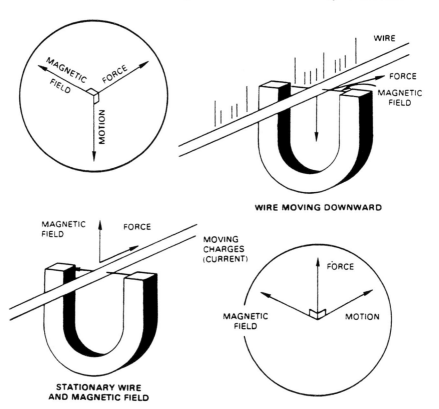

current. In the lower half of the diagram where the magnet is stationary and
the wire is stationary, when a current moves through the wire to the right,
there is a perpendicular upward force on the electron. Since there is no
conducting path upward, the wire is tugged upward along with the electrons of
the charged particles. The relationship between magnetic fields and
electrical fields can be summarized by saying that moving charges experience a
force that is perpendicular to the magnetic field lines that they traverse.

    The fact that a magnetic field induces an electrical field and a moving
electrical field produces a magnetic field is how an electromagnetic wave is
produced. Consider an electrical charge vibrating back and forth at a certain
frequency. The charge, because it is a moving charged particle, will produce
an electrical field around it. The moving charge, if it vibrates back and
forth, creates a magnetic field. However, the magnetic field is also changing
or moving; and the moving magnetic field produces an electrical field. Thus,
the two fields are mutually induced. The changing magnetic field induces an

electrical field which induces a magnetic field, etc., and electromagnetic
waves are produced.

Consider first the initial magnetic field induced by the moving charge.
This changing magnetic field induces a changing electrical field, which in
turn induces a magnetic field. The magnitude of this further induced magnetic
field depends not only on the vibrational rate of the electrical field but
also on the motion of the electrical field or the speed at which the induced
field emanates from the vibrating charge. The higher the speed, the greater
the magnetic field it induces. At low speeds, electromagnetic regeneration
would be short lived because the slow-moving electrical field would induce a
weak magnetic field which in turn would induce a weaker electrical field. The
induced fields become successively weaker, causing the mutual induction to die
out. But what about the energy in such a case? The fields contain energy
given to them by the vibrating charge. If the fields disappear with no means
of transferring energy to some other form, energy would be destroyed.
Low-speed emanation of electrical and magnetic fields is incompatible with the
law of conservation of energy. At emanating speeds too high, on the other
hand, the fields would be induced to ever-increasing magnitudes with a
crescendo of ever-increasing energies--again clearly in contradiction with the
conservation of energy. At some critical speed, however, mutual induction
would continue indefinitely with neither a loss nor a gain in energy. This.
critical speed without loss or gain of energy is 186,000 miles per second--the
speed of light. Thus, energy in an electromagnetic wave is equally divided
between electrical and magnetic fields that are perpendicular. Both fields
oscillate perpendicular to the direction of the wave propagation. (Figure
5.1.8)

Figure 5.1.8

Representation of electromagnetic wave.

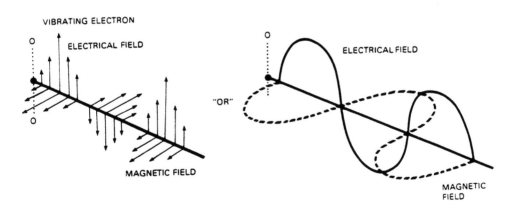

Electromagnetic Spectrum

In 1885 H. R. Hertz showed that radiation of electromagnetic energy can occur at any frequency. All electromagnetic waves travel at the same speed in a vacuum. The waves are different from one another in their frequency and wavelength. The relationship between velocity, frequency, and wavelength is as follows:

$$C = f\lambda$$

where C denotes velocity, f denotes frequency, and λ denotes wavelength.

If the speed or velocity of electromagnetic waves is constant, then when the frequency changes, the wavelength must change. The higher the frequency of the vibrating charge, the shorter the wavelength.

Figure 5.1.9 shows the electromagnetic spectrum. It extends from radio waves to gamma waves. In all sections of the electromagnetic spectrum, the waves are the same in nature; they differ only in frequency and wavelength.

Figure 5.1.9

Electromagnetic spectrum.

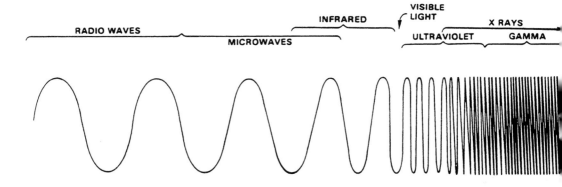

Electromagnetic waves in principle can have any frequency from zero to infinity. The classification of electromagnetic waves according to frequency is called the "electromagnetic spectrum." Electromagnetic waves with frequencies of the order of several thousand hertz (kilocycles/sec) are classified as radio waves. The VHF (very high frequency) television band starts at about 15 million hertz (megacycles/sec). Still higher frequencies are called "microwaves" followed by infrared waves often called "heat waves." Further still is visible light which makes up only one percent of the measured electromagnetic spectrum. Beyond light, the higher frequencies extend into the ultraviolet, X-ray, and gamma-ray regions. There is no sharp distinction between these regions which actually overlap each other. The spectrum is simply broken up into these arbitrary regions for classification.

The Quantum Theory

Around 1885 light was thought to be wave-like and not particle-like. However, in 1887 Hertz noticed that an electrical spark would jump more readily between charged fields when their surfaces were illuminated by the light from another spark. This observation is commonly known as the "photoelectric effect." The arrangement for the photoelectric effect can be seen in Figure 5.1.10.

Figure 5.1.10

Photoelectric effect.

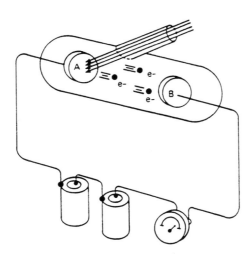

Light shining on the negatively charged photosensitive metal plate liberates electrons, which are attracted to the positive plate, producing a measurable current. This photoelectric effect could not be explained by the electromagnetic wave theory of light. The brightness of light in no way affected the energies of the ejected electrons. If light was accepted to be electromagnetic radiation, then the stronger electric fields of bright light would surely interact with electrons, causing them to eject at greater speeds and, thus, greater energies. Yet, this was not the case. No increase in electron kinetic energy was detected. A weak beam of ultraviolet light produced a given number of electrons but much higher kinetic energies. This was puzzling; the wave theory of light could not explain this phenomenon.

In an attempt to bring experimental observations into agreement with theory, Max Planck published his quantum hypothesis. He found that the problem with the electromagnetic theory of light lay with the assumption that energy is radiated continuously. He postulated that electromagnetic energy is absorbed or emitted in discrete packets or quanta, referred to as photons. Planck postulated that the energy states of electrons in atoms are quantized; i.e., electrons can only vibrate with certain discrete amounts of energy. An electron farther away from the nucleus has a greater potential energy with respect to the nucleus than the electron nearer the nucleus; the furthermost electron is at a higher energy level. When an electron in an atom is raised to a higher energy level, the atom is said to be <u>excited</u>. The higher level of the electron is only momentary. The electron loses its temporarily acquired energy when returning to a lower energy level. (Figure 5.1.11)

Figure 5.1.11

Energy levels.

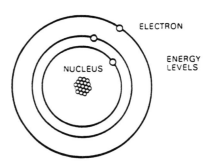

Radiation occurs when an electron makes the transition from a higher energy state to a lower energy state; i.e., when the atom becomes de-excited. This energy is in quanta. The electron moves in discrete steps from higher levels to lower levels. Each element has its own number of electrons; each element also has its own characteristics of energy levels. An electron's dropping from a higher energy level to a lower energy level in an excited atom emits energy in photons or quanta with each jump. So for each element, the amount of energy will be different.

Planck postulated that the energy of the resulting quanta of radiation would be equal to the difference in the energy state of the atom. Further, he postulated that the frequency of the emitted radiation is proportional to this energy difference. Planck's equation can be written as

$$E = hf$$

where E denotes the energy of the photon, f denotes the frequency of radiation, and h is the proportionality factor called <u>Planck's constant</u>.

Thus, a photon or quantum of infrared radiation has a very small energy; a quantum of green light, a small energy; and a quantum of ultraviolet light, a larger energy. The greater the radiation frequency of the quantum, the greater the energy.

With Planck's theory, the nature of light was seen to be dualistic--it had wave-like properties and particle properties (quanta or photons being released upon de-excitation). It is customary to discuss the wave-like properties of light when the propagation of light is discussed, and it is customary to use the particle theory when the interaction of light with matter is discussed. Light may be thought of as radiant energy transported in photons which are carried along by a wave field.

The Emission Spectra

Every element has its own characteristic pattern of electron levels. An electron dropping from higher to lower energy levels in an excited atom emits a photon with each jump. Many frequency characteristics of an atom are emitted corresponding to the many paths the electron may take when jumping from level to level. These frequencies combine to give light from each excited atom its own characteristic color. This unique pattern can be seen when the light is sent through a prism.

Each component color is focused at a definite position according to its frequency and form. If the light given off by a sodium vapor lamp is analyzed, a single yellow line is produced. If the width of the ray of yellow light could be narrowed, it would be found that the line is composed of two very close lines. These lines correspond to the two predominant frequencies of light emitted by the excited sodium atoms. The rest of the spectrum is dark. (There are many other lines too dim to be seen with the naked eye.)

This situation is not unique in sodium. Examining the light from a mercury vapor lamp reveals two strong yellow lines close together (but in different positions than those of sodium), a very intense green line, and several blue and violet lines. Similar but more complicated patterns of lines are found in light emitted by a neon tube. The light emitted by every element in a vapor state produces its own characteristic pattern of lines. These lines correspond to the electron transitions between atomic energy levels and are characteristic of each element as are the fingerprints of people.

Incandescence

Light emitted from a neon tube is red because the average difference in neon energy level is proportional to the frequency of red light. Light emitted by a common incandescent lamp, however, is white. All frequencies of visible radiation are emitted. Does this mean that tungsten atoms making up the lamp filament are characterized by an infinite number of energy levels? The answer is a definite "no." If the filament were vaporized and then excited, the tungsten gas would emit a finite number of frequencies, producing an overall bluish color. The frequency of light emitted by atoms depends not only upon the energy levels within the atom but also on the spacings between neighboring atoms themselves. In a gas, the atoms are far apart. Electrons undergo transition between energy levels within the atom quite unaffected by the presence of neighboring atoms. But when the atoms are closely packed, as in a solid, the electrons of the outer orbits make transitions not only within the energy levels of the parent atoms but also between the levels of neighboring atoms. These energy level transitions are no longer well defined but are altered by interactions between neighboring atoms, resulting in an infinite variety of energy level differences, thence, an infinite number of radiation frequencies. And this is why tungsten filament light is white.

Mercury vapor light is bright and less expensive than incandescent lamps. Most of the energy in incandescent lamps is converted to heat, while most of the energy put into mercury vapor lamps is converted to light. As the filament in a tungsten filament lamp becomes heated, wider energy level transitions take place, and higher frequencies of radiation are emitted. A hotter filament produces a whiter light.

Fluorescence and Fluorescent Lamps

Atoms absorb light as well as emit light. An atom will most strongly absorb light having the same frequency or frequencies to which it is tuned, the same frequency it emits. For example, when a beam of white light passes through a gas, the atoms of the gas absorb selected frequencies. This absorbed energy is reradiated in all directions instead of in the directions of the incident light.

Some atoms become excited when absorbing a photon of light. Ultraviolet light has more energy per photon than lower frequency light. Many substances undergo excitation when illuminated by ultraviolet light. When a substance excited by ultraviolet light emits visible light upon de-excitation, this action is called fluorescence. What happens in some of these materials is that a photon of ultraviolet light collides with an atom of the material and gives up its energy in two parts. Part of the energy goes into heat, increasing the kinetic energy of the entire atom. The other part of the energy goes into excitation, boosting the electron to a higher orbit. Upon de-excitation, this part of the energy is released as a photon of light. Since some of the energy of the ultraviolet photon is converted to heat, the photon emitted has less energy and, therefore, lower frequency than the ultraviolet photon. That is, the secondary photon of light that is released is of less energy than the primary photon since some energy goes to heat; thus, it is of a lower frequency. Light emitted from fluorescent lamps is produced by primary and secondary excitation processes. The primary process is excitation of a gas by electron bombardment; and the secondary process is excitation by ultraviolet photons, fluorescence. The common fluorescent lamp consists of a cylindrical gas tube with electrodes at each end. (See Figure 5.1.12.) As in the neon sign tube, electrons are boiled off from the electrodes and forced to vibrate back and forth at high speeds within the tube by an AC voltage; and the tube is filled with very low-pressure mercury vapor which is excited by the impact of high-speed electrons. .As the energy levels in the mercury are relatively far apart, the resulting emission of light is of very high frequency, mainly ultraviolet light. This is the primary excitation process. The secondary process occurs when the ultraviolet light impinges upon a thin coating of powdery material made up of phosphors on the inner surface of the glass tube. The phosphors are excited by the absorption of the ultraviolet photon and give off a multitude of lower frequencies in all directions that combine to produce white light. Different phosphors can be used to produce different colored lights.

Figure 5.1.12

Fluorescent lamp.

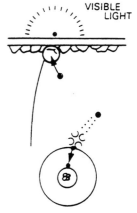

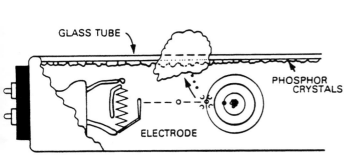

1. Electrode emits electron at high speed.
2. Collides with atom (usually mercury atom).
3. Collision causes excitation. Upon de-excitation, a photon is released (ultraviolet light).
4. Ultraviolet photon hits phosphor crystals where excitation takes place.

5. Upon de-excitation, a photon is released, producing visible light.

Comparing Different Light Sources

The process of excitation and de-excitation (and the release of photons) explains how light is emitted. Mercury vapor lamps, fluorescent lamps, and incandescent lamps all work on the same principle.

Incandescent lamps produce extremely white light. The hotter the filament, the whiter the light. However, the hotter they burn, the weaker they get and the more wear and tear on the filament, thus decreasing the life of the lamp.

High-pressure mercury lamps are about twice as efficient as filament lamps because less energy is converted into heat. One of the disadvantages of high-pressure mercury lamps is the delay in starting and restarting them. Several minutes are required for the lamps to reach full brightness. In cases of power interruption, the lamps will not restart until the arc tube has cooled sufficiently for the mercury vapor to condense (about five minutes). This disadvantage can be overcome by installing a filament lamp along with a mercury lamp.

Fluorescent lamps (low-pressure mercury lamps) are about three times as efficient as filament lamps. A coating on the glass filters out the radiation that would be harmful to the eyes or to the skin. In the past, fluorescent lamps were started with a starter that heated the electrodes at the end of the tube. Modern lamps are started with a ballast; they have sufficient voltage to start the lamp immediately. Fluorescent bulbs give long life, about 7500 hours. The lamp is affected by the number of starts. Lamps will last longer if started less frequently.

When deciding what type of lamp to use, one has to look at both efficiency and cost. Where costs are low, a shorter lamp life would be sufficient. Where lamps are costly or the labor costs of replacing them are high, a longer-life lamp is more economical.

Incandescent filament lamps come in various shapes and sizes. The lamp bulbs are designated by a letter code followed by a numeral. The letter indicates the shape (straight, S; flame, F; globe, G; general service, A; tubular, T; pear shape, PS; parabolic, PAR; and reflector, R). The number indicates the size--the diameter of the bulb in eighths of an inch. Thus, a T-12 lamp is a tubular lamp that is 12/8 inches or 1.5 inches in diameter. Incandescent lamps also come with different kinds of bases: disc, candelabra, intermediate, mogul, bayonet, bipost, etc.

Mercury vapor lamps are designated by ASA nomenclature; e.g., H33-1-CL/C, where H denotes mercury; 33-1, the ballast number; CL, arbitrary letters designating physical characteristics of the lamp such as bulb size, shape, material, and finish; and C indicates the color of the light.

2. Light and Seeing/Design of a Lighting System

The last chapter discussed the nature of light. Light was seen as radiant energy transported in photons that are carried by a wave field. In this chapter, the eye is discussed. Also discussed are some objective factors in the seeing process. The chapter ends by introducing some terms used by illumination engineers.

Behavior of Light

In the last chapter, the origin of light was discussed. This chapter discusses briefly the behavior of light after it leaves the source. Three . basic characteristics of light will be discussed. The first characteristic is:

Light travels in a straight line unless it is modified or redirected by means of a reflecting, refracting, or diffusing medium.

When light travels, it travels in a straight line. When it is incident upon a surface, part of the light is reflected. On a metallic surface, almost 100 percent of the light is reflected; while on a clear glass surface, only a small portion is reflected. The ratio of light reflected from a surface to that incident upon it is called reflectance.

The law of reflectance is simply stated as: The angle of incidence is equal to the angle of reflection. (See Figure 5.2.1.)

Figure 5.2.1

Law of reflection.

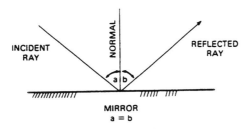

509

Reflections may be of several types; the most common are specular (see Figure 5.2.2), diffuse (see Figure 5.2.3), spread reflection (see Figure 5.2.4), and mixed reflection (see Figure 5.2.5), which is a combination of diffuse and spread reflection.

Figure 5.2.2   Figure 5.2.3

Specular reflection.   Diffuse reflection.

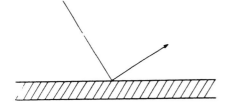   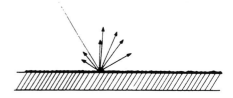

Figure 5.2.4

Spread reflection.

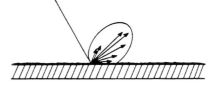

Figure 5.2.5

Mixed reflection.

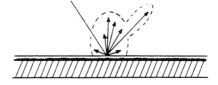

Refraction is the "bending" of light as it passes from one transparent medium to another. The speed at which light travels through these materials is what makes light bend. The speed of light is consistent in space. However, light has a lesser speed in a transparent medium. In water, light travels 75 percent of its speed compared to a vacuum; in glass, about 67 percent, depending upon the type of glass; in a diamond, about 41 percent. When light emerges from these media, it again travels at its original speed. This concept may be troublesome because from what is known about energy, this may seem like strange behavior. If a bullet is fired through a board, the bullet slows when passing through the board and emerges at a speed less than its incident speed. It loses some of its kinetic energy while interacting with the fibers and splinters in the board. But things are different with light. To understand the behavior of light, the individual photons of light that make up a beam and the interaction between the photons and the molecules they encounter must be considered. Incident photons interact with the electrons of molecules. Orbiting electrons can be thought of as attached to little springs. These electrons will resonate at certain frequencies and can be forced into vibration over the range of frequencies. This range varies for different molecules. In clear glass, for example, the range extends over the entire visible region. When a photon is incident upon a transparent medium such as glass, it is absorbed by a molecule at the surface. An electron in the absorbing molecule is set in vibration at a frequency equal to that of the incident photon. This vibration then causes the emission of the second photon of identical frequency. It is a different but indistinguishable photon. The second photon travels at 186,000 miles per second until it quickly is absorbed by another molecule in the glass, whereupon an electron is set in vibration re-emitting a different but indistinguishable photon of its own. This absorption/re-emission process is not an instantaneous event. Some time is required for the process; and, as a result, the average speed of light through the material is less than 186,000 miles per second. That is, the photon that enters the glass is not the same photon that leaves the glass.

Light bends when it passes obliquely from one medium to another. This is called refraction. It is the slowing of light upon entering the transparent medium that causes the refraction. (See Figure 5.2.6.)

The straight line travel of light can also be altered by a diffusing material. Light traveling through a transparent or translucent material is said to be transmitted, such as light traveling through a clear glass plate. When light leaves the material, it may become diffuse. (See Figure 5.2.7.) The degree of diffusion depends upon the type and density of the material. Most luminaires are made so that the light leaving the luminaire becomes diffuse.

The second characteristic of light is:

Light waves pass through one another without alteration of either.

That is, a beam of red light will pass directly through a beam of blue light unchanged in direction and color.

Figure 5.2.6

Refraction of light.

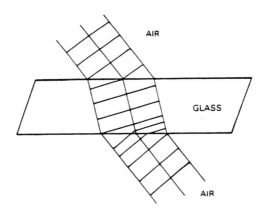

Figure 5.2.7

Diffusing glass.

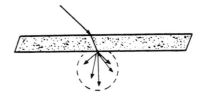

The third characteristic of light is:

Light is invisible in passing through space unless some medium, such as dust or water, scatters it in the direction of the eye.

The scattering of light is similar to the phenomenon of resonance in sound and forced vibration. Atoms and molecules behave like tuning forks and selectively scatter waves of the appropriate frequency. A beam of light falls upon an atom and causes the electrons to vibrate. The vibrating electron in turn radiates light in different directions. An example of scattering is a searchlight beam sweeping across the sky at night. Such beams are seen by light being scattered by particles (dust or water droplets) in the atmosphere

The Human Eye

Figure 5.2.8 shows the structure of the eye. Light passes through the cornea (a protective coating over the front of the eye). Light next passes

Figure 5.2.8

The human eye.

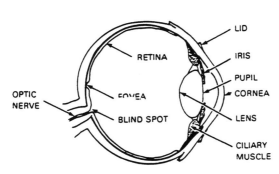

through the pupil, an opening in the iris that can be widened or narrowed to let more or less light in by contractions in the muscles of the iris, the colored portion of the eye. Light passes through the pupil into the lens, a transparent capsule behind the iris whose shape can be changed in order to focus objects at various distances. The lens is controlled by the ciliary muscle, which is ring shaped and changes the curvature of the lens. The light is then focused through the lens into the inner lining of the back of the eyeball, the retina. There the light stimulates receptor cells that transmit the information to the brain via the optic nerve.

More than six million cones and 100 million rods are distributed in the retina. Rods are slim nerve cells--receptors--which are sensitive to low levels of illumination. Rods have no color response. They are found only on the outside of the foveal region, increasing in number with the distance from the fovea. The outer portion of the retina is composed chiefly of rods which do not afford distinct vision but are highly sensitive to movement and flicker. When light strikes a rod, it causes the breakdown of a chemical rhodopsin (visual purple). This photosensitive chemical triggers activity in the optic nerve and, subsequently, in the brain.

Cones are the receptors that make possible the discrimination of fine detail and the perception of color. Cones are insensitive at low levels of illumination. The cones are found mainly near the center of the retina, with the greatest concentration at the fovea. A few cones are mixed with rods all the way to the outer edges of the retina, but the center of the eye is the most color-sensitive portion. The cones also contain a photosensitive chemical that breaks down when struck by light waves.

The eye has the ability to adapt to a wide variety of illumination levels. Adaptation involves a change in the size of the pupils along with photochemical changes in the rods and cones. In dim light--low levels of illumination--the chemicals in the rods and cones are built up faster than they are broken down by light stimulation. The greater the concentration of these chemicals, the lower the visual threshold. Thus, the adaptation to darkness is a matter of building up a surplus of rhodopsin in the rods and other chemicals in the cones.

The cones adapt quickly in the dark (10 minutes or so), but the rods ada slowly and continue to adapt even after 30 minutes or more of darkness. The are only rough estimates since the length of time of adaptation depends upon the previous state of adaptation and the magnitude of the change. When completely adapted, the rods are much more sensitive to light than the cones Thus, to see a dim light in pitch darkness, one should not look directly at since the center of the eye contains only the less sensitive cones. By looking away from the object, the image will fall on the edge of the retina where the rods are. This manner of viewing affords a higher likelihood of seeing the dim light. Since the rods work in dim light and the cones do not vision in very dim light is entirely colorless. Although vision is colorles in dim light, the eye becomes relatively sensitive to energy at the blue end of the spectrum and almost blind to red.

Visual acuity is the ability to discriminate the details in the field of vision. The normal field of vision extends approximately 180° in the horizontal plane and 130° in the vertical plane (60° above the horizontal an 70° below). One way the ability to discriminate detail in the field of visi can be measured is by using the familiar eye chart. Standard perfect vision is often called "20/20 vision." If a person stands 20 feet away from the ey chart and sees the material on the chart clearly, he or she is seeing normal and is said to have 20/20 vision. If the person does not see normally, some of the material will be blurred. If a person standing 20 feet away from the chart sees what a person with normal vision sees at 50 feet, the person has 20/50 vision. If a person has 20/10 vision, he sees things 20 feet away as sharply as a person with normal vision sees them at 10 feet.

Part of the retina, the "blind spot," has no visual acuity. This spot i the point at which the nerves of the eye converge to form the optic nerve. The optic nerve extends through the back wall of the eyeball and connects th eye to the brain. People are usually unaware of the blind spot; they compensate for this blind spot in their vision primarily by moving their hea and making use of their other eye.

The four most common causes of defective vision are astigmatism, the inability to bring horizontal lines and vertical lines into focus at the same time; myopia, where objects focus in front of the retina--nearsightedness; hypermetropia, where objects focus behind the retina--farsightedness; and presbyopia, loss of elasticity of the lens with age. All of these visual defects can usually be corrected by properly fitted corrective glasses or lenses.

Variables in the Seeing Process

What makes an object easy to see? Investigations have shown that adequa seeing depends upon at least four variables. These are the size of the object, the contrast of the object with its background, the brightness of th object, and the time available to see the light.

The obvious factor in seeing an object is its size. The size of the object depends upon the visual angle. The larger an object in terms of its visual angle--the angle subtended by the object at the eye--the more readily it can be seen. The familiar eye test chart illustrates this principle. The person who brings a small object closer to his eyes in order to see it more clearly is unconsciously making use of the size factor by increasing the visual angle. (See Figure 5.2.9.)

Figure 5.2.9

Size of object--visual angle of object.

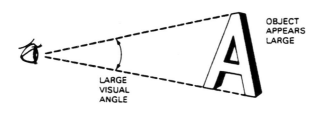

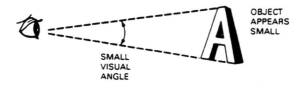

Along with the size of the object is visual acuity. Visual acuity, expressed as the reciprocal of the visual angle in minutes, is a measure of the smallest detail that can be seen. Since visual acuity increases markedly with increase in illumination, light is sometimes said to act as a magnifier, making visible small details that could not be seen with less light.

The second factor involved in seeing objects is contrast. Contrast primarily refers to two factors--color contrast and brightness contrast. Color contrast refers to the contrast in color between the object to be seen and its immediate background. For a given set of conditions, visibility is at its highest when the contrast is at a maximum. Black print on white paper is much more visible than the same print on grey paper. (See Figure 5.2.10.) Brightness contrast is the contrast in brightness between the object and its immediate background.

The third factor in seeing is brightness. The luminance or brightness of an object depends upon the intensity of the light striking it and the proportion of that light reflected in the direction of the eye. A white surface will have a much higher luminance than a black surface receiving the same illumination. However, by adding enough light to a dark surface, it is possible to make it as "bright as the white one." The darker an object or visual task, the greater the illumination necessary for greater illuminance and, under like circumstances, for equal visibility. In addition, the brightness between the object and its immediate background should be approximately the same. Different ratios in brightness between the object and the background can cause problems for the viewer.

The fourth factor in seeing is time. Seeing is not an instantaneous process--it requires time. The eye can see very small detail under very low levels of illumination if sufficient time is allotted and eyestrain is ignored. However, more lighting is required for quick seeing. The time factor is particularly important when the visual object is in motion. High lighting levels actually make moving objects appear to move more slowly and greatly increase their visibility.

Size, luminance, contrast, and time are mutually interrelated and interdependent. Within limits, deficiency in one can be made up by an adjustment in one or more of the others. In most cases, size is a fixed factor of the visual task, with luminance, contrast, and time subject to some degree of modification. Of these, luminance and contrast are usually most directly under the control of the illuminating engineer. Properly employed, they can be of tremendous aid in overcoming unfavorable conditions, small size, and limited time for seeing.

To see the interrelation among the four factors, consider the following:

A. Small objects must have a high contrast to be seen.
B. Low contrast objects must be large in size.
C. As brightness increases, contrast and size can be decreased.
D. When more time is available for seeing objects, the size can be smaller and the contrast lower.
E. In most situations, the object is fixed, contrast is usually fixed, and the time for seeing is fixed; thus, brightness is most often the variable under the control of the engineer.

Terminology Used in the Science of Light

There are some terms related to the science of light with which everyone working with light should be familiar.

Luminous Flux (F). Luminous flux is the total radiant power emitted from a light source that is capable of affecting the sense of sight. Actually, it is more precisely defined as the time rate of flow of light (or luminous energy). In ordinary practice, the time element can be neglected, and luminous flux is commonly considered a definite quality. Luminous flux is measured in units of a lumen where one lumen is defined as the luminous flux emitted from a $1/60$ cm^2 opening in a standard source and included within a solid angle of I steradian. The standard source consists of a hollow enclosure maintained at the temperature of solidification of platinum, about $1773°C$. A solid angle in steradians is given by:

$$\Omega = \frac{A \cos \theta}{R^2}$$

Where Ω denotes a solid angle, A denotes surface area, and R denotes distance (or radius of a sphere), where R is perpendicular to the surface, A, and θ represents the angle from the center of the sphere to the surface area (A).

A solid angle can be graphically illustrated as in Figure 5.2.11.

Figure 5.2.10   Figure 5.2.11

Contrast.   Definition of a solid
                                       angle in steradians.

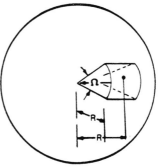

If $\theta = 0°$, that is, the surface area is perpendicular to the center of the sphere, then $\cos \theta = 1$ and $\Omega = A/R^2$.

In the definition of a lumen, then, one steradian can be defined as the solid angle subtended at the center of a sphere by an area A on its surface that is equal to the square of its radius R. It can be shown that there are 4π steradians in a complete sphere.

$$\Omega = \frac{A}{R^2}$$
$$= \frac{4\pi R^2}{R^2}$$
$$= 4\pi \text{ steradians}$$

A <u>lumen</u> is often defined as the flux falling on a surface one square foot in area, every part of which is one foot from a point source having a luminous intensity of one candela (candlepower) in all directions. Luminous intensity is a term not yet defined.

Luminous Intensity. Luminous intensity of a light source is the luminous flux emitted per solid angle:

$$Intensity = Flux/\Omega$$

The unit for intensity is the lumen per steradian called a candela or candlepower, as it was called when the international standard was defined in terms of the quantity of light emitted by the flame of a certain candle. (This initial standard was replaced by the platinum standard.) This standard candle had a luminous intensity in a horizontal direction of approximately one candela. If a light from a candle with the candlepower of 1 fell on a surface of one square foot, where every part of the surface was one foot from the candle, the amount of flux would be one lumen. Note from the above equation that

$$Flux = Intensity \times \Omega$$

If the light source is an isotropic source (one which emits light uniformly in all directions), then the total flux emitted would be

$$Flux = 4\pi \; Intensity$$

since the total solid angle for an isotropic source is 4π steradians.

Example

If a spotlight one foot away from a wall had a bulb with a candlepower of 1 candela and the beam covered an area of 1 square foot of the wall, what would the luminous intensity of the spotlight be?

Solution

Total flux emitted by the 1 candela bulb is

$$
\begin{aligned}
Flux &= 4\pi \; intensity \\
&= (4\pi)(1 \; candela) \\
&= 12.56 \; lumens \quad (flux \; is \; measured \; in \; lumens)
\end{aligned}
$$

The light is concentrated into a solid angle given by

$$
\begin{aligned}
\Omega &= \frac{A}{R^2} \\
&= \frac{1 \; ft^2}{(1 \; ft)^2} \\
&= 1 \; steradian
\end{aligned}
$$

And the intensity of the beam is given by

$$Intensity = Flux/\Omega$$

$$= \frac{12.56 \text{ lumens}}{1 \text{ steradian}}$$

$$= 12.56 \text{ candela} \quad (\text{intensity is measured in candela})$$

Note that the unit of intensity, candela (lumens/steradian) and the unit of flux (lumen) are the same dimensionally because the solid angle in steradians is dimensionless. Also note that flux and intensity will be equal when $\Omega = 1$ steradian (i.e., when $A = R^2$).

Illumination. Illumination is the density of luminous flux on a surface area; i.e.,

Illumination = Flux/Area

When flux is measured in lumens and area is measured in square feet, then illumination is expressed in lumens per square feet. The lumens per square feet is sometimes called the foot-candle. If a lumen is defined as the flux falling on a surface area of one square foot, where every part of the surface is one foot from a point source having a luminous intensity of 1 candela (candlepower), then it is obvious that one lumen uniformly distributed over one square foot of surface provides the illumination of one foot-candle. Visually, a foot-candle is the illumination at a point, X, on a surface which is one foot from and perpendicular to a uniform point source of one candela. (See Figure 5.2.12.) In this special case where the incident light is perpendicular to the surface, it can be shown that

$$\text{Illumination} = \frac{\text{Intensity}}{\text{Distance}^2}$$

The relationship

$$\text{Illumination} = \frac{\text{Lumens (flux)}}{\text{Area}}$$

is important and will be used during the discussion of the lumen method of designing a lighting system.

Luminance. Luminance (sometimes called photometric brightness) is a measure of the brightness of a surface, when viewed from a particular direction, emitting or reflecting one lumen per square foot. Luminance is direction-specific and is often measured in foot-lambert units.

Reflectance. Reflectance is a measure of how much light is reflected from a surface. It is the ratio of luminance to illumination.

$$\text{Reflectance} = \frac{\text{Luminance}}{\text{Illumination}}$$

Figure 5.2.12

Foot-candle.

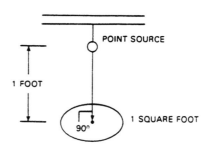

The Measurement of Light

Foot-candle Measurements. Illumination measurements are most commonly
made with one of several types of foot-candle meters embodying a
light-sensitive, barrier-layer cell. (See Figure 5.2.13.) This type of cell
consists essentially of a film of light-sensitive material mounted on a
metal-based plate and covered by a very thin translucent layer of metal
spattered on its outer surface. Light striking the cell surface causes the
semiconducting, light-sensitive material to emit electrons that are picked up
by the metal collector in contact with the translucent front electrode. A
potential difference is thus set up between the collector and the base plate;
and, when a microammeter is connected between them, it measures the current
generated by the cell. Since the current is proportional to the intensity of
the incident light, the meter can be calibrated to read directly in
foot-candles. Portable meters are made in a number of types and with a wide
range of sensitivity for various applications. Although portable,
light-sensitive cell meters are simple and highly convenient to use, most of
them are not designed to be precision instruments. Careful handling and
frequent calibration will help to maintain reliability. Ordinary measurements
made in the field should not be expected to have an accuracy greater than $\pm$ 5%
under the most favorable conditions. In addition, all light-sensitive cells
have certain inherent characteristics that the user must understand if he or
she is to obtain the best possible results:

A.   The instrument must be color corrected because the response of the
     light-sensitive cells to the various wavelengths of the visible
     spectrum is quite different from that of the human eye.

B.   They must be cosine corrected; that is, adjusted for the angle of the
     reflected light.

C.   All light-sensitive cells exhibit a certain amount of fatigue; that
     is, a tendency for the meter indication to drop off slowly over a
     period of minutes until a constant reading is reached. This effect
     is most noticeable at high foot-candle values, particularly if the

Figure 5.2.13

Illumination meter.

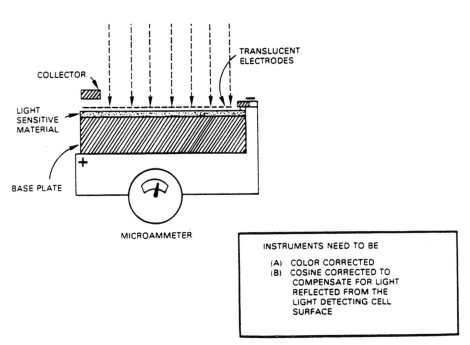

cell has just been previously in the dark for some time or exposed to a much lower level of illumination. Before any measurements are recorded, therefore, the meter should be given as long an adaptation period as may be necessary at the foot-candle level to be measured. In addition, there is a constant need to have the instrument calibrated.

Brightness or luminance is measured using a photoelectric tube. The instrument is aimed at the surface to be measured, and a lens focuses the image on a small area on the tube which produces a current proportional to luminance. The current is read on a microammeter calibrated in foot-lamberts.

Brightness is also measured by a visual luminance meter. This uses an optical system to bring the eyes of the observer side by side to the surface to be measured and a comparison field inside the meter.

Luminance can be measured with a foot-candle meter providing the reflectance of the surface is known. This is because illuminance equals luminance divided by reflectance.

Reflectance can be measured by a cell-type foot-candle meter. There are two procedures that can be used. The more accurate procedure requires a piece

of matte material at least one foot square, the reflectance of which is
known. White blotting paper, at about 80 percent reflectance, is suitable.
The blotting paper is placed against the surface to be measured, and the mete
is held two to four inches away with the cell facing the paper, reading A.
The blotting paper is then removed without moving the meter, and the reading
is noted. The reflectance of the surface is reading B divided by reading A
times 0.80. In all measurements of this sort, special care must be taken to
maintain all conditions, especially the position of the meter, constant for
both readings of a pair.

Light Survey Procedures

"How to Make a Lighting Survey," developed by the Illuminating Engineering
Society, provides detailed information on conducting a lighting survey. A se
of instructions and a form are included with this information.

The survey includes reporting on the following information:

1. Description of the illuminated area:

    a. Room dimensions
    b. Color
    c. Reflectance
    d. Conditions of room surface
    e. Temperature surrounding the lights

2. Description of the general lighting system:

    a. Quantities
    b. Conditions
    c. Wattages
    d. Lamps
    e. Distribution
    f. Spacings
    g. Mountings

3. Description of any supplementary lighting that might be used.

4. Description of instruments to be used.

5. Illumination measurement:

    a. Operator must be aware not to cast shadows.
    b. Operator must be careful not to reflect additional light from
        clothing.
    c. Test surfaces should be as close as possible to the working
        plane. If there is no definite working plane, take measurements
        on a horizontal plane 30 inches above the floor.

6. Luminance measurements.

Evaluation of Results. Data resulting from a light survey can be used to compare the illumination levels for compliance with the recommended levels; to compare the luminance with compliance luminance levels; to determine luminance ratios for visibility and safety; to determine indications of comfort and pleasantness in the area; to determine deficiencies in the area; and to determine a maintenance schedule--that is, a good housekeeping schedule.

3. Lighting Design

Introduction

In the last chapter, the four factors of seeing industrial tasks--size, contrast, brightness, and time--were discussed. Also discussed were common lighting terminology and the behavior of light when it leaves the source.

This chapter discusses the design of a lighting system. The design of any lighting system involves the consideration of many variables: What is the purpose of the lighting--is it lighting for critical seeing, lighting for selling, or lighting for decoration? How severe is the seeing task, and for what length of time is it to be performed? What are the architectural and decorative requirements, together with the constructional limitations, of the area? What economic considerations are involved? The answers to such questions as these determine the amount of light that should be provided and the best means for providing it. Since individual tastes and opinions vary, especially in matters of appearance, no one solution of a lighting problem will be the most desirable under all circumstances. However, there are certain basic rules governing adequate lighting and the quality of that lighting. Two factors that must be considered in designing a lighting system are the quantity of light and the quality of light reaching the seeing task.

Quantity of Light

The most obvious consideration in designing a lighting system is the adequacy of the light on the seeing task. Research has shown that illumination of thousands of foot-candles is required to see dark, low-contrast tasks as easily as light-colored tasks of high contrast under low levels. However, there are other factors involved. These factors suggest that for any task the minimum number of foot-candles is 30.

The Illuminating Engineering Society published a document entitled "IES Lighting Handbook--Application Volume", 1981, which contains a complete table of illuminance ranges recommended for certain kinds of tasks. A page from this document can be found in Table 5.3.1.

Evidence providing a sound basis for definite illuminance recommendations is not easy to obtain. Much work in this field has been done over a period of many years, using various methods and various criteria of visual performance. On the basis of such research, the Illuminating Engineering Society has made illuminance recommendations for a wide variety of representative industrial operations and other visual activities.

The illumination recommended in the IES Lighting Handbook is to be provided on the work surface, whether it is horizontal, vertical, or oblique. Where there is no definite area, it is assumed that the illumination is measured on a horizontal plane 30 inches above the floor. The values given are not to be construed as initial foot-candles provided by a new installation; they are

Table 5.3.1

Currently recommended illuminance categories and illuminance values for lighting design--target maintained levels.

I. Illuminance Categories and Illuminance Values for Generic Types of Activities in Interiors

Type of Activity	Illuminance Category	Ranges of Illuminances		Reference Work-Plane
		Lux	Footcandles	
Public spaces with dark surroundings	A	20–30–50	2–3–5	General lighting throughout spaces
Simple orientation for short temporary visits	B	50–75–100	5–7 5–10	
Working spaces where visual tasks are only occasionally performed	C	100–150–200	10–15–20	
Performance of visual tasks of high contrast or large size	D	200–300–500	20–30–50	Illuminance on task
Performance of visual tasks of medium contrast or small size	E	500–750–1000	50–75–100	
Performance of visual tasks of low contrast or very small size	F	1000–1500–2000	100–150–200	
Performance of visual tasks of low contrast and very small size over a prolonged period	G	2000–3000–5000	200–300–500	Illuminance on task obtained by a combination of general and local (supplementary lighting)
Performance of very prolonged and exacting visual tasks	H	5000–7500–10000	500–750–1000	
Performance of very special visual tasks of extremely low contrast and small size	I	10000–15000–20000	1000–1500–2000	

II. Commercial, Institutional, Residential and Public Assembly Interiors

Area/Activity	Illuminance Category	Area/Activity	Illuminance Category
Air terminals (see Transportation terminals)		Barber shops and beauty parlors	E
Armories	C'	Churches and synagogues	(see page 7-2)*
Art galleries (see Museums)		Club and lodge rooms Lounge and reading	D
Auditoriums Assembly Social activity	C' B	Conference rooms Conferring Critical seeing (refer to individual task)	D

Banks (also see Reading)
Lobby
  General
  Writing area
Tellers' stations
	
	C
	D
	E³
		Court rooms
		Seating area
		Court activity area
		Dance halls and discotheques
			
			C
			E
			B

By permission of the Illuminating Engineering Society.   Source: IES Lighting Handbook, 1981 Application Volume.

recommended minimum foot-candles at any point on a task at any time. This means that the installation must be so designed that the collection of dirt on luminaires, lamps, walls and ceilings and the normal depreciation of light output of the lamps themselves will not at any time lower the illumination below the recommended levels. In order to ensure the minimum levels, one should design a lighting system with higher levels than those indicated in the tables. One can look at the minimum levels specified in the document as being the levels on the task when the lighting systems on the room surfaces have depreciated to their lowest level before maintenance procedures are affected (cleaning, relamping, painting, etc.). In addition, the recommended levels do not take into account the wearing of goggles. If goggles are worn, the levels of illumination should be increased in accordance with the absorption of the goggles. The levels specified in the document again should be viewed as minimum levels. They are not to be construed as standards. They are suggested levels. However, one can use the tables to identify what level-- what quantity of illumination--is needed for any specified task.

The quantity of light also depends upon the distribution of the luminaires. In light for seeing or light for production and inspection, it is usually desirable to position the luminaire to provide reasonably uniform general illumination over the entire area. The ratio of maximum foot-candles under the luminaires to the minimum between them should never be greater than 2:1; and for best results, it should be nearer to unity. Units with wide distribution characteristics can be spaced farther apart for the same mounting height than those with more concentrated distributions. Maximum spacing-to-mounting height or ceiling-height ratios for various types of equipment are supplied by the manufacturers.

Quality of Light

In addition to the quantity of light, one must consider the quality of light when designing a lighting system. Quality of light refers to glare, brightness ratio, diffusion, and color.

Glare is the effect of brightness differences within a visual field sufficiently high to cause annoyance, discomfort, or loss of visual perception; while brightness is the intensity of light emitted, transmitted, or reflected from a given surface. Basically, there are two kinds of glare: glare caused by a bright light source which is sometimes called direct glare; and glare by bright reflections, sometimes called reflected glare. There are generally considered to be two forms of glare--discomfort glare and disability glare--each of which may be caused by a bright light source or by bright reflections on room surfaces. Discomfort glare, as its name implies, produces discomfort and may affect human performance but does not necessarily interfere with visual performance or visibility. In some cases, extremely bright sources can even cause pain. Disability glare does not cause pain but reduces the visibility of objects to be seen. An example is the reduced visibility of objects on a roadway at night caused by glare of bright oncoming headlights.

Direct glare results from high brightness light sources or luminaires in the field of view that are not sufficiently shielded or cover too great an

area. It is also possible that direct glare can result from improperly shaded
windows.

An industrial environment, then, will be relatively comfortable if there
is no direct glare; and seeing will be unimpaired if there is no disability
glare. The effects of direct glare can be avoided or minimized by mounting
the luminaires as far above or away from the normal lines of sight as
possible. In general, this can be done by shielding luminaires to at least 25
degrees down from the horizontal and preferably down to 45 degrees. In other
words, brightness of bare lamps should not be seen when looking in the range
of sight straight ahead up to 45 degrees above the horizontal.

Direct glare from windows can be minimized by properly shielding the
sources of daylight with adjustable shades, blinds, or louvers.

Reflected glare is bright areas on shiny surfaces that become annoying.
Light sources between the vertical and 45 degrees from the vertical contribute
to reflected glare. Luminaires with lens that polarize light (lens that
transmit light waves which vibrate in only one direction) tend to reduce
reflected glare in many cases. Reflected glare can also be reduced by
adjusting the position of the seeing task and by controlling the distribution
pattern of lighting fixtures.

In addition to the above information about glare, the following should be
considered:

1. Glare is influenced by characteristics of the room and the use of
    luminaires. This is particularly true when considering reflected
    glare.

2. Luminaire brightness that is comfortable in a small office where the
    lighting units are out of range of vision may be excessive in larger
    rooms where the luminaires farthest away may approach the line of
    vision.

3. Luminaires that do not have objectionable high brightness may, if
    mounted in large groups, present a total picture that is
    uncomfortable. This usually results when some type of fluorescent
    luminaires are mounted across the line of sight in an area with
    relatively low ceilings.

4. The color of walls and ceilings is extremely important. This is
    particularly true with reflected glare. Since specular reflection is
    directional, it is frequently possible to prevent reflected glare by
    positioning the light source, the work surface, or the worker so that
    the reflected light will be directed away from the eyes. Reflected
    glare may also be controlled by means of large-area, low-brightness
    sources, and by using light colors with dull, nonglossy reflected
    finishes on furniture and working surfaces.

The next concept to consider when dealing with quality of light is the
brightness ratio or brightness contrast. Brightness is sometimes called

luminance or photometric brightness. The brightness ratio refers to the different levels of brightness in the area of a task and the immediate background surrounding the area. Even though the differences in brightness between a surrounding area and the task may not be severe enough to cause glare, the differences in brightness may be detrimental to the lighting quality. If there is a difference in brightness between the task area and the surrounding background, the eyes will continuously have to adapt between the task and the surrounding area. It takes some time for the eyes to do this kind of adaptation; and, therefore, the visibility of the task will be affected. In addition, brighter surroundings tend to attract the eyes away from the task. The eyes function more efficiently and comfortably when the luminance within the visual environment is not too different from that of the seeing task. To reduce the effect, maximum luminance ratios are recommended as shown in Table 5.3.2. A ratio of the brightness of the task to that of the immediate surroundings of 3 to I is generally acceptable. Ratios no greater than 10 to I anywhere in the field of vision are desirable, and 30 to I or 40 to I is the maximum permissible.

As an aid in achieving these reduced luminance ratios, the reflectance upon room surfaces and equipment should be as listed in Table 5.3.3.

The third factor influencing the quality of light is diffusion. Diffusion is light coming from many directions as opposed to light coming from one direction. Diffusion is measured in terms of the absence of sharp shadows. The degree or absence of diffusion depends upon the type of work being performed. Perfectly diffuse light is ideal illumination for many critical seeing tasks; for example, in schools and offices. Where polished metal surfaces must be viewed, a highly diffused light is essential to prevent annoying specular reflections. In other cases, direct lighting may be more important or desirable than diffuse lighting; for example, surface irregularities that are almost invisible under diffuse light may be clearly revealed in light directed at a grazing angle. Diffusion is achieved by multiple lighting sources, by having a large number of low brightness luminaires, by indirect or partially indirect lighting in which the ceilings and walls become secondary sources, and by light-colored, matte finishes on ceilings, walls, furniture, and even on the floors. A quality lighting system will have luminaires spaced so that the ratio of the intensity below the luminaires to the intensity between the luminaires is 1 to 1. Ratios of 1.5 to 1 are acceptable, and the maximum is 2 to 1.

The fourth factor to consider when discussing the quality of light is color. Color is the sensation produced in the eye in response to light in certain portions of the dichromatic spectrum (wavelengths of 3800 to 7200 angstroms; to convert angstroms to inches multiply by 3.937×10^{-9}). The eye is more sensitive to energy emitted at certain wavelengths than at others. The effectiveness of energy emitted at a given wavelength in producing a response in the eye is indicated by the relative luminosity factor. (See Figure 5.3.1.)

A source of light might be emitted in (1) a narrow band of one or two frequencies (line spectrum), (2) a continuous spectrum containing various quantities of all frequencies in the visibility spectrum (such as tungsten

Table 5.3.2

Recommended maximum luminance ratios.

		Environmental Classification		
		A	B	C
1.	Between tasks and adjacent darker surroundings	3 to 1	3 to 1	5 to 1
2.	Between tasks and adjacent lighter surroundings	1 to 3	1 to 3	1 to 5
3.	Between tasks and more remote darker surfaces	10 to 1	20 to 1	*
4.	Between tasks and more remote lighter surfaces	I to 10	1 to 20	*
5.	Between luminaires (or windows, skylights, etc.) and surfaces adjacent to them	20 to 1	*	*
6.	Anywhere within the normal field of view	40 to 1	*	*

*Luminance ratio control not practical.

A.   Interior areas where reflectances of entire space can be controlled in line with recommendations for optimum seeing conditions.

B.   Areas where reflectances of immediate work area can be controlled. but control of remote surroundings is limited.

C.   Areas (indoor or outdoor) where it is completely impractical to control reflectances and difficult to alter environmental conditions.

Source: The Industrial Environment: Its Evaluation and Control.

lamps), or (3) an equal energy spectrum containing equal amounts of energy at each wavelength in the visible spectrum.

Color is often described by a temperature, where the temperature compares the color of a light source with the color of a black box heated to various temperatures (usually measured in degrees Kelvin). Designation of color by temperature is usually limited to colors with continuous spectrum characteristics because black bodies do not emit colors comparable to those with line-band radiation.

Table 5.3.3

Recommended reflectance values
applying to environmental classifications
A and B.

	Reflectance* (percent)
Ceiling	80 to 90
Walls	40 to 60
Desk and bench tops, machines and equipment	25 to 40
Floors	Not less than 20

*Reflectance should be maintained as near as practical
to recommended values.

Source: The Industrial Environment: Its Evaluation and Control.

Figure 5.3.1

Relative luminosity factor.

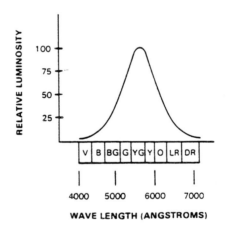

Objects appear to be a certain color because they have the ability to absorb light energy of particular wavelengths. The characteristic of the reflected light determines the color of the object.

For performance of ordinary visual tasks, no one color light source has any advantage over any other. However, color must be considered a key factor in specialized applications. For example, minor color differences are best distinguished when an object is viewed under a light with low energy in the spectral region of the object's maximum reflectivity.

Color may also be important for psychological reasons. Certain colors convey a feeling of warmth, and others appear cool. The design of a lighting system must recognize psychological and traditional factors in achievement of quality for a particular seeing task.

Luminaire Classification

Luminaires are designed to control the source of light so that it can be better used for a given seeing task. The materials used in luminaires are designed to reflect, refract, diffuse, or obscure light. Luminaires are classified into two general types, general and supplemental. General lighting luminaires are subdivided as shown in Figure 5.3.2.

Indirect Lighting. Ninety to 100 percent of the light output of the luminaire is directed toward the ceiling at an angle above the horizontal. Practically all the light effective at the work plane is redirected downward by the ceiling and, to a lesser extent, by the side walls. Since the ceiling is in effect a secondary lighting source, the illumination produced is quite diffuse in character. Because room finishes play such an important part in redirecting the light, it is particularly important that they be as light in color as possible and be carefully observed and maintained in good condition.

The ceiling should always have a matte finish if reflected images of light sources are to be avoided. For comfort, the ceiling luminance must be within the prescribed limits. Diffuse lighting is usually desirable because it gives even distribution and minimum shadows and minimum reflected glare.

Semi-Indirect Lighting. Sixty to 90 percent of the light output of the luminaire is directed toward the ceiling at angles above the horizontal while the balance is directed downward. Semi-indirect lighting has most of the advantages of the indirect system but is slightly more efficient and is sometimes preferred to achieve a desirable luminance ratio between the ceiling and the luminaire at high-level installations. The diffuse medium employed in these luminaires is glass or plastic of lower density than that employed in indirect equipment.

General Diffuse or Indirect Lighting and Direct-Indirect Lighting. Forty to 60 percent of the light is directed downward at angles below the horizontal. The major portion of the illumination produced on ordinary working planes is a result of light coming directly from the luminaire. There is, however, a substantial portion of the light directed to the ceiling and

Figure 5.3.2

Classififcation of luminaires.

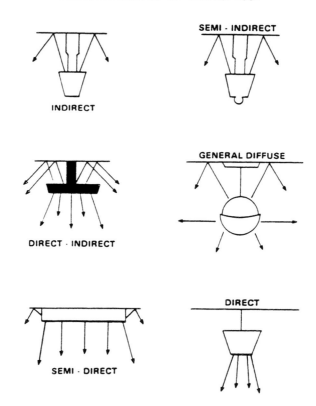

the side walls. The difference between the general diffuse and
direct-indirect lighting classification is the amount of light produced in a
horizontal direction. The general diffuse type is exemplified by the
enclosing globe (lamp) which distributes light nearly uniformly in all
directions, while the direct-indirect luminaire produces very little light in
a horizontal direction due to the density of its side panels.

Semi-Direct Lighting. Sixty to 90 percent of the light is directed
downward at angles below the horizontal. The light reaching the normal
working plane is primarily the result of the light coming directly from the
luminaire, not from the ceiling or from the walls. There is a relatively
small indirect component, the greatest value of which is that it brightens the
ceiling around the luminaire, with the resultant lowering of the brightness
contrasts.

Supplementary Lighting. The supplementary lighting category of luminaire
is also subdivided. These luminaires are used along with the general lighting
system but are localized near the seeing tasks to provide the higher levels or

quality of light not readily obtainable from the general lighting system.
They are divided into five major subtypes, from S-I to S-V, based upon their
light distribution and luminance characteristic.   Each has a specific group of
applications, as shown in Figure 5.3.3.

Figure 5.3.3

Supplementary luminaires.

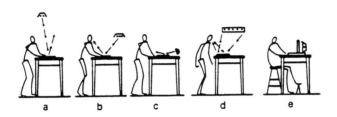

Examples of Placement of Supplementary Luminaires: (a) Luminaire located
to prevent reflected glare--reflected light does not coincide with angle of
view. (b) Reflected light coincides with angle of view. (c) Low angle lighting to
emphasize surface irregularities. (d) Large-area surface and pattern are
reflected toward the eye. (e) Transillumination from diffuse sources.

Lighting Systems or Illumination Methods

The illumination produced by any one of the five types of luminaire
systems may be further classified according to the distribution of light
throughout the area. Whether the lighting is general, localized general, or
supplementary depends upon the location of equipment and its distribution
characteristics.

General Lighting. General lighting is the arrangement of lighting
equipment so that a uniform level of illumination is produced.   Factors
affecting uniform distribution of light are:

a.   the physical characteristics of the room
b.   the level of illumination desired
c.   the appearance of the finished installation

Uniform lighting can be obtained using the lumen method (described later)
which gives the number of luminaires needed to provide a certain quantity of
light.   After the number of luminaires is computed, the approximate location
can be made so that the total number of luminaires can be adjusted to be
evenly divisible by the number of rows.   The exact distance between fixtures
is determined by dividing the length of the room by the number of luminaires
in a row, allowing for about one-third of this distance between the wall and
the first unit.   In a similar manner, the distance between the rows is the
width of the room, divided by the number of rows, with about one-third of the

distance left between the side of the wall and the first row. In high-ceiling industrial areas, these recommended distances may be up to one-half of the luminaire spacing.

Localized General Lighting. Localized general lighting is the positioning of general lighting equipment with reference to particular work areas where high intensities are necessary, with the spill light from the same luminaires usually providing sufficient illumination for adjacent areas. Luminaires of a direct, semi-direct, or direct-indirect type are usually employed for this purpose since a substantial direct component is essential where it is desirable to concentrate most of the light on the restricted area beneath the luminaire; that is, the work plane.

Supplementary Lighting. Supplementary lighting is the provision of relatively high intensity at specific work points by means of direct lighting equipment used in conjunction with general localized illumination. It is frequently necessary where specialty-seeing critical tasks are involved and where it is not feasible to provide the desired intensity by either general lighting or localized general lighting. It is also used where light of directional quality is required for certain inspection tasks. Equipment used for this purpose varies in distribution characteristics depending upon the area to be covered, by the distance from the equipment location to the work-point, and the foot-candles required. When using supplementary lighting, care must always be exercised to keep a reasonable relationship between the intensities of the general illumination and the supplementary lighting, since an excessive luminance ratio between the work point and its surroundings creates an uncomfortable seeing condition.

Other Factors to Consider When Designing a Lighting System

When designing a lighting system, one must consider the quantity of light, the quality of light, the type of light (that is, direct or indirect), and the type of lighting system (e.g., supplementary, general localized, or general). In addition, other factors should be considered. Such factors are:

1. The choice of light source
   - Filament
   - Mercury vapor
   - Fluorescent

2. Heat produced from the source

3. Efficiency of the lamp or light source

4. Electrical features
   - Use equipment that conforms to the industrial specifications
   - Use adequate type of wiring and circuits

5. Mechanical structure of the support of the fixtures

6. Appearance/decoration

One of the other characteristics to consider when designing a lighting system is the maintenance of the luminaires. There are three things to look at in maintenance of luminaires.

1. The light source

2. The luminaire

3. The room surface

The life of the light source is a maintenance problem. Length of life is different for filament, mercury vapor, and fluorescent lamps. Filament lamps have the least length of life. Mercury vapor and fluorescent last longer; however, near the end of their life, they produce only about 75 percent of their original output. It is frequently found to be economical to establish a replacement program in which new lamps are installed before the old ones have reached the end of their life; that is, the 75 percent of their original output. Such a program can be best carried out by systematically replacing the lamps in a specific area after they have burned a predetermined number of hours. This procedure is commonly termed "group relamping." This method has an advantage in that it results in less variation in the illumination level effectiveness in the area.

The second factor to consider in maintenance of the system is the luminaires. Luminaires do not function efficiently when they are covered with dirt. The amount of dirt depends upon the characteristics of the environment, the room area, and the type of activity being conducted in the room. The reason dirt interferes with the luminaire is that the light must travel through the layer of dirt; and because dirt changes the distribution characteristics of the equipment, it is necessary to take this into consideration when the lamp is to provide a direct beam of light--the dirt makes the resulting light diffuse. Because maintenance of the luminaires and the dust accumulating on them is a problem, one must consider these problems before selecting the type of luminaire. One should look for such things as how difficult the unit is to handle, its weight, its size, its accessibility or inaccessibility. One must also look to see if the luminaire is hinged or otherwise secured to the main body of the fixture. For purposes of cleaning, it is an advantage to be able to remove the lamps and reflecting equipment readily. The normal cleaning heights of the luminaires must also be considered. They can be cleaned at regular heights usually from stepladders. However, where ceilings are high or the floor area beneath the luminaires is inaccessible, telescoping ladders with extension platforms may be required. These are frequently necessary for use in machine shops and large auditoriums. In these conditions, the possibility of catwalks or messenger cables should be considered. The cleaning schedule depends upon how dirty the environment is. If the cleaning coincides with the replacement schedule, the labor costs will be reduced.

The third factor to consider in maintenance is the room surface. If the lighting system is indirect lighting, the dirt on the room surfaces may affect the quality of light. A reduction in the reflection factor due to dirt has less effect in a direct system than in an indirect or partly indirect system. The necessity for cleaning or refinishing room surfaces varies with conditions. In areas where the dirt sticks to the surface, walls and ceilings should be reconditioned once or twice a year. Where the dirt condition is less severe or where air-cleaning systems are employed, room surfaces may be permitted to go several years between servicing.

Lumen Method of Lighting Design

Introduction

The following characteristics of designing a good lighting system have been discussed: the quality of light; the quantity of light; luminaire classification; illumination system; and the maintenance of luminaires, room surfaces, and light sources.

There are two types of calculations that can be used in designing a lighting system. One is the lumen method; the other is the point-by-point method. The lumen method is appropriate for generalized lighting only. It is a way for computing the average illumination throughout the entire room. The procedure is not very good when general localized or supplementary lighting- is used. In these cases, one must compute the illumination at the point where the actual seeing task is located. The average illumination throughout the room is meaningless in this case. In the case of generalized localized lighting or supplementary lighting, the point-by-point method is used to calculate the quantity of illumination. The point-by-point method will not be discussed in this text.

The first step in the lumen method is to analyze the seeing task and the working environment. One should ask himself the following questions:

1. How should the task be portrayed by the light?
2. Should the lighting be diffuse or directional or some combination of both?
3. Are shadows important?
4. Is color important?
5. What is the area atmosphere and, therefore, the type of maintenance characteristics that will be needed?
6. What are the economics of the lighting system?

From the answers to the above questions, one can determine the following two things:

1. What level of illumination is needed for the task. (This can be determined by looking at the recommended standards.)
2. The type of luminaires that are needed (that is, direct or indirect) and the required maintenance considerations.

Once the type of luminaires that are going to be used and the amount of illumination needed have been determined, then it is possible to calculate the number of luminaires needed to produce that illumination using the technique that follows.

The Formula

The lumen method is based on the definition of a foot-candle equaling one lumen per square foot; thus

$$\text{Foot-candles} = \frac{\text{Lumens striking area}}{\text{Square feet of area}}$$

By knowing the initial lumen output of each lamp (published by the lamp manufacturer), the number of lamps installed in the area, and the square feet of area, one can calculate the lumens per square foot generated initially in an area. However, this value differs from the foot-candles in the area. This difference occurs because some lumens are absorbed in the luminaire and also because of such factors as dirt on the luminaire and the gradual depreciation in lumen output of the lamp. (Recall that fluorescent lamps operate at only about 75 percent of their original output at the end of their life.) These factors plus others are taken into consideration in the lumen method formula which is as follows:

$$\text{Foot-candles} = \frac{\text{Lamps per luminaire x lumens per lamp x coefficient of utilization x light loss factor}}{\text{Area per luminaire}}$$

By manipulating this equation, one can determine the number of luminaires needed. This is as follows:

$$\text{Number of luminaires} = \frac{\text{Foot-candles x area}}{\text{Lamps per luminaire x lumens per lamp x coefficient of utilization x light loss factor}}$$

Or one can calculate the number of lamps needed:

$$\text{Number of lamps} = \frac{\text{Foot-candles x area}}{\text{Lumens per lamp x coefficient of utilization x light loss factor}}$$

And the number of luminaires can be computed as follows:

$$\text{Number of luminaires} = \frac{\text{Number of lamps}}{\text{Lamps per luminaire}}$$

Knowing the type of luminaires and the number or quantity of light needed, the next step is to use the formula: that is, to apply the formula to the problem to determine the number of luminaires that are needed to cover the area. To use the formula, it is necessary for the user to understand conceptually some of the quantities in it; for example, the coefficient of utilization and the light loss factor.

Coefficient of Utilization

The coefficient of utilization is the ratio of the lumens reaching the work area (assume a horizontal plane 30 inches above the floor) to the total lumens generated by the lamps. It is a factor that takes into account the efficiency and distribution of the luminaires, luminaire mounting height, room proportions, and reflectance of walls, ceilings and floors. (Note: Because of multiple reflections within a room, some light passes downward through the imaginary work plane more than once. Under some circumstances, this may cause the coefficient of utilization to be larger than 1.)

In general, the higher and narrower the room, the larger the percentage of light absorbed by the walls and the lower the coefficient of utilization. Rooms are classified according to shape by ten room-cavity ratio numbers. The room-cavity ratio is computed using the following formula:

$$\text{Room-cavity ratio} = \frac{5h \ (\text{room length} + \text{room width})}{\text{room length} \times \text{room width}}$$

where h is the height of the cavity.

A more conveniently used formula is the following:

$$\text{Room-cavity ratio} = \frac{10h}{\text{room width}} \times \text{Gaysunas ratio}$$

The Gaysunas ratio comprehends the influence of room length and varies with the ratio of the room length to the room width. The Gaysunas number is selected from Table 5.3.4.

Table 5.3.4

Gaysunas ratio.

Room Length Room Width	Gaysunas Ratio
1.00	1.0
1.25	9/10
1.50	5/6
2.00	3/4
2.50	7/10
3.00	2/3
4.00	5/8
5.00	6/10
∞	1/2

Source: Westinghouse Lighting Handbook.

One must compute the room-cavity ratio before looking up the coefficient of utilization. A room can be broken up into three cavity areas: the ceiling-cavity area, the distance between the ceiling and the luminaire plane; the room-cavity area, the distance between the luminaire plane and the work plane; and the floor-cavity area, the distance between the floor and the work plane.

In effect, then there can be a ceiling-cavity ratio, a room-cavity ratio, and a floor-cavity ratio. All these cavity ratios are computed using the formula given previously.

Assume a room 20 feet by 40 feet by 12 feet high with the luminaires installed 2 feet from the ceiling and the work plane 2.5 feet from the floor. The ceiling-cavity ratio would be equal to

$$\text{Ceiling-cavity ratio} = \frac{10h}{\text{room width}} \times \text{Gaysunas ratio}$$

where h is the distance between the ceiling and the luminaire plane; in this case, 2 feet.

From the table of Gaysunas ratios, the Gaysunas ratio for room length/room width of 2.00 is 3/4. Substituting 2 feet for h and 3/4 for the Gaysunas ratio in the formula above, the ceiling-cavity ratio would be equal to:

$$\text{Ceiling-cavity ratio} = \frac{10 \times 2 \text{ ft}}{20 \text{ ft.}} \ (3/4)$$

$$= 0.75$$

The floor-cavity ratio would be equal to

$$\text{Floor-cavity ratio} = \frac{10h}{\text{room width}} \times \text{Gaysunas ratio}$$

where h is the distance of the work plane from the floor; in this case, 2.5 feet. The Gaysunas ratio remains the same. Substituting in the formula, the floor-cavity ratio would be equal to

$$\text{Floor-cavity ratio} = \frac{10 \times 2.5 \text{ ft}}{20 \text{ ft}} \ (3/4)$$

$$= 0.94$$

The room-cavity ratio also can be computed using the same formula:

$$\text{Room-cavity ratio} = \frac{10h}{\text{room width}} \times \text{Gaysunas ratio}$$

where h equals the distance of the room cavity, the distance between the work plane and the luminaire plane. In this case, h would be 7.5 feet, and the Gaysunas ratio would remain the same.

Substituting these values in the formula gives

$$\text{Room-cavity ratio} = \frac{10 \times 7.5 \text{ ft}}{20 \text{ ft}} \quad (3/4)$$

$$= 2.81$$

It should be pointed out that tables are available to compute the cavity ratios. One of these tables is shown in Table 5.3.5. The calculations just completed can be determined using this table. For example, from the table for room width 20 feet, room length 40 feet and ceiling cavity 2 feet, the ceiling-cavity ratio is equal to about 0.75.

The ceiling-cavity ratio is used to look up the coefficient of utilization. However, before the room-cavity ratio can be used for this purpose, the reflectance of the ceiling and of the walls must be known. They are two ceiling reflecting values that are important: the actual reflectance of the ceiling and the effective ceiling reflectance. The effective ceiling reflectance is actually an adjustment of the actual ceiling reflectance, using the ceiling-cavity ratio. For example, a room is 20 feet by 40 feet by 12 feet high, the actual ceiling reflectance is 80 percent, and the reflectance of the walls is 50 percent. Although the actual ceiling reflectance is 80 percent, this must be adjusted for the fact that the lights will be installed 2 feet from the ceiling. This will change the reflectance. To compute the effective ceiling reflectance, a table such as the one provided in Table 5.3.6 must be used. For the example where the ceiling-cavity ratio is 0.75 and theactual ceiling reflectance is 80%--which on the table is called the base reflectance--and the wall reflectance is 50%, the effective ceiling reflectance would be between 69% and 71%, or about 69.68%.

Once the effective ceiling-cavity reflectance is known, the coefficient of utilization can be determined from a table, such as is shown in Table 5.3.7. Notice that to look up the coefficient of utilization the following information must be known: the type of luminaire, the type of distribution of that luminaire, the effective ceiling-cavity reflectance, the wall reflectance, and the room-cavity ratio. For example, using the first luminaire on the table, the coefficient of utilization can be found for an effective ceiling-cavity reflectance of 80%, wall reflectance of 50%, and a room-cavity ratio (RCR) equal to 5. The coefficient of utilization is 0.50. (Note: The ceiling-cavity reflectance in the table refers to the effective ceiling-cavity reflectance.) The categories of luminaires as they are indicated on the table will be discussed later.

For ceiling-mounted luminaires or recessed luminaires, the ceiling-cavity reflectance is the same as the actual ceiling reflectance; that is, one does not need to compute the ceiling-cavity ratio and adjust the ceiling reflectance by the ceiling-cavity ratio. But for suspended luminaires, it is necessary to determine the effective ceiling-cavity reflectance as has been done in the example.

Table 5.3.5

Room-cavity ratios.

Room Dimensions		Cavity Depth																			
Width	Length	1.0	1.5	2.0	2.5	3.0	3.5	4.0	5.0	6.0	7.0	8	9	10	11	12	14	16	20	25	30
8	8	12	19	25	31	37	44	50	62	75	87	100	112	125							
	10	11	17	22	28	34	39	45	56	67	79	90	101	112	124						
	14	10	15	20	25	29	34	39	49	59	69	79	88	98	108	118					
	20	9	13	17	22	26	31	35	44	52	61	70	79	87	96	105	122				
	30	8	12	16	20	24	28	32	40	47	55	63	71	79	87	95	111				
	40	7	11	15	19	22	26	30	37	45	52	60	67	75	82	90	105	120			
10	10	10	15	20	25	30	35	40	50	60	70	80	90	100	110	120					
	14	9	13	17	21	26	30	34	43	51	60	69	77	86	94	103	120				
	20	7	11	15	19	22	26	30	37	45	52	60	67	75	82	90	105	120			
	30	7	10	13	17	20	23	27	33	40	47	53	60	67	73	80	93	107			
	40	6	9	12	16	19	22	25	31	37	44	50	56	62	69	75	87	100	125		
	60	6	9	12	15	17	20	23	29	35	41	47	52	58	64	70	82	93	117		
12	12	8	12	17	21	25	29	33	42	50	58	67	75	83	92	100	117				
	16	7	11	15	18	22	26	29	36	44	51	58	66	73	80	87	102	117			
	24	6	9	12	16	19	22	25	31	37	44	50	56	62	69	75	87	100	125		
	36	6	8	11	14	17	19	22	28	33	39	44	50	56	61	67	78	89	111		
	50	5	8	10	13	16	18	21	26	31	36	41	46	52	57	62	72	83	103		
	70	5	7	10	12	15	17	20	24	29	34	39	44	49	54	59	68	78	98	122	
14	14	7	11	14	18	21	25	29	36	43	50	57	64	71	79	86	100	114			
	20	6	9	12	15	18	21	24	30	36	42	49	55	61	67	73	85	97	121		
	30	5	8	10	13	16	18	21	26	31	37	42	47	52	58	63	73	84	105		
	42	5	7	10	12	14	17	19	24	29	33	38	43	48	52	57	67	76	95	119	
	60	4	7	9	11	13	15	18	22	26	31	35	40	44	48	53	62	70	88	110	
	90	4	6	8	10	12	14	17	21	25	29	33	37	41	45	50	58	66	83	103	124
17	17	6	9	12	15	18	21	24	29	35	41	47	53	59	65	71	82	94	118		
	25	5	7	10	12	15	17	20	25	30	35	40	44	49	54	59	69	79	99	124	
	35	4	7	9	11	13	15	17	22	26	31	35	39	44	48	52	61	70	87	109	
	50	4	6	8	10	12	14	16	20	24	28	32	35	39	43	47	55	63	79	99	118
	80	4	5	7	9	11	12	14	18	21	25	29	32	36	39	43	50	57	71	89	107
	120	3	5	7	8	10	12	13	17	20	24	27	30	34	37	40	47	54	67	84	101
20	20	5	7	10	12	15	17	20	25	30	35	40	45	50	55	60	70	80	100	125	
	30	4	6	8	10	12	15	17	21	25	29	33	37	42	46	50	58	67	83	104	125
	45	4	5	7	9	11	13	14	18	22	25	29	32	36	40	43	51	58	72	90	108
	60	3	5	7	8	10	12	13	17	20	23	27	30	33	37	40	47	53	67	83	100
	90	3	5	6	8	9	11	12	15	18	21	24	27	31	34	37	43	49	61	76	92
	150	3	4	6	7	8	10	11	14	17	20	23	25	28	31	34	40	45	57	71	85
24	24	4	6	8	10	12	15	17	21	25	29	33	37	42	46	50	58	67	83	104	125
	32	4	5	7	9	11	13	15	18	22	26	29	33	36	40	44	51	58	73	91	109
	50	3	5	6	8	9	11	12	15	18	22	25	28	31	34	37	43	49	62	77	92
	70	3	4	6	7	8	10	11	14	17	20	22	25	28	31	34	39	45	56	70	84
	100	3	4	5	6	8	9	10	13	16	18	21	23	26	28	31	36	41	52	65	77
	160	2	4	5	6	7	8	10	12	14	17	19	22	24	26	29	34	38	48	60	72

Table 5.3.6

Effective cavity reflectance.

Top section

Base Refl. %		90							80							70							60							50						
Wall Refl. %		90	80	70	50	30	10	0	90	80	70	50	30	10	0	90	80	70	50	30	10	0	90	80	70	50	30	10	0	90	80	70	50	30	10	0
0.2		89	88	88	86	85	84	82	79	78	78	77	76	74	72	70	69	68	67	66	65	64	60	59	58	58	56	55	53	50	50	49	48	47	46	44
0.4		88	87	86	84	81	79	76	79	77	76	74	72	70	68	69	68	67	65	63	61	58	60	59	57	54	52	50		50	49	48	47	45	43	42
0.6		87	86	84	80	77	74	73	78	76	75	71	68	65	63	69	67	65	63	59	57	54	60	58	57	55	51	50	46	50	48	47	45	43	41	38
0.8		87	85	82	77	73	69	67	78	75	73	69	65	61	57	68	66	64	60	59	53	50	59	57	56	54	48	46	43	50	48	47	44	40	38	36
1.0		86	83	80	75	69	64	62	77	74	72	67	62	57	55	68	65	62	58	53	50	47	59	57	55	51	45	43	41	50	48	46	43	38	36	34
1.5		85	80	76	68	61	55	51	75	72	68	61	54	49	46	67	62	59	54	46	42	40	59	55	52	46	40	37	34	50	47	45	40	34	31	26
2.0		83	77	72	62	53	47	43	74	69	64	56	48	41	38	66	60	56	49	40	36	33	58	54	50	43	35	31	29	50	46	43	37	30	26	24
2.5		82	75	68	57	47	40	36	73	67	61	51	42	35	32	65	60	54	45	36	31	29	58	53	47	39	30	25	23	50	46	41	35	27	22	21
3.0		80	72	64	52	42	34	30	72	65	58	47	37	30	27	64	58	52	42	32	27	24	57	52	46	37	28	23	20	50	45	40	32	24	19	17
3.5		79	70	61	48	37	31	26	71	63	55	43	33	26	24	63	57	50	38	29	23	21	57	50	44	35	25	20	17	50	44	39	30	22	17	15
4.0		77	69	58	44	33	25	22	70	61	53	40	30	22	20	63	55	48	36	26	20	17	57	49	42	32	23	18	14	50	44	38	28	20	15	12
5.0		75	59	53	38	28	20	16	68	58	44	35	25	18	14	61	52	44	31	22	16	12	56	48	40	28	20	14	11	50	42	35	25	17	12	09
6.0		73	61	49	34	24	16	11	66	55	44	31	22	15	10	60	51	41	28	19	13	09	55	45	37	25	17	11	07	50	42	34	23	15	10	06
8.0		68	55	42	27	18	12	06	62	50	38	25	17	11	05	57	46	35	23	15	10	05	53	42	33	22	14	08	04	49	40	30	19	12	07	03
10.0		65	51	36	22	15	09	04	59	46	33	21	14	08	03	55	43	31	19	12	08	03	51	39	29	18	11	07	02	47	37	27	17	10	06	02

Bottom section

Base Refl. %		40							30							20							10							0						
Wall Refl. %		90	80	70	50	30	10	0	90	80	70	50	30	10	0	90	80	70	50	30	10	0	90	80	70	50	30	10	0	90	80	70	50	30	10	0
0.2		40	40	39	38	36	36		31	31	30	29	28	27		21	20	20	20	19	19	17	11	11	11	10	10	09	09	02	02	02	01	01	00	
0.4		41	40	39	38	36	34	34	31	31	30	29	28	26	25	22	21	20	20	19	18	16	12	11	11	11	09	08		04	03	03	02	01	00	
0.6		41	40	39	37	33	32	31	32	31	30	28	26	25	23	23	21	21	19	18	17	15	13	13	12	11	08	08	08	05	05	04	03	02	01	
0.8		41	40	38	36	33	31	29	32	31	30	28	25	23	20	24	22	21	19	18	16	14	15	14	13	11	08	07		07	06	05	04	02	01	
1.0		42	30	38	34	32	29	27	33	32	30	27	24	22	20	25	23	22	19	17	15	13	16	14	13	12	08	07		08	07	06	04	02	01	
1.5		42	39	37	32	28	24	22	34	33	30	25	22	18	17	26	24	22	18	16	13	11	18	16	15	12	10	07	06	11	10	08	06	03	01	
2.0		42	39	36	31	25	21	19	35	33	29	24	20	16	14	28	25	23	18	15	11	09	20	18	16	13	09	06	05	14	12	10	07	04	01	
2.5		43	39	35	29	23	18	15	36	32	29	23	18	14	12	29	26	23	18	14	10	08	22	20	17	13	09	05	04	16	14	12	08	05	02	
3.0		43	39	35	27	21	16	13	37	33	29	22	17	12	10	30	27	23	17	13	09	07	24	21	18	13	09	05	03	18	16	13	09	05	02	
3.5		44	39	34	26	20	14	12	38	33	29	21	15	10	09	32	27	23	17	12	08	05	26	22	19	13	09	05	03	20	17	15	10	05	02	
4.0		44	38	33	25	18	12	10	38	33	28	21	14	09	07	33	28	23	17	10	07	07	27	23	20	14	09	04	02	22	18	15	10	05	02	
5.0		45	38	31	22	15	10	07	39	33	28	19	13	08	05	35	29	24	16	10	06	04	30	25	20	14	08	04	02	25	21	17	11	06	02	
6.0		44	37	30	20	13	08	05	39	33	27	18	11	06	04	36	30	24	16	10	05	03	31	26	21	14	08	03	01	27	23	18	12	06	02	
8.0		44	35	28	18	11	06	03	40	33	26	16	09	04	02	37	30	23	15	08	03	01	33	27	21	13	07	03	01	30	25	20	12	06	02	
10.0		43	34	25	15	08	05	02	40	32	24	14	08	03	01	37	29	22	13	07	03	01	34	28	21	12	07	02	01	31	25	20	12	06	02	

Table 5.3.7

Coefficients of utilization.

COEFFICIENTS OF UTILIZATION

LUMINAIRE	DISTRIBUTION	Spacing Not to Exceed	Ceiling Cavity Walls	80%			50%			10%			0%
				50%	30%	10%	50%	30%	10%	50%	30%	10%	0%
			RCR	Coefficients of Utilization									
Category III Ventilated Dome Reflector	0 ← I → 79	1.3 Mounting Height	1	85	82	79	79	77	75	73	72	71	69
			2	74	69	65	70	66	62	65	62	59	58
			3	65	60	54	62	57	53	57	54	51	49
			4	58	51	46	55	49	45	51	47	44	42
			5	50	44	38	47	42	37	45	40	36	35
			6	44	38	33	43	36	32	40	35	32	30
			7	40	33	28	38	33	28	36	32	27	26
			8	36	29	24	34	28	24	32	27	23	22
			9	33	25	20	31	25	20	29	24	20	18
			10	29	22	18	28	22	18	26	21	18	17
Category I R-52 Filament Reflector Lamp Wide Dist –500- and 750-Watt	0 ← I → 100	1.5 Mounting Height	1	108	105	102	110	99	97	94	93	91	89
			2	98	93	89	93	89	86	88	85	82	80
			3	89	83	78	85	80	76	80	76	73	71
			4	81	74	68	77	72	67	73	69	65	64
			5	73	66	60	70	64	59	66	63	58	56
			6	67	59	53	64	58	52	61	56	52	50
			7	60	52	47	58	51	46	55	50	46	45
			8	54	46	40	52	45	40	49	44	40	38
			9	48	40	35	46	39	35	44	38	34	33
			10	43	36	30	42	35	30	40	34	30	28
Category I R-57 Filament Reflector Lamp Narrow Dist –500- and 750-Watt	0 ← I → 100	6 Mounting Height	1	110	108	105	104	102	100	97	96	95	93
			2	102	98	94	97	94	91	91	89	88	86
			3	95	90	85	91	87	83	86	83	81	79
			4	88	82	78	85	80	76	81	77	75	73
			5	82	76	71	79	74	70	76	72	69	67
			6	77	70	66	74	69	65	72	68	64	63
			7	71	65	61	69	64	60	67	63	60	58
			8	66	60	56	65	59	55	63	58	55	54
			9	62	55	51	60	55	51	59	54	50	49
			10	58	51	47	56	51	47	55	50	46	45

Table 5.3.7 (Continued)

Category III										
Ventilated Porcelain Enamel Low Bay 400-W Phos Coated Vapor Lamp — Mounting Height 12'										
1	81	78	76	76	74	72	71	69	68	67
2	73	69	65	69	66	63	64	62	60	59
3	65	60	56	62	58	55	58	55	53	51
4	59	53	49	56	52	48	53	50	47	45
5	53	47	43	51	46	42	48	44	41	40
6	48	42	38	46	41	37	44	40	37	35
7	43	37	33	41	36	32	39	36	32	31
8	39	33	29	38	32	28	36	32	28	27
9	36	30	26	34	29	25	33	28	25	24
10	32	27	23	31	26	23	30	25	22	21

Category III										
18" Ventilated Alum. High Bay Conc Dist 400-W Clear Vapor Lamp — Mounting Height 7'										
1	93	90	88	85	83	82	76	75	74	72
2	86	82	79	79	77	74	72	70	69	67
3	79	75	71	74	70	68	68	65	64	62
4	74	69	65	69	65	62	64	61	59	57
5	68	63	59	64	60	57	60	57	54	53
6	63	58	54	60	56	52	56	53	50	49
7	58	53	49	56	51	48	52	49	46	45
8	55	49	45	52	47	44	49	45	43	41
9	50	45	41	48	43	40	45	42	39	38
10	47	41	38	45	40	37	42	38	36	35

Category III										
18" Ventilated Alum High Bay Spread Dist 400-W Coated Vapor Lamp — Mounting Height 12'										
1	88	86	84	80	80	77	71	70	69	67
2	81	77	74	75	79	70	67	65	64	62
3	74	70	66	69	72	62	62	60	58	56
4	68	63	59	64	65	57	58	55	53	51
5	63	57	53	59	60	51	54	51	49	47
6	58	52	48	54	55	46	50	47	44	43
7	53	47	43	50	50	42	46	43	40	39
8	48	43	39	46	45	38	42	39	36	35
9	44	39	35	42	41	34	39	35	33	31
10	41	35	31	39	37	30	36	32	28	28

Category III										
24" Ventilated Porcelain Enamel 1000-W Phosphor Coated Vapor Lamp — Mounting Height 13'										
1	86	83	80	78	76	73	68	67	65	63
2	77	72	68	70	66	63	61	59	57	55
3	68	62	57	62	60	55	55	52	49	47
4	61	55	49	56	51	47	50	46	43	41
5	55	48	42	50	45	41	45	41	38	36
6	49	42	37	45	39	35	40	36	33	31
7	43	36	31	40	34	30	36	31	28	26
8	39	32	28	36	30	26	31	28	25	23
9	35	28	24	33	27	23	29	25	22	20
10	32	25	21	29	24	20	26	22	19	17

Table 5.3.7 (Continued)

COEFFICIENTS OF UTILIZATION

LUMINAIRE	DISTRIBUTION	Spacing Not to Exceed	Ceiling Cavity		Reflectances										
			Walls		80%			50%			10%			0%	
			RCR		50%	30%	10%	50%	30%	10%	50%	30%	10%	0%	
					Coefficients of Utilization										
Category III — 55, 90, 135 & 180 Watt Low Pressure Sodium Asymmetrical Reflector	●←|→ 77	3⁺ × Mounting Height	1		80	76	73	75	72	70	69	67	66	64	
			2		69	64	59	65	60	57	60	57	54	52	
			3		59	53	48	56	51	46	52	48	45	43	
			4		52	45	40	49	43	39	46	41	38	36	
			5		46	38	33	43	37	32	40	35	31	30	
			6		40	33	27	38	31	27	35	30	26	25	
			7		35	28	23	33	27	22	31	26	22	20	
			8		31	24	20	30	24	19	28	23	19	17	
			9		28	21	17	27	21	17	25	20	16	15	
			10		26	19	14	24	18	14	23	18	14	13	
Category III — 55, 90, 135 & 180 Watt Low Pressure Sodium Symmetrical Reflector	●←|→ 76	2⁺ × Mounting Height	1		80	77	74	75	73	71	69	68	66	65	
			2		70	66	61	66	63	59	62	59	57	55	
			3		62	56	51	59	54	50	55	51	48	47	
			4		55	49	44	52	47	43	49	45	42	40	
			5		49	42	37	46	41	37	44	39	36	34	
			6		44	37	32	41	36	32	39	34	31	29	
			7		39	32	28	37	31	27	35	30	27	25	
			8		35	29	24	33	28	24	32	27	23	22	
			9		32	25	21	30	25	21	29	24	20	19	
			10		29	22	18	28	22	18	26	21	18	17	
Category III — 24" Ventilated Alum High Bay Dist 1000-W Phos Ctd Vapor Lamp	↖←|→ 72	1.0 × Mounting Height	1		91	88	86	84	82	80	75	74	73	71	
			2		83	78	75	77	73	71	70	67	66	64	
			3		75	69	65	70	65	62	64	61	58	56	
			4		68	62	57	63	58	55	58	55	52	50	
			5		61	55	50	57	52	48	53	49	46	44	
			6		55	49	44	52	47	43	48	44	41	39	
			7		50	43	38	47	41	37	43	39	36	34	
			8		45	39	34	43	37	33	39	35	32	30	
			9		41	34	30	39	33	29	36	32	28	27	
			10		37	31	27	35	30	26	33	28	25	24	

Table 5.3.7 (Continued)

Category III — 24" Ventilated Alum High Bay, 1000-W Phos Coated Vapor Lamp

Spacing: 1.2 ← | → 1.2   Mounting Height: 1.3 × Mounting Height

RCR										
1	90	88	86	81	80	78	71	70	70	67
2	83	79	76	76	73	71	67	66	64	62
3	77	72	68	70	67	64	63	61	59	57
4	71	66	62	66	62	59	59	57	55	53
5	65	60	56	61	57	53	55	52	50	48
6	60	55	50	56	52	48	52	48	46	44
7	55	50	46	52	47	44	48	44	42	40
8	51	45	41	48	43	40	44	41	38	37
9	47	41	38	44	40	37	41	38	35	34
10	44	38	34	41	37	33	38	35	32	31

Category III — 2 T-12 Lamps — Any Loading, For T-10 Lamps — C U × 1.02

Spacing: 1.0 ← | → 1.2   Mounting Height: 1.3 × Mounting Height

RCR										
1	88	84	81	79	77	74	69	68	66	64
2	77	71	66	70	65	62	61	59	56	54
3	68	61	56	61	56	52	54	51	48	46
4	60	52	47	54	49	44	48	44	41	39
5	52	45	39	48	42	37	43	38	35	33
6	47	39	34	43	37	32	38	34	30	28
7	42	34	29	38	32	28	34	30	26	24
8	37	30	25	34	28	24	31	26	22	21
9	33	26	21	31	25	21	28	23	19	18
10	30	23	19	28	22	18	25	20	17	15

Category II — 2 T-12 Lamps — Any Loading, For T-10 Lamps — C U × 1.02

Spacing: 1.2 ← | → 1.1   Mounting Height: 1.3 × Mounting Height

RCR										
1	84	81	78	77	75	73	65	64	62	59
2	75	70	65	68	64	60	57	55	53	50
3	66	60	56	60	55	51	51	48	45	42
4	59	52	47	53	48	43	45	42	38	36
5	52	45	40	46	41	37	40	36	33	30
6	47	40	35	42	36	31	36	31	28	26
7	42	35	30	38	32	27	32	28	24	22
8	38	31	26	34	28	23	29	24	21	19
9	34	27	22	30	25	20	26	21	18	16
10	31	24	20	26	22	18	24	19	16	14

Category II — 2 T-12 Lamps — Any Loading, Center Shield For T-10 Lamps — C U × 1.02

Spacing: 1.0 ← | → 1.3   Mounting Height: 1.3 × Mounting Height

RCR										
1	84	81	78	70	72	70	61	60	59	56
2	75	70	65	59	62	59	55	53	51	48
3	66	60	56	51	54	51	49	47	44	42
4	59	52	47	43	47	43	44	41	38	36
5	52	45	40	37	41	37	39	36	33	31
6	47	40	35	32	36	32	36	32	29	27
7	42	35	30	28	32	28	32	28	25	23
8	38	31	26	24	28	24	29	25	22	20
9	34	27	22	21	25	21	26	22	19	17
10	31	24	20	18	22	18	23	19	17	15

Table 5.3.7 (Continued)

COEFFICIENTS OF UTILIZATION

Category III

3 T-12 Lamps — 430 or 800 MA
For T-10 Lamps — C U · 1.02

Spacing Not to Exceed: 1.3 × Mounting Height

RCR	Reflectances — Coefficients of Utilization									
Ceiling Cavity	80%			50%			10%			0%
Walls	50%	30%	10%	50%	30%	10%	50%	30%	10%	0%
1	86	83	80	78	76	73	69	67	66	64
2	75	70	66	69	65	61	61	58	56	54
3	67	60	55	61	56	52	54	51	48	46
4	59	52	47	54	49	44	48	45	41	39
5	52	45	39	48	42	38	43	39	35	33
6	46	39	34	43	37	32	38	34	30	28
7	41	34	29	38	32	28	34	30	26	25
8	37	30	25	34	28	24	31	26	23	21
9	33	26	22	31	25	21	28	23	20	18
10	30	23	19	28	22	18	25	21	17	16

Category II

3 T-12 Lamps — 430 or 800 MA
For T-10 Lamps — C U · 1.02

Spacing Not to Exceed: 1.3 × Mounting Height

RCR	Reflectances — Coefficients of Utilization									
Ceiling Cavity	80%			50%			10%			0%
Walls	50%	30%	10%	50%	30%	10%	50%	30%	10%	0%
1	85	82	79	76	73	71	64	63	62	59
2	75	70	65	67	63	59	57	55	52	50
3	66	60	55	59	54	50	51	48	45	42
4	59	52	46	52	47	43	45	41	38	36
5	51	44	39	46	40	36	40	36	33	30
6	46	39	33	41	35	31	36	31	28	26
7	41	34	29	37	32	27	32	28	24	23
8	37	30	25	33	27	23	29	24	21	19
9	33	26	21	30	24	20	26	21	18	16
10	30	23	19	27	21	18	23	19	16	14

Category V

2 T-12 Lamps — 430 MA
For 800 MA — C U · .96

Spacing Not to Exceed: 1.5 × Mounting Height

RCR	Reflectances — Coefficients of Utilization									
Ceiling Cavity	80%			50%			10%			0%
Walls	50%	30%	10%	50%	30%	10%	50%	30%	10%	0%
1	70	66	63	62	59	57	52	51	49	47
2	60	54	50	53	49	46	45	42	40	37
3	52	46	41	46	41	38	39	36	33	31
4	46	39	34	41	36	32	35	31	28	26
5	40	33	28	36	30	26	31	27	24	22
6	36	29	24	32	26	22	27	23	20	18
7	32	25	21	29	23	19	25	21	17	16
8	29	22	18	26	20	17	22	18	15	13
9	26	19	15	23	18	14	20	16	13	11
10	23	17	13	21	16	12	18	14	11	10

Table 5.3.7 (Continued)

Category V — 2 T-12 Lamps — 430 MA, Prismatic Lens 1' Wide — For T-10 Lamps — C U · 1 02 (1 2 · Mounting Height)

1	63	61	59	59	58	56	55	54	53	52
2	57	54	51	54	51	49	50	49	47	46
3	51	48	44	49	46	43	46	44	42	41
4	46	42	39	44	41	38	42	39	37	36
5	42	37	34	40	36	34	38	35	33	32
6	38	34	30	37	33	30	35	32	29	28
7	35	30	27	33	29	27	32	29	26	25
8	31	27	24	30	26	23	29	26	23	22
9	28	24	21	27	23	20	26	23	20	19
10	26	21	18	25	21	18	24	20	18	17

Category V — 2 T-12 Lamps — 430 MA, Prismatic Lens 2' Wide — For T-10 Lamps — C U · 1 01 (1 2 · Mounting Height)

1	73	71	68	69	67	66	64	62	61	60
2	66	62	59	62	59	57	58	56	55	53
3	59	55	51	56	53	50	53	50	48	47
4	53	48	45	51	47	44	48	45	43	41
5	48	43	39	46	42	39	44	40	38	36
6	44	38	34	42	37	34	40	36	33	32
7	39	34	30	38	33	30	36	32	30	28
8	36	30	26	34	30	26	33	29	26	25
9	32	27	23	31	26	23	29	25	23	21
10	29	24	20	28	23	20	27	23	20	19

Category V — 55 Watt Low Pressure Sodium Surface Mount Security Fixture (2 · Mounting Height)

1	68	64	60	58	56	53	48	46	44	42
2	58	52	47	50	46	42	41	38	36	33
3	50	44	38	43	38	34	35	32	29	27
4	44	38	32	38	33	29	31	28	25	23
5	39	32	27	34	29	25	28	24	21	19
6	35	28	23	30	25	21	25	21	18	16
7	31	25	20	27	22	18	23	19	16	14
8	28	22	18	25	20	16	21	17	14	12
9	26	20	15	22	18	14	19	15	12	11
10	23	17	14	21	16	12	17	14	11	09

Category V — 55 Watt Low Pressure Sodium 2' · 2' Security Fixture (2 · Mounting Height)

1	66	64	62	62	60	59	57	56	56	54
2	60	56	53	56	54	51	53	51	49	48
3	53	49	46	51	48	45	48	46	44	42
4	49	44	41	46	43	40	44	41	39	38
5	44	39	36	42	38	35	40	37	34	33
6	40	35	31	38	34	31	36	33	30	29
7	36	31	27	34	30	27	33	29	26	25
8	32	27	24	31	27	24	29	26	23	22
9	29	24	21	28	24	21	27	23	21	19
10	26	22	18	25	21	18	24	21	18	17

Table 5.3.7 (Continued)

COEFFICIENTS OF UTILIZATION

LUMINAIRE	DISTRIBUTION	Spacing Not to Exceed	Ceiling Cavity	Reflectances										
				80%			50%			10%			0%	
			Walls	50%	30%	10%	50%	30%	10%	50%	30%	10%	0%	
			RCR	Coefficients of Utilization										
Category V — 4 T-12 Lamps — 430 MA — Prismatic Lens 2' Wide — For T-10 Lamps — C.U. × 1.02		1.2 × Mounting Height	1	66	64	62	62	61	59	58	57	56	55	
			2	60	56	53	56	54	52	53	51	49	48	
			3	54	50	46	51	48	45	48	46	44	43	
			4	49	44	41	46	43	40	44	41	39	38	
			5	44	39	35	42	38	35	40	37	34	33	
			6	40	35	31	38	34	31	36	33	31	29	
			7	36	31	28	35	30	27	33	30	27	26	
			8	32	28	24	31	27	24	30	26	24	23	
			9	29	24	21	28	24	21	27	23	21	20	
			10	27	22	19	26	23	20	25	21	18	17	
Category V — 6 T-12 Lamps — 430 MA — Prismatic Lens 2' Wide — For T-10 Lamps — C.U. × 1.03		1.2 × Mounting Height	1	60	58	56	56	55	54	52	51	50	49	
			2	54	51	48	51	49	47	48	46	45	44	
			3	49	45	42	46	43	41	44	41	40	39	
			4	44	40	37	42	39	36	40	37	35	34	
			5	40	35	32	38	35	32	36	33	31	30	
			6	36	32	29	35	31	28	33	30	28	27	
			7	33	28	25	32	28	25	30	27	25	24	
			8	30	25	22	28	25	22	27	24	22	21	
			9	27	22	19	26	22	19	25	21	19	18	
			10	24	20	17	23	20	17	22	19	17	16	

Table 5.3.7 (Continued)

Category V

8 T-12 Lamps — 430 MA
Prismatic Lens 4' × 4'
For T-10 Lamps — C.U × 1.02

1.3 × Mounting Height

1	59	57	55	55	54	52	51	50	49	48
2	53	50	47	50	48	46	47	45	44	43
3	48	44	41	45	42	40	43	40	39	38
4	43	39	36	41	38	35	39	36	34	33
5	39	35	31	37	34	31	35	32	30	29
6	35	31	28	34	30	28	32	29	27	26
7	32	28	25	31	27	25	29	26	24	23
8	29	25	22	28	24	22	27	24	21	20
9	26	22	19	25	21	19	24	21	19	18
10	24	20	17	23	19	17	22	19	17	16

Category V

4 T-12 Lamps — 430 MA
Prismatic Lens 2' Wide
For T-10 Lamps — C.U × 1.02

1.2 × Mounting Height

1	56	54	52	52	50	49	47	46	45	44
2	50	47	45	47	44	42	43	41	40	39
3	45	41	38	42	39	37	39	37	35	34
4	41	37	34	38	35	32	35	33	31	30
5	37	32	29	34	31	28	32	29	27	26
6	33	29	26	31	28	25	29	27	24	23
7	30	26	23	29	25	22	27	24	22	20
8	27	23	20	26	22	20	24	21	19	18
9	25	20	18	23	20	17	22	19	17	16
10	22	18	16	21	18	15	20	17	15	14

Table 5.3.7 (Continued)

COEFFICIENTS OF UTILIZATION

Luminaire: Category V — 2 T-12 Lamps — 430 MA, 1' Wide Prismatic Wrap-Around
Spacing Not to Exceed: 1.2 Mounting Height

	Reflectances									
Ceiling Cavity	80%			70%			50%			0%
Walls	50%	30%	10%	50%	30%	10%	50%	30%	10%	0%
RCR				Coefficients of Utilization						
1	68	65	63	65	63	61	61	60	58	
2	60	56	53	58	55	52	55	52	49	
3	54	49	45	52	48	45	50	46	43	
4	49	43	40	47	43	39	45	41	38	
5	44	38	34	43	38	34	40	36	33	
6	40	34	30	39	34	30	37	32	29	
7	36	31	27	35	30	26	33	29	26	
8	32	27	24	32	27	23	30	26	23	
9	29	24	21	29	24	20	27	23	20	
10	27	22	18	26	21	18	25	21	18	

Luminaire: Category V — 4 T-12 Lamps — 430 MA, 2' Wide Prismatic Wrap-Around
Spacing Not to Exceed: 1.3 Mounting Height

	Reflectances									
Ceiling Cavity	80%			70%			50%			0%
Walls	50%	30%	10%	50%	30%	10%	50%	30%	10%	0%
RCR				Coefficients of Utilization						
1	66	64	61	64	62	60	61	59	57	
2	59	55	52	57	54	51	55	52	49	
3	53	48	45	52	48	44	49	46	43	
4	48	43	39	47	42	39	45	41	38	
5	43	38	34	42	37	34	40	36	33	
6	39	34	30	38	34	30	36	32	29	
7	35	30	26	34	30	26	33	29	26	
8	32	27	23	31	26	23	30	26	23	
9	28	24	20	28	23	20	27	23	20	
10	26	21	18	25	21	18	25	20	17	

Luminaire: Category I — 2 Lamp Strip — Any Loading
Spacing Not to Exceed: 1.6 Mounting Height

	Reflectances									
Ceiling Cavity	80%			70%			50%			0%
Walls	50%	30%	10%	50%	30%	10%	50%	30%	10%	0%
RCR				Coefficients of Utilization						
1	83	79	75	79	76	72	73	70	67	
2	71	65	60	68	62	57	62	58	54	
3	62	55	49	59	53	47	53	49	44	
4	55	47	41	52	45	39	48	42	37	
5	48	40	34	46	38	33	42	36	31	
6	43	35	29	41	33	28	38	31	26	
7	38	30	25	36	29	24	34	27	23	
8	34	26	21	33	25	21	30	24	19	
9	30	23	18	30	23	18	27	21	17	
10	28	21	16	27	20	15	25	19	15	

Table 5.3.7 (Continued)

Category	Distribution	Mounting	No.								
Category V — 1 Lamp – Any Loading, 2' Wide, 1' Deep Prismatic Lens		12' Mounting Height	1	.64	.62	.60	.63	.61	.59	.60	.59	.57
			2	.58	.55	.52	.57	.54	.51	.55	.52	.50
			3	.52	.48	.45	.51	.47	.44	.49	.46	.44
			4	.47	.42	.39	.46	.42	.39	.45	.41	.38
			5	.42	.37	.34	.42	.37	.34	.40	.36	.34
			6	.38	.33	.30	.38	.33	.30	.37	.32	.30
			7	.35	.30	.26	.34	.30	.26	.33	.29	.26
			8	.31	.26	.23	.31	.26	.23	.30	.26	.23
			9	.28	.23	.20	.28	.23	.20	.27	.23	.20
			10	.26	.21	.18	.25	.21	.18	.25	.21	.18

Category	Distribution	Mounting	No.								
Category VI — 2 Lamp — Any Loading, Opaque Sides		1.5' Mounting Height	1	.68	.65	.62	.59	.56	.54	.42	.41	.39
			2	.59	.54	.51	.51	.48	.44	.37	.35	.32
			3	.52	.46	.42	.45	.40	.37	.32	.29	.27
			4	.46	.40	.35	.40	.35	.31	.28	.25	.23
			5	.40	.34	.30	.35	.30	.26	.25	.22	.20
			6	.36	.30	.26	.31	.27	.23	.22	.20	.17
			7	.32	.26	.22	.28	.23	.19	.20	.17	.14
			8	.29	.23	.19	.25	.20	.17	.18	.15	.13
			9	.26	.20	.17	.23	.18	.15	.17	.13	.11
			10	.24	.18	.15	.21	.16	.13	.15	.12	.10

Category	Distribution	Mounting	No.								
Category VI		1.5 to 2.0' Mounting Height above Diffuser	1	For cavities that are painted white use 70% effective ceiling cavity reflectance			.60	.58	.56	.58	.56	.54
			2				.53	.49	.45	.51	.47	.43
			3				.47	.42	.37	.45	.41	.36
			4				.41	.36	.32	.39	.35	.31
			5	For cavities that are obstructed or have lower reflectances use 50% effective ceiling cavity reflectance			.37	.31	.27	.35	.30	.26
			6				.33	.27	.23	.31	.26	.23
			7				.29	.24	.20	.28	.23	.20
			8				.26	.21	.18	.25	.20	.17
			9				.23	.19	.15	.23	.18	.15
			10				.21	.17	.13	.21	.16	.13

Luminous Ceiling — 50% Transmission, 80% Cavity Reflectance

Category	Distribution	Description	No.								
Category VI		Cove 12 to 18 inches below ceiling. Reflectors with fluorescent lamps increase coefficients of utilization 5 to 10%. Cove Without Reflector	1	.42	.40	.39	.36	.35	.33	.25	.24	.23
			2	.37	.34	.32	.32	.29	.27	.22	.20	.19
			3	.32	.29	.26	.28	.25	.23	.19	.17	.16
			4	.29	.25	.22	.25	.22	.19	.17	.15	.13
			5	.25	.21	.18	.22	.19	.16	.15	.13	.11
			6	.23	.19	.16	.20	.16	.14	.14	.12	.10
			7	.20	.17	.14	.17	.14	.12	.12	.10	.09
			8	.18	.15	.12	.16	.13	.10	.11	.09	.08
			9	.17	.13	.10	.15	.11	.09	.10	.08	.07
			10	.15	.12	.09	.13	.10	.08	.09	.07	.06

By permission of North American Philips Lighting Corporation.

NOTE: The coefficients of utilization determined in the examples presented will be applicable for areas having 20 percent floor-cavity reflectance. If the actual floor-cavity reflectance differs substantially from 20 percent, a correction may be necessary depending upon the accuracy desired. Correction factors for floor-cavity reflectance of 10 percent and 30 percent are given in Table 5.3.8. The effective floor-cavity reflectance is determined in the same manner and using the same tables as were used in determining effective ceiling-cavity reflectance. For 30 percent effective floor-cavity reflectance, multiply by the appropriate factor found in the table. For 10 percent effective floor-cavity reflectance, divide by the appropriate factor found in the table.

In the calculations included in this chapter, correction will not be made for floor-cavity reflectance. The floor-cavity reflectance will be assumed to be 20 percent. However, you should be aware that such adjustments can and should be made, depending upon the accuracy required.

Table 5.3.8

Correction factor for effective floor-cavity reflectances other than 20 percent.

Room-Cavity Ratio	Percent Effective Ceiling-Cavity Reflectance											
	80			70			50			10		
	Percent Wall Reflectance											
	50	30	10	50	30	10	50	30	10	50	30	10
1	1.08	1.08	1.07	1.07	1.06	1.06	1.05	1.04	1.04	1.01	1.01	1.01
2	1.07	1.06	1.05	1.06	1.05	1.04	1.04	1.03	1.03	1.01	1.01	1.01
3	1.05	1.04	1.03	1.05	1.04	1.03	1.03	1.03	1.02	1.01	1.01	1.01
4	1.05	1.03	1.02	1.04	1.03	1.02	1.03	1.02	1.02	1.01	1.01	1.00
5	1.04	1.03	1.02	1.03	1.02	1.02	1.02	1.02	1.01	1.01	1.01	1.00
6	1.03	1.02	1.01	1.03	1.02	1.01	1.02	1.02	1.01	1.01	1.01	1.00
7	1.03	1.02	1.01	1.03	1.02	1.01	1.02	1.01	1.01	1.01	1.01	1.00
8	1.03	1.02	1.01	1.02	1.02	1.01	1.02	1.01	1.01	1.01	1.01	1.00
9	1.02	1.01	1.01	1.02	1.01	1.01	1.02	1.01	1.01	1.01	1.01	1.00
10	1.02	1.01	1.01	1.02	1.01	1.01	1.02	1.01	1.01	1.01	1.01	1.00

Source: Westinghouse Lighting Handbook

The Light Loss Factor

The other factor in the formula that needs to be explained is the light loss factor.

From the day the new lighting is energized, the illumination is in the process of continually changing as the lamp ages, as the luminaire accumulate dirt and dust, and as the effect of other contributing factors is felt. Some contributing loss factors may, in some instances, tend to increase the illumination; but their net effect is nearly always to cause a decrease in illumination. The final light loss factor is the product of all contributing loss factors; it is the ratio of the illumination when it reaches its lowest level at the task just before corrective action is taken to the initial level if none of the contributing loss factors were considered. In this context, the initial illumination is that which would be produced by lamps producing initially rated lumens. (NOTE: Lamp manufacturers rate filament lamps in accordance with lumen output when the lamp is new. Vapor discharge lamps, including fluorescent, mercury and other common types, are rated in accordanc with their output after 100 hours of burning.)

There are eight contributing loss factors that must be considered. Some of these must be estimated; others can be evaluated on the basis of extensive test data or published information. Of the eight factors, only four factors can be obtained from published information. The remaining four factors have to be estimated. Only the four common factors that can be located in test data or by manufacturers' published data will be discussed here. These four factors will be considered the only four factors contributing to the light loss factor.

1. <u>Ballast performance</u>. Fluorescent lamps as well as some other lamps include a ballast which serves as (1) an autotransformer to step up supply voltage (e.g., 120, 208, 240, 277, etc. volts) to the necessary starting valu (e.g., 255 or 500 volts) and (2) a choke to limit the current through the lamp. Ballast consists of a core and coil which stabilize the operation of the lamps; a power capacitor which corrects the power factor and reduces the load on the electrical distribution system; a radio interference-suppressing capacitor which reduces feedback of radio frequency energy to the power line; and a compound which fills all voids inside the ballast case, improving heat dissipation and reducing sound.

The Certified Ballast Manufacturers (CBM) Association specification for fluorescent lamps requires the ballast to operate a fluorescent lamp at 95 percent of the output of the lamp when operated on a reference ballast. A reference ballast is the laboratory standard used by lamp manufacturers in establishing lamp ratings. For ballast bearing the CBM label, use a factor o 0.95. For ballast not bearing the CBM label, lumen output is usually lower. Lamp life is also usually shortened. Consult with the ballast manufacturer for this light loss factor

2. <u>Luminaire reflectance and transmission changes</u>. This effect is usually small but may be significant over a long period of time for luminaires with inferior finishes or plastic. Comprehensive data are usually not available.

3. Lamp lumen depreciation. The gradual reduction in lumen output of a lamp as it burns through life is more rapid for some lamps than for other lamps. The contributing light loss factor for fluorescent lamps is usually expressed as a ratio of the lumen output of the lamp at 70 percent of rated life to the initial (100) hour value. Since the life is influenced by burning hours per start, the contributing loss factor is usually expressed as a function of burning hours per start, even though it is actually a function of lamp burning hours. The lamp lumen depreciation for fluorescent filament and mercury lamps can usually be found in manufacturers' data. As an example, Table 5.3.9 is a listing of fluorescent lamps.

Table 5.3.9

Fluorescent lamp data.

Lamp Ordering Abbreviation [1]	Approx. Watts	Base	Lamp Lumen Depreciation (LLD) [2]			Rated Initial Lumens [3]
			Hours per Start			
			6	12	18	
Pre-Heat-Rap. St.						
F40CW	40	Med Bipin	88	87	86	3150
F40T10/CW/99	40	Med Bipin	86	84	83	3200
FB40CW/6	40	Med Bipin	85	83	81	2950
Slimline						
F48T12/CW	38 5	Single Pin	88	87	86	3000
F72T12/CW	56	Single Pin	88	87	86	4550
F96T12/CW	73 5	Single Pin	88	87	86	6300
High Output						
F48T12 CW HO	60	Rec D C	85	84	83	4200
F72T12/CW/HO	85	Rec D C	85	84	83	6650
F96T12/CW/HO	110	Rec D C	85	84	83	9000
Very High Output						
F48T12/CW/VHO	110	Rec D C	80	79	78	6900
F72T12 CW/VHO	160	Rec D C	80	79	78	11.100
F96T12/CW/VHO	215	Rec D C	80	79	78	15.500
F96T12 CW/VHOII	215	Rec D C	80	79	78	15.500

[1] For Standard Cool White lamp Other colors must have proper designations
[2] Lamp Lumen Depreciation values apply to Standard Cool White Standard Warm White and White lamps at 70% of rated life
[3] Values apply to Standard Cool White For other colors multiply by the following factors White and Standard Warm White. 1 04. Daylight. 86. Cool Green. 92. Warm White Deluxe and Cool White Deluxe. 75

Using Table 5.3.9, it is found that a fluorescent lamp--a high-output lamp F96T12/CW/HO--would have a lamp lumen depreciation of 0.85 if it burns six hours per start; 0.84 if it burns 12 hours per start; and 0.83 if it burns 18 hours per start.

4. Luminaire dirt depreciation.   This factor varies with the type of luminaire and the atmosphere in which it is operating. Luminaires are divided into six categories. The category for each luminaire has its own set of dirt depreciation curves. The dirt depreciation curves are as follows:

Figure 5.3.4

Dirt depreciation.

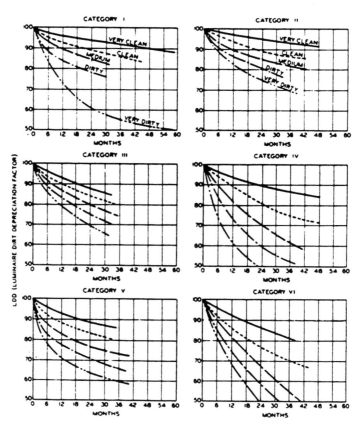

By permisssion of North American Philips Lighting Corporation.

After determining the category, the luminaire dirt depreciation factor can be read from one of the five curves for each category. The point on the curve should be selected on the basis of the number of months between cleaning the luminaires. The particular curve selected should be based on dirt content and atmosphere. For example, in category II, if cleaning were every 24 months and the conditions were very dirty, the luminaire dirt depreciation factor would be about 0.75.

The total light loss factor is determined by multiplying the separate four factors together. For example, if a lamp had a ballast performance of 0.95, luminaire reflectance of 0.98, lamp lumen depreciation of 0.85, and luminaire dirt depreciation of 0.70, the combined light loss factor would be 0.55.

Using the Formula. Recall that the formula for the number of lamps is as follows:

$$\text{Number of lamps} = \frac{\text{Foot-candles x area}}{\text{Lumens per lamp x coefficient of utilization x light loss factor}}$$

where the number of luminaires is as follows:

$$\text{Number of luminaires} = \frac{\text{Number of lamps}}{\text{Lamps per luminaire}}$$

Problem. Assume a small office 20 feet by 40 feet with 12.5 foot ceilings is to be illuminated for regular office work. The reflectance of the ceiling is 80% (actual reflectance, not effective reflectance), and reflectance of the walls is 50%. The luminaires will be installed 2 feet from the ceiling, and the work plane is 2.5 feet from the floor. The luminaires will have opaque sides and are category VI lamps. Assume that the environment will be considered clean and that the luminaires will be cleaned every 12 months. The ballast will meet the requirements of the Certified Ballast Manufacturers. From this information, compute the number of lamps and the number of luminaires that will be needed to provide a sufficient quantity of light.

Solution. The first task is to determine the number of foot-candles that are recommended for regular office work. According to "Recommended Levels of Illumination," published by the Illuminating Engineering Society, regular office work requires a minimum of 100 foot-candles.

The second step is to determine the coefficient of utilization. To do this, the room-cavity ratio and the ceiling-cavity ratio must be computed. The room-cavity ratio would be

$$\text{Room-cavity ratio} = \frac{10h}{\text{room width}} \times \text{Gaysunas ratio}$$

Using 8 feet for h and a Gaysunas ratio of 3/4, the room-cavity ratio is 3.0. (If the table is used to compute the room-cavity ratio, the room-cavity ratio from the table is 2.9 with an 8-foot cavity depth.)

The ceiling-cavity ratio is computed as follows:

$$\text{Ceiling-cavity ratio} = \frac{10 \times 2 \text{ ft}}{20} \quad (3/4)$$

$$= 0.75$$

Using the room-cavity ratio and the ceiling-cavity ratio, the effective cavity reflectance of the ceiling can be found using the Effective Cavity Reflectance Table, Table 5.3.6. The table shows that for an 80% base (actual ceiling) and a 50% wall reflectance, the cavity reflectance is between 69% for 0.8 cavity ratio and 71% for 0.6 cavity ratio; so for this room, the ceiling-cavity reflectance is approximately 70%. Using the effective ceiling reflectance as 70% and the wall reflectance of 50%, use the Coefficient of Utilization Tables (Table 5.3.7) to look up the coefficient of utilization. This is done by finding the luminaire that is in category VI with a 75% distribution of light hitting the ceiling for a room-cavity ratio of 3.0, a ceiling effective cavity reflectance of 70% and a wall reflectance of 50%. The coefficient of utilization is then 0.45.

The next step is to determine the light loss factor. The first consideration in determining the light loss factor is the ballast performance. Although the ballast performance is not indicated in the data given, it has a CBM label, so assume the ballast performance is 0.95. The second factor to consider in computing the light loss factor is the luminance reflectance and transmission changes which were not given. Assume that to be about 0.98. Next, consider the lamp lumen depreciation. Assume that the luminaire takes a F96T12/CW/HO lamp that will burn 12 hours per start. Using the lamp data for fluorescent lamps, Table 5.3.9, the lamp lumen depreciation factor would be 0.84. The next factor to consider is the dirt depreciation factor. This can be computed from the appropriate dirt depreciation curves. For a category VI lamp for a 12 month replacement, it would be around 0.86 under the clean condition. This means that the total light loss factor would be

$$0.95 \times 0.98 \times 0.84 \times 0.86 = 0.67$$

The next thing needed in order to use the formula is the lumens per lamp. This can be found using the lamp data provided in the lamp data table (Table 5.3.9). For F96T12/CW/HO lamp, the rated initial lumens is 9000. Substituting these values in the basic formula gives

$$\text{Number of lamps} = \frac{\text{Foot-candles} \times \text{area}}{\text{Lumens per lamp} \times \text{coefficient of utilization} \times \text{light loss factor}}$$

$$\text{Number of lamps} = \frac{100 \text{ foot-candles} \times 20 \text{ ft} \times 40 \text{ ft}}{9000 \text{ lumens} \times 0.45 \times 0.67}$$

$$= 29.48 \text{ lamps or 30 lamps}$$

The number of luminaires can be computed using the following formula:

$$\text{Number of luminaires} = \frac{\text{Number of lamps}}{\text{Number of lamps per luminaire}}$$

Substituting in the equation gives approximately 15 luminaires (use 14). Fourteen 2-lamp luminaires can be installed in seven rows of two luminaires mounted crosswise in the room. Ordinarily, it is preferable for the luminaires to be mounted so that the lowest candlepower is projected in the direction of most of the workers in the area. This may require that some luminaires be mounted parallel to the line of sight of most workers. Other luminaires should be mounted perpendicular to the line of sight. This particular luminaire has low candlepower from all viewing directions, but it does tend to create a high ceiling brightness. However, the bright ceiling is shielded from view by the luminaires if they are mounted perpendicular to the line of sight. Since in this room the predominant line of sight is most likely to be parallel to the length of the room, it is suggested that the luminaires by mounted perpendicular to the room length.

Summary of Steps Involved in Computing Lumen Method

Step 1. Determine the required level of illumination using the recommenations of the Illuminating Engineering Society.

Step 2. Determine type of luminaire.

   a.   Distribution
   b.   Category
   c.   Lumens
   d.   Lamp lumen depreciation
   e.   When replaced
   f.   Environmental conditions

Step 3. Determine coefficient of utilization

   a.   Compute room-cavity ratio.
   b.   Compute ceiling-cavity ratio.
   c.   Compute floor-cavity ratio.

   NOTE: Use either

$$\frac{5h \ (\text{room length} + \text{room width})}{\text{room length x room width}}$$

   or

$$\frac{10h}{\text{room width}} \ \text{x Gaysunas ratio}$$

   d.   Determine effective cavity reflectances using Effective Cavity Reflectances Table.

Compute ceiling-cavity reflectance
(If floor-cavity reflectance other than 20%, use correction table.)

NOTE: Compute floor-cavity reflectance same as room-cavity
reflectance to determine if less than 20%.

e.   Use effective ceiling-cavity reflectance, room-cavity reflectance
wall reflectance, and look up coefficient of utilization in table
for selected luminaire.

Step 4.   Determine light loss factor (LLF).

a.   Ballast performance (0.95 if certified ballast) = _____
b.   Luminaire reflectance and transmission changes = _____
c.   Lamp lumen depreciation = _____
d.   Luminaire dirt depreciation (determined from LLD curves) = _____
e.   LLF - a x b x c x d = _____

Step 5.   Use formula.

$$\text{Number of lamps} = \frac{\text{Foot-candles x area}}{\text{Lumens per lamp x coefficient of utilization x light loss factor}}$$

NOTE: Coefficient of utilization was computed in Step 3. Light loss
factor computed in Step 4.

Step 6.   Determine number of luminaires.

Step 7.   Determine layout.

a.   Spacing not to exceed (see Coefficient of Utilization Table).
b.   Draw layout.

4. References

Baumeister, Theodore, ed. Mark's Standard Handbook for Mechanical Engineers,
7th ed. New York: McGraw-Hill Book Company, 1967.

Hewitt, Paul G. Conceptual Physics . . . A New Introduction to Your
Environment. Boston: Little, Brown, and Company, 1974.

North American Philips Lighting Corporation, Lighting Handbook. Bloomfield.
NJ: North American Philips Lighting Corporation, 1984.

Patty, Frank A. Industrial Hygiene and Toxicology, 2d ed., 2 vol. New York:
Interscience Publishers, Inc., 1958.

Trippens, Paul E. Applied Physics. New York: McGraw-Hill Book Company, 1973.

U. S. Department of Health, Education and Welfare, Public Health Service.
Center for Disease Control, National Institute for Occupational Safety
and Health. Recognition of Occupational Health Hazards, Student Manual,
1974.

___. The Industrial Environment: Its Evaluation and Control.
Washington: U. S. Government Printing Office, 1973.

Westinghouse Electric Corporation, Lighting Handbook. Bloomingfield, NJ:
Westinghouse Electric Corporation, Lamp Division, 1974.

Section 6

Radiation

1. Principles of Nonionizing Radiation

Introduction

   In prior chapters, the principles of visible radiation (light) have been discussed. As discussed, light has characteristics of both wave and particles, and a light wave is energy released from a de-excitation of an orbital electron. Further, energy released is in discrete units or quanta of energy referred to as photons. Each wave in the visible spectrum has a characteristic wavelength, frequency, and photon energy. These characteristics can be correlated by using the following formula:

$$C = f\lambda$$
   where
       $3 \times 10^8 \, m/sec$
       C = the speed of light (3×10^{10} cm/sec)
       f = the frequency of oscillation per second
       λ = the wavelength (centimeters)
and by the equation
       $E = hf$
   where
       E = the photon energy (joules)
       h = Planck's constant (6.624×10^{-34} joule-seconds)
       f = the frequency of oscillation per second (Hz)

The importance of the visible radiation is that the eye is sensitive to this specific range of the electromagnetic spectrum.

   To expand on this, all ranges of the electromagnetic spectrum are fundamentally the same in that they are produced by moving electrical charges. Where light is produced by the movement of electrons, other ranges of electromagnetic radiation are formed by the movement of molecules, electrons, neutrons, etc. All of these radiations have the same basic properties as visible radiation, and all are referred to as "electromagnetic radiation."

Radiation--Overview

   Radiation is the emission of particles or energy in wave form. Radiation varies in wavelength and frequency. The electromagnetic spectrum is divided into regions, depending upon the wavelength and frequency of the radiation being discussed. Figure 6.1.1 illustrates the electromagnetic spectrum and shows the various regions that will be discussed. Specifically, the discussion will emphasize radio frequencies, microwaves, infrared, ultraviolet, X-radiation, and gamma radiation. The upper region (shorter wavelength) is of particular concern to the physicist and scientist who describe radiation in terms of wavelength (angstrom, centimeters, microns, millimeters, and nanometers). The lower region (longer wavelengths) has been explored by the communications scientists and engineers, who prefer to describe electromagnetic radiation in terms of frequency (Hertz, megahertz, cycles, kilocycles, megacycles, and gigacycles).

Units of Measure. Before discussing each of the regions of the electromagnetic spectrum, it is appropriate to review the units of measure that are used. The wavelength is the distance from peak to peak of a wave and is usually expressed in centimeters. The frequency refers to the number of oscillations per second, usually expressed in Hertz (Hz) or cycles per second as presented in Table 6.1.1.

Table 6.1.1

Physical units.

Unit	Symbol	Equivalent
Wavelength		
centimeter	cm	1 cm
micrometer	μm	10^{-4} cm
nanometer	nm	10^{-7} cm
angstrom	A	10^{-8} cm
Frequency		
hertz	Hz	1 cps
cycles per second	cps	1 cps
kilocycle	kc	1000 cps
megacycle	Mc	10^6 cps
gigacycle	Gc	10^9 cps

The energy of electromagnetic radiation is expressed in terms of joules or electron volts. A joule is the work done when a constant force of one newton moves a body one meter. An electron volt is the energy acquired by an electron as it passes through a potential difference of one volt. To relate the two units, one electron volt (eV) is equal to 1.602×10^{-19} joules. If the energy is expressed over a given area, the energy density is being considered. Finally, power of electromagnetic radiation refers to an energy over time, usually expressed in watts (W).

Radiation also exists that is not electromagnetic in nature but is made up of particles. This type of radiation is formed from radioactive decay or nuclear reactions. The particles possess the high energy necessary to cause radiation. This particular radiation (alpha, beta, neutrons) will be discussed in later chapters.

Figure 6.1.1

The electromagnetic spectrum.

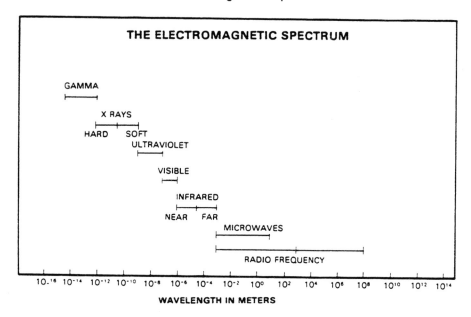

Often unit prefixes (Table 6.1.2) are used to express the magnitude of the unit; e.g., 1 μm = 1 x 10^{-4} cm.

Table 6.1.2

Table of unit prefixes.

Multiples and Submultiples	Prefix	Symbols
1,000,000,000,000 = 10^{12}	tera-	T
1,000,000,000 = 10^{9}	giga-	G
1,000,000 = 10^{6}	mega-	M
1,000 = 10^{3}	kilo-	k
100 = 10^{2}	hecto-	h
10 = 10	deka-	da
0.1 = 10^{-1}	deci-	d
.01 = 10^{-2}	centi-	c
.001 = 10^{-3}	milli-	m
.000001 = 10^{-6}	micro-	μ
.000000001 = 10^{-9}	nano-	n
.000000000001 = 10^{-12}	pico-	p

Radiation can be divided into two types: ionizing and nonionizing. The difference between the two types of radiation is based upon the energy level of the radiation. <u>Ionization</u> is defined as the removal of electrons from an atom forming both a positive and negative ion. <u>Nonionization</u>, then, will refer to energy available in sufficient quantity to excite atoms or electrons but not sufficient to remove electrons from their orbitals. It is known that approximately 10 electron volts (eV) is required to cause ionization of an oxygen or hydrogen molecule. With 10 electron volts as a lower limit for ionizing energy level, the equations

$$E = hf$$
and
$$C = f\lambda$$

can determine the minimum wavelength which would have sufficient energy to cause ionization.

$$E = hf$$
$$C = f\lambda$$

$$E = \frac{Ch}{\lambda}$$

or

$$\lambda = \frac{hC}{E}$$

then

$$h = 6.602 \times 10^{-34} \text{ joule-sec}$$
$$C = 3.0 \times 10^{10} \text{ cm/sec}$$
$$E = 10 \text{ eV} \times 1.602 \times 10^{-19} \text{ joules/eV}$$

$$\lambda = \frac{(6.602 \times 10^{-34} \text{ J-sec})(3.0 \times 10^{10} \text{ cm/sec})}{(10 \text{ eV})(1.602 \times 10^{-19} \text{ J/eV})}$$

$$\lambda = 1.24 \times 10^{-5} \text{ cm}$$

Therefore, electromagnetic radiation with a wavelength greater than 1.24 x 10^{-5} centimeters will not cause ionization and will be classified as nonionizing radiation. This will include the areas of the spectrum as follows: ultraviolet, visible, infrared, and radio frequencies.

Nonionizing Radiation--General

Nonionizing radiation is defined as radiation with sufficient energy to cause excitation of electrons, atoms, or molecules, but insufficient energy to cause the formation of ions (ionization).

Electromagnetic radiation is caused by the movement of charges and is association with a vibrating electrical field with accompanying magnetic field. The waves vary with proportional wavelength, frequency, and intensity. The radiation can act as discrete particles (quanta of energy), but they also have basic wave properties. It should be noted that there are no distinct dividing lines between regions on the electromagnetic spectrum. The regions that have been identified are arbitrarily established based upon general properties, but the distinction in region is not finite.

Nonionizing radiation comes from a variety of sources. The emission of electromagnetic radiation may be designed, as in a microwave oven unit or radio transmitter antenna. Or, the nonionizing radiation may be an unwanted byproduct such as the formation of infrared radiation in arc welding or in the processing of molten metal. The production of nonionizing electromagnetic radiation varies according to the frequency of the radiation. For example, radio frequencies are formed from the oscillation of electric current; infrared radiation is emitted from heated bodies and reflects the rotational movement of atoms; and visible radiation is the electron transition between energy levels. Specific sources of each type of nonionizing radiation will be discussed further in later chapters.

Even though nonionizing radiation does not cause the formation of ions, excessive levels of nonionizing radiation do present a potential health hazard in the working environment. The eye is the most sensitive organ to electromagnetic radiation injury; however, it is not equally sensitive to all wavelengths. Figure 6.1.2 illustrates the sensitivity of the eye to the various wavelengths. Even though it is not equally sensitive to all wavelengths of electromagnetic radiation, it can be a good indicator of exposure because of its sensitivity.

Nonionizing radiation will affect other parts of the body through different means. For example, if the body absorbs nonionizing radiation, it will potentially have a thermal effect and cause heating of the tissue. It is also possible for nonionizing radiation to have a photochemical effect; i.e., chemical changes in the body caused by the radiation. An example of this would be the development of pigment in the skin from exposure to ultraviolet radiation; i.e., a suntan. It has also been shown that excessive exposure to ultraviolet radiation may catalyze or stimulate growth of carcinogenic cells (cancer).

Nonionizing Radiation--Specific Regions

This section of the chapter deals with the characteristics, sources, biological effects, and permissible exposure limit values for ultraviolet, infrared, and radio frequency regions of the electromagnetic spectrum. In this and other discussions of permissible exposure limit values it must be noted that such recommended or mandatory values change with time. Therefore, when faced with practical problems, the industrial hygiene engineer must consult current references to obtain up-to-date values of concern. Because of their wide use, the region of microwaves will be dealt with specifically, and the use of lasers will also be presented.

Ultraviolet Region. The ultraviolet region is the highest energy of the nonionizing radiation group. It is normally divided into three segments.

Figure 6.1.2

Eye sensitivity.

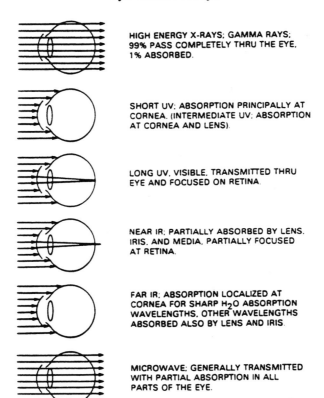

HIGH ENERGY X-RAYS; GAMMA RAYS;
99% PASS COMPLETELY THRU THE EYE.
1% ABSORBED.

SHORT UV; ABSORPTION PRINCIPALLY AT
CORNEA. (INTERMEDIATE UV; ABSORPTION
AT CORNEA AND LENS).

LONG UV, VISIBLE, TRANSMITTED THRU
EYE AND FOCUSED ON RETINA.

NEAR IR; PARTIALLY ABSORBED BY LENS.
IRIS, AND MEDIA, PARTIALLY FOCUSED
AT RETINA.

FAR IR; ABSORPTION LOCALIZED AT
CORNEA FOR SHARP H_2O ABSORPTION
WAVELENGTHS, OTHER WAVELENGTHS
ABSORBED ALSO BY LENS AND IRIS.

MICROWAVE; GENERALLY TRANSMITTED
WITH PARTIAL ABSORPTION IN ALL
PARTS OF THE EYE.

1. Vacuum--This region is representative of ultraviolet radiation with wavelengths of less than 160 nanometers. Because it is completely absorbed by air, vacuum ultraviolet radiation can only exist in a vacuum.

2. Far--This region of ultraviolet radiation represents the region with a wavelength of 120 to 320 nanometers. Radiation with wavelengths < 220 nanometers is poorly transmitted through air. Radiation above 200 nanometers is absorbed by the atmospheric ozone layer.

3. Near--The final region is that which extends from 320 to 400 nanometers. This region transmits through air but only partially through glass. Figure 6.1.3 illustrates the ultraviolet spectrum as discussed.

The most critical range is between 240-320 nanometers (actinic region) because ultraviolet has the higher biological effect in this range.

Figure 6.1.3

UV spectrum.

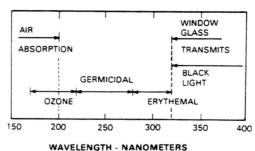

WAVELENGTH - NANOMETERS

The primary source of ultraviolet radiation is the sun. Ultraviolet radiation is also emitted from incandescent or fluorescent lighting sources, welding operations, plasma torches, and laser operations. Typically, solar radiation on a midsummer day in the temperate latitudes causes a daily ultraviolet exposure (λ less than 400 nanometers) equal to approximately 2×10^{-3} J/cm^2. Of that, only 10^{-5} J/cm^2 is reasonably effective. (This concept will be further explained.)

Ultraviolet radiation has a number of uses because of its various properties. The most common application of ultraviolet radiation is in the production of visible light from fluorescent lamps. The fluorescent lamp bulb consists of a phosphor-coated glass tube that contains a small amount of mercury vapor. An electrical discharge travels through the mercury vapor in the tube, generating ultraviolet radiation. The ultraviolet radiation is absorbed by the phosphor coating on the inside of the tube, causing the phosphor to fluoresce. This fluorescence produces longer electromagnetic wavelengths (visible) energy. Because the ultraviolet radiation is absorbed by the phosphor coating, incandescent and fluorescent lamps used for general lighting purposes emit little or no ultraviolet radiation and are generally not considered as a potential hazard.

Because of basic absorption properties of ultraviolet radiation with respect to certain bacteria and molds, ultraviolet radiation has been used as a germicide. In Figure 6.1.4, the absorption properties of ultraviolet in E. coli are illustrated. Because of this, ultraviolet has been used in the prevention and cure of rickets, killing of bacteria and molds, and for other therapeutic effects.

The "black light" properties of ultraviolet radiation have found use in industry in such things as blueprinting, laundry mark identification, and dial illumination of instrument panels. These applications generally are based on the same principle of fluorescence as described for fluorescent light. A substance (laundry marking) that is not visible to the eye in the presence of visible light, when exposed to ultraviolet radiation, will fluoresce, producing visible energy which then can be seen.

Figure 6.1.4

UV action spectra.

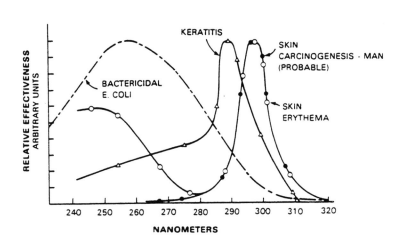

The most common exposure to ultraviolet radiation is from the sun. Persons continually working in the sunlight are continuously exposed to ultraviolet radiation and may develop tumors. Electric welding lamps and germicidal lamps are the most common source of ultraviolet radiation aside from the sun.

The primary biological effect of ultraviolet radiation is upon the skin and eyes. If the skin absorbs an adequate amount of ultraviolet radiation, the skin will redden (erythema). Different wavelengths of ultraviolet radiation have different effects. The general range of ultraviolet radiation that will cause erythema (skin reddening, blisters) is from 240 to 320 nanometers. The maximum effect is at a wavelength of 296.7 nanometers with a secondary peak effect at 250 nanometers. This is also illustrated in Figure 6.1.4 in what is known as the standard erythemal curve, indicated by the skin erythema scale.

The signs and symptoms that may be observed are dependent upon the dose received. Minimal dose may cause simple reddening, where a moderate dose may cause the formation of blisters or even peeling of skin (disquamation). The time required for the onset of symptoms is also dependent upon the dosage. It may range from two to several hours. The peak effect is usually visible 12 to 24 hours after exposure. If the ultraviolet source is removed, the symptoms will subside. If the skin is exposed to continuous ultraviolet radiation, a protective mechanism develops for subsequent exposures. The skin increases the pigmentation in the upper layer which acts as a screen to the ultraviolet radiation. This is commonly known as the "suntan."

The dosage required to cause erythema varies according to the pigmentation content of the skin; for example, Negroid skin may require two to three times

as much ultraviolet radiation as the average Caucasian skin to cause
erythema. Further, untanned skin would require less ultraviolet radiation to
cause erythema. In general, the erythemal-causing dose of ultraviolet
radiation for the average Caucasian is in the range of 0.02-0.03 J/cm^2.

Ultraviolet radiation can also affect the eye. If the exposure is above
the threshold limit value (TLV), inflammation of the conjunctiva
(conjunctivitis) or inflammation of the cornea (keratitis) may occur. The
cornea is probably the most vulnerable because of two factors. First, it is
avascular, which means that it contains very few blood vessels. Because there
are few blood vessels, the cornea has difficulty dissipating the heat that
would be generated through the absorption of ultraviolet radiation. Second,
there is an abundance of nerve endings in the cornea. This would increase the
intensity of pain of the overexposure. It has been found that maximum damage
to the eye occurs when the wavelength is in the area of 288 nanometers.

If an exposure above the TLV of ultraviolet radiation occurs, common signs
and symptoms of the problem will be inflammation of the conjunctiva, cornea,
or eyelid. The individual may also experience pain and an abnormal
intolerance of light. It is also possible that as a reflex protective action
the eyelids will close tightly (blepharospasms), and the individual will have
difficulty opening his eyes. The time required for the onset of symptoms is
dependent upon the dosage. It may take from 30 minutes to 24 hours for the
symptoms to appear. Once the ultraviolet source has been removed, symptoms
will regress after several days with no permanent damage.

A common example of ultraviolet radiation exposure to the eyes is welder's
"flash burn." This occurs when, during a welding operation, a welder does not
fully protect his eyes against the ultraviolet radiation. In this instance,
the individual will exhibit signs and symptoms previously mentioned and will
have difficulty with vision. However, as mentioned, the symptoms will regress
after several days with no permanent damage.

Unlike the skin, the eye has no mechanism to establish an increased
tolerance to repeated exposures of ultraviolet radiation. Therefore, it is
possible for problems such as welder's flash burn to occur repeatedly if
exposure levels are not reduced.

Another biological effect caused by ultraviolet radiation is the
fluorescence of the vitreous fluid of the eye. If the wavelength of
ultraviolet radiation approximates 360 nanometers, the vitreous humor
fluoresces, causing diffuse haziness and decreased visual acuity. This
"internal haze" is strictly a temporary condition and has no detrimental
effects and should disappear when exposure ceases. However, because of the
decreased visual acuity, the individual being affected by this problem may
become anxious because of his reduced vision.

It is presumed that continuous exposure to ultraviolet radiation is
related to skin cancer. This is presumed because of the increased number of
cases of skin cancers found in outdoor workers who are constantly exposed to
ultraviolet radiation. Further, there is even a more significant increase in
the number of cases of skin cancer when outdoor workers are simultaneously

exposed to chemicals such as coal tar derivatives, benzopyrene, methylcholanthrene, and other anthracene compounds. It is further assumed that industrially-induced skin cancer cases have not been reported because the dosages required to cause cancer are in excess of the dosages required to cause skin and eye burns. Therefore, the pain would be intolerable; and the individual would remove himself from the source before an adequate dosage to cause cancer would be reached. With outdoor workers, however, the ultraviolet radiation is continuous over an extended period of time and may catalyze cancer development.

One final biological effect that has proved of value is that ultraviolet radiation in the range of 160 nanometers is absorbed by nucleoproteins, which in turn cause irreparable damage to certain types of bacteria. As previously discussed, low-pressure mercury discharge lamps are used as bactericides. While this type of procedure provides an adequate method for destruction of bacteria in certain processes, the ultraviolet radiation which acts as a bactericide can also cause erythema and conjunctivitis.

Some indirect, nonbiological effects of ultraviolet radiation have also been discovered and are of concern. It has been found that certain wavelengths of ultraviolet radiation can dissociate certain molecular structures to form toxic substances. For example, ultraviolet radiation (λ less than 250 nanometers) can cause dissociation of molecular oxygen to form ozone (O_3). A wave of less than 160 nanometers can cause dissociation of molecular nitrogen, which in turn reacts to form nitrogen oxide; and if the wavelength is less than 290 nanometers, the ultraviolet radiation can cause decomposition of chlorinated hydrocarbons, e.g., carbon tetrachloride, trichloroethylene, to form toxic gases such as hydrochloric acid and phosgene. This is of value in that care must be taken to evaluate the substances which are being used in an area which may have ultraviolet radiation.

Exposure Criteria. The threshold limit values (TLV's) recommended by the American Conference of Governmental Industrial Hygienists (ACGIH) refer to the ultraviolet in the spectral region between 200 and 400 nanometers and represent conditions under which it is believed that nearly all workers may be repeatedly exposed without adverse effects. The values presented apply to ultraviolet radiation from arcs, gas and vapor discharges, fluorescent and incandescent sources, and solar radiation. The values present a guide in the control of exposure to continuous sources where the exposure duration is not less than 0.1 second.

The TLV for occupational exposure to ultraviolet radiation incident upon the skin or eye where irradiance values are known and exposure time is controlled are as follows:

1. For the near ultraviolet spectral region (320 to 400 nanometers), total irradiance incident upon the unprotected skin or eye should not exceed 1 mW/cm^2 for periods greater than 10^3 seconds (approximately 16 minutes), and for exposure times less than 10^3 seconds should not exceed 1 J/cm^2.

2. For the actinic ultraviolet spectral region (200 to 315 nanometers), radiation exposure incident upon the unprotected skin or eye should not exceed values presented in Table 6.1.3 within an 8-hour period.

In many instances, the individuals in the working environment will be exposed to a broad-band source of ultraviolet radiation. Because the erythemal effect of ultraviolet radiation is not the same for all wavelengths within the spectrum, it is necessary to weigh the exposure by wavelength according to the spectral effectiveness curve. The following weighting formula can be used to determine the effective irradiance of a broadband source.

$$E_{eff} = \Sigma E_\lambda S_\lambda \Delta\lambda$$

where

E_{eff} = the effective irradiance relative to a monochromatic source at 270 nanometers in W/cm^2 $(J/s/cm^2)$

E_λ = the spectral irradiance in W/cm^2 per nanometer

S_λ = the relative spectral effectiveness (unitless)

$\Delta\lambda$ = the band width in nanometers

Table 6.1.3

Relative spectral effectiveness by wavelength.

Wavelength (nm)	TLV (mJ/cm^2)	Relative Spectral Effectiveness S_λ
200	100	0.03
210	40	0.075
220	25	0.12
230	16	0.19
240	10	0.30
250	7.0	0.43
254	6.0	0.5
260	4.6	0.65
270	3.0	1.0
280	3.4	0.88
290	4.7	0.64
300	10	0.30
305	50	0.06
310	200	0.015
315	1000	0.003

Once the effective irradiance relative to a monochromatic source has been determined, the permissible exposure time in seconds for exposure may be computed by dividing 0.003 J/cm^2 by the effective irradiance in W/cm^2. The exposure time may also be determined by using Table 6.1.4 which provides exposure time corresponding to effective irradiance in μW/cm^2.

Visible Light

Because Section 5 deals with visible light, it will not be discussed in this section.   If there are any questions, please refer to the section on Illumination.

Infrared Radiation

Infrared (IR) radiation is found at the lower end of the visible spectrum.   It includes the wavelength range of 750 nanometers to 0.1 centimeters.   The IR region is divided into two regions; the near region represents the wavelength of 750 nanometers to 5.0 micrometers, and the far region represents the wavelengths from 5 micrometers to 0.1 centimeters.

Table 6.1.4

Permissible ultraviolet exposure.

Duration of Exposure Per Day	Effective Irradiance E_{eff} (μW/cm^2)
8 hrs	0.1
4 hrs	0.2
2 hrs	0.4
1 hr	0.8
30 min	1.7
15 min	3.3
10 min	5
5 min	10
1 min	50
30 sec	100
10 sec	300
1 sec	3,000
0.5 sec	6,000
0.1 sec	30,000

Exposure to infrared radiation can occur from any surface which is at a higher temperature than the receiver.   Infrared radiation may be used for any heating application where the principal product surface can be arranged for exposure to the heat sources.   Transfer of energy or heat occurs whenever radiant energy emitted by one body is absorbed by another. The electromagnetic spectrum wavelengths longer than those of visible energy and shorter than those of radar waves are used for radiant heating. The best energy absorption of white, pastel-colored, and translucent products is obtained by using wavelength emissions longer than 2.5 micrometers. The majority of dark-pigmented and oxide-coated materials will readily absorb wavelength emissions from 0.75 to 9.0 micrometers. Water vapor and visible aerosols such as steam readily absorb the longer infrared wavelengths.

Sources of infrared radiation are primarily those pieces of equipment which are designed to provide a commercial heating source using infrared radiation. However, in any process which requires the extreme heating of metals or glass to a melting point, e.g., 2100°F, infrared radiation will be formed. Examples of this include molten metals or glass or any type of welding arc process.

The basic application of infrared radiation is in the production of heat and heating materials. Depending upon the absorption qualities of the absorbing material and the surrounding environment, infrared radiation can be used to provide rapid rates of heating if desired. Typical industrial applications of infrared radiation include such things as:

1.   Drying/baking of paints, varnishes, or enamels
2.   Heating of metal parts for brazing, forming, thermal aging
3.   Dehydration of textiles, vegetables, sand molds
4.   Localized controlled heating of any desired absorbing material

Although not a direct application of infrared radiation, a common source of infrared radiation is from furnaces and similar heated bodies which are working with molten glass and metals. Most arcing processes (welding) also produce a significant amount of infrared radiation.

Infrared radiation is perceptible as a sensation of warmth on the skin. The increase in tissue temperature upon exposure to infrared radiation depends upon the wavelength, the total amount of energy delivered to the tissue, and the length of exposure. Infrared radiation in the far wavelength region is completely absorbed in the surface areas of the skin. Exposure to IR radiation in the region between 0.75 and 1.5 micrometers can cause acute skin burns and increased persistent skin pigmentation.

The short wavelength region of the infrared is capable of causing injuries to the cornea, iris, retina, and lens of the eye. Excessive exposure of the eyes to luminous radiation, mainly visible and IR radiation, from furnaces and similar hot bodies has been said for many years to produce "glass blower's cataract" or "heat cataract." This condition is an opacity of the rear surface of the lens. Generally, the signs and symptoms of infrared radiation exposure are similar to that of ultraviolet radiation exposure. The symptoms include skin burns, vasodilation of the capillary beds, erythema, blistering of the skin, pain, and potential increased pigmentation. The difference between the two, however, is that exposure to infrared radiation has no latent period, and symptoms will appear immediately. Because of this, extended exposure to intense infrared radiation is minimized because the pain produced by the exposure forces the individual to remove himself from that environment.

Threshold Limit Values. Because overexposure of infrared radiation to the skin causes pain and the individual will remove himself from the environment, the primary concern is overexposure of the eyes to infrared radiation. Further, it has been determined that the damage is dependent upon the wavelength absorbed, the intensity of the wave, and the duration of the exposure. As these relate to the threshold phenomenon, it would appear that a maximum permissible dose (TLV) of 0.4–0.8 J/cm^2 could limit the occurrence of acute radiation effects.

The American Conference of Governmental Industrial Hygienists, in its 1983–1984 List of Threshold Limit Values, has published a list of proposed TLV's for light and near-infrared radiation in the wavelength range of 400 nanometers to 1400 nanometers, which represent conditions under which it is believed that nearly all workers may be exposed without adverse effect. These values should be used as guides in the control of exposure to light and should not be regarded as a fine line between safe and dangerous levels.

The Threshold Limit Values for occupational exposure to broad band light and near-infrared radiation for the eye apply to exposure in any eight-hour workday and require knowledge of the spectral radiance (L_λ) and total irradiance (E) of the source as measured at the position(s) of the eye of the worker. Such detailed spectral data of a white light source is generally only required if the luminance of the source exceeds 1 cd cm^{-2}. At luminances less than this value, the TLV would not be exceeded.
The TLV's are:

1. To protect against retinal thermal injury, the spectral radiance of the lamp weighted against the function R (Table 6.1.5) should not exceed:

$$\sum_{400}^{1400} L_\lambda R_\lambda \Delta\lambda \leq 1/\alpha \ t^{0.5}$$

where L_λ is in $W \ cm^{-2}sr^{-1}$ and t is the viewing duration (or pulse duration if the lamp is pulsed) limited to 1 μs to 10 s, and α is the angular subtense of the source in radians. If the lamp is oblong, α refers to the longest dimension that can be viewed. For instance, at a viewing distance r = 100 cm from a tubular lamp of length l = 50 cm, the viewing angle is:

$$\alpha = l/r = 50/100 = 0.5 \ rad$$

2. To protect against retinal photochemical injury from chronic blue-light exposure, the integrated spectral radiance of a light source weighted against the blue-light hazard function B (Table 6.1.5) should not exceed:

$$\sum_{400}^{1400} L_\lambda tB_\lambda \Delta\lambda \leq 100 \ J{\bullet}cm^{-2}sr^{-1} \quad (t \leq 10^4s)$$

$$\sum_{400}^{1400} L_\lambda B_\lambda \Delta\lambda \leq 10^{-2} \ W{\bullet}cm^{-2}sr^{-1} \quad (t > 10^4s)$$

The weighted product of L_λ and B_λ is termed L(blue). For a source radiance L weighted against the blue-light hazard function [L(blue)] which exceeds 10 mW•cm^{-2}•sr^{-1} in the blue spectral region, the permissible exposure duration t_{max} in seconds is simply

$$t_{max} = 100 \text{ J•cm}^{-2}\text{sr}^{-1}/L(blue)$$

The latter limits are greater than the maximum permissible exposure limits for 440 nm laser radiation because a 2–3 mm pupil is assumed rather than a 7 mm pupil for the laser TLV. For a light source subtending an angle α less than 11 mrd (0.011 radian), the above limits are relaxed such that the spectral irradiance weighted against the blue-light hazard function B_λ should not exceed E(blue).

$$\sum_{400}^{1400} E_\lambda t B_\lambda \Delta\lambda \leq 10 \text{ mJ•cm}^{-2} \quad (t = 10^4 s)$$

$$\sum_{400}^{1400} E_\lambda B_\lambda \Delta\lambda \leq 1\mu W \text{•cm}^2 \quad (t \geq 10^4 s)$$

For a source where the blue light weighted irradiance E(blue) excee 1µW•cm^{-2}, the maximum permissible exposure duration t_{max} in seconds is:

$$rt_{max} = 10 \text{ mJ•cm}^{-2}E(blue)$$

3. Infrared Radiation: To avoid possible delayed effects upon the len of the eye (cataractogenesis), the infrared radiation ($\lambda > 770$ nm) should be limited to 10 mW•cm^{-2}. For an infrared heat lamp or any near-infrared source where a strong visual stimulus is absent, the near-infrared (770–1400 nm) radiance as viewed by the eye should be limited to:

$$\sum_{770}^{1400} L_\lambda \Delta\lambda = 0.6/\alpha$$

for extended duration viewing conditions. This limit is based upon 7 mm pupil diameter.

Radio Frequencies

As with the other regions of radiation discussed, radio frequencies obey the general laws of electromagnetic radiation. The radio frequencies range from a frequency of 1×10^{-3} to 3×10^{13} Hertz or cycles per second. This would translate into a wavelength of 3×10^{-3} to 1×10^8 meters.

Radio frequencies have the capability of inducing electrical currents in conductors. Further, they may also induce the displacement of current in semiconductors, thus transforming radiant energy to heat. By transforming th frequency to an electrical current, patterned energy may be transferred such as with radio or television. If the radio frequency encounters a semiconductor, then the radio frequency can be used as a heat source.

Radio frequencies are generally polarized and form two zones or fields. The near field (Fresnel zone) is representative of the area around the source in which the radio frequency wave has a unique distribution because the waves emitted interact with the source itself. The size of the field is a function of the wavelength emitted and the area of the source (antenna). The radius of the Fresnel zone can be calculated using the formula

$$R = A/2\lambda$$

where

R = radius of the field (cm)
A = area of the antenna (cm^2)
λ = wavelength (cm)

Table 6.1.5

Spectral weighting functions for assessing retinal
hazards from broad-band optical sources.

Wavelength (nm)	Blue-Light Hazard Function Bλ	Burn Hazard Function Rλ
400	0.10	1.0
405	0.20	2.0
410	0.40	4.0
415	0.80	8.0
420	0.90	9.0
425	0.95	9.5
430	0.98	9.8
435	1.0	10
440	1.0	10
445	0.97	9.7
450	0.94	9.4
455	0.90	9.0
460	0.80	8.0
465	0.70	7.0
470	0.62	6.2
475	0.55	5.5
480	0.45	4.5
485	0.40	4.0
490	0.22	2.2
495	0.16	1.6
500–600	$10^{[(450-\lambda)/50]}$	1.0
600–700	0.001	1.0
700–1049	0.001	$10^{[(700-\lambda)/505]}$

In the Fresnel zone, the energy is transmitted by both the electric and magnetic vectors. This energy can be measured in terms of volts/meter for the electric vector and amps/meter for the magnetic field. However, measurement of field strength in the Fresnel zone is a very complicated process because of the interaction with the source.

The far field (Fraunhofer zone) is the outer field. Energy in this field is transmitted by the electric vector only and is measured in terms of volts/meter. Because there is no interaction with the source, measurements in the Fraunhofer zone are more easily taken. Generally, meters are calibrated in the Fraunhofer zone.

Threshold limit values for radio frequencies are usually expressed in terms of power density (watts/m^2). The field strength (volts/m) can be converted to power density using the formula

$$P = \frac{E^2}{120\pi}$$

where
P = power density (watts/m^2)
E = energy density (volts/m)

The common sources of radio frequency include telecommunications, high radio frequency heating instruments, and scientific instruments.

The application of radio frequency radiation can be divided into two basic areas, that of heating absorbing materials and communications. Radio frequency heating is used in a wide variety of industrial applications. For example, radio frequency radiation may be used for such things as hardening gear teeth, cutting tools, and bearing surfaces. It may also be used for soldering and brazing. Applications in the field of wood working include such things as bonding plywood, laminating, and general gluing procedures. It is also used for such applications as molding plastics, vulcanizing rubber, and setting twist in textile materials.

There are basically two types of radio frequency heaters, induction and dielectric. Induction heaters are used when the absorbing material to be heated is some type of conductor. In the induction heater, the absorbing material is brought near an induction coil which is connected to a source of high-frequency power. The absorbing material will resist the flow of induced high-frequency current and thus be heated. The dielectric heater is used for nonconducting materials; e.g., rubber, wood, plastics, leather. With this type of heater, the absorbing material is placed between plates of a capacitor connected to a source of high-frequency power. In the radio frequency field developed, the molecules of the absorbing material become agitated and the material heats because of molecular friction. The most commonly used application of the radio frequency capability is the microwave oven.

Radio frequency radiation is also commonly associated with communications. The radio frequency wave is used to carry a signal which can be received and converted to some form of discernible message. All radio communications, broadcasting, and even the use of radar, fall in the spectrum of radio frequency electromagnetic radiation.

The effect of radio frequency varies greatly in individuals. The primary effect of radio frequencies on an individual is the thermal effect. For the radio frequency to have an effect on the body, the body must have a diameter of at least 1/10 of the wavelength. Therefore, any wavelength greater than 20 meter will have no thermal effect on the body. The body acts as a semiconductor. As discussed, the electromagnetic radiation is transformed to heat in a semiconductor. The absorption and transformation of the radiation to heat is dependent upon the water content, and the depth of penetration of the radio frequency is dependent upon the fatty tissue content. Radio frequencies display an interesting property in that they may be reflected atinterfaces of dielectrically nonhomogeneous layers, giving rise to "a standing wave." This causes a concentration of the energy. The various layers of the skin exemplify this phenomenon. Because the layers are dielectrically nonhomogeneous, standing waves can be produced and the energy of the waves concentrated. Further, the rate of energy absorption and heat accumulation is dependent upon such factors as field strength and power density; the length of exposure; the environmental temperature and humidity; the type of clothing worn; the type of body layers, e.g., fat versus muscle; and the reflection of the waves.

Specific regions of the body that are sensitive to temperature are more critically affected by radio frequency radiation. For example, the lens of the eye can be affected because of its difficulty in dissipating heat. Thus, cataracts may form from radio frequency exposure. Radio frequency exposure to the male reproductive organs causes a temperature increase which critically affects the sperm cells in the testes. Less androgen is produced and, thus, the level of sex hormone decreases. Finally, because the central nervous system consists of thick bones and has a high fatty content, the penetration of radio frequency is facilitated, but heat dissipation is hindered. Further, the spherical shape of the spinal column and skull cavity may cause reflections and concentration of the energy. Therefore, radio frequency radiation must be monitored in areas where the energy and power density could reach the TLV.

Radio frequency radiation can also have nonthermal effects that may be detrimental. First, because of the effect of the electric and magnetic fields in combination, particles greater than 15 micrometers in diameter having an electrical charge will polarize in the Fresnel zone. Because there are no histological structures in the body that are greater in diameter than 15 micrometers, polarization does not occur in human tissue; but the potential does exist. Radio frequency radiation can also demonstrate a demodulating effect. This effect involves organs of the body that display modulating electrical activity: i.e., the heart and central nervous system. The exposure of these organs to radio frequency causes a change in amplitude and peak frequency in electrocardiograms and electroencephalograms. This effect does not appear to have any permanent effects and is eliminated when the radiofrequency exposure is removed. Finally, radio frequency radiation can have an effect on molecular structure. In essence, the radiation causes excitation of molecules and a potential for molecular polarization. Although the molecular structure is not changed, this effect can exert a catalytic action upon some chemical and enzymatic reactions: i.e., making molecules more receptive to certain types of chemical reactions.

Experts in the USSR have established health standards with respect to radio frequency radiation. Their standards have discriminated between various radio frequencies. For example, for radio frequencies between 3 and 30 megahertz, any radio frequency radiation source which is used for inductance heating should not exceed 20 volts/m (electrical field) or 5 amps/ (magnetic field). If the source is being used for dielectric heating or broadcasting in that given frequency range, the energy density should not exceed 20 volts/m. For the range of 30 to 300 megahertz, the energy densities should not exceed 5 volts/m. Finally, for the range of 300 to 300,000 megahertz, exposure should not exceed 10 microwatts/cm^2 for a continuous exposure over an average working day; 100 microwatts/cm^2 for a 2-hour exposure per 24-hour period; or 1 milliwatt/cm^2 for a 15- to 20-minute exposure per 24-hour period.

Each of the regions of nonionizing radiation have been briefly presented in the previous section. The remaining two sections will deal with nonionizing radiation that is not specifically represented on the electromagnetic radiation spectrum. First will be the use of microwaves. Microwaves are essentially a subgroup of the radio frequencies just discussed. The second section will deal with lasers. Lasers are essentially a special application of electromagnetic radiation and as such are not specifically represented on the electromagnetic spectrum. However, lasers play an increasingly important role in the industrial environment and present some special potential health and safety hazards that should be presented. Because the American Conference of Governmental Industrial Hygienists (ACGIH) has established Threshold Limit Values for radio frequency radiation in conjunction with microwave radiation, these health standards will be discussed after the material on microwaves.

Microwaves

Radio frequencies above 1000 megahertz are classified as microwaves. Microwaves demonstrate the basic properties of all other electromagnetic radiations. They have the capability of being transmitted over long distances through air and rain. They follow a quasi line-of-sight path with minimal diffraction spreading. Microwaves may be readily generated with high power densities. Because of their unique absorption properties in dielectric insulators, microwaves lead to uniform heat disposition in many materials. Microwaves are strongly reflected and can be contained by metallic surfaces.

There are basically two types of microwave units. The first type is a continuous wave microwave unit. This type of unit generates a microwave on a continuous basis with no interruptions in the production of the wave. The second type is a pulse wave unit. In this unit, the wave is produced for a short period of time (10^3 microseconds). The advantage of the pulsed wave unit over the continuous wave unit is that greater power levels can be obtained with the pulsed wave unit.

Specific uses of microwave frequencies have been established by the Federal Communications Commission. Typical uses of microwave radiation are presented in Table 6.1.6.

The FCC has also established specific frequencies for use in communication. General bands have also been established. For example, three common bands have been designated "S," "X," and "K" bands; and these bands have a wavelength of 10, 3, and 1.2 centimeters respectively.

Table 6.1.6

Microwave band designations.

Designation		Wave-length	Frequency	Application
Very high frequency (VHF)	Ultra-short (meter)	10-1 m	30-300 MHz	FM broadcast, television, air traffic control, radionavigation
Ultra high frequency (UHF)	Decimeter	1-0.1 m	0.3-3 GHz	Television, citizens band, microwave point-to-point, microwave ovens, telemetry, tropo scatter, and meteorological radar
Super high frequency (SHF)	Centimeter	10-1 cm	3-30 GHz	Satellite communication, airborne weather radar, altimeters, shipborne navigational radar, microwave point-to-point
Extra high frequency (EHF)	Millimeter	1-0.1 cm	30-300 GHz	Radio astronomy, cloud detection radar, space research, HCN (hydrogen cyanide) emission

The two practical sources of the microwave are the klystron and the magnetron. The klystron is designed to generate low power levels in the neighborhood of 1 watt. The magnetron has the capability of generating much higher power levels in the neighborhood of 1 kilowatt on a continuous wave basis. Microwaves are produced by the deceleration of electrons in an electrical field. As the electrons slow down, kinetic energy is released in the form of microwaves.

The klystron has six basic components (see Figure 6.1.5). These components include evacuated glass tube, electron-emitting cathode, accelerating grid (anode), two metal ring-like microwave cavities referred to as a "buncher" and a "catcher," an accelerating grid, and coaxial feed line.

The operation of the klystron is relatively simple. A stream of high speed electrons is produced at the cathode. The electrons travel toward the anode; as they pass through the accelerating grid, they increase their speed. In the buncher cavity, the electrons are modulated by a microwave field into bunches.

When the bunched electrons pass the catcher grind, the electrons slow down and microwave radiation is released; and the microwaves are removed by the coaxial cable. Finally, the electrons are captured at the anode. The specific radiation released is dependent upon the dimensions of the tube, the dimensions of the cavity, and the velocity of the electrons.

Figure 6.1.5

Klystron microwave source.

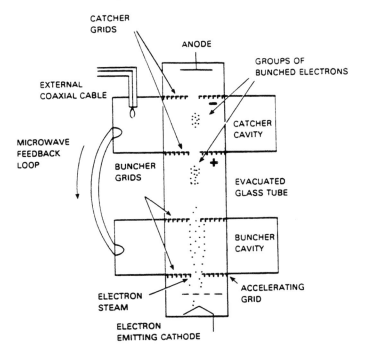

The magnetron operates on the same principle as the klystron but is a much higher energy source. With the magnetron, the electron beam travels in a circular orbit within a magnetic field. In the magnetron, there are a multiple number of cavities (6 or more), and the same cavities bunch the electrons and catch the electrons (Figure 6.1.6). The ability of the magnetron to function with high currents and with many cavities gives it greater power capability than the klystron. It is also easier to cool, which is a limiting factor in the klystron.

Figure 6.1.6

Magnetron-microwave generator.

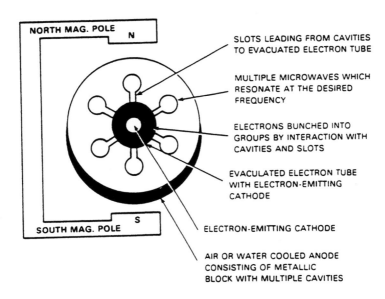

SLOTS LEADING FROM CAVITIES
TO EVACUATED ELECTRON TUBE

MULTIPLE MICROWAVES WHICH
RESONATE AT THE DESIRED
FREQUENCY

ELECTRONS BUNCHED INTO
GROUPS BY INTERACTION WITH
CAVITIES AND SLOTS

EVACUATED ELECTRON TUBE
WITH ELECTRON-EMITTING
CATHODE

ELECTRON-EMITTING CATHODE

AIR OR WATER COOLED ANODE
CONSISTING OF METALLIC
BLOCK WITH MULTIPLE CAVITIES

Biological Effects. The biological effects attributed to microwaves are similar to the biological effects caused by radio frequency. One special concern is that the thermal heating of an exposed tissue takes place throughout the volume and does not originate from the surface as with some of the other electromagnetic radiations discussed. The depth of penetration is dependent upon the frequency of the wave and the type of tissue relative to water content. For example, fat layers and bone have low water content and therefore low absorption of microwave energy. However, the skin and muscles have high water content and therefore high absorption of energy. With microwaves, the thermal effects are more significant than nonthermal effects. However, in any case, both the thermal and nonthermal effects of microwave radiation are the same as for radio frequencies.

Threshold Limit Values. These Threshold Limit Values (TLV's) refer to radiofrequency (RF) and microwave radiation in the frequency range from 10 kHz to 300 GHz, and represent conditions under which it is believed workers may be repeatedly exposed without adverse health effects. The TLV's shown in Table 6.1.7 are selected to limit the average whole-body specific absorption rate (SAR) to 0.4 W/kg in any six minutes (0.1 hr) period for 3 MHz to 300 GHz (see Figure 6.1.7). Between 10 kHz and 3 MHz, the average whole body SAR is still limited to 0.4 W/kg, but the plateau at 100 mW/cm^2 was set to protect against shock and burn hazards.

Since it is usually impractical to measure the SAR, the TLV's are expressed in units that are measurable, viz, squares of the electric and

Table 6.1.7

Radiofrequency/microwave threshold limit values.

Frequency	Power Density (mW/cm^2)	Electric Field Strength Squared (V^2/m^2)	Magnetic Field Strength Squared (A^2/m^2)
10 kHz to 3 MHz	100	377,000	2.65
3 MHz to 30 MHz	900/f^2*	3770 x 900/f^2*	900/(37.7 x f^2*
30 MHz to 100 MHz	1	3770	0.027
100 MHz to 1000 MHz	f*/100	3770 x f*/100	f*/37.7 x 100
1 GHz to 300 GHz	10	37,700	0.265

*f = frequency in MHz

Figure 6.1.7

Threshold limit values for radiofrequency/microwave
radiation in workplace (whole-body SAR < 0.4 W/kg).

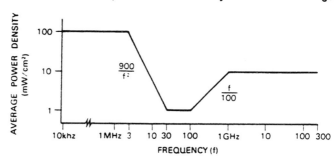

By permission of the American Conference of Governmental Industrial Hygienists

magnetic field strengths, averaged over any 0.1 hour period. This can be
expressed in units of equivalent plane wave power density for convenience.
The electric field strength (E) squared, magnetic field strength (H) squared,
and power density (PD) values are shown in Table 6.1.7. For near field
exposures, PD cannot be measured directly, but equivalent plane wave power
density can be calculated from the field strength measurement data as follows:

PD in mW/cm^2 = E^2/3770

where,

E^2 is in volts squared (V^2) per meter squared (m^2)

and   PD in mW/cm^2 = 37.7 H^2

where,

H^2 is in amperes squared (A^2) per meter squared (m^2).

These values should be used as guides in the evaluation and control of exposure to radiofrequency/microwave radiation, and should not be regarded as a fine line between safe and dangerous levels.

Lasers

The term "laser" is an acronym for "light amplification by stimulated emission of radiation." The laser can use ultraviolet, infrared, visible, or microwave (maser) radiation.

The laser is a device that produces a concentrated light beam with the following properties. First, the light beam is coherent. This means that the beam is highly uniform in phase over an extended area, allowing for a narrow directional beam over long distance. Second, the beam is monochromatic, meaning that the emitted radiation has a very narrow wavelength band. Finally, the power density can be very high. This comes about because the beam is coherent and monochromatic.

There are a variety of laser sources available, depending upon the power and wavelength of interest. These sources are usually categorized according to the type of instrumentation used, whether it be ruby crystal, gaseous, or injection-type laser.

In general, every laser has three basic elements. The first element is an optical cavity, consisting of at least two mirrors, one of which is partially transmissive. The second component is some type of active laser medium. This is a material that can be excited from an unenergized ground state to a relatively long-lived excited state. The third element of a laser is some means of "pumping." This pumping procedure is necessary for supplying the excitation energy to the active laser medium.

As an example, the ruby laser, as shown in Figure 6.1.8, will be presented. This consists of a high voltage power that feeds into an electrical pulse-forming network. This pulse-forming network produces short pulses of very high electrical current that feed into a xenon flash lamp. A flash lamp trigger pulse is also produced. The flash lamp produces a short and very intense optical pulse that is absorbed by the ruby rod.

The ruby rod is a crystal of aluminum oxide with about 0.05% chromium oxide. It is the chromium oxide that gives the ruby its pink color and acts as the active laser material.

The ruby laser is excited by optical pumping which lifts the system from the ground state of the chromium ion to one of the wide absorption bands. These absorption bands are optically wide in comparison to the sharp photon wavelength later emitted.

Figure 6.1.8

Laser

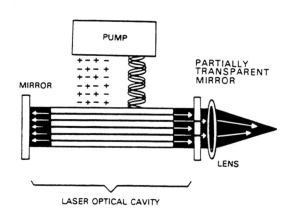

LASER OPTICAL CAVITY

Once these absorption bands are excited, they quickly drop to a lower energy level by a radiation-free transition. This lower energy level is actually split into two levels which are close together in energy. One of them is very long lived with a life of T = 3 milliseconds. One photon can be emitted by each state. The longer wavelength photon, which comes from the long-lived state, is more numerous. These photons that are emitted in a rapid pulse much shorter than the lifetime of the state give the high power of the ruby laser.

The ends of the ruby crystal act as the optical cavity. Once the critical level is reached, the presence of photons stimulates emission of other photons, and chromium ions return to their ground state again. Simultaneous emission of the photons forms the coherent light. This light is then transmitted through the transmission mirror-like end of the ruby crystal tube. The entire sequence described requires approximately one-thousandth of a second. The coherent wave is produced because the critical level of photons required for stimulated emission is reached.

The ruby crystal is but one type of laser: solid crystal with impurities. Depending upon the wavelength or obtainable power of interest, a variety of types of lasers are available. Table 6.1.8 lists the common types of lasers.

As with microwave units, laser units may also operate in the pulse or continuous wave mode. Again, as with microwaves, the advantage of the pulse mode is the tremendous increase in power density that is obtainable.

The power produced by the laser is measured in terms of joules per second or watts. If the time of the pulse is decreased, then the watts or energy is increased. Further, if the power density is defined as the power per unit area, then if the area is reduced, power density increases. Assume that a

Table 6.1.8

Most common types of lasers.

Laser Type	Example	Mode of Operation	Power per Pulse	CW Power
Solid host	Ruby (Chromium)	Pulsed or	1000 megawatts	1 watt
	Neodymium YAG	Rapid Pulse Mode	10 megawatts	100 watts
	Neodymium Glass	Same		
Gas Laser (Neutral Atom)	Helium Neon	CW		up to 100 milliwatts
Ion Gas Laser watts.	Argon	CW		1 to 20 watts
Molecular Gas Laser	Carbon Dioxide	CW		10 to 5000 watts
Molecular Gas Laser	Nitrogen	Pulsed or Rapid Pulse Mode		250 milliwatts
Semiconductor Diode	Gallium Arsenide	Pulsed or CW	1 to 20 watts	
Chemical Laser	HCl	CW or Pulsed		
Liquid Laser	Organic Dye Laser (tuneable)	Pulsed	1 megawatt	

laser produces a peak power of 1 joule. (Note: One joule is enough energy to operate the average home iron for approximately three-tenths of a second.) Further, assume that the pulse of the power is reduced to 10^{-3} seconds and that through a series of lenses the power is focused on a one square millimeter area. With the capability of shortening the pulse and focusing on a minute finite area, then the power density (W/m^2) becomes:

$$\frac{1 \text{ joule}/10^{-3} \text{ sec}}{10^{-3} \text{ m}^2} = 1 \times 10^6 \text{ joules/sec} \cdot m^2 = 10^9 \text{ W/m}^2$$

which is equal to 10^6 watts/m². As can be seen, the ability of the laser to focus on a finite area with a short pulse of energy increases the power density generated.

As mentioned, the capability of the laser to present a coherent beam that
may be focused on a small spot is of great advantage. Aside from the
coherence, the ability of the laser beam to maintain a parallel beam increases
its great potential. For example, a laser beam may be divided into two
regions based upon its beam divergence (Figure 6.1.9). The first region is
the parallel region and is defined as:

$$L = D^2/2.44\lambda$$

where

    L = the parallel region (cm)
    D = the beam divergence (cm)
    λ = the wavelength of the laser wave (cm)

Figure 6.1.9

Beam divergence.

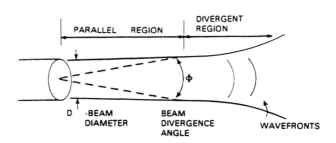

For example, if infrared radiation of a wavelength equal to 10^{-4} cm and a
beam diameter of .1 cm was used, then the parallel region would be
approximately 41 cm. The divergence region would then begin at that point.
With beam divergence, the intensity of the wave begins to decrease. The
energy lost, however, is very small. For the example wavelength, the beam
divergence angle after the parallel region is only 0.85 milliradians.
Therefore even over large distances, the laser beam will maintain its
integrity to a great degree. The calculation of the parallel region and the
divergent region is not so important as the concept that the laser beam has
the capability of maintaining a coherent parallel wave over long distances.

The application of laser radiation is quite varied. The construction
industry has found great use for the helium neon (He-Ne) gas laser. Because
of the culmination of the beam, the laser can be used to project a reference
line for construction equipment in such operations as dredging, tunneling, and
pipe laying. Figure 6.1.10 illustrates a typical procedure for laying a
pipeline with the laser providing a reference beam.

Because of the high energy content of the laser beam, it has been used
also for such things as welding and machining of fine parts. Also, because of
their tremendous energy, lasers have a potential use in the drilling of
tunnels through rock.

Figure 6.1.10

Cable installation.

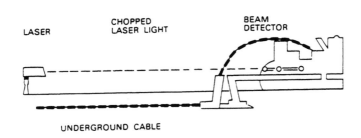

The laser beam can also be used to transmit communication signals. Theoretically, it will be possible for a laser to transmit as many messages as all communication channels now in existence. The major obstruction to the use of lasers in this application is the lack of the laser's ability to penetrate fog, rain, or snow.

Biological Effects. Because of the high power density outputs of the laser, the eye and the skin seem most vulnerable. Effect to the eyes depends on the type of laser beam: that is, its wavelength, output, power, beam divergence, and the pulse repetition frequency created by the unit. Damage to the eye caused by the laser beam is extremely critical because the lens of the eye further focuses the laser beam on the fovea. This focusing by the lens of the eye increases the power density of the laser to several magnitudes greater than the actual laser beam output. The general effect of laser beam radiation is thermal in nature. It may cause heating of the retina and cornea, depending upon the wavelength. Laser radiation which operates in the visible light spectrum affects the retina and retinal pigment. However, because the eye is sensitive to visible radiation, high intensities of laser radiation in this region will stimulate the protective reflex of the eye and will prevent long durations of exposure. However, when the laser operates in the infrared or ultraviolet regions, the eye is not sensitive to these wavelengths and therefore no protective reflex will be stimulated. Therefore, damage may be greater. In general, it can be stated that damage to the eye in the form of retinal burns may occur if the beam power density is greater than 1 milliwatt/cm^2.

Threshold Limit Values

The threshold limit values are for exposure to laser radiation under conditions to which nearly all workers may be exposed without adverse effects. The values should be used as guides in the control of exposures and should not be regarded as fine lines between safe and dangerous levels. They are based on the best available information from experimental studies.

The TLV's expressed as radiant exposure or irradiance in this section may be averaged over an aperture of 1 mm except for TLV's for the eye in the spectral range of 400-1400 nm, which should be averaged over a 7 mm limiting aperture (pupil); and except for all TLV's for wavelengths between 0.1-1 mm where the limiting aperture is 10 mm. No modification of the TLV's is permitted for pupil sizes less than 7 mm.

The TLV's for "extended sources" apply to sources which subtend an angle greater than α (Table 6.1.9) which varies with exposure time. This angle is not the beam divergence of the source.

Table 6.1.9

Limiting angle to extended source
which may be used for applying extended
source TLV's.

Exposure Duration(s)	Angle α (mrad)	Exposure Duration(s)	Angle α (mrad)
10^{-9}	8.0	10^{-2}	5.7
10^{-8}	5.4	10^{-1}	9.2
10^{-7}	3.7	1.0	15
10^{-6}	2.5	10	24
10^{-5}	1.7	10^{2}	24
10^{-4}	2.2	10^{3}	24
10^{-3}	3.6	10^{4}	24

The TLV's for skin exposure are given in Table 6.1.10. The TLV's are to be increased by a factor (C_A) as shown in Figure 6.1.11 for wavelengths between 700 nm and 1400 nm. To aid in the determination of TLV's for exposure durations requiring calculations of fractional powers, Figures 6.1.12 through 6.1.18 may be used.

Since there are few experimental data for multiple pulses, caution must be used in the evaluation of such exposures. The protection standards for irradiance or radiant exposure in multiple pulse trains have specific limitations as discussed in the ACGIH 1983-84 List of TLV's (p. 71).

Figure 6.1.11

TLV correction factor for λ = 700-1400 nm*.

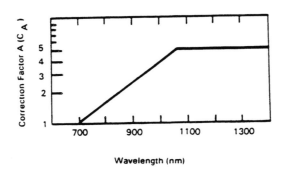

Wavelength (nm)

* For λ = 700-1400 nm, C_A = $10^{[0.002 (\lambda - 700)]}$.
  For λ = 1050-1400 nm, C_A = 5.

By permission of the American Conference of Governmental Industrial Hygienists.

Table 6.1.10

TLV for skin exposure from a laser beam.

Spectral Region	Wave Length	Exposure Time, (t) Seconds	TLV
UV	200 nm to 400 nm	10^{-9} to 3×10^4	Same as Table 4*
Light &	400 nm to 1400 nm	10^{-9} to 10^{-7}	$2\ C_A \times 10^{-2}$ J $\bullet$ cm^{-2}
IR-A	400 nm to 1400 nm	10^{-7} to 10	$1.1\ C_A\ ^4$ t J $\bullet$ cm^{-2}
IR-A	400 nm to 1400 nm	10 to 3×10^4	$0.2\ C_A$ W $\bullet$ cm^{-2}
IR-B & C	1.4μm to $10^3\mu$m	10^{-9} to 3×10^4	Same as Table 4*

C_A = 1.0 for λ = 400-700 nm; see Figure 2* for λ = 700 to 1400 nm.

*Reference data in ACGIH - TLV's and BEI for 1983-84.

Figure 6.1.12

TLV for intrabeam (direct viewing of
laser beam 400-700 nm).*

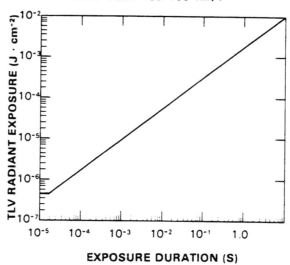

Figure 6.1.13

TLV for intrabeam (direct viewing of
CW laser beam 400-1400 nm).*

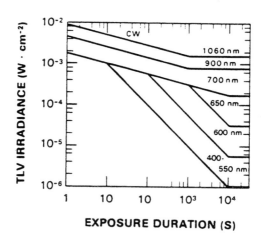

* By permission of the American Conference of Governmental Industrial
Hygienists.

Figure 6.1.14

TLV for laser exposure of skin and eyes for far-infrared
radiation (wavelengths > 1.4 μm).*

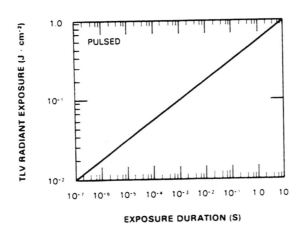

EXPOSURE DURATION (S)

Figure 6.1.15

TLV for CW laser exposure of skin and eyes for far-infrared
radiation (wavelengths > 1,4 μm).*

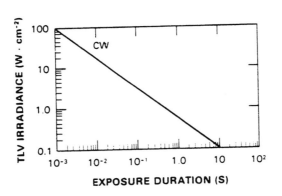

EXPOSURE DURATION (S)

* By permission of the American Conference of Governmental Industrial
Hygienists.

Figure 6.1.16

TLV for extended sources or diffuse reflections
of laser radiation (400-700 nm).*

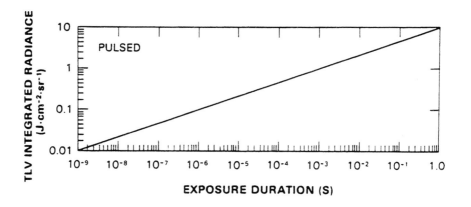

Figure 6.1.17

TLV for extended sources of diffuse reflections of
laser radiation (400-1400 nm).

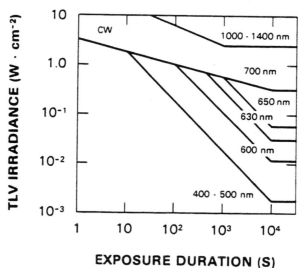

* By permission of the American Conference of Governmental Industrial
Hygienists.

Figure 6.1.18

Multiplicative correction factor for repetitively pulsed
lasers having durations of < 10^{-5} second.*

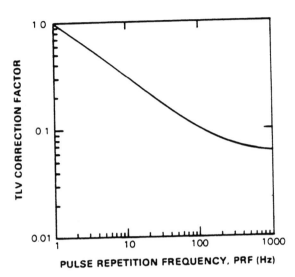

PULSE REPETITION FREQUENCY, PRF (Hz)

* TLV for a single pulse of the pulse train is multiplied by the correction
  factor. Correction factor for PRF > 1000 Hz is 0.06.

By permission of the American Conference of Governmental Industrial Hygienists.

Summary

In general, the discussion in this section has concerned the
characteristics, sources, application, biological effects, and established
threshold limit values for electromagnetic regions of the spectrum including
ultraviolet, infrared, and radio frequency. The specific areas of microwaves
and lasers have also been discussed. Future sections will be devoted to the
applications related to hazards and the control of these nonionizing
radiations.

2. Control of Nonionizing Radiation

In this chapter, the recognition and control of ultraviolet radiation, microwave radiation, and lasers will be discussed. Because the measurement and control of the other types of electromagnetic radiation discussed in the previous chapter are similar to those for ultraviolet and microwave radiation, these specific types of radiation have been selected because of their common application in industry.

Ultraviolet Radiation

Ultraviolet radiation covers the range from 10 to 400 nanometers. This range has been divided into regions based upon their effect on man. Figure 6.2.1 illustrates these specific regions. For example, wavelengths in the keratitic region have the greatest effect upon the cornea. Wavelengths in the erythemal region cause pronounced skin reddening and blisters, and wavelengths in the actinic region (200-315 nanometers) have a generally adverse effect on man.

Figure 6.2.1

The ultraviolet region.

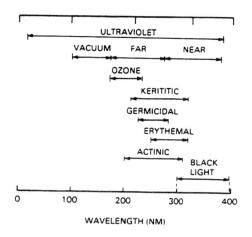

WAVELENGTH (NM)

As discussed, the primary source of ultraviolet radiation is the sun. Industrial sources of ultraviolet radiation are from black-light lamps, carbon arcs, welding arcs, high-pressure mercury vapor, and low-pressure mercury vapor sources.

When measuring ultraviolet radiation exposure, the measurements must reflect the relative effectiveness by wavelength of the ultraviolet radiation. This can be accomplished in two ways. First, a filtering system that mimics the actinic curve (Figure 6.2.2) will minimize the air and account for the relative effectiveness by wavelength.

Figure 6.2.2

Instrument response vs. relative effectiveness.

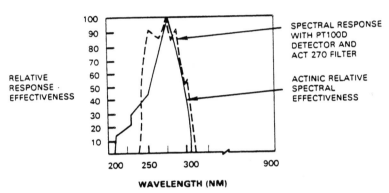

The second procedure that can be used if the ultraviolet is a broad-band source is to take measurements at specified wavelengths and then calculate the effective irradiance. This is done by measuring the specific band widths, then calculating the exposure for each, and finally adjusting according to the relative actinic spectral effectiveness. Once this is done, the sum of all exposures for all widths is calculated. The formula is as follows:

$$E_{eff} = \Sigma\ E_\lambda S_\lambda \Delta\lambda$$

where

E_{eff} = effective irradiance (W/cm^2)
E_λ = spectral irradiance ($W/cm^2/nm$)
S_λ = relative actinic spectral effectiveness
   (Value taken from Table 6.1.3)

$\Delta\lambda$ = band width (nm)

To date, broad-based measuring devices for measurement of ultraviolet energy are not readily available. However, devices for measuring specific wavelengths are available. The two major classes of detectors--photon and thermal--are based upon the interaction of the ultraviolet radiation with the detector. Photoelectric monitoring devices use a phototube and

photomultiplier to monitor ultraviolet radiation. When the ultraviolet
radiation interacts with the metal target of the phototube, electrons are
ejected and counted on the photomultiplier. The number of electrons ejected
is proportional to the ultraviolet radiation present.

Photovoltaic measuring devices work on the principle of the production of
a voltage difference in the device caused by ultraviolet absorption. The
devices are usually semiconductors, such as selenium photocells or silicon
solar cells. Each of these devices is valuable because special consideration
can be given to the type of target used, since various metals have different
reactive capabilities with various wavelengths of ultraviolet radiation.

One particularly useful device for measuring ultraviolet radiation is the
thermopile. This device operates on the principle of the production of
voltage by increased temperature caused by ultraviolet absorption. The change
in voltage is proportional to ultraviolet radiation.

Since available photocells and filter combinations do not always closely
approximate the ultraviolet biological action spectrum (Figure 6.2.2), it is
necessary to calibrate each photocell and meter for the specific use. Special
care must be taken to control ambient conditions during the calibration
process. Filtering combinations may also allow for the discrimination of
wavelengths. This discrimination is necessary because of the variation in
effect of the various wavelengths of ultraviolet radiation.

Some instruments used will read the power density (W/m^2) directly, while
others may give readings that require conversion to a power density value by a
calibration factor. This calibration factor is instrument dependent and is
supplied by the manufacturer, if necessary. Then, given the distance from the
source of the reading and the average time of personnel exposure, exposure can
be calculated and then compared to the threshold limit value. For example,
using a photometer a reading of 0.5 microamps is taken at 90 cm. (90 cm is
the mean body/eye distance of the worker.) If the worker is exposed to the
radiation for approximately 15 minutes per 8-hour shift, is the TLV exceeded?
(Assume the calibration factor = 90.6 microwatts/cm^2/μamp and the filters
corrected to 270 nm.)

Solution

$$0.5 \ \mu amps \times 90.6 \mu W/cm^2/\mu amp = 45.3 \ \mu W/cm^2$$

$$\frac{45.3 \ \mu J}{sec-cm^2} \times \frac{15 \ min}{8 \ hr} \times \frac{60 \ sec}{min} = \frac{40.77 \ mJ}{cm^2-8 \ hr}$$

TLV = 3.0 mJ/cm^2 for 8-hr day

The TLV is exceeded.

Extending this example further, what is the maximum exposure time per 8-hour
period that the employee could work in this environment at the specified

distance? The solution to this problem may be found by dividing the TLV, 3.0 mJ/cm^2, by the actual exposure rate, or 45.3 mJ/cm^2/sec.   The calculation would be:

$$\frac{3.0 \text{ mJ}}{\text{cm}^2} \times \frac{\text{sec-cm}^2}{45.3 \times 10^{-3} \text{ mJ}} = 66.2 \text{ sec}$$

As previously mentioned, readings can be taken for specified band widths of ultraviolet radiation and then the effective irradiance calculated.   The following example illustrates this procedure:

Wavelength	Reading (μW/cm^2)
200	0.081
220	0.091
240	0.18
260	0.18
280	0.27
300	0.36

Solution

$E_{eff} = \Sigma E_\lambda S_\lambda \Delta\lambda$

$E_{200} = 0.08 \ \mu\text{W} \bullet \text{cm}^{-2} \times 0.03 \ \text{mm}^{-1} \times 20 \ \text{nm} = 0.048 \ \text{W/cm}^2$

$E_{220} =$	$0.09 \times 0.12 \times 20$	$= 0.216$
$E_{240} =$	$0.18 \times 0.30 \times 20$	$= 1.080$
$E_{260} =$	$0.18 \times 0.65 \times 20$	$= 2.340$
$E_{280} =$	$0.27 \times 0.88 \times 20$	$= 4.752$
$E_{300} =$	$0.36 \times 0.30 \times 20$	$= \underline{2.160}$
E_{total}		$= 10.596 \ \mu\text{W/cm}^2$

Using the TLV table for 15 minutes (Table 6.1.4), TLV $= 1.7 \ \mu$W/cm^2. Therefore, the exposure is 3.2 times the permissible level at the distance of the measurements.

When taking measurements for ultraviolet radiation exposure, certain factors must be considered to avoid errors of major magnitude. First, the monitoring instrument must match the spectral output of the ultraviolet radiation source. Further, the spectral output and measurement must be compared to the relative spectral efficiency as previously described. Second, certain types of devices require periodic calibration for the specified ultraviolet source. Solarization or aging of the lenses, especially with long usages or following measurements of high-intensity ultraviolet radiation, causes shifts in the instrumentation. Third, atmospheric conditions must be considered. Water vapor in the atmosphere will reduce the readings of ultraviolet radiation by absorbing the ultraviolet radiation. Although there is no specific calibration or correction factor for atmospheric conditions, this must be considered when taking measurements. Fourth, the meters and probes used are directional, and it is necessary to ensure that measurements are taken in all directions. Fifth, readings can be affected by the reflection of ultraviolet radiation from nearby sources or by high-intensity visible light. Because of this, efforts must be made to reduce the presence of visible light and potential reflection of ultraviolet radiation when taking readings. Finally, readings should be taken at the approximate distance from the source that the personnel would be exposed. This is because of the "inverse square law" where the exposure rate is reduced by $1/\text{distance}^2$.

Personnel Protection. When protecting personnel against ultraviolet radiation, the primary concern is exposure to the skin and eyes. There are basically three protective tools that can be used: time, distance, and shielding.

The use of time as a protective tool is rather self-explanatory. By decreasing the time of exposure, the total exposure to the personnel is decreased. Therefore, when analyzing any potential ultraviolet radiation hazard, it is important to know the time of exposure per given workday or per week to calculate potential personnel exposure. In many instances, the analysis of the task being performed may indicate procedural changes which would reduce the exposure time to the personnel.

The second tool that may be used is distance. The intensity of the radiation is decreased by the square of the change in distance (inverse-square law). For example, if a reading of 15 μW/cm^2 is taken at 1 meter, the reading would then be expected to be 3.75 μW/cm^2 at 2 meters or $15/2^2$. If one were interested in the reading at 3 meters, then the expected reading would be $15/3^2$ or 1.66 μW/cm^2. The distance may not be an important factor because of the type of work involved. For example, it would be difficult for a welder to be moved a greater distance from the potential source because it is necessary for him to be close to perform the welding. When working with distance as a tool, two factors must be considered. First, all measurements should be taken at the distance that approximates the worker distance. If, for example, the hands are normally closer to the ultraviolet source, measurements should be taken at various distances for hands and mean body distance. Second, efforts should be made to maximize the distance and thus minimize the exposure to personnel between the personnel and the ultraviolet source. This may be done through the use of tongs to handle materials, automation, etc.

Shielding. The use of shielding is a procedure whereby the exposure to the personnel is reduced by placing an absorbing material between the personnel and the ultraviolet source. With ultraviolet radiation, this can be done using three types of shielding--enclosures, protective clothing, and eye protection.

Enclosures minimize the exposure to persons working directly with an ultraviolet source and also to personnel in the vicinity of the ultraviolet source. The selection of enclosure material is dependent upon the wavelength and the properties of the wavelength involved: e.g., reflectance and absorption characteristics. For example, clear glass is opaque to ultraviolet radiation, yet transparent to visible light; while a red opaque filter is opaque to visible light, yet transparent to an ultraviolet source. Any area that includes an enclosure should be adequately marked and labeled as a radiation area.

Protective clothing can be worn to minimize ultraviolet exposure. In almost all instances, heavy clothing will absorb the ultraviolet radiation before it reaches the personnel. Examples of protective clothing are items such as gloves, coats, overalls, and face shields. Again, the type of clothing to be worn is dependent upon the radiation source and the type of radiation being emitted. In all instances, however, dark clothing should be worn to avoid the reflectance of the radiation.

Protective eye shields are commonly used to shield the eyes against radiant energy. The selection of filters is based upon the type, wavelength, and intensity of the radiation to be attenuated. Various filters transmit differently for different wavelengths. Table 6.2.1 illustrates the various types of filters that can be used for ultraviolet and infrared radiation, while Table 6.2.2 presents recommended filter lens for welding. Emphasis should be placed on the fact that most ultraviolet sources are broad-band sources and that each band must be analyzed for the selection of proper filtering. In many instances, the filtering selected for a given wavelength may be inadequate for other wavelengths which are present.

When evaluating an ultraviolet radiation source for hazards, associated nonradiation hazards must be considered. First, instruments producing ultraviolet radiation may require high voltage for operation and thus produce a possible electrical hazard. Further, the presence of high voltage may also precipitate the extraneous production of X-radiation (discussed in Chapter 3). Second, the ultraviolet radiation reacts with oxygen in the atmosphere to produce ozone (TLV of O_3 = 0.1 ppm) which is an extremely toxic substance. Therefore, it is necessary to maintain adequate ventilation in areas where ultraviolet radiation is present. Ultraviolet radiation also reduces chlorinated hydrocarbons (trichloroethylene) to toxic substances. The ultraviolet radiation may also cause the formation of nitrogen oxides. Further, heating processes which form ultraviolet radiation may also form toxic fumes if the procedures involve base metals including elements such as zinc, fluorine, beryllium, lead, and cadmium. Because of this, efforts must be made to analyze materials that are involved in the procedure and chemicals that may be found in the work environment. Every effort should be made to minimize or eliminate potentially toxic substances from the working area. This can be done by evaluating the location of the ultraviolet source and also by providing adequate ventilation systems.

When surveying an area for ultraviolet radiation exposure, a diagram of the area should be prepared indicating:

1.   The ultraviolet radiation source.

2.   Personnel location.

3.   Protective devices presently in use: signs, screens, ventilation systems, etc.

Table 6.2.1

Transmittances and tolerances in transmittance of various shades of filter lenses.

Shade No.	Optical Density Min.	Std.	Max.	Luminous Transmittance Max. (per cent)	Std. (per cent)	Min. (per cent)	Maximum Infrared Transmittance (per cent)	Maximum Spectral Transmittance in the Ultraviolet and Violet for Four Wavelengths (millimicrons) 313 (per cent)	334 (per cent)	365 (per cent)	405 (per cent)
1.5	0.17	0.214	0.26	67	61.1	55	25	0.2	0.8	25	65
1.7	0.26	0.300	0.36	55	50.1	43	20	0.2	0.7	20	50
2.0	0.36	0.429	0.54	43	37.3	29	15	0.2	0.5	14	35
2.5	0.54	0.643	0.75	29	22.8	18.0	12	0.2	0.3	5	15
3.0	0.75	0.857	1.07	18.0	13.9	8.50	9.0	0.2	0.2	0.5	6
4.0	1.07	1.286	1.50	8.50	5.18	3.16	5.0	0.2	0.2	0.5	1.0
5.0	1.50	1.714	1.93	3.16	1.93	1.18	2.5	0.2	0.2	0.2	0.5
6.0	1.93	2.143	2.36	1.18	0.72	0.44	1.5	0.1	0.1	0.1	0.5
7.0	2.36	2.571	2.79	0.44	0.27	0.164	1.3	0.1	0.1	0.1	0.5
8.0	2.79	3.000	3.21	0.164	0.100	0.061	1.0	0.1	0.1	0.1	0.5
9.0	3.21	3.429	3.64	0.061	0.037	0.023	0.8	0.1	0.1	0.1	0.5
10.0	3.64	3.857	4.07	0.023	0.0139	0.0085	0.6	0.1	0.1	0.1	0.5
11.0	4.07	4.286	4.50	0.0085	0.0052	0.0032	0.5	0.05	0.05	0.05	0.1
12.0	4.50	4.714	4.93	0.0032	0.0019	0.0012	0.5	0.05	0.05	0.05	0.1
13.0	4.93	5.143	5.36	0.0012	0.00072	0.00044	0.4	0.05	0.05	0.05	0.1
14.0	5.36	5.571	5.79	0.0004	0.00027	0.00016	0.3	0.05	0.05	0.05	0.1

NOTE: The values given apply to class I filter glass. For class II filter lenses, the transmittances and tolerances are the same, with the additional requirement that the transmittance of 589.3 millimicrons shall not exceed 15 per cent of the luminous transmittance. Some of the headings in this table have been changed to conform with NBS Letter Circular LC857.

Spectral-Transmissive Properties and Use of Eye-Protective Glasses. Reprinted from National Bureau of Standards Circular

4.   Potential nonradiation hazards--location of ultraviolet source near
     degreasing area, lack of ventilation system.

When surveying an area, the sample form found in Figure 6.2.3 can be used
as a basis for the survey.

Table 6.2.2

Filter lens shade numbers for various welding
and cutting operations (welder and helpers).

Type of Operation	Recommended Shade Number
Resistance welding, and for protection against stray light from nearby welding and cutting (if persons are out of the danger zone)	Clear or filters up to No. 2
Torch brazing and soldering	3 to 4
Light oxygen cutting and gas welding (to 1/8 inch)	4 or 5
Oxygen cutting, medium gas welding (1/8 to 1/2 inch) and arc welding up to 30 amps	5 or 6
Heavy gas welding (over 1/2 inch) and arc welding and cutting from 30 to 75 amps	6 or 8
Arc welding and cutting from 70 to 200 amps	10
Arc welding and cutting from 200 to 400 amps	12
Arc welding and cutting exceeding 400 amps	14

Note: Flash goggles should be worn under all arc-welding helmets,
       particularly for gas-shielded metal arc welding.

Adapted from Welding Handbook, 5th ed, American Welding Society.

Although the form is specifically defined for use with a specific
measurement device, the information to be collected on the form provides an
adequate summary of the information needed to evaluate an ultraviolet
radiation source. A summary of the components of the form is as follows:

1.   USING ORGANIZATION--Company or division responsible for the
     ultraviolet source.

Figure 6.2.3

Ultaviolet radiation survey.

ULTRAVIOLET RADIATION SURVEY

GENERAL INFORMATION			
USING ORGANIZATION		ADDRESS	
TYPE OF EQUIPMENT		INTENDED USE	

MANUFACTURER	MODEL	SERIAL NUMBER	OTHER

WELDER ONLY	GAS	CURRENT	VOLTAGE	FILLER	MATERIAL

HAZARD DETERMINATION

MONITORING INSTRUMENT		PROBE	FILTER

ATTACHMENT	WAVELENGTH RANGE

INSTRUMENT READING	DISTANCE TO SOURCE	D/R	KEY	EXPOSURE TIME	· EXCEEDS STANDARD	
					YES	NO

ENVIRON- MENT

PHOTOSENSITIZING AGENTS NOTED: YES____ NO____

PERSONNEL

BACKGROUND
SAFETY TRAINING
UNAWARE ONLOOKER
OTHER

PERSONAL PROTECTION

IN USE

SIGNS	SKIN CREAM	PARTITIONS
EYE PROTECTION	CLOTHING	OTHER
RESTRICTED AREA	CURTAINS	
GLOVES	ENCLOSURES	

RECOM- MENDED

SURVIVED BY   DATE

2. ADDRESS--Self-explanatory.

3. TYPE OF EQUIPMENT--Ultraviolet radiation source: e.g., welder, germicidal lamp, xenon lamp.

4. INTENDED USE--Purpose of the source: e.g., research, construction, material testing, etc.

5. MANUFACTURER--Model, serial number, and identification specifications of the ultraviolet source.

6. WELDER ONLY--Refers to the operating parameters if a welder is used.
    a. GAS--List gases used for welding operation.
    b. VOLTAGE/CURRENT--If electric welder is used.
    c. FILLER--Welding rods and material used.
    d. MATERIAL--Material being welded, including coating.

7. MONITORING INSTRUMENT--Device used to monitor ultraviolet source.

8. PROBE--Detector used.

9. FILTER--Type of filtering system used.

10. ATTACHMENTS--Attenuator, screen, beam splitters, etc.

11. WAVELENGTH RANGE--Sensitivity range of the monitoring system.

12. INSTRUMENT READING

13. DISTANCE TO SOURCE--Distance from measuring point to source.

14. D/R--Whether it is a direct or reflected reading.

15. KEY--Key location in diagram developed.

16. EXPOSURE TIME--Average exposure time per workday.

17. EXCEEDS STANDARD--Comparison of instrument reading to exposure standard.

18. ENVIRONMENT--A drawing of the potential exposure area including ultraviolet radiation source, point of measurement, personnel location (time of exposure per workday), nonradiation hazards, protective devices, and presence of photosensitizing agents.

19. PERSONNEL--The type of personnel usually involved in the area of the ultraviolet source, their location, and exposure time per day should be recorded.

20. PERSONNEL PROTECTION--Existing protection devices which are presently being used and any recommended protection devices that could be added including such things as painting the walls to reduce reflection.

21.   SURVEY BY/DATE--The signature and date of the surveyor conducting t
analysis.

Lasers

Lasers provide a unique hazard because of the high concentration of ener
that can be placed on a point target. As with ultraviolet radiation, the
primary concern is with exposure to the skin and eyes. The eyes present an
interesting problem in that the already concentrated ray of energy may be ev
more concentrated by the focusing capability of the lens of the eye, as
presented in Figure 6.2.4. Part A of the figure illustrates parallel rays o
a laser being focused to a point image by the eye. Part B illustrates rays
from an extended source (as from a conventional lamp or rays from a diffuse
reflection of a laser beam) produce a sizable (and less dangerous) image at
the retina. Therefore, threshold limit values have been established for the
eye and the skin.

Figure 6.2.4

Observing laser light.

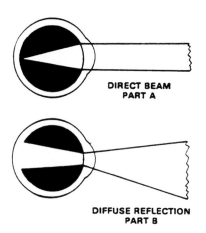

The requirements for periodic analysis and measurement of laser beams are
minimized because of the accuracy of the manufacturers' specifications,
design, and engineering; the problems and complexity of radiometric
measurement techniques; and in general, the high cost of detectors. It is
possible, however, to calculate the beam intensity (I-J/cm^2) at a selected
range. To do this, the power output (E-Watts), the range of interest (r-cm),
beam divergency (ϕ-radians), and initial beam diameter (a-cm) must be
known. To calculate the beam intensity, the following formula is used:

$$I = \frac{Ee^{-ur}}{[\pi/4(a + r\phi)]^2}$$

NOTE: e^{-ur} where r is the range of interest and u is an atmospheric
attenuation factor (cm^{-1}) related to atmospheric attenuation
which can be ignored if the range is less than 10 kilometers.

Example

A typical laser has an initial beam diameter of 2.54 cm, power output of
5 mW, and a beam divergence of 0.1 mrad (10^{-4} rad). What is the beam
intensity at 60 cm?

Solution

$$I = \frac{E}{[\pi/4(a + r\phi)]^2}$$

$$I = \frac{5.0 \times 10^{-3}W}{[\pi/4(2.54 + 60(10^{-4}))]^2}$$

$$= 1.25 \times 10^{-3}W/cm^2$$
$$= 1.25 \ mW/cm^2 \ at \ 60 \ cm$$

The calculation may then be further carried out to determine if the TLV level
is exceeded if the wavelength and typical exposure time are known. If it is
assumed that this particular laser beam operates at 312 nm and a typical
exposure is for 1 minute, then the exposure may be found to be:

$$TLV = 250 \ mJ/cm^2$$

$$\frac{250 \ mJ}{cm^2} \times \frac{sec\text{-}cm^2}{1.25 \ mJ} = 200 \ seconds$$

$$60 \ sec < 200 \ sec$$

The TLV is not exceeded.

By using the same equation, (a) substituting the threshold limit value per
unit time and (b) solving for time, it is possible to calculate the maximum
viewing time at a given distance.

$$I = \frac{E}{[\pi/4(a + r\phi)]^2}$$

$$I = \frac{J}{sec\text{-}cm^2} \qquad Assume \ I_t = TLV$$

$$I = \frac{I_t}{t} \qquad where \ t = time \ (sec)$$

$$\frac{I_t}{t} = \frac{E}{[\pi/4(a + r\phi)]^2}$$

$$t = (I_t/E)[(\pi/4)(a + r\phi)]^2$$

Further, if the equation is rearranged to solve for r, a minimum safe viewing distance can be calculated for a given exposure time.

$$t = (I_t/E)[(\pi/4)(a + r\phi)]^2$$

$$\frac{E \cdot t}{I_t} = [(\pi/4)(a + r\phi)]^2$$

$$(E \cdot t/I_t)^{1/2} \times 4/\pi = a + r\phi$$

$$r = \frac{(E \cdot t/I_t)^{1/2} \times (4/\pi) - a}{\phi}$$

To use any of the formulas, it is necessary to know the operational wavelength of the laser, the TLV, and the average viewing time or distance.

Example

A typical laser operating at 312 nm has an initial beam diameter of 1.5 cm, a power output of 2.25 mW, and a beam divergence of 0.1 milliradians. Calculate:

A. Maximum direct viewing time for an 8-hour period if the average viewing distance is 50 cm.

B. Minimum viewing distance if the average viewing time is 3 minutes p 8-hour period.

$$TLV_{312 \text{ nm}} = 250 \text{ mJ/cm}^2/8 \text{ hr}$$

Solution

A. $t = (I_t/E) [(\pi/4)(a + r\phi)]^2$
$I_t = 150 \text{ mJ/cm}^2$
$E = 2.25 \text{ mW}$
$a = 1.5 \text{ cm}$
$r = 50 \text{ cm}$
$\phi = 10^{-4} \text{ radians}$

$$t = (250 \text{ mJ} \cdot \text{cm}^{-2}) \times (1/2.25 \text{ sec} \cdot \text{mJ}^{-1}) \times [\pi/4 \ (1.5 \text{ cm} + 50 \text{ cm} \ (10^{-4}))]^2$$

$$= 155.2 \text{ sec} = 2.59 \text{ minutes}$$

B.
$$r = \frac{(E \bullet t / I_t)^{1/2} \times (4/\pi) - a}{\phi}$$

$I_t = 250$ mJ/cm^2
$E = 2.25$ mW
$a = 1.5$ cm
$t = 180$ sec
$\phi = 10^{-4}$ radians

$$r = \frac{[(2.25 \text{ mJ} \bullet \text{sec}^{-1} \times 1/250 \text{ cm}^2 \text{mJ}^{-1} \times 180 \text{ sec})^{0.5} (4/\pi)] - 1.5 \text{ cm}}{10^{-4}}$$

$$r = \frac{(1.27 \text{ cm} \times 4/\pi) - 1.5 \text{ cm}}{10^{-4}} = \frac{1.62 - 1.5 \text{ cm}}{10^{-4}} = 1200 \text{ cm}$$

This example illustrates the importance of properly controlling laser operation. If the direct viewing time is increased by 25 seconds (180 sec - 155 sec), the safe viewing distance varies from 50 cm to 1206 cm: a 24-fold increase.

A variety of detectors may be used to monitor laser intensity. These detectors are selected based upon the laser wavelength, its pulse duration, and the power intensities it generates. Generally, the two categories of laser detectors are thermal and photon. The photon devices operate on the principle of measuring the rate at which light quanta are absorbed. Examples of this type of detector are the photoelectric, photoconductive, and photovoltaic monitoring devices. Thermal devices measure the effect of heat and temperature change on a material when absorbing light energy. Examples of this type of device include the calorimeter, bolometer, thermocouple, and thermopile.

Average power measurements of continuous wave laser systems are usually with the conventional thermopile or photovoltaic cell. A typical thermopile will detect signals in the power range of from 10 mW to 100 mW. Many calorimeters and virtually all photographic methods measure total energy, but they can also be used for measuring power if the time history of the radiation is known.

When measuring laser intensities, the aperture stop of the device should closely approximate a pupil opening of 7 mm in distance. Calibration of the detector is required based upon the type of laser and wavelength involved. The spectral response of measurement devices should always be specified since the ultimate use of the measurements is the correlation with the spectral response of the biological tissue receiving the radiation insult.

The control of laser hazards is based primarily upon educating operating personnel, providing warnings to unsuspecting persons in the laser area, and general engineering designs that minimize hazards. For purposes of discussion, lasers have been classified based upon their potential hazard as identified in Table 6.2.3.

Table 6.2.3

NIOSH laser classification guide.

Class	Potential Hazard
I	Incapable of creating biological damage
II	Low-power—Beam may be viewed directly under carefully controlled conditions
III	Medium power—Beam cannot be viewed.
IV	High-power—Direct and diffusely reflected beam cannot be viewed or touch the skin.
V	Class II, III, IV which are completely enclosed so no radiation can leak out.

General operating requirements have also been established for each of the classes. Generally, a protective housing and interlock system which prevents human access during operation must be included as part of the laser design. Classes III and IV must have a key-activated master control which prevents the laser from being operated unless the key-activated switch is used. Classes II, III, and IV must give some type of visible or audible indication when the laser is emitting. Further, Classes II, III, and IV must have controls which are located outside the beam area. Finally, the viewing optics used in any laser system must reduce emission to below the threshold limit value. More specific requirements by classes are presented in Figure 6.2.5.

Aside from the aforementioned guidelines, the following guidelines are presented for consideration when developing a laser facility.

1. The laser should be attended at all times during operation.

2. Only personnel educated in the operation of the laser and in potential hazards should be permitted in the laser area.

3. Untrained personnel should not be permitted in the laser area.

4. Laser equipment and the laser area should be properly posted.

5. Direct viewing of the laser should not be done using binoculars or telescopes.

6. The laser should not be aimed at occupied areas without appropriate shielding.

7. Methods of confining laser plumes and laser-induced vaporization should be used.

8. Nonreflecting surfaces should surround the laser area.

9. Any laser beam that must pass through glass should pass through perpendicularly to minimize the amount of beam reflectance.

10. The maximum range of the beam direction should be controlled and minimized to within the shielded area.

11. Combustible solvents and materials should be stored away from the laser.

12. Potential nonlaser hazards should be evaluated, including:

    a. Voltage sources and leads
    b. X-radiation from high-voltage sources
    c. Ozone generation from high-voltage sources and ultraviolet radiation
    d. Underground electrical equipment, including laser heads and work stations
    e. Toxic materials
    f. Combustible materials
    g. Chemically active materials
    h. Cryogenic fluids
    i. Inert purging gases
    j. Flash-lamp explosion
    k. Radiation other than laser beam
    l. Violent interactions during the interactions of the laser radiation and materials: e.g., explosions, fires, chemical reactions, brilliant plumes
    m. Mechanical failures
    n. Interlock failures
    o. Accidental discharging of the laser
    p. Invisibility of ultraviolet and infrared laser beams
    q. Potential human fallibility

13. Protective eyewear should be provided in any instances where the potential exposure is above $1 \ \pi W/cm^2$.

14. Periodic (annual) medical examinations, including eye examination, should be performed on all personnel working with or near the laser.

Eye protection should be provided whenever exposure levels may exceed $1 \ \pi W/cm^2$. The protective eyewear should prevent direct observation of the beam and also observation of the reflected beam; that is, side panels should be used. The protective eyewear should also be made of curved lens material such that the beam may not be reflected off the eyewear. Protective eyewear is developed based upon the wavelength of the laser beam, the optical density necessary to reduce the intensity of the beam to an acceptable level, the potential maximum output of the laser beam, the visible transmittance of the filtering system, and the filter damage threshold; i.e., level at which the filter is damaged by high energy lasers.

Generally, protective eyewear for lasers is based upon two concepts. First, the use of filters for absorption of specific spectral regions and

Figure 6.2.5

Special requirements by class.

Class of Laser			
I	II	III	IV
No requirement	Posting of signs in area	Well-controlled area	Restricted entry to facility--interlock
	Control of beam direction	No specular surfaces	Fail-safe system
		Terminate beam with diffuse material and minimum reflection	Alarm system
			Panic button
		Eye protection for direct beam viewing	Good illumination-- 150 footcandles
			Light-colored diffuse room surfaces
			Operated by remote control
			Designed to reduce fire hazard, buildup of fumes, etc.

second, selective reflection from a dielectric coating of a given percent of the beam. Figure 6.2.6 illustrates the method of construction of the eyewear using the dielectric coating procedure.

Table 6.2.4 illustrates typical laser eye-protection goggles based upon the manufacturers' information. As can be seen, the appropriate eyewear is based upon the various factors previously described; e.g., wavelength, visibl light transmission, and optical density.

Medical Surveillance. Medical examinations should be given to all personnel working with or near the laser unit. The examination should includ ophthalmologic examinations and dermatologic examinations by experienced personnel. Persons with the following conditions should not be permitted to work near lasers: eye disease, skin problems, chronic pulmonary or cardiovascular disease, chronic emotional and mental illness, hypothyroidism, diabetes, and pregnancy. In general, strict guidelines should be established with respect to the medical surveillance of personnel working with lasers.

Figure 6.2.6.

Eyewear construction.

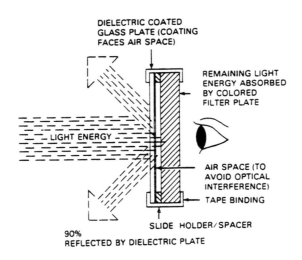

DIELECTRIC COATED
GLASS PLATE (COATING
FACES AIR SPACE)

REMAINING LIGHT
ENERGY ABSORBED
BY COLORED
FILTER PLATE

LIGHT ENERGY

AIR SPACE (TO
AVOID OPTICAL
INTERFERENCE)

TAPE BINDING

SLIDE HOLDER/SPACER

90%
REFLECTED BY DIELECTRIC PLATE

Microwaves

The general hazard in dealing with microwave and other radio frequency
radiation is the absorption of microwave causing a general temperature
increase at the exposure site or overall body temperature. Microwaves also
have the capability of potential cataract formation, and some experts believe
that microwaves have a potential effect on the central nervous system.

When measuring microwaves, the near and far fields of the microwave must
be considered. In the near field, the electrical and magnetic field are
perpendicular to each other and may potentially interact with the microwave
source. In the far field, there is no interaction between the electric,
magnetic, and the source of the wave. The radius of the near field or the
distance from the antenna to the intersection of the near and far field can be
calculated as follows:

$$radius = a/2\lambda$$

where
a = the antenna
λ = the wavelength

With microwaves, it is possible to calculate the power densities in the
near and far fields and to calculate a minimum safe approach distance in the
far field. To estimate the power density (W) in the near field, the following
formula is used:

$$W = 4P/A$$

Table 6.2.4

Laser eye protection goggles based on manufacturer's information.

$$\text{OPTICAL DENSITY} = \log_{10} \frac{1}{\text{Transmittance}}$$

Manufacturer or Supplier	Catalogue Number	Argon 4880 Å	HeNe 6328 Å	Ruby 6943 Å	GaAs 8400 Å	Nd 10600 Å	CO₂ 10.6 µ	UV <4000 >3000 Å	Coated Filter	Approx. Cost $	No. of glass filters & thickness of each	Visible Light transmission	Useful Range Å
American Optical Co.	SCS—437,*	0.15	0.20	0.36	1	5	High	No	No	55	1, 3.5 mm	90 %	10600
	SCS—440												10600
	580, 586°	0.2	2	3.5	4	2.7	—	>0.2	No	35, 25*1, 3.5 mm		27.5%	—
	581, 587°	0.6	4.1	6.1	5.5	3	—	>1.6	No	35, 25*1, 3.5 mm		9.6%	6328
	584	0	1	5	13	11	High	>0.6	No	55	2, 2 mm	46 %	10600
	585	0.3	2	8	21	17	High	>0.6	No	55	2, 2 mm	35 %	6943-10600
	598*	13	0	0	0	—	—	>14	No	25*	1, 3 mm	23.7%	4550-5150
	599	11	0	0	0	—	—	>14	No	35	1, 2.5 mm	24.7%	4550-5150
	680	0	0	0	0	0	50	No	No	35	1, 2.7 mm	92 %	10600
	698	13	1	4	11	8.5	High	>14	No	55	2, 2&3mm	5 %	10600 and 5300
Bausch & Lomb	5W3754	15	0.2	0	0	0	≦35	20	Yes	39	1, 7.9 mm	4.3%	3300-5300
	5W3755	4	0	0	0	0.1	≦35	10	Yes	39	1, 7.9 mm	57 %	4000-4600
	5W3756	0.8	12	15	5.6	4.8	≦35	3	Yes	39	1, 6.4 mm	6.2%	6000-8000
	5W3757	0.9	4.5	7.7	12	5.7	≦35	2	Yes	39	1, 7.1 mm	4.7%	7000-10000
	5W3758	1.9	1.8	2.2	4.8	7.5	≦35	2	Yes	39	1, 7.6 mm	3 %	10000-11500
Control Data Corp.	TRG-112-1	—	5	12	30	30	—	No	No	50	1, 6 mm	22 %	6943
	TRG-112-2	10	0	0	0	0	—	No	No	50	1, 6 mm	31 %	4880
	TRG-112-3	5	2	6	15	15	—	No	No	50	2, 3 mm	5 %	6943-4880
	TRG-112-4	—	—	—	—	—	High	No	No	50	1, 5 mm	92 %	106000
Fish-Schurman Corp.	FS650AL/18	0.34	3.8	10	>10	>10	—	No	No	30	1, 6 mm	30 %	6943, 8400, 106000
Glendale Optical Co.	NDGA**	1	0.5	2	16	16	High	>20	No	25	Plastic	60 %	8400, 10600
	R**	0.4	2.2	6.3	0.4	0.0	High	5	No	25	Plastic	19 %	6943
	NH**	0.4	5	2.5	0.6	0.5	High	>10	No	25	Plastic	19 %	6328
	A**	15	0	0	0	0	High	>12	No	25	Plastic	59 %	4880, 5143
	NN**	0	0	0	0	0	High	>12	No	25	Plastic	70 %	3320, 3370
Spectrolab	—	8	5	9	13	12	0	8	Yes	115	2, 3.2 mm	<5 %	Broadband

*Spectacle Type.
°°Available in goggles or spectacle type.

CAUTION
1. Goggles are not to be used for viewing of laser beam. The eye protective device must be designed for the specific laser in use.
2. Few reliable data are available on the energy densities required to cause physical failure of the eye protective devices.
3. The establishment of engineering controls and appropriate operating procedures should take precedence over the use of eye protective devices.
4. The hazard associated with each laser depends upon many factors, such as output power, beam divergence, wavelength, pupil diameter, specular or diffuse reflection from surfaces.

where

W = power density (mW/cm²)
P = power output (mW)
A = effective area of the antenna (cm²)

If the above values are known, then the power density can be calculated. If the calculated power density is less than the TLV, then the near field is safe for occupancy. If the calculated W is greater than the TLV, then it must be assumed that the calculated level is present in all parts of the near field.

The far field power density is calculated by

$$W = \frac{AP}{\lambda^2 r^2}$$

where
  W = power density (mW/cm^2)
  A = effective antenna area (cm^2)
  P = average power output (mW)
  λ = wavelength (cm)
  r = distance from antenna (cm)

Rearranging this equation, it is possible to calculate a safe distance.

$$r = [(AP)/\lambda^2 W]^{1/2}$$

where
  r = safe distance (cm)
  A = effective antenna area (cm^2)
  P = average power output (mW)
  λ = wavelength (cm)
  W = power density (mW/cm^2)

Most survey instrumentation is designed to measure the far field and is calibrated in units of milliwatts per cm^2. Generally, this type of calibration is adequate for the measurements being taken to evaluate microwave hazards. The actual measurement of microwave radiation in the near field is much more complicated.

Generally, microwave survey instruments consist of a probe, meter and amplifier, and a power source as illustrated in Figure 6.2.7. The microwave instrumentation should be portable, rugged, and easily readable; and the probe should be directionally independent.

Microwave detectors are generally divided into two categories: thermal and electrical. Thermal detectors operate on the principle of absorption of microwave radiation causing a change in resistance (bolometer). For example, a thermistor is a semiconductor in which resistance decreases as the temperature increases. A barretter operates on the same principle; only the resistance increases as the temperature increases. Another type of thermal detector is the thermocouple, which has been discussed previously. This particular device produces a voltage difference when heated. One final detector that has not been discussed is an air pressure system. This type of detector measures the pressure changes in a confined gas when exposed to microwave radiation and the gas is heated. The problem with thermal detection devices is that they are sensitive to ambient temperature changes.

Electrical detectors, such as a diode or rectifier, are used to convert radio frequency current into direct current. This type of system is extremely sensitive and is used where a low level of microwave radiation may be present.

Figure 6.2.7

Microwave survey instruments.

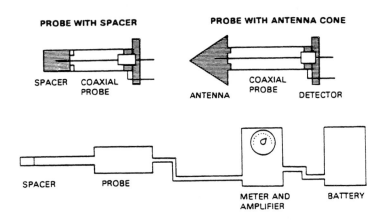

Except for the air pressure system, all detectors require some type of antenna (probe) to convert the wave radio frequency to wire-conducted radio frequency. The probes are typically wavelength specific; however, it may be possible to have a wide-band detector. When used, the probe must be parallel to the field during the reading to avoid field disturbance caused by the probe. Usually, the instruments and attached probe are calibrated for specific use upon purchase.

When taking measurements and calculating the exposure for microwave radiation, a similar procedure as outlined for ultraviolet radiation may be followed. Measurements should be taken periodically in any area of potential wave leakage or personnel exposure. A floor plan and outline of the work environment, equipment and personnel involved should be prepared. The calculation of exposure is also done as for ultraviolet radiation and should include such factors as exposure level, time, and distance from the source. However, a spectrum of relative biological effectiveness does not exist for microwave radiation as with ultraviolet radiation. Therefore, the calculatio of exposure is simplified.

Hazard Control. Hazards are generally best controlled by engineering design: e.g., location of the antenna, appropriate shielding within the device, and the preparation of safe operating procedures. When surveying for potential hazards, the following should be given consideration as potential hazard sources:

1.   Improper installation.

    a.   Poor location
    b.   Lack of proper grounding of low frequency supply
    c.   Inadequate or inoperative interlocks, controls, relays, and fus
    d.   Inadequate shielding of radio frequency areas and circuits

2.   Unsafe operating practices.

   a.   Unauthorized personnel operating equipment
   b.   Unauthorized adjustments of control
   c.   Lack of attention while operating equipment
   d.   Reaching into hoppers and conveyors to adjust or extract pieces
      while microwave is in operation
   e.   Failure to shut down equipment and report operating defects such
      as faulty operating sequence, relays that stick, circuit
      breakers that do not open or close properly, interlocks that
      fail or are blocked out
   f.   Feeding of brazing or soldering alloys during the heating cycle

3.   Faulty maintenance practices.

   a.   Poor maintenance schedule
   b.   Unauthorized repairmen
   c.   Failure to shut off power and use lockout procedures before
      servicing
   d.   Not discharging capacitors
   e.   Failure to short high-voltage leads to ground before working on
      equipment
   f.   Improper tools and failure to pick up tools after job
   g.   Lack of final check, after repairs and adjustments have been
      made, before energizing equipment

The use of protective clothing as identified with ultraviolet radiation is
not necessarily needed with microwave radiation except in special instances
where engineering design does not provide adequate protection for the
personnel. Shielding materials and enclosures may be considered in
environments where microwave radiation is present. The calculation and
development of the shielding is similar in principle as previously described
for ultraviolet radiation. Sample attenuation of potential shielding material
for microwave radiation may be found in Table 6.2.5. Finally, as with all
potential radiation sources, areas with microwave and radio frequency
radiation should be properly posted to advise personnel of potential hazards.

Table 6.2.5

Attenuation factors (shielding).

Material	Frequency			
	1-3 GHz	3-5 GHz	5-7 GHz	7-10 GHz
60 x 60 mesh screening	.01	.003	.006	.01
32 x 32 screening	.016	.006	.006	.016
16 x 16 window screen	.016	.01	.01	.006
1/4" mesh (hardware cloth)	.016	.032	.06	.1
Window glass	.63	.63	.50	.45
3/4" pine sheathing	.63	.63	.63	.45
8" concrete block	.01	.006	.002	.001

Presented at American Industrial Hygiene Conference, 1967; Palmisano, W., U.S. Army Environmental Hygiene Agency, Edgewood Arsenal, MD.

Summary

In this chapter, an introduction to the management and control of nonionizing radiation has been discussed. Specifically, ultraviolet radiation, lasers, and microwave radiation have been presented. The intent of this chapter is to provide an overview of the topic of control of nonionizing radiation.

3. Principles of Ionizing Radiation

This chapter is dedicated to the basic properties of ionizing radiation. The discussion will include a review of atomic structure, radioactivity, the types of radiation, the biological effects of ionizing radiation, and the established maximum permissible doses for the various types of ionizing radiation.

Atomic Structure

Over one hundred chemical elements exist on the earth. These elements provide the basic ingredients in all material things. An atom is the smallest particle of an element that possesses the chemical properties of that element. Each atom is composed of three fundamental particles that are most easily described in terms of two physical properties--electric charge and mass. The first particle is a proton. The <u>proton</u> has a positive charge (+1) and a mass of approximately one atomic mass unit (amu). The identity of the chemical element is based on the number of protons. The second particle is a <u>neutron</u>. This particle has no charge and a mass of approximately one amu. The proton and neutron contribute most of the mass of an atom and reside in a small volume called the "nucleus." The third particle is an <u>electron</u>. The electron has a negative charge (-1) and a mass of approximately 5.4×10^{-4} amu. The electrons exist in orbit around the nucleus. Each orbit represents a higher energy level for the electron.

An atom is said to be electrically neutral if the number of protons in the nucleus is equal to the number of electrons orbiting the nucleus. An atom with a surplus or deficit of orbital electrons will be negatively or positively charged respectively and is called an <u>ion</u>. The number of neutrons found in the nucleus is related to the number of protons, but there is not a direct correlation between protons and neutrons as there is in an electrically neutral atom. Figure 6.3.1 illustrates the particles of an atom for helium.

Radioactivity

As stated, in the nucleus of an atom with a given number of protons, nuclear stability exists with a specific number of neutrons. It is assumed that the neutrons provide stability in the nucleus by acting as a "nuclear cement" that counteracts the repulsive forces and increases the attractive forces of the positively charged protons confined in a small area. It is entirely possible, however, that an atom exists having a different number of

Figure 6.3.1

Components of the atom.

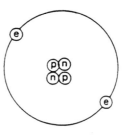

p = PROTON

n = NEUTRON

e = ELECTRON

neutrons, other than the number that causes stability, for the same number of protons. When an element has the same number of protons but a different number of neutrons, the element with the excess neutrons is referred to as an isotope. Figure 6.3.2 shows the element hydrogen with its isotopes. In each of the atoms--hydrogen, deuterium, and tritium--the number of protons and electrons remains the same (one of each) and the number of neutrons varies. As shown, hydrogen is the stable atom; deuterium is a stable isotope of hydrogen; and tritium is a radioactive isotope of hydrogen.

Figure 6.3.2

Isotopes of hydrogen.

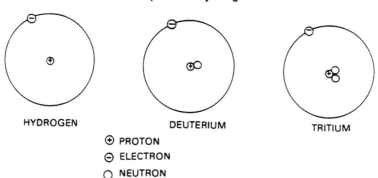

HYDROGEN   DEUTERIUM   TRITIUM

⊕ PROTON
⊖ ELECTRON
○ NEUTRON

With respect to nomenclature, the symbol for each of these isotopes is as follows:

Hydrogen: $_1H^1$
Deuterium: $_1H^2$--Hydrogen-2; ^2H
Tritium: $_1H^3$--Hydrogen-3; ^3H

In the first type of nomenclature, the subscript to the left of the element symbol indicates the number of protons in the element. The superscript to the right of the element symbol indicates the atomic weight of the isotope. Because the atomic weight attributed to the orbital electrons is usually considered insignificant (5.4×10^{-4} amu), the number of neutrons in the isotope being discussed can be calculated by subtracting the atomic weight from the number of protons. Therefore, using this approach, the number of neutrons in the isotope $_{92}U^{238}$ would be 146. The remaining two nomenclature forms merely list the element and atomic weight. These are important concepts because many elements have a number of isotopes, and these isotopes are present in the literature in any one of the preceding formats.

Because the isotope of an element has an improper combination of protons and neutrons, the nucleus of the atom is at a higher energy level and is said to be unstable. The term, radioactivity, refers to this improper combination of protons and neutrons that is in an unstable energy state. In an effort to find a more stable state, the atom will spontaneously transform, emitting some type of radiation to release energy. This is analogous to an orbital electron going from a higher energy orbital to a lower energy orbital and, in doing so, giving off light energy. In the instance of radiation being emitted from the nucleus, however, the radiation (energy) may be emitted as:

1. Alpha particle--A high-energy particle composed of two protons and two neutrons. It has a mass of 4 amu and a charge of +2.

2. Beta particles--Electrons emitted by the nuclei which may be positively or negatively charged. The mass of a beta particle is insignificant.

3. Gamma radiation--Bundles (photons) of electromagnetic radiation.

4. A combination of the above emissions.

Alpha Particles. The alpha particle originates in the nucleus of a radioactive atom. It is composed of two protons and two neutrons. It has a mass of four atomic mass units (amu) and a charge of +2. Because of its structure, it is the same as the nucleus of a helium atom.

Depending upon the radionuclide source, the energy of an alpha particle varies and may be as high as 10 million electron volts (MeV). Because of its energy, the alpha particle causes more ionization (formation of ions in an absorbing material) than a beta or gamma radiation would in an absorbing material. However, because of its large mass and positive charge, the distance the alpha particle can travel is very short. For example, the general range of an alpha particle in air is approximately 4 inches. It can be stopped by a film of water, sheet of paper, or other paper-thin materials. Because of its short range, the danger in alpha particle radiation is not penetration through the skin but entrance of alpha particle emitters into the body through the respiratory or digestive systems.

The emission of alpha particles occurs through the radioactive decay of the larger elements. An example of an alpha source is Thorium-232 or Uranium-238. As discussed, if an alpha particle is emitted, the atomic weight and atomic number of the emitting radionuclide are altered. Referring to the sample radioactive decay (Figure 6.3.3), the alteration of the elements can be seen each time an alpha particle is emitted.

Once emitted, the alpha particle will attract two electrons to form a helium atom. Because the alpha particle causes the removal of two electrons from other atoms or molecules, the alpha particle is said to cause direct ionization (Figure 6.3.3).

Figure 6.3.3

Alpha particle interaction.

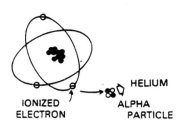

IONIZED   ALPHA
ELECTRON   PARTICLE

Beta Particles. The beta particle, as with the alpha particle, originates in the nucleus of a radioactive atom. The beta particle is an electron emitted during radioactive decay. The beta particle can be positively or negatively charged; but in either case, the atomic mass of the beta particle is negligible when considering the change in atomic weight of the radionuclide. The energy level associated with a beta particle is usually in the range of 0.017 to 4.0 million electron volts (MeV).

As previously stated, the beta particle may be positively or negatively charged. If the beta particle has a positive charge, it is referred to as a positron. In the formation of a positron, a proton in the nucleus assumes the properties of a neutron, and the beta particle is emitted with a positive charge. Because a proton is lost in the process, when a positron is emitted the atomic number of the element decreases by one. However, because only themass of an electron is emitted, the atomic mass of the element remains the same. For example, when the element Zinc-65 ($_{30}Zn^{65}$) emits a positron, the new element which would be produced because of the loss of a proton would be copper ($_{29}Cu^{65}$). Once the positron is emitted, it will collide or interact with an electron in the medium and be annihilated. Upon annihilation, gamma radiation is emitted.

If the beta particle emitted is negative, then it is referred to as a negatron or high-speed electron. In the nucleus, a neutron assumes the basic properties of a proton, and a negatron is emitted. Because a proton is added to the nucleus, the atomic number increases by one, and a new element is formed. Once emitted, the high-speed electron will interact with the medium and cause direct ionization along with the formation of X-radiation. An example of beta decay that involves the emission of negatrons may be observed in the radioactive decay series (Figure 6.3.4). As shown in Table 6.3.1, each time a negatron is emitted, the atomic mass remains the same while the atomic number increases by one. Because each element is defined by its atomic number, each time a negatron is emitted, a new element is formed.

Table 6.3.1

Positron versus negatron.

Beta	Description	Charge	Mass (amu)	Energy Level	Effect of Emission
Positron	High-speed electron with positive charge	+1	0.00054	Up to several MeV	Z number decreases by 1
Negatron	High-speed electron with negative charge	-1	0.00054	Up to several MeV	Z number increases by 1

The penetration capability of the beta particle is somewhat greater than the alpha particle. This is due to the smaller mass and charge of the beta particle. For example, the average range of a beta particle in air is less than six feet; in wood, 1.5 inches; in human tissue, 0.1-0.5 inches. Beta particles can be stopped by material of low atomic weight; e.g., aluminum. In general, this is the type of shielding material used when dealing with beta radiation.

As with alpha radiation, beta radiation causes direct ionization. Further, as discussed, the interaction of the positron with the medium causes the formation of gamma radiation; and the interaction of a negatron with the medium causes the formation of X-radiation. Because of its relatively short range, the beta particle provides a minimum hazard. However, because of the potential formation of secondary gamma and X-radiation with somewhat longer range, the beta particle is a greater external radiation hazard than the alpha particle.

Gamma Radiation. Gamma radiation is a short-wave electromagnetic radiation. It originates from the nucleus; but emission of gamma radiation does not cause any change in the element's properties, atomic number, or atomic weight. Gamma radiation is emitted because the nucleus is in an unstable, excited state; and the emission of gamma radiation releases energy and causes the nucleus to fall to a more stable energy level.

The energy level associated with gamma radiation is the highest electromagnetic radiation that will be discussed. The energy level of gamma radiation is dependent upon the radionuclide source but usually falls within the range of 0.15 to 4 million electron volts. The source of gamma radiation is the radioactive decay of radioisotopes and the destruction of positrons as previously described.

Because gamma radiation has no mass or charge, is a wave, and has a relatively high energy content, gamma radiation has the potential for very deep penetration. This capability of deep penetration presents a tremendous health problem in the working environment. For example, to dissipate the energy of 1 millielectron volt of gamma radiation to one-half its original energy level, it would be necessary to have a shield of 0.5 inches of steel. Considering that potential energy levels of gamma radiation can reach one million times this value, gamma radiation is an obvious problem.

The photons associated with gamma radiation interact with atoms and molecules of the absorbing material in three ways.

1.   Photoelectric effect--Incident photons cause the ejection of orbital electrons. These electrons possess energy equal to the difference between the photon energy and the electron binding energy. As shell vacancies are corrected, X-radiation is formed. Also, the resultant electron may interact to form X- or gamma radiation.

2.   Compton effect--Incident photon gives up part of energy to orbital electrons. The electrons may recoil and be rejected. Further, the degraded photon may interact further with other electrons.

3.   Pair production--High-energy photon interacts with electric field surrounding a charged particle (nucleus). The interaction causes the formation of an electron and positron of equal energy. When the positron and electron collide or slow down, X- or gamma radiation is formed.

There are approximately 240 radionuclides (radioactive isotopes) which undergo this spontaneous transformation (radioactive decay) to reach a more stable energy level. Depending upon the type of emission, the isotope may undergo a change and, in essence, form a new element or new isotope. If, for example, an alpha or beta particle is emitted, a new element would be formed because protons are either gained or lost. If a neutron is emitted, the element is the same; but a new isotope is formed. If gamma radiation is emitted, then the element would remain the same; but the energy level in the nucleus would be lower.

It is entirely possible that, as radioactive decay occurs, the new isotope that is formed is also in an unstable state. It too would then undergo a spontaneous transformation, emit some type of radiation, and form a new element. Each of the new radionuclides formed from the spontaneous transformation is referred to as a "daughter product." Spontaneous transformation and the production of daughter products will continue until the chain of events forms a stable isotope or element. The decay change presented in Figure 6.3.4 illustrates the decay of Uranium-238 ($_{92}U^{238}$) to Lead-206 ($_{82}Pb^{206}$) through a series of alpha and beta emissions.

The steps in the decay process are shown in the diagram, where each nucleus that plays a part in the series is shown by a circle. The vertical

Figure 6.3.4

Uranium-238 decay.

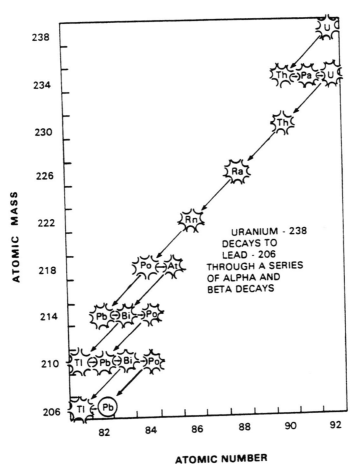

column containing the circle indicates its atomic number, and the horizontal
column indicates the atomic mass. Each arrow that slants downward toward the
left shows an alpha emission (two protons and two neutrons), and each arrow
that points to the right shows a beta emission (electron). Notice that some
of the nuclei in the series can decay in more than one direction. This is but
one of four similar radioactive series that can occur in nature. Because of
this chaining effect of radioactive decay, it is possible for the total
radioactivity to increase beyond the radioactivity present in the original
isotope.

The radioactive decay rate of a radionuclide is measured in terms of a
characteristic time, the half-life. The half-life of a radioactive material
is the time needed for half of the active atoms of any given quantity to
decay. Isotope X, for example, has a half-life of 24 hours. This means that
half of any given specimen of Isotope X will be converted to some other
element by the end of 24 hours. Then, in the next 24 hours, half of the
remaining Isotope X will decay, leaving only one-fourth of the original number
of Isotope X atoms. Therefore, the number of atoms decaying is proportional
to the number of atoms present. This is constant for any radionuclide.
Figure 6.3.5 illustrates a typical half-life scheme ($T^{1/2}$) for an isotope
having a half-life value of 24 hours. As can be seen by the illustration, by
the end of the third half-life, the radioactivity has dropped to approximately
one-eighth of its original activity; and by the end of the seventh half-life
period, the activity has decreased to less than one percent of the original
activity. Using this illustration, one can see that the longer the half-life
value, the smaller the amount of radiation that will be released at any given
time.

Figure 6.3.5

Decay of radioactive material.

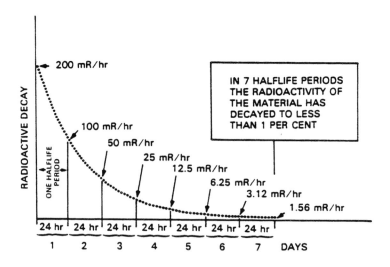

There are two other types of ionization radiation which are important but are not formed by radioactive decay. The two forms of radiation to be discussed are X-radiation and neutrons.

X-radiation. X-radiation is also electromagnetic radiation. It is similar in property to gamma radiation and interacts with absorbing materials in a similar manner, but it does not have as high an energy level as gamma radiation.

X-radiation originates outside the nucleus. In general, the principle behind the formation of X-radiation is that high-speed electrons (negatrons) are slowed down or stopped. In the process of slowing down, the electrons give up energy in the form of X-radiation. The quantity of energy released is dependent upon the speed of the electron and the characteristics of the medium (striking target). Generally, there are two types of radiation formed: bremstrahlung, which is caused by deflection of electrons traveling near a nucleus; and characteristic, which is produced in energetic transitions between orbital electron levels.

X-radiation is generally produced by machine, although some X-radiation is emitted from the collision of negatrons during the process of radioactive decay.   The machine necessary to produce X-radiation has basically three components (Figure 6.3.6): (1) cathode (electron source), (2) anode (target), and (3) potential difference between the cathode and the anode in a vacuum. In the machine, a potential difference is established between the cathode and the anode. The electrons travel through the vacuum at high speeds until they strike the target (anode). The energy released from their collision is in the form of X-radiation.

Figure 6.3.6

X-ray machine.

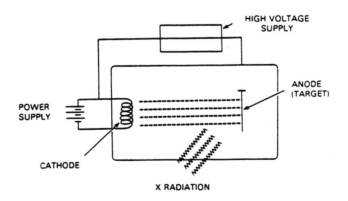

The penetrating capability of X-radiation is dependent upon the wavelength of the radiation. X-radiation with a short wavelength (approximately 0.001-0.1 nm in length) is called "hard" X-radiation. This type of radiation has the capability to penetrate several inches of steel. X-radiation with longer wavelength (0.1-1.0 nm) is called "soft" and is less penetrating than hard X-radiation. The range of penetration of X-radiation is dependent upon the energy of the radiation and the type of medium it is penetrating. For example, the half-value layer (thickness required to reduce incident radiation by 0.5) is several inches of concrete. As previously discussed, the interaction with the target medium is the same for X-radiation as with gamma radiation.

Neutrons. The final type of ionizing radiation to be discussed is the neutron. The neutron particle originates from the nucleus. It has an atomic mass of 1 amu and a charge of 0. The energy level usually associated with neutrons is greater than gamma or X-radiation but is less than alpha or beta radiation. However, because of the zero charge on the neutron, the neutron has a greater penetrating capability than the alpha or beta particle.

Neutrons are formed in basically two ways. First, it is possible to bombard a light element, e.g., beryllium or lithium, with alpha particles or gamma radiation and increase the energy in the nucleus so that a neutron will be emitted. The second source is the fission of isotopes of uranium or plutonium. This fission is caused by neutron bombardment and results in the production of more neutrons. Because the reaction is produced by neutrons and results in the production of neutrons, a chain reaction may be established such that the neutrons resulting in the fission of a given uranium or plutonium isotope cause the fission of more isotopes. Because of this, the principle of criticality evolves. There is a minimum level of concentration required of the radioisotope to allow the chain reaction to begin. This is usually referred to as the "critical level." If the critical level is not exceeded, the chain reaction will not occur. If, however, the critical level is exceeded, a chain reaction may be produced by the fission of a single plutonium atom.

Neutrons are developed through nuclear reactions as described above or are mechanically produced through the use of accelerators such as the Van de Graff or the Cockroft-Walton generator.

The interaction of neutrons with a target medium is dependent upon the energy level of the neutron. Neutrons of a high energy level (fast neutrons) collide with the nuclei of the absorbing material and lose energy in a billiard-ball-like collision. Neutrons with less energy (slow/thermal neutrons) are captured by the absorbing nuclei. In either case, alpha, beta, or gamma radiation is emitted. Because ionization is secondary, the calculation of neutron dose is difficult.

The penetrating capability of the neutron is dependent upon the energy level, characteristics of the medium, and type of collision which occurs. The average distance the neutron of a given energy level will travel before some type of interaction is referred to as mean free path (mfp). The probability of an interaction in three mean free paths is equal to 0.95. As an example, in human tissue, the mean free path of a neutron may vary from 0.25 to several inches.

Table 6.3.2 summarizes the ionizing radiation discussed, and Figure 6.3.7 illustrates the relative penetrating capability of the types of ionizing radiation.

Units of Measure

When discussing radioactivity and the energies involved, the following units of measure will be of value. When reviewing the terms, place emphasis on the concepts of each term rather than the actual numerical value.

Units of Energy. In physics, the standard unit of energy is the joule. The joule represents the work done when a constant force of one newton moves a body a distance of one meter in the direction of the force. Energies of atomic and nuclear phenomena are usually given in terms of electron volts (eV). One electron volt is the kinetic energy acquired by an electron after being accelerated through a potential difference of one volt. Energies encountered in radioactive decay processes are usually expressed in terms of thousands of electron volts (KeV) or millions of electron volts (MeV). For example, the energy of Cesium-137 gamma radiation is 0.667 million electron volts. If necessary, it is possible to convert joules to electron volts using the factor:

$$1,000,000 \text{ electron volts (eV)} = 1.602 \times 10^{-13} \text{ joules (J)}$$

Units of Activity. The measure of the rate of radioactive decay is given in terms of activity. The activity reflects the number of radioactive atoms emitting ionizing radiation. The special unit of activity is the curie (Ci) and is defined in terms of events per unit time, disintegrations per minute, or counts per minute. The numerical value for a curie is as follows:

$$1 \text{ curie (Ci)} = 3.7 \times 10^{10} \text{ disintegrations per second}$$

When discussing a quantity of radioisotopes, the quantity is discussed with respect to the amount of activity of that quantity. Therefore, it would be more appropriate to state that a quantity of uranium is "an amount of uranium with an activity of 500 curies" rather than "500 curies of uranium."

Exposure. The roentgen (R) is the special unit of exposure. This unit refers specifically to the measure of the amount of charge produced in air by gamma or X-radiation. Numerically, one roentgen corresponds to the production of about 2×10^9 ion pairs per centimeter^3 of dry air at standard temperature and pressure. Exposure rate is the time derivative of exposure and is usually expressed in terms of roentgens per hour, roentgens per minute, or milliroentgens per hour, etc. The exposure rate constant (Γ) is the exposure rate per curie of radioisotope at 1 meter. The values of Γ are tabulated in the literature for many gamma emitters.

Absorbed Dose. The absorbed dose (D) is the energy imparted by ionizing radiation to absorbing matter per unit mass of absorbing material. The

Table 6.3.2

Properties of ionizing radiation.

Type	Source	Description	Charge	Mass (amu)	Energy	Radiation Hazard	Necessary Shielding
Alpha	Natural and manmade isotopes	Helium nucleus-- causes direct ionization	+2	4	2-9 MeV	Internal hazard only	Thin sheet of paper
Beta	Most radio-active isotopes	Electron (+ or -) ionizes 1/100 as heavily as alpha	+1	.00054	Up to several MeV	Internal or external danger	Thick sheet of cardboard
Gamma	Natural isotopes-- nuclear reactions	High energy electromagnetic radiation	0	0	Up to several MeV	Dangerous--deep penetration	Heavy shielding -- e.g., inches of lead
X	Slowing of electrons	High energy electromagnetic radiation--less than gamma	0	0	Up to several MeV	Dangerous--deep penetration	Heavy shielding
Neutrons	Nuclear reactions	Uncharged particles	0	1	Up to several MeV	Hazardous	Thick shielding composed of light elements

Figure 6.3.7

Ionizing penetration.

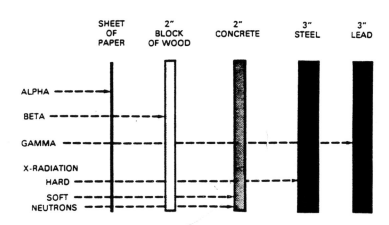

standard unit of absorbed dose is the <u>rad</u> and is defined as
1 rad = 10^{-2} joules/Kg. The absorbed dose rate is the time derivative of
absorbed dose and reflects the given absorbed dose over a given period of
time. It is usually expressed in terms of millirads per hour, rads per
second, etc.

Dose Equivalent. Because of the specific biological effects and actions
of radiation upon human tissue, the measure of exposure or even absorbed dose
does not present completely the measurement of ionizing radiation. For
example, each type of ionizing radiation has a different penetrating
capability. Alpha particles will have no detrimental effect to the body
unless they enter the body through some means other than penetrating through
the skin; whereas, gamma radiation easily penetrates the protective layer of
the skin and can cause severe internal damage. Further, certain radionuclide
sources, if introduced to the body, will migrate to certain areas of the
body. An example of this is the radioisotope of calcium. Because of their
properties and involvement in the development of bone tissue, most
radioisotopes with properties similar to that of calcium will tend to
concentrate in the body in the bone areas. Because of this, one cannot
evaluate the problem of radiation based upon a whole-body exposure. Finally,
the effect of the various types of radiation on different parts of the body
will vary. For example, areas of the hands, arms, and feet are less sensitive
to radiation exposure than other areas such as the eyes, internal organs, or
the reproductive organs.

To deal with these variations, a standard unit of dose equivalent has been
developed. It attempts to take into consideration the above-mentioned
factors. Generally, the unit, known as the <u>rem</u>, is equivalent to the exposure
(R) or the absorbed dose (rad) multiplied by the quality factor. Although not
absolute, it will be assumed that this quality factor (QF) corrects for the

relative biological efficiency of the different types of radiation (RBE). The exact QF varies according to the source of radionuclide, area of exposure, and type of ionizing radiation. However, to calculate the dose equivalent, the following values may be used for purposes of determining the rem value, given exposure or absorbed dose.

Calculation of dose equivalent.
[rem = rad (or R) x QF]

Type	QF
X-radiation	1.0
Gamma radiation	1.0
Beta radiation	1.0
Alpha radiation	20.0
Neutron (fast)	3.0
Neutron (slow)	10.0
Fission fragments	20.0

An example of the calculation is as follows:

Example

If the absorbed dose reading from a $_{88}Ra^{226}$ (alpha emitter) is found to be 0.05 mrad/hr at a distance of 1 meter, what is the dose equivalent for an exposure lasting 8 hours?

Solution

$$rem = rad \times QF$$

$$= \frac{0.05 \text{ mrad}}{hr} \times \frac{20 \text{ mrem}}{mrad}$$

$$= \frac{1.0 \text{ mrem}}{hr}$$

$$rem/8 \text{ hr} = \frac{1.0 \text{ mrem}}{hr} \times 8 \text{ hr} = 8.0 \text{ mrem}$$

Although the quality factor (QF) is not exact, it can be used to calculate the dose equivalent given the exposure or absorbed dose rate for low level sources. In later sections, the importance of dose equivalent will be presented.

Fluence. When evaluating particulate radiation (alpha, beta, neutron) it may be useful to know the number of particles entering a cross section of a given area. The unit used to express this value is fluence (Φ) and is expressed in terms of "particles per centimeter^2." If the sum of the energies of the particles that enter the cross sectional unit is to be discussed, then the unit is energy fluence (ψ) and is expressed in terms of "millielectron volts per centimeter^2."

Flux Density. If the fluence is to be determined over a given period of time and rate calculated, then this rate of fluence per unit time is referred to as flux density (ϕ). This is usually expressed in terms of "particles per centimeter^2 per second"; e.g., neutrons per centimeter^2 per second. The energy flux density is the energy fluence of a given period of time and is expressed in million electron volts per centimeter^2 per second.

Each of the terms presented in this section will be used throughout the remainder of the sections on ionizing radiation. It is not necessary to memorize all numerical values, but it is important to understand the concept behind each unit of measurement.

Biological Effects of Ionizing Radiation

The fundamental property of ionizing radiation relates to the transfer of energy when the radiation passes through material. Absorption of the energy may cause ionization (the expulsion of orbital electrons from the atom or molecule) or excitation of the orbital electrons to a higher energy state. The ions formed in turn react with other atoms and molecules in the absorbing material, causing potential changes in those molecules and the absorbing structure. Because ionizing radiation causes changes at the atomic and molecular level, the effects of ionizing radiation to the cells will be discussed initially; and then the overall systems function will be discussed.

The energy required to cause cell death is very small. A lethal dose of radiation dissipates approximately one-millionth the amount of energy dissipated by the cell during its normal daily function. Thus, a lethal dose affects only one of 2.0×10^7 molecules in a cell.

In the cell, ionizing radiation has two actions. First, if the ionizing radiation irradiates critical molecules of the cell, e.g., DNA or mitochondria, immediate cell death will occur. An indirect action can also occur by the irradiation of water molecules. This irradiation forms active products, e.g., H_2O_2, OH^-, O_2H^-, which react with other molecules within a cell and cause damage or death. Because irradiation is random at the cell level, the indirect action is more significant than the direct action. In general, radiation causes the following: immediate cell death, cell damage that prevents growth or causes the formation of cell mutations, or reduction of cell function and ultimately body function.

All forms of ionizing radiation produce some type of injury to the cell. Tissue reaction is dependent upon the density of the ionization in the radiation path; i.e., linear energy transfer. Particulate radiation (alpha, beta) produces more damage per energy absorbed, and thus a high relative biological efficiency and a greater linear energy transfer factor (amount of energy transferred per linear penetration). Electromagnetic radiation, because of its high penetration capability, causes more diffuse ionization. It should be noted that the particulate radiation is more damaging if allowed to enter the body (internal radiation hazard). Because particulate radiation has a small penetrating capability, the protective layers of the skin tend to provide a barrier to prevent the penetration of particulate radiation through the skin.

The response of an individual to radiation is dependent upon the dosage o the radiation; the amount and type of tissue irradiated, e.g., localized versus whole-body irradiation; and the length of time of exposure. A localized exposure; e.g., to the hands and arms, will cause damage to the specific irradiated site or organ. However, it is possible for a local exposure to cause systemic changes. Whole-body irradiations tend to cause systemic-type illnesses. Signs and symptoms such as nausea, vomiting, skin erythema, intestinal bleeding, and diarrhea are common to whole-body irradiation. The following effects would be observed in man after acute whole-body doses of penetrating radiation:

1. 0-25 rad--no observable effect.

2. 25-50 rad--minor temporary blood changes.

3. 50-150 rad--possible nausea and vomiting, along with reduced white blood cell count.

4. 150-300 rad--exaggeration of above symptoms plus diarrhea, malaise, and loss of appetite.

5. 300-500 rad--exaggeration of above symptoms, plus hemorrhaging and loss of hair (depilation). About 50 percent of the untreated exposed population will die at 450-500 rad level.

6. Above 500 rad--Most of the above symptoms will appear sooner in more severe form. Survival chances diminish rapidly with higher doses.

Acute high-level doses or moderate doses over longer periods of time can produce effects later in life. The most notable effects include increased risk of cancer or leukemia; nonspecific life span shortening, i.e., acceleration of aging process; and harmful mutations that may be transmitted to future generations. In general, exposure to ionizing radiation causes a decrease in the efficiency of cell activity to the point that cell function is diminished and may ultimately cause cell death. To minimize the effect of ionizing radiation in the occupational environment, maximum levels of ionizing radiation exposure have been established.

Industrial Uses of Ionizing Radiation

For many years following the basic investigations in the field of radioactivity, the primary use of ionizing radiation was in the medical field and little progress was made in integrating ionizing radiation in industrial areas. Recent advances, such as fission and fusion techniques, have brought about the availability of economic radionuclides that are rapidly being introduced into the industrial field.

In most countries, only a small percentage of the total work force is involved in the industrial use of ionizing radiation. With few exceptions, the use of ionizing radiation has been remarkably free of radiation accident and injury. However, because of the potential hazard, much consideration must be given to the health and safety aspects as well as to the actual industrial applications of ionizing radiation. The following are examples of uses of ionizing radiation in the industrial environment.

Radiation Gauges. Ionizing radiation penetrates or is reflected by matter; and, with a suitable detector, it is possible to extract useful information from the transmitted or reflected beam. Because the intensity of radiation used is small, the beam is nondestructive and lends itself to automation. Some uses of a radiation gauge include the determination of sheet metal thickness, the density of metals or fluids, or the calculation of moisture content.

There are two types of gauges in use. The first is a transmission gauge that monitors the radiation penetrating a given substance. When using this type of gauge, the factors that will vary the transmission reading include the density and composition of the target material. The second type of gauge is a reflection-type gauge. It is more sensitive and in many instances may be the only practical solution. An illustration of a "backscatter" or reflection-type radiation gauge is given in Figure 6.3.8.

Figure 6.3.8

Reflection-type thickness gauge.

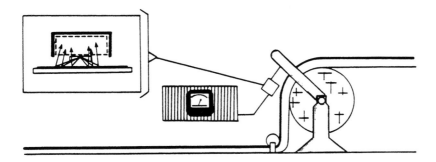

In these gauges, beta emitters are used in conjunction with a reflecting or backing material such that the backscatter electron intensity is linearly proportional to the thickness of the substance to be checked over a given range. These gauges are finding wide application because of the increasing industrial importance of thin films and coatings.

If the gauges automatically control the process, e.g., metal sheet rolling, then a greater accuracy can be obtained than with conventional control methods. Table 6.3.3 illustrates the increase in quality control when using a radiation gauge with automatic control versus a conventional type control sampling method.

Table 6.3.3

Process quality control comparison.

Industry	Application	Conventional Control (Normal sampling method)	Process Control (95% Correlation) Radiation Gauge With Manual Control	Radiation Gauge With Automatic Control
Paper	Fourdrinier paper machine	±12%	±10%	±3%
Metals	Tandem cold roll mill	±10%	±7%	±1.5%
Rubber	Sheeting calender	±10%	±6%	±3.2%
Rubber	Tire fabric calender	±6.5%	±5.5%	±3.5%
Plastics	Calender	±7%	±3.5%	±2.5%
Impregnation	Saturation dip coater	Automatic control provided an improvement factor of 2.5 over conventional		
Abrasive	Abrasive maker	Automatic control provided an improvement factor of 2 over conventional		

(From Crompton, C. E.)

The three types of ionizing particles in common use in radiation gauges are photons (X or gamma), beta (normally negative electrons), and neutrons (fast and thermal). A common source for industrial radiation gauge is a sealed source of Strontium-90 of up to 1 curie activity. All radiation sources made for such use must meet rigid specifications regarding resistance to temperature, pressure, impact, vibration, and puncture. Safety experience with such sources has been favorable; even gauges exposed to intense heat and fires have evidenced little or no leakage. Their locations and layout are normally such that external exposure of personnel is minimal. However, all sources should be periodically checked for leakage and maintained by qualified personnel.

Radiography and Fluoroscopy. Radiography is defined as the production of a shadow image of the internal structure of an object on a permanent record, usually by some type of film and template. The primary types of ionizing radiation used include photons (X or gamma) or neutrons (fast or thermal).

Radiography provides a close inspection during and after fabrication of materials or structure. Welds in nuclear power plants or high pressure pipelines, critical joints in the foundation of large buildings, and engines in large jet planes are only a few examples in which such a radiographic section plays a critical part. Industrial radiography comprises both field radiography and stationary radiography. Both are based on the same principle; but in field radiography the source of radiation is taken to the specimen, while in stationary radiography the specimen is taken to the source of radiation.

Fluoroscopy works on the same principle as radiography with the exception that the shadow image is presented temporarily on a screen. It is most appropriate for use in industry as a quality control tool for mass produced components, such as turbine blades and transistors, and for the inspection of such items as cables. Fluoroscopy is about four times less sensitive than radiography; therefore, it can be used only where such low sensitivity can be tolerated and is usually backed up by radiography.

In either of the above techniques, the primary hazard is the radiation source that is being used as part of the procedure.

X-Ray Diffraction and Fluorescent Analysis. It has been known for many years that the planes in a molecular crystal lattice will diffract X-radiation in a set three-dimensional pattern. Using this information, if X-radiation is emitted through a molecular structure and the diffraction pattern determined, it is then possible to evaluate the crystal state of the material. Further, it is also possible to determine the actual content of the material based upon the absorption and emission properties of ionizing radiation of that material.

The procedure of crystals for broadcast transmitters, watch movements, silicone and germanium semiconductors are all aided by the determination of crystal structure through X-ray diffraction techniques. The determination of crystalline structure of a finished product, such as a turbine blade or nuclear reactor vessel, provides information on the soundness and freedom from stress which are important in predicting the useful life of the product.

The personnel hazards are of a specialized nature. The greatest hazard is associated with very fine, intense X-ray beams. Further, the electron accelerating voltage is normally in the range of 30,000 to 50,000 volts. It is possible, therefore, that the primary beam of X-radiation may have an intensity as high as 7000 roentgens per second; and any part of the body held

in the beam for only fractions of a second would receive such a dose. Beside
the risk of exposure to the primary beam, a hazard also exists of exposure to
a beam scatter off the specimen or analyzing crystal, which could be quite
intense. Much less intense, but still strong enough to make further shielding
precautions advisable, is the scattered radiation around joints, around
shielding, and in general when the radiation is scattered at least twice.

The prime requisite for the safe operation of an X-ray diffraction and
fluorescent unit consists of proper training and supervision of operation
personnel. Accidents frequently occur when operators place their fingers and
hands in the primary beam to remove samples, forgetting that the beam is on.

Electron-Beam Equipment. The development of reliable electron guns and
electron optics using electric and magnetic fields has led to many interesting
and important industrial applications of electron beams. Two of them,
electron-beam evaporators and electron-beam welders, take advantages of the
unique ability of a defined electron beam to introduce a large amount of heat
at a specified point or area in a specimen. Two other applications, electron
microscopes and scanning electron microscopes, take advantage of the fact that
the electron beam can behave like a light wave and is capable of an extremely
high resolving power.

The electron-beam evaporator uses the heat generated when an electron beam
from a cathode strikes a target after being accelerated by application of a
high-potential, concentrated biomagnetic or electric field acting as an
electromagnetic "lens." The power emitted by the electron beam is absorbed as
heat at the surface of the target, causing the target surface to evaporate at
a rate that may be controlled by varying the voltage and the current of the
electron source. Metals such as tungsten and molybdenum and nonmetals such as
quartz and aluminum oxide may be evaporated in this way. The evaporated metal
is then used to provide thin antistatic coatings on glass or plastic and, in
general, to meet other needs in the field of solid-state and laser
technology. The hazards normally associated with electron-beam evaporators
are the production of X-radiation, the high energy levels of electron beams,
and the high voltage required to accelerate the electrons.

Electron-beam welders operate much like electron-beam evaporators using
higher voltages and tighter focusing to concentrate the beam at a point on the
target. The advantage of electron-beam welding versus conventional welding
that the work piece is heated from the inside, thereby eliminating the
distortion often associated with conventional welding techniques. The hazards
associated with the electron-beam welder are similar to those of the
electron-beam evaporator with the added hazard of higher voltages; those
required by the welder are in the range of 150,000 volts rather than the
13,000 to 20,000 volts required by the evaporator.

Electron microscopes are used in research and industrial applications where
resolving power approaching the ultimate possible is required. An optical
microscope is limited by the wavelength of visible light which may be taken as
500 cm. In the electron microscope, however, the theoretical limit is a
function of the electron beam accelerating voltage.

The basic components of an electron microscope are the electron gun, composed of a cathode and anode, and the condensing magnetic lens, specimen state, objective magnetic lens, projection magnetic lens, and viewing screen. The electron beam from the cathode is accelerated to the anode and concentrated into a parallel beam by the condensing lens. The beam then passes through the specimen. The energy of the electrons must be sufficient to penetrate the specimen, and accelerating voltages of 50,000 to 60,000 are commonly used. Passing through the objective lens, a magnified image is formed at the intermediate lens which converges the electron beam before passing through the final magnification stage. The final image can usually be viewed through observation ports on a fluorescent screen. Magnification as high as 200,000 times and a point resolution of 0.4 nanometers are now available on commercial models.

As with any of the electron beam devices, the hazards associated with the electron microscope are similar. The unit should be monitored for leakage of X-radiation, and precautions should be taken when dealing with the high voltage of the unit.

Activation Analysis. In this technique of chemical analysis, the test material is irradiated by one of several different types of uncharged or charged particles. A probability exists that in the reaction the target nuclei will be transformed into unstable or radioactive nuclei, the number of which depends upon the number of bombarding projectiles, the number of target nuclei, and the cross section of the reaction. Once radioactive, the target material will begin emitting ionizing radiation. Each radionuclide has a distinct pattern of X- and gamma radiation emission. Once an analysis of the emission is performed, then the identity and quantity of the elements present may be determined.

Radioactive Tracers. Isotopes have the same chemical properties whether they are radioactive or not. Therefore, it is possible to substitute a known quantity of radioactive isotope in a given material or process and then "trace" its progress. An example of the use of these tracers in product improvement is the study of the effect of various lubricating oil combinations on the wear of pistons in engines and cylinders. In this application, a piston ring was irradiated and was used on a piston in a cylinder of an internal combustion engine. The amount of activity in the lubricant was determined by counting and the location of wear was determined by auto-radiography. This study permitted the development of improved lubricants in a relatively short time.

Another example of the use of tracers is to determine wetting, detergency, absorption, and durability. To improve the accuracy of a radiochemical separation, one can add a known quantity of radionuclide to a mixture with an unknown quantity of a radionuclide of the same element, for example Strontium-85 to a Strontium-90 mixture, and determine quantitatively the amount of Strontium-90 in the mixture.

Still another example of the use of tracers is in determining the volume of complex reservoirs in hydrology by utilizing a technique known as "isotope dilution." A known volume of radioisotope at a known concentration is added to a complex mixture or reservoir. If one assumes a perfect mixture and a sample is taken, it is possible to determine the volume of the reservoir by taking a known volume of sample and measuring its isotope concentration. Fr this, the actual volume of the entire reservoir or complex mixture may be extrapolated.

The tagging of a product in transit is an example of the use of radioactive tracers in the petroleum industry. In one application, various radioactive tracers are used to tag the input water in water flooding projects. Finally, in the field of solid-state technology, minute concentrations of metals and nonmetals can have profound effects on a semiconductor, and radioactive tracers are used as the only practical method of identifying behavior of trace elements found in reagents used in semiconductor fabrication.

Aerosol Fire Detectors. One of the most sensitive detectors of combustible gases and smoke relies on the use of radioactive materials. In this system, two ionization chambers, each containing a radioactive foil, ar used. One is sealed and the other is open to the ambient air. These two chambers are connected to a cold-cathode, gas-discharge tube. In the absenc of air contaminants, the gas discharge tube does not fire. If the air becom contaminated with combustible gases and smoke particles, the tube fires, actuating an electromagnetic relay which sounds the alarm. The hazard associated with this device is minimal because of the size of the sealed source.

Luminescent Dials. One of the oldest applications of ionizing radiation involves the use of radium as a source of radiation in a self-luminous compound. If a compound of phosphor (zinc sulfide) is bombarded with ionizi particles, the phosphor scintillates, causing it to "glow." The hazards associated with self-luminous compounds are present in all stages of the process, including the preparation of the compound, painting and assembly, a inspection. In each stage, steps must be taken to minimize personnel contac

Large Radiation Sources. The use of large radiation sources has achieve practicality with the advent of inexpensive radionuclides and engineering design advances in accelerators. One application of large radiation sources is radiation processing. This is the use of ionizing radiation to produce a biological or chemical change. Routine uses of radiation processing in industry include sterilization of medical supplies, an enzyme for laundry us synthesis of ethyl bromide, controlled degradation of polyethylene oxide polymer, irradiation of wood-plastic composites, and control of anthrax bacillus in sheep hides and wood. Table 6.3.4 indicates industrial applications of radiation processing.

The second use of large radiation sources is a thermoelectric generator. The ionizing radiation is used as a heat source, and thermoelectric converte to convert the heat to electricity. The primary hazards involved are the presence of gamma and X-radiation, and neutrons produced by the procedure.

A third potential use of large source radiation is in nuclear explosions They may be used in the construction industry for excavating and tunneling, the mining industry for breaking up ore, and in the petroleum industry for stimulation of gas fields. Although most industrial uses of radionuclides emphasize the safety and health protection of the working personnel, when using large radiation sources, protection of the general public must also be considered.

Agricultural Uses

Agricultural uses of ionizing radiation may be categorized into two groups. The first use is the irradiation of living tissue with the intent of modifying the matter. Examples of this use include irradiation of potatoes to inhibit sprout production, the sterilization of fruit, or irradiation of seeds to cause mutations in an effort to develop various strains of the plant. With these uses, machine sources as well as naturally occurring radioisotopes are used.

Widely used radioisotope sources in agriculture and research include:

1.   Multikilocurie gamma sources for food disinfection, pasteurization, and sterilization.

2.   Beta and less intensive gamma sources used in radiography, thickness and density and level gauges.

3.   Alpha sources used in electrostatic discharges, gauges, and electronic warning devices.

4.   Isotope accelerators used for neutron activation analysis of soil, metals, and protein.

As in industrial uses, tracers are used to evaluate biological phenomena. All types of radiation are used in agriculture. Alpha particles are used to study cellular disposition. Beta particles are used in evaluation of metabolic processes, pathways of fertilizer and nutrient deposition; and finally, X- and gamma radiation are used to evaluate processes similar to the use of beta particles.

Medical Uses

Medical uses for ionizing radiation may also be grouped into two categories. The first category is the application of X-radiation. Most people are familiar with its common use in the development of a film outline of bones, teeth, and calcified structures, along with the internal organs. Further, injection or ingestion of X-radiation opaque substance into the body provides outlines of the desired organ. For example, barium sulfate is ingested to provide a film of the intestinal tract.

The medical profession has also found various uses of radionuclides, primarily in diagnosis and therapy. When the radioactive isotopes of elements that are normally found in various areas of the body are introduced via injection or ingestion, it is possible to chart the path and deposition of specific elements and compounds throughout the body. For example, if an analysis of the activity of the thyroid gland were of interest, then radioactive iodine would be used since iodine tends to migrate to the thyroid gland; if the kidney were of interest, radioactive mercury migrates to the kidney just as iodine does to the thyroid gland. Certain types of cancers ma

Table 6.3.4

Some applications of ionizing radiation in industry.

A = Research B = Pilot Plants C = Production	Industrial Process*												
	1	2	3	4	5	6	7	8	9	10	11	12	13
Sewage Treatment	A												
Semiconductors													A
Flooring							A	B		A		A	
Furniture							A	B		A		A	
Hides and Hair	C		C	C	C								
Textile							B	A		B	A	B	
Adhesives							A	A			A		A
Rubber							A	A		B	B		A
Spices		A	A	A	A								
Paints and Coatings								B		B	A	A	A
Membranes	A						A	A		B		B	
Chemical Synthesis								A	A	B			
Fuels									A				A
Lubricants									A				A
Wood-Plastic Composites							A	B		A		A	
Plastic Piping							A	A		A		A	
Heat Shrinking Tubing							B	B		A			
Enzymes		A	A		A								
Cosmetics	B	A	A		A								
Pharmaceutical	A	A	A		A								
Medical Supplies	C				A								
Foods	B	A	A	B	A	B							

*
1 = Sterilization	8 = Polymerization
2 = Pateurization	9 = Scission
3 = Salmonella Control	10 = Free Radicals
4 = Insect Disinfestation	11 = Curing
5 = Disinfection	12 = Grafting
6 = Sprout Inhibition	13 = Testing and Evaluation
7 = Cross LInking	

Source: Gamma Industries, Inc.

be identified by noting that the cancerous cells do not absorb or use the same elements of the body as do normal, healthy tissues. Therefore, if a radioactive isotope were introduced into a given area and the cells did not absorb the radioisotope as would be expected, then the location of the cancer could be identified.

The uses of radionuclides in therapy are rather well known. Because of the biological effects of ionizing radiation, it is possible to expose nondesirable (cancerous) cells to specific types of ionizing radiation that will not affect normal tissue; and the effect of the ionizing radiation will be to cause cell damage and death to the cancerous tissues.

Hazards. In general, each of the industrial, agricultural, or medical uses has basically the same hazard. In those instances where a naturally occurring radioisotope is being used, specific exposures to that isotope is the primary problem. In those instances where high voltage equipment is needed to create the radiation, e.g. X-radiation, then an alternate problem of potential high-voltage danger should be considered. Radioisotopes may be used for specific types of radiation, e.g., alpha source, but the isotope selected may also emit gamma or beta radiation. Care must be taken to evaluate properly the extraneous as well as desired radiation.

Maximum Permissible Dose

In an effort to minimize the effect of ionizing radiation exposure, the following maximum permissible dose (MPD) levels have been established. The dose levels are presented in units of dose equivalents (rem).

Using the MPD values presented in Table 6.3.5, it will be possible to calculate the exposure levels in the working environment that will not exceed the MPD level.

Efforts have also been made to convert the equivalent dose maxima to actual concentrations of radionuclides that may be present in the working environment, specifically in the air and water. Handbook #69, "Maximum Permissible Body Burdens and Maximum Permissible Concentrations of Radionuclides in Air and Water for Occupational Exposure," specifically identifies the maximum permissible burdens and permissible concentrations for each of the radionuclides presently being used in the working environment. The handbook also identifies the critical organ affected by that radionuclide. In essence, the handbook has converted the maximum permissible dose equivalent to a concentration of a specific radionuclide based upon the energy levels of the emissions of the nuclide. Table 6.3.6 is an excerpt from Handbook #69.

Table 6.3.5

MPD equivalent recommendations.

	Maximum Weekly Dose (rem)	Maximum 13-Week Dose (rem)	Maximum Yearly Dose (rem)	Maximum Accumulative Dose (rem)
Occupational Exposure				
Whole Body	0.23	3.0	12.0	5(N-18)*
Skin		10.0	30.0	
Hands, feet		25.0	75.0	
Forearms, ankles		10.0	30.0	
Non-Occupational Exposure	0.01			
Emergency Situation				
Whole Body	?0			
Hands and forearms	?0 additional			

*Assume personnel of age greater than 18 yrs.

Table 6.3.6

Maximum permissible body burdens and maximum permissible concentrations of radionuclides in air and in water for occupational exposure.

Radionuclide and type of decay	Organ of reference (critical organ in boldface)	Maximum permissible burden in total body $q(\mu c)$	Maximum permissible concentrations			
			For 40 hour week		For 168 hour week	
			$(MPC)_w$ μc/cc	$(MPC)_a$ μc cc	$(MPC)_w$ μc/cc	$(MPC)_a$ μc cc
	(Insol) **GI (LLI)**		2×10^{-3}	4×10^{-7}	8×10^{-4}	10^{-7}
	Lung			2×10^{-6}		6×10^{-7}
$_{34}Se^{75}(\epsilon,\gamma)$	**Kidney**	90	9×10^{-3}	10^{-6}	3×10^{-3}	4×10^{-7}
	Total Body	100	0.01	10^{-6}	3×10^{-3}	5×10^{-7}
(Sol)	Liver	100	0.01	2×10^{-6}	4×10^{-3}	5×10^{-7}
	Spleen	200	0.02	3×10^{-6}	8×10^{-3}	10^{-6}
	GI (LLI)		0.07	2×10^{-5}	0.03	6×10^{-6}
				10^{-7}		4×10^{-7}
(Insol)	**Lung**		8×10^{-3}	10^{-7}	3×10^{-3}	5×10^{-7}
	GI (LLI)			10^{-6}		
$_{34}Br^{82}(\beta^-,\gamma)$ (Sol)	**Total Body**	10	8×10^{-3}	10^{-6}	3×10^{-3}	4×10^{-7}
	GI (SI)		8×10^{-3}	2×10^{-6}	3×10^{-3}	6×10^{-7}
(Insol)	GI (LLI)		10^{-3}	2×10^{-7}	4×10^{-4}	6×10^{-7}
	Lung			6×10^{-7}		2×10^{-7}
$_{36}Kr^{85m}(\beta,\gamma)$ (Immersion)	**Total Body**			6×10^{-6}		10^{-6}
$_{36}Kr^{85}(\beta^-)$ (Immersion)	**Total Body**			10^{-5}		3×10^{-6}
$_{36}Kr^{87}(\beta^-,\gamma)$ (Immersion)	**Total Body**			10^{-6}		2×10^{-7}

Summary

In this chapter, the atom, radioactivity, and the process of radioactive decay have been briefly discussed. Five types of ionizing radiation, including alpha, beta, gamma, X-, and neutron have been examined. The basic biological effects of ionizing radiation, applications of ionizing radiation, and the established maximum permissible dose levels for the working environment have been presented.

4. Instrumentation

Introduction

Radiation detection instruments monitor the effect of ionizing radiation on a given material. For example, the ions produced in a given volume of gas can be measured, and the ions will be proportional to the energy absorbed by the gas. No single instrument performs acceptably under all conditions and requirements. Therefore, no single instrument can monitor and discriminate between all types of radiation at the various energy levels. In this chapter, the most commonly used radiation detectors will be discussed, including:

    Ionization chambers
    Proportional counters
    Geiger-Mueller (G-M) counters
    Scintillation detectors
    Photographic devices
    Solid-state and activation devices

Specific applications of these detectors in personnel monitoring devices, including film badges, pocket dosimeters, and pocket ion chambers, will also be presented.

The obvious purpose of monitoring radioactivity in the working environment is to ensure that the exposure rate and absorbed dose for any given individual are less than the maximum permissible dose (MPD) equivalents established as a minimum standard. However, the response recorded on a detector is due to the energy absorbed by the detector itself; and in some instances the detector does not have the same properties as human tissue. It is possible to select a detector and probe that can provide readings proportional to the absorbed dose that would be experienced by an employee in a given environment. Generally, however, the response of the instruments is not exactly equivalent to the response of human tissue receiving the same amount of energy. This is due primarily to the secondary ionization that would normally occur in human tissue but does not necessarily occur in the detector. For purposes of this discussion, however, it may be assumed that the response of the detector is equivalent to the absorbed dose unless otherwise stated.

The absorbed dose for an individual can rarely be determined directly, if at all. An estimation made by using some type of detector must be acceptable. Realizing the absorbed dose cannot be determined and that an estimation must be used, the maximum permissible dose equivalent values that have been previously presented take into consideration that an estimation will be used and, therefore, MPD values are conservative. These values have been conservatively established to the extent that an error in actual reading of ±30% could be tolerated. In most instances, the instruments selected, if appropriately matched to the environment and type of radiation of interest, will fall within this range. In general, the accuracy of the detectors for photon energies tends to be somewhat better than for particulate radiation.

If the detection instruments are calibrated according to the manufacturer's recommendation for the environment and radiation type of interest, no further effort is usually necessary to increase the accuracy of the instrument. However, if the readings should approximate the maximum permissible dose equivalent established, it is important that the most accurate readings possible be obtained. If the MPD value is approximated, the individual receiving this exposure may receive different medical treatment based upon the amount of exposure that has been calculated. Therefore, to ensure appropriate treatment, the most accurate reading possible should be obtained. For readings that are well above or well below the MPD value, the need for accuracy is not as great.

Instrumentation

This section deals with the most common radiation detection and monitoring devices presently being used.

Ionization Chamber Instruments. The ionization chamber is an instrument that monitors the change in a gas caused by ionizing radiation. Ionizing radiation falls on the gas contained in the chamber and forms ions that migrate toward the cathode and anode within the chamber and are collected there. The potential voltage difference that is created because of the migration of the primary ions is measured. This potential difference is proportional to the quantity of ionizing radiation that falls upon the chamber.

This instrument can be used to measure relatively high levels of radiation. It can measure both particulate and electromagnetic radiation. The ionization chamber responds to any ionization produced in the chamber itself. It does not have the capability of discriminating between radiation types and specifically between particles of different linear energy transfer (alpha versus beta).

The ionization chamber is usually 190 to 320 cubic centimeters in volume. In general, the larger the chamber, the greater the sensitivity and required operational voltage. It can be designed to measure all types of radiation. The chamber is usually open to the atmosphere and requires corrections for ambient temperature and pressure. Sealed chambers are also available; they do not require corrections for the ambient temperature and pressure but may have reading changes because of leakage or absorption and adsorption on inside surfaces of the gas within the chamber. The thickness of the wall of the chamber is of critical importance. The thickness must approximate the maximum range of the ionized particles produced by the ionizing radiation. Table 6.4.1 illustrates the various wall thicknesses required, based upon the energy of the radiation.

The chambers can also be designed to be air or tissue equivalent.   If the chamber is designed to be air equivalent, then the readings reflect exposure rates.   If the chambers are designed to be tissue equivalent, then the properties of the chamber simulate human tissue and the readings are calibrated to measure absorbed dose.

Table 6.4.1

Thicknesses of ionization chamber walls required for establishment of electronic equilibrium (ICRU, 1964).

Photon energy (MeV)	Thickness ($g \bullet cm^{-2}$)
0.02	0.0008
0.05	0.0042
0.1	0.014
0.2	0.044
0.5	0.17
1	0.43
2	0.96
5	2.5
10	4.9

The primary advantage of the ionization chamber instrument is that it is simple, rugged device that reliably determines absorbed dose or exposure.   The disadvantage of this instrument is that special designs or modifications are required for the instrument to discriminate well between the types of radiation.   Because of this, it is necessary to have a general knowledge of the radiation spectrum being evaluated.

Proportional Counter Instruments.   THe proportional counter (Figure 6.4.1 functions on the same principle as the ionization chamber.   However, the voltage on the collection plates is increased such that as the primary ions approach the collection plates, secondary ionization occurs.   This secondary ionization and the ions produced from it contribute to the ion current pulse that is registered on the meter.   This process is referred to as "gas amplification."   This gas amplification process increases the sensitivity of the proportional counter over a simple ionization chamber by a factor of 10^3 to 10^4 times.   Even though gas amplification does occur, there still remains a proportionality between the counter current and energy fluence rate of the radiation which enters the proportional counter.

The proportional counter is more useful in measuring particle radiation than photon radiation.   It has the capability of measuring both alpha and beta radiation and can discriminate between the two types if they are simultaneously present.   If the chamber is lined with a boron film or filled

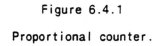

Figure 6.4.1

Proportional counter.

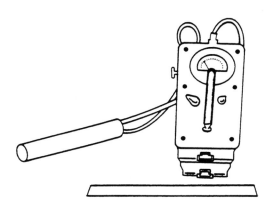

with BF_3 gas, then thermal neutrons can also be monitored. Fast neutrons of low energy level may also be measured with this instrument. Because of the proportionality between the counter and the energy entering the chamber, it is possible to use the proportional counter for spectrometry.

The selection of the type of gas and wall construction for the proportional counter chamber is dependent upon the purpose and type of measurements that are to be made. As with the ionization chamber, the proportional counter chamber can be designed to be air or tissue equivalent. Further, by changing the thickness of the wall, one can get an indication of the absorbed dose at various levels in human tissue.

The primary advantages of the proportional counter are its discrimination capabilities. For example, it is possible for the counter to eliminate the effects of gamma radiation while counting neutrons and to negate the effects of beta when counting alpha. Its primary advantage is its high sensitivity with relative high accuracy and counting efficiency. The disadvantages of this unit include the insulation requirements around the components to prevent miscellaneous radiation from entering the components. Also, in some instances, inaccuracies in the readings may occur due to losses of absorbed energy. These losses may decrease accuracy by as much as 50%.

Geiger-Mueller (G-M) Counter. The Geiger-Mueller counter (Figure 6.4.2) is used extensively as a sensitive radiation detector. The G-M counter operates much like the ionization chamber and proportional chamber, with the exception that the applied voltage is increased still further so that all gas atoms in the chamber undergo secondary ionization. Because of the extensive secondary ionization, the sensitivity is greatly increased. However, the electrical pulse current generated internally is not generally proportional to the type of ionizing event, and it cannot be directly related to either absorbed dose or exposure. Therefore, the G-M counter is used primarily as a detector of potential radiation hazard but cannot usually be used as a monitoring device.

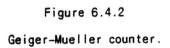

Figure 6.4.2

Geiger-Mueller counter.

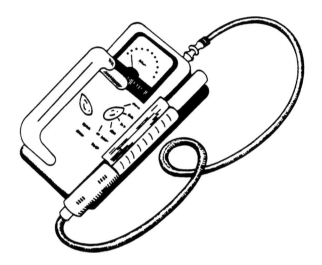

The G-M counter is used primarily to detect the existence of low-level radiation, especially in the range of 0-20 milliroentgens per hour. Under special conditions, the G-M counter can be modified to yield a response that is proportional to the exposure over a limited range of photon energies, but primarily it is used as a detection device for low-energy beta and gamma radiation. The G-M counter has the capability of monitoring gamma radiation in the presence of neutrons.

The G-M counter is made in a variety of shapes, sizes, and compositions. These factors must be matched to the environment and the type of radiation that is to be monitored. In some instances, the sensitivity to beta radiation is dependent upon the angle of incidence of radiation; that is, the G-M counter is direction-dependent. Survey procedures that are used to detect radiation must take into consideration the directional factor of the G-M counter.

One characteristic of the G-M counter that also must be considered is the so-called "dead time." Dead time, which ranges from approximately ten to several hundred microseconds, is the time required for the ion avalanche to be initiated, to travel along the anode, and to be quenched, leaving the counter ready for a new count. Because of the G-M counter designs and the massive secondary ionization caused by ionizing radiation and high voltage, time is required for the instrument to respond to the ionization in the chamber, initiate the avalanche, and then have the chamber return to a neutral state so that ionization may again occur. The halting of the avalanche is accomplished by the inclusion of an inert gas in the ion chamber. This gas is commonly referred to as a "quenching gas."

The G-M counter should <u>not</u> be used if it is anticipated that the count rate will be greater than 1000 cpm (counts per minute). Because the G-M counter is energy dependent, an increased radiation level will cause a decrease or blockage of the meter reading. This occurs because the mechanics of a G-M counter cannot operate with such a high level of ionizing radiation. In this instance, the G-M counter may show a "no field" or no ionizing radiation present when, in fact, the field is very high. In the instance where meter blockage occurs, no count will be registered. If the meter is not blocked, at least one count every few seconds will occur because of typical background radiation present in the environment. Therefore, if no counts register during the first few seconds, the counter is either inoperative or blocked. In this case, a less sensitive detector should be used, such as an ionization chamber. For the same reason, G-M counters should not be used for the measurement of short, high-intensity pulses since this may also cause meter blockage.

The primary advantage of the G-M counter is that the unit is typically portable, generally stable and rugged, and has a high sensitivity. The disadvantages of this unit are that the readings cannot be directly related to absorbed dose or exposure but merely indicate the presence of ionizing radiation. Further, because of the presence of a high radiation field, the meter may block and read "no field" at 1000 cnts/min. Finally, most G-M counters have a directional sensitivity, requiring a sweeping-type motion during any survey process.

<u>Scintillation Detector</u>. The scintillation detector (Figure 6.4.3) works on a different principle than the ionization chamber instruments previously discussed. With the scintillation detector, the ionizing radiation interacts with a phosphor or crystal that is capable of producing light. When the ionizing radiation falls on the scintillation counter, the crystal is excited and emits light. The light produced registers on a photomultiplier and is converted to electrical impulses. The electrical impulses are then magnified and registered on a microammeter. The number and size of the electrical impulses recorded are related to the energy deposited in the scintillator chamber.

The scintillation detector has basically three components. The scintillator itself is a photo-sensitive crystal, plastic, or liquid that, when exposed to ionizing radiation, will emit light. The photomultiplier collects the light and converts it to electrical impulses. The final component of the system is the electronic counting equipment that registers and records the electrical current produced. The scintillation detector is most useful in the evaluation of the alpha and low level gamma radiation. With a sodium iodide crystal, gamma radiation may be measured in the presence of beta. Also, the instrument may be modified so that beta radiation may be measured in the presence of high-energy gamma. Further, soft X-rays may also

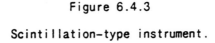

Figure 6.4.3

Scintillation-type instrument.

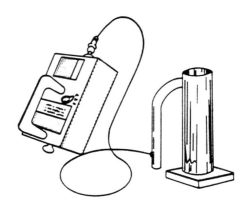

be monitored using this instrument. Alpha particles using a cesium iodide
crystal can be evaluated. To avoid the problem of the window of the chamber
absorbing alpha particles, the radioactive sample can be placed in the
scintillation chamber and a direct reading taken without interference from the
window.

     The primary advantage of this type of instrument is its sensitivity. It
is possible to monitor low-energy sources in the range of 5 μR/hr above
background radiation. It can discriminate between different types and
energies of radiation and has a relatively high counting efficiency; i.e.,
alpha and beta particle monitoring approached 100% efficiency. Finally, the
unit can be used as a spectrometer so that a mixture of several radionuclides
can be analyzed quantitatively and qualitatively. This can be done because of
the direct relationship between the pulse shape and height and the type and
energy of the radiation being monitored.

     One problem with this unit is that the photomultiplier and crystals are
relatively fragile. The unit can be designed as a portable unit, but care
must be taken not to damage the internal parts of the unit. Further, some
crystals used are easily damaged by moisture and humidity and will cause
erroneous readings because of environmental conditions. Care must be taken
also to keep the scintillator and photomultiplier in a light-tight case to
ensure that erroneous readings are not taken. The instrument is usually
designed to provide this light-tight case. However, because of wear and use,
extraneous light can enter the system and cause erroneous readings.

     Photographic Devices. Photographic capabilities can also be used to
monitor ionizing radiation. Photographic devices can be designed to provide a
reasonably accurate and permanent record of cumulative exposure. Photographic
films are available that are sensitive to the various types of ionizing

radiation. The ionizing radiation interacts with the silver halide in the photographic emulsion on the film. The silver is ionized and then attracted to negatively charged sensitivity centers on the crystals in the film emulsion. At this point, the silver ions produced are reduced to a free silver compound. When the film is processed, the silver ions are removed; and the free silver stays attached to the film. The quantity of silver that remains is proportional to the exposure of ionizing radiation.

The range of the film and the type of radiation to which it is sensitive are dependent upon the characteristics of the emulsion, the filtration that might be used, the processing technique, and the type and quality of exposing radiation. In general, the range of the emulsion is usually 10:1.

The primary use of the photographic device is in personnel monitors. These are commonly used as "film badges." Figure 6.4.4 is an illustration of a film badge.

Figure 6.4.4

Radiation film badge.

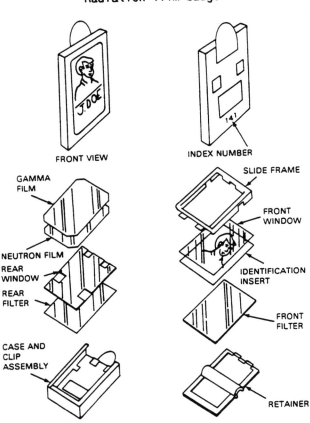

Film badges generally are used to monitor beta, neutron, X-, and gamma radiation. Because the film must be maintained in a light-tight casement, only beta energy of greater than 0.2 MeV can penetrate the film casement. This also eliminates the possibility of using the film badge to monitor alpha radiation.

Usually the film badges are quite small. They require no power supply to operate, and special holders and packs have been devised to monitor various parts of the body; e.g., wrists and fingers. In many instances, larger film casements and film processes have been used to monitor ionizing radiation.

Using the photographic devices as a monitoring process is relatively expensive and is not generally cost effective for less than two hundred people. Usually film badges are changed every two to four weeks and then processed. However, in some areas if radiation is either very critical or noncritical, they may be changed weekly or quarterly, as the system requires. A potential problem in using the film badge and not changing the badge on a biweekly or monthly basis is that high levels of accidental exposure may be undetected for long periods of time; e.g., if the film badges are changed on a quarterly basis.

Use of the film badge provides some distinct advantages. It provides a permanent record of radiation exposure and can be used on large populations of individuals. Film badges can be designed to discriminate between types of radiation and, because of their size and stability, can be used to monitor whole-body as well as individual parts of the body: e.g., fingers. However, there are some problems with using the film badge that should be considered. First, the film badge and exposure of ionizing radiation to the film badge is dependent upon the direction of the incident radiation. Therefore, if the film badge is not appropriately placed with respect to the potential source and the individual receiving the exposure, the readings on the film badge will be incorrect. Second, it is difficult to assess the absorbed dose and dose equivalent to within 20 to 50 percent for simple radiation fields. In those areas where a complex or multi-course radiation field may exist, the error may be even greater. Third, calibration and processing of the film is somewhat complex. Because of the variations in the reactivity of the film emulsions from batch to batch, it is necessary to expose some of the film to a standardized radiation source and use this as the standard for that particular batch. This variation in sensitivity of the emulsions can cause problems in interpretation and calibration of the film system.

Finally, some film emulsions are reactive to water vapor, causing potential error in readings. Therefore, it is necessary to carefully contain all film badges in moisture-tight casements.

Solid-State and Activation Devices. Any solid material that, when radiated, exhibits a property whose response is a function of the energy absorbed may in principle be used as a radiation device. Aside from the properties already discussed, other physical properties that have been considered include coloration, photoluminescence, thermoluminescence, and photoconductivity. Of these, thermoluminescent, photoluminescent, and semiconductor detectors are also in common use.

Thermoluminescent detectors are useful in measuring X- and gamma radiation and high-energy beta particles. The thermoluminescent material, when exposed to radiation, is ionized and "holes" develop in the lattice structure of the material. In essence, these "holes" are areas in the lattice where an electron has been removed by the ionizing radiation. When the material is heated, this provides adequate energy for the electrons to shift in the material and fill the holes. As this recombination occurs, light is emitted. The quantity of light emitted is proportional to the ionizing radiation exposure that originally caused the change in the lattice structure. Typically, materials such as calcium chloride, lithium chloride, and calcium phosphate are used for thermoluminescent detectors.

The advantage of these detectors is that they can be quite small, e.g., 0.1-1 gram. They are rugged and durable and provide monitoring over a wide range (10 milliroentgens, 10^5 roentgens). The reading provided usually is within +5-10 percent, and the detector is reusable. The disadvantage of this type of detector is that an instrument is required to "read" the device. This reading device heats the detector and then records the light emitted. One problem that does exist with the use of thermoluminescent detectors is that of fading. The heat at room temperature may cause recombination and thus a reduction in the signal. For example, calcium sulphate readings may decrease by as much as 30 percent after eight hours and as much as 65 percent after eight days. Because of this problem, it is necessary to read the detector as soon as possible after potential exposure.

Photoluminescent devices work on a similar principle as thermoluminescent devices, with the exception that rather than exposing the detector to heat to cause the emission of light, the photoluminescent device is exposed to ultraviolet light, thus causing light emission. Photoluminescent devices have the same advantages as the thermoluminescent devices including the long range and portability. They also share common problems in that a device is required to read the detector and fading may occur.

One final type of device that may be encountered is a device based upon the semiconductor principle. With this device, an exposure to ionizing radiation causes a change in conductivity of the subject material. This change in conductivity is then measured and, in some instances, is proportional to the exposure dose. This type of device can be used to measure alpha, beta, X-, or gamma radiation. In general, it acts as a solid ionization chamber with the exception that the range is from 10^{-6} to 10^4 roentgens per hour. The major problem with this type of device is that the semiconductor may be temperature sensitive.

Personnel Monitoring Devices

Because of the importance of personnel monitoring, this section reviews the major types of detection devices used for personnel monitoring.

Film Badges. Film badges were previously discussed. As mentioned they are designed to provide a reasonably accurate and permanent record of cumulative exposure. They can be used to monitor whole-body or parts of the body as required. The primary problem as mentioned with the film badges is the complexity and time required for film processing.

Pocket Dosimeter. The pocket dosimeter is widely used in radiation monitoring. The dosimeter works on the principle of an ion chamber. It has the capability of indicating accumulated exposure to radiation at any given time and can be read by the individual without any type of reading instrument. However, the pocket dosimeter does not provide a permanent record of exposure; but it may be recharged which will reset the monitor to zero for reuse. The pocket dosimeter is prepared with a radiation scale to a maximum of 200 milliroentgens.

Pocket Chamber. The pocket chamber is also commonly used in monitoring radiation. It is similar in size and shape to a fountain pen. It, as with the pocket dosimeter, works on the principle similar to an ion chamber. The pocket chamber will indicate accumulated exposure to radiation at any time, but it requires a separate unit to read the device. As with the pocket dosimeter, it is calibrated in terms of milliroentgens and also requires recharging to reset the unit for repeated usages.

Choice and Use of Instruments

The factors that affect the selection of a particular instrument for use in monitoring ionizing radiation include the directional dependence of the instrument, the response rate and range, the susceptibility of the instrument to the environmental interference, and the precision and accuracy of calibration as required by the user. Table 6.4.2 outlines generally the typical use of each of the devices discussed.

It will be necessary, however, to evaluate each individual setting to determine the specific instrument that would be appropriate for monitoring that environment.

Table 6.4.2

Types of detectors used
for various types of radiation.

Type of Detector	Type of Radiation
Proportional or Scintillation Counter	Alpha
Geiger-Mueller Tube or Proportional Counter	Beta, Gamma
Ionization Chamber	X- and Gamma
Proportional Counter	N_f
Proportional Counter	N_t

5. Control of Ionizing Radiation

Identification of Radiation Safety Problems

Ionizing radiation cannot be felt, seen, heard, tasted, or smelled. This gives it a mysterious quality. However, unknown radioactive isotopes can be identified and measured with the instruments described in the last chapter. Ionizing radiation can be adequately monitored and properly controlled.

Areas where radiation dose rates may be excessive can be guarded during exposure time by suitable methods: erecting barriers and warning signs, stationing attendants to keep personnel out of restricted localities and, in extreme cases, completely closing the areas. Safe exposure times and safe operating practices can be established through measurement and control and by profiting from experience.

Work with radiation can and should be so planned and managed that radiation exposure of employees and the general public is kept to a minimum. No radioactive material that can result in exposures above the established levels should be released through contaminated air or water, through loss of control over contaminated waste materials, equipment or shipments, or by employees unknowingly leaving the place of work with contamination of their persons, clothing, or shoes.

When examining the work environment for a potential radiation safety problem, many factors must be considered. First, the type of work in which the employee is involved must be evaluated. The potential level of exposure for working near the processing of feed materials for nuclear reactors is much greater that that which would be present in the area of an alpha-emitting static eliminator or beta ray thickness gauge. Further, radiation fields occurring with X-ray machines can be much more controlled than an unsealed radioisotope source. It is also dependent upon how involved the employee is with the process. For example, employees involved with the application of radioactive compounds, such as that applied to luminous instrument dials, would be in much closer contact with the radioactive source than an individual who is monitoring radioactive tracers used as labels in large pipeline distribution systems.

The second consideration that must be made is the source of the radiation. The amount and type of radiation is important. As mentioned, those radioactive sources that are instruments or machines can be turned off, whereas radioisotopes will emit radiation constantly. Also, each radionuclide has a radio toxicity per unit activity that varies from nuclide to nuclide.

659

Further, sealed sources are not nearly so dangerous as unsealed sources. Finally, if the radioisotope is in the form of a radioactive metal that is going through some type of machining process, a major problem will be the spread of loose material--e.g., flaking, grinding chips--and the contamination of the employee.

If the operational factors are considered, the required level of radiation protection and potential problems that might arise can be determined. The operational factors that should be evaluated include such things as:

1. The area involved (square feet), number of rooms and buildings.

2. Number of employees potentially exposed to the radiation and the location of those employees.

3. The chemical and physical states of the radioactive material and its use.

4. Potential incidents that are likely to occur that would increase the potential exposure to the employees.

5. Nonradiation hazards that might be involved; that is, high voltage, toxicity of chemical substances.

6. The nature of the probable exposure to the employees; that is, whether or not the exposure would be a controlled or supervised release such as through some type of disposal procedure, accidental release that may not be sensed by warning devices, or a violent release of dust droplets or gases--such as through fire or explosion--that may carry radioactive contamination.

7. The inherent danger of the materials and procedure being implemented.

8. The probability of detection of a potentially harmful radioactive situation by routine surveys and monitoring.

9. Possible effects of a radiation accident on operation; for example, loss of production, loss of space, and cleanup costs.

Finally, consideration must be given to the potential employee exposure. Efforts should be made to calculate the maximum dosage, given a specific type of incident, that the employee might receive. This should be done for both external and internal radiation potentials.

If the above factors are given consideration in the development of an overall radiation safety analysis, then potential employee exposure will be minimized.

Authorization for Radionuclide Use

Generally, the use of radionuclides and radiation-producing instruments (X-ray machines) is licensed through the Federal government or state health departments. The Nuclear Regulatory Commission (NRC) has established guidelines for the licensing of radionuclide users. Table 6.5.1 indicates the minimum quantity for radioactive materials that must be licensed through the NRC. Because of the variation in state requirements, licensing procedures should be investigated if radionuclide sources are to be used.

In general, any request for license requires the following information: the type and potential use of radionuclide along with the maximum quantities; the training and experience of the users; the laboratory facilities, handling equipment, and the monitoring procedures; disposal procedures, if necessary; and an outlined radiation-protection program.

Although the above requirements need to be met only if NRC licensure is being sought, these requirements for licensure provide a good general outline of the components of a radiation safety program.

Table 6.5.1

Sample licensure.

Radionuclide	Minimum Quantity for Radioactive Materials Sign in Room (μCi)	Minimum Quantity for Radioactive Materials Label (μCi)
Calcium-25	100	10
Carbon-14	1,000	100
Cesium-137 and Barium-137	100	10
Chlorine-36	100	10
Chromium	10,000	1000
Cobalt-60	10	1
Copper-64	1,000	100
Gold-198	100	100
Hydrogen-3	10,000	1000
Iodine-125	10	1
Iodine-131	10	1
Iron-55	1,000	100
Iron-59	100	10
Phosphorus-32	100	10
Potassium-42	100	10
Radium-226	0.1	0.01
Sodium-24	100	10
Strontium-90 and Yttrium-90	1	0.1
Zinc-65	100	10
Unidentified, but not α emitter	1	0.1
Unidentified α emitter	0.1	0.01

Protection from Radiation Hazard

There are three basic tools that can provide protection against a radiation source. These are time, distance, and shielding. The goal of the protection is to prevent overexposure from external radiation and to minimize the entry of radionuclides into the body, or minimize internal radiation.

Time. As an element of protection, time is almost self-explanatory. Radiation occurs at a rate of roentgens (or rads) per hour. Therefore, the shorter the time of exposure, the smaller the radiation dose received by the personnel. Figure 6.5.1 illustrates this concept.

Figure 6.5.1

Time vs. radiation exposure.

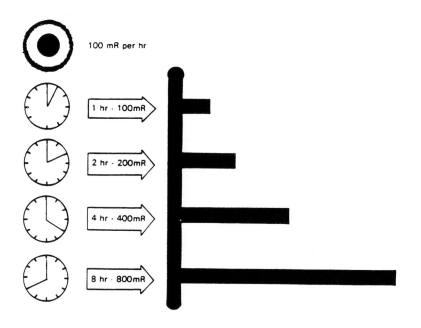

100 mR per hr

1 hr - 100mR

2 hr - 200mR

4 hr - 400mR

8 hr - 800mR

According to the figure, if someone is in an area where the radiation level from penetrating external radiation is 100 mR/hour, then in one hour 100 mR would be received. After two hours, the exposure dose would be 200 mR. Therefore, if work procedures can be reviewed and analyzed such that the time of exposure is minimized, then the exposure dose received by the employee is also minimized. Time also plays an important role with respect to protection when considering the factor of "half-life." If an exposure potential is high in a given area and the radioactive source has a short half-life, it is possible to just wait for radioactive decay to occur; and the activity of the radionuclide will be reduced. As can be seen in Figure 6.3.5, at the end of seven half-lives the activity is reduced to one percent of the original activity. It is possible to calculate the loss of activity due to radioactive decay if the original activity and date of measure are known.

The decrease of activity is equal to $(1/2)^n$, where n is equal to the number of half-lives that have passed since the last known measurement.

Example

An isotope user acquired from a national laboratory a surplus Co-60 source in June, 1977. The source was last measured for activity in January, 1970. At that time, the source had an activity of 40 mR/hr at 10 cm.
What is the anticipated exposure rate at 10 cm in June, 1977?

Solution

January 1970 to June 1977 = 7.5 years
Half-life of Co-60   = 5.3 years
Half-life transpired   = 7.5/5.3 = 1.415 half lives
Using $(1/2)^n$ $(1/2)^{1.415}$ = 0.375

$$\text{Exposure rate (June 1977)} = \frac{40 \text{ mR}}{\text{hr}} \times 0.375 = \frac{15 \text{ mR}}{\text{hr}}$$

For convenience, tables for $(1/2)^n$ have been developed for use as illustrated in Table 6.5.2.

Table 6.5.2

Powers of one-half for attenuation and decay calculations, $(1/2)^{n*}$.

n	0.0	0.1	0.2	0.3	0.4	0.5	0.6	0.7	0.8	0.9
0	1.000	0.933	0.871	0.812	0.758	0.707	0.660	0.616	0.578	0.536
1	0.500	0.467	0.435	0.406	0.379	0.354	0.330	0.308	0.287	0.268
2	0.250	0.233	0.217	0.203	0.190	0.177	0.165	0.154	0.144	0.134
3	0.125	0.177	0.109	0.102	0.095	0.088	0.083	0.077	0.072	0.067
4	0.063	0.058	0.054	0.051	0.047	0.044	0.041	0.039	0.036	0.034
5	0.031	0.029	0.027	0.025	0.024	0.022	0.021	0.019	0.018	0.017
6	0.016	0.015	0.014	0.013	0.012	0.011	0.010			

* "n" is the number of half-value layers or half-lives.

Distance. The second tool used for protection against radiation exposure is distance. The exposure rate is reduced by a factor of one divided by the square of the distance between the employee and the source. This is referred to as the "inverse-square law." Figure 6.5.2 demonstrates the effect of the inverse-square law on the intensity of radiation.

If there is a point source of radiation giving off 1000 units of penetrating external radiation at one foot, a worker would receive only one-fourth as much, or $(1/2)^2$, if the distance is doubled to two feet. If the distance is tripled, the dose is reduced to one-ninth, or $(1/3)^2$.

For example, if it is known that the radiation level is 0.1 R/hr at one foot, what would the exposure be if the worker was moved to a distance of fiv feet? Using the inverse-square law, the radiation level at five feet would b equal to 1.0 R/hr divided by $(5)^2$, or 0.04 R/hr. The advantage of distance as a protective tool when working with radiation can be seen from this example. The example illustrates the valuable use of tools such as long tongs. One important point that must be mentioned is that the distance of measurement and the units used in the "inverse-square law" must be equivalent that is, if exposure levels are determined at X feet, the variations in distance must also be calculated in feet.

Figure 6.5.2

Distance vs. radiation exposure.

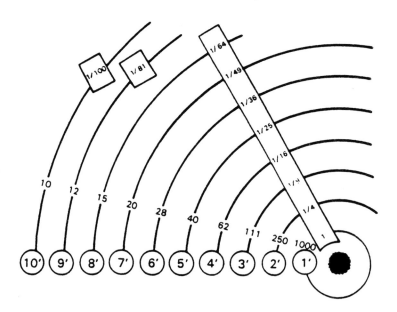

Shielding. The third tool to be used in protection against radiation is shielding. Shielding reduces radiation to the employee by placing a radiation-absorbing barrier between the source and the employee to be protected. The selection of the shielding is dependent upon the type and quantity of the radionuclide present. Table 6.5.3 illustrates some typical shielding materials used for the various types of radiation. The arrangement of the materials in the table is in the general order of increased thickness required to be an adequate shield.

Table 6.5.3

Typical shielding materials for radionuclides.

| | Shielding Material | | |
	Permanent	Temporary	Additional Clothing
Alpha	Unnecessary	Unnecessary	Unnecessary
Beta	Lead, copper, iron, aluminum	Iron, aluminum, plastics, wood	Leather, rubber, plastic, cloth
Gamma, X-rays	Lead, iron, copper, lead glass, heavy aggregate concrete, aluminum, ordinary concrete, plate glass, wood, water, paraffin	Lead, iron, lead glass, aluminum, concrete blocks, water, wood	Lead fabrics (but not for "hard" gamma)

Care must be taken to ensure that the location and shape of the shield limits radiation in all directions which may provide potential exposure to all employees; e.g., floor, ceiling. Thickness of the shielding required is relatively independent of the distance from the source or object. However, to minimize the size of the shield and to maximize protection, the shield should be as close to the source as possible as illustrated in Figure 6.5.3.

By placing the shield in close proximity to the source, incident radiation is minimized, and the expenditure for the shield is also reduced. Shields may be cylindrical or box shaped, depending upon local needs. Local shields are often built of lead bricks or concrete blocks, as presented in Figure 6.5.4.

A major concern in developing local shielding with any type of block or brick is that radiation may leak through the cracks in the blocks, or incident radiation may be reflected off walls or even the shield itself. In many instances, the radioactive source is so active that the shielding limits the employee to approaching the radioactive source from a distance or by remote control (Figure 6.5.5).

Gamma Radiation Shielding. The purpose of shielding is to reduce the radiation exposure to an acceptable level; the shield absorbs the radiation. Gamma radiation is photon energy with a high penetrating capability; and,

Figure 6.5.3

Shielding placement.

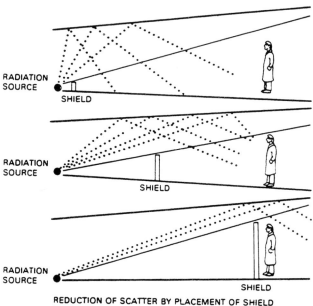

REDUCTION OF SCATTER BY PLACEMENT OF SHIELD
CLOSE TO EITHER SOURCE OR PERSON TO BE SHIELDED

therefore, materials of high density--including lead, iron, and concrete--are
used as shielding materials. The absorption of gamma radiation by a shield is
an exponential function related by the equation

$$I = I_0 e^{-\mu x}$$

where I is the exposure rate (R/hr) after passing through the shield, I_0 is
the initial exposure rate (R/hr) at the shield, μ is the absorption
coefficient of the shielding materials (cm^{-1}), and x is the shield thickness
(cm). The absorption coefficient is a function of the energy level of the
radiation and the properties of the shielding materials. Often the absorption
coefficient is expressed as a mass attenuation coefficient (cm^2/g)
(Table 6.5.4). To calculate μ, given the mass attenuation coefficient, it
is necessary to divide the mass attenuation coefficient by the density of the
shielding material. Therefore, shielding requirements or effects of a given
shield can be calculated.

The effect of shielding is also often expressed in terms of half value
layers (HVL). The half value layer is the thickness of a specified shielding
material to reduce the exposure rate from a specific radiation source by a
factor of 0.5. For example, in 2.6 half value layers, the number of photons
will be reduced $(0.5)^{2.6}$ or 0.165 of the original number entering the

Figure 6.5.4

Materials for shielding.

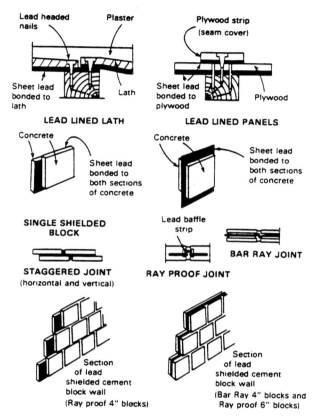

specified shield. Using $(0.5)^n$ or Table 6.5.2, it is possible to calculate the number of half value layers required for a desired attenuation of the radiation. It also allows for the calculation of a given attenuation for a certain thickness of a shield. Table 6.5.5 illustrates some typical half value layers for five isotopes. The calculation of HVL is similar to the calculation of the effect of half life: i.e., attenuation shield = $(0.5)^{HVL}$.

An example may further explain the shielding calculation.

<u>Example</u>

    Calculate the thickness of a lead shield necessary to reduce the exposure rate from 10.0 R/hr to 2.5 R/hr from a Cc-60 source.

Figure 6.5.5

Master-slave manipulation.

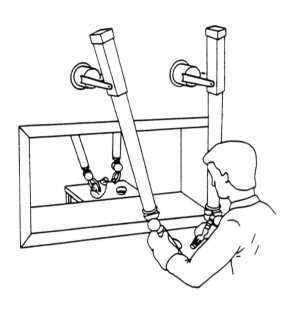

Table 6.5.4

Mass attenuation coefficients.

Photon Energy MeV	Mass Attenuation Coefficient in cm^2/g for--				
	Aluminum	Iron	Lead	Water	Concrete
0.01	26.3	173	133	5.18	26.9
0.02	3.41	25.5	85.7	0.775	3.59
0.05	0.369	1.94	7.81	0.227	0.392
0.1	0.171	0.370	5.40	0.171	0.179
0.5	0.0844	0.0840	0.161	0.0968	0.087
1.0	0.0613	0.0599	0.0708	0.0707	0.0637
5.0	0.0284	0.0314	0.0424	0.0303	0.0290
10.0	0.0231	0.0298	0.0484	0.0222	0.0231

Source: "Radiological Health Handbook,"   U.S. DHEW, Public Health
          Service, 1970.

Table 6.5.5

Data for gamma-ray sources.

Radio-isotope	Atomic Number	Half Life	Gamma Energy (MeV)	Half-Value Layer Conc. (in)	Steel (in)	Lead (in)	Lead (cm)	Tenth-Value Layer† Conc. (in)	Steel (in)	Lead (in)	Lead (cm)	Specific Gamma-Ray Constant $\frac{R\ cm^3/m*}{Ci-h}$
Cesium-137	55	27 y	0.66	1.9	0.64		0.65	6.2	2.1		2.1	3.2
Cobalt-60	27	5.24 y	1.17, 1.33	2.6	0.82		1.20	8.2	2.7		4.0	13.0
Gold-198	79	2.7 d	0.41	1.6	--		0.33	5.3	--		1.1	2.32
Iridium-192	77	74 d	0.13 to 1.06	1.7	0.50		0.60	5.8	1.7		2.0	5.0¶
Radium-226	38	1622 y	0.047 to 2.4	2.7	0.88		1.66	9.2	2.9		5.5	8.25§

From "NCRP Report No. 34," National Council on Radiation Protection and Measurements, Washington, D.C., 1971.

†Approximate values obtained with large attenuation.
*These values assume that gamma absorption source is negligible. Value is R/millicurie-hour at 1 cm can be converted to R/Ci-h at 1 meter by multiplying the number in this column by 0.10.
¶This value is uncertain.
§This value assumes that the source is sealed within 0.5 mm thick platinum capsule, with units of R/mgh at 1 cm.

Solution

HVL Method

$$\text{Attenuation required} = \frac{2.5 \text{ R/hr}}{10.0 \text{ R/hr}} = 0.25$$

Calculate HVL necessary

$$(0.5)^{HVL} = 0.25$$

$$HVL = \frac{\log 0.25}{\log 0.5} = \frac{-0.602}{-0.301} = 2 \text{ HVL}$$

$$2 \text{ HVL} \times \frac{1.25 \text{ cm Pb}}{HVL} = 2.5 \text{ cn Pb}$$

I/I_0 Method

$$I = I_0 e^{-\mu x}$$
$$x = -\ln(I/I_0)/\mu$$
$$I = 2.5 \text{ R/hr}$$
$$I_0 = 10.0 \text{ R/hr}$$

Using table

$$\mu = 0.060 \text{ cm}^2/\text{g} \times 11.34 \text{ g/cm}^3 = 0.680 \text{ cm}^{-1}$$
$$\text{Note: Pb (density)} = 11.34 \text{ g/cm}^3$$

$$x = \frac{-\ln(2.5/10.0)}{0.68 \text{ cm}^{-1}} = 2.04 \text{ cm}$$

Example

An unshielded source of Cesium-137 has an exposure rate of 0.1 mR/hr. What would be the exposure rate if a 3 centimeter lead shield were placed around the source? (HVL: Cesium-137 = 0.64 cm lead (Pb), MeV: Cs-137 = 0.66 MeV)

Solution

HVL Method

The solution to this example is rather straightforward. The HVL of these gamma photons is 0.65 cm. The number of HVL in a 3 cm shield would then be equal to 3.0   0.65 or 4.62 half value layers. Using Table 6.5.2, n is equal to 4.62, which when extrapolated would indicate an attenuation coefficient of approximately 0.41. Therefore, the exposure rate with a 3 cm lead shield surrounding the source would be equal to 0.1 mR/hr x 0.041 or 4.1 μR/hr.

I/I$_o$ Method

$$I = I_o e^{-\mu x}$$
$$I = ?$$
$$I_o = 0.1 \text{ mR/hr}$$
$$X = 3 \text{ cm}$$
$$\mu = 0.105 \text{ cm}^2/g \times 11.34 \text{ g/cm}^3 = 1.19 \text{ cm}^{-1} \text{ (from table)}$$
$$I = 0.1 \text{ mR/hr} \times e^{-(1.19 \times 3)}$$
$$I = 2.82 \text{ R/hr}$$

In the previous example, the calculated values as determined by the two methods are somewhat different. More important, the effect as calculated by the I/I$_o$ method is significantly less.   This is because the formula, I = I$_o$e$^{-\mu x}$, does not take into consideration a "buildup" phenomenon.   In matter being traversed by a beam of electromagnetic radiation, there is actually a higher intensity of photons at any point in the matter than would be predicted by the equation.   This is true because of the presence of X-radiation and secondary or scattered photons produced as the radiation penetrates the matter.   The increase in exposure rate, buildup (B), is not easily calculated but must be considered when determining shielding requirementsN A factor B is included in the attenuation equation I = BI$_o$e$^{-\mu x}$, with the tabulated values of B for specific conditions available in the literature.   Table 6.5.6 illustrates the dose buildup factor for a point isotropic source. Using such a table, the factor B can be included in the shielding calculation.

Example

   Calculate the exposure rate (I) for the previous example allowing for the buildup factor.

Solution

$$I = BI_o e^{-\mu x}$$
$$I_o = 0.1 \text{ mR/hr}$$
$$\mu = 0.105 \text{ cm}^2/g \times 11.34 \text{ g/cm}^3 = 1.19 \text{ cm}^{-1}$$
$$x = 3.0 \text{ cm Pb}$$

Using table 6.5.6 for

$$\mu x = 1.19 \text{ cm}^{-1} \times 3.0 \text{ cm} = 3.57$$
$$\text{MeV for Cs-137} = 0.66 \text{ MeV}$$
$$\text{Interpolating, } B = 1.79$$
$$I = 1.78 \times 0.1 \text{ mR/hr} \times e^{-(3.57)}$$
$$I = 5.04 \text{ } \mu R/hr$$

One final calculation that can be made when examining gamma radiation is that of projecting the potential exposure rate at a given distance of a gamma source. To make this calculation, it is necessary to know the type of radionuclide, the relative energies of that nuclide, and its activity.   The

Table 6.5.6

Dose buildup factor (B) for a point isotropic source.

Material	MeV	μX*						
		1	2	4	7	10	15	20
Water	0.255	3.09	7.14	23.0	72.9	166	456	982
	0.5	2.52	5.14	14.3	38.8	77.6	178	334
	1.0	2.13	3.71	7.68	16.2	27.1	50.4	82.2
	2.0	1.83	2.77	4.88	8.46	12.4	19.5	27.7
	3.0	1.69	2.42	3.91	6.23	8.63	12.8	17.0
	4.0	1.58	2.17	3.34	5.13	6.94	9.97	12.9
	6.0	1.46	1.91	2.76	3.99	5.18	7.09	8.85
	8.0	1.38	1.74	2.40	3.34	4.25	5.66	6.95
	10.0	1.33	1.63	2.19	2.97	3.72	4.90	5.98
Aluminum	0.5	2.37	4.24	9.47	21.5	38.9	80.8	141
	1.0	2.02	3.31	6.57	13.1	21.2	37.9	58.5
	2.0	1.75	2.61	4.62	8.05	11.9	18.7	26.3
	3.0	1.64	2.32	3.78	6.14	8.65	13.0	17.7
	4.0	1.53	2.08	3.22	5.01	6.88	10.1	13.4
	6.0	1.42	1.85	2.70	4.06	5.49	7.97	10.4
	8.0	1.34	1.68	2.37	3.45	4.58	6.56	8.52
	10.0	1.28	1.55	2.12	3.01	3.96	5.63	7.32
Iron	0.5	1.98	3.09	5.98	11.7	19.2	35.4	55.6
	1.0	1.87	2.89	5.39	10.2	16.2	28.3	42.7
	2.0	1.76	2.43	4.13	7.25	10.9	17.6	25.1
	3.0	1.55	2.15	3.51	5.85	8.51	13.5	19.1
	4.0	1.45	1.94	3.03	4.91	7.11	11.2	16.0
	6.0	1.34	1.72	2.58	4.14	6.02	9.89	14.7
	8.0	1.27	1.56	2.23	3.49	5.07	8.50	13.0
	10.0	1.20	1.42	1.95	2.99	4.35	7.54	12.4
Lead	0.5	1.24	1.42	1.69	2.00	2.27	2.65	(2.73)
	1.0	1.37	1.69	2.26	3.02	3.74	4.81	5.86
	2.0	1.39	1.76	2.51	3.66	4.84	6.87	9.00
	3.0	1.34	1.68	2.43	2.75	5.30	8.44	12.3
	4.0	1.27	1.56	2.25	3.61	5.44	9.80	16.3
	5.1087	1.21	1.46	2.08	3.44	5.55	11.7	23.6
	6.0	1.18	1.40	1.97	3.34	5.69	13.8	32.7
	8.0	1.14	1.30	1.74	2.89	5.07	14.1	44.6
	10.0	1.11	1.23	1.58	2.52	4.34	12.5	39.2

*μX = mass absorption coefficient (μ/ρ) x shield thickness (cm) x
    shield density (g/cm^2).

NOTE: For concrete, use an average of aluminum and iron;
    e.g., B (concrete) = [B(iron) + B(Al)]/2.

Source: "Radiological Health Handbook," U.S. DHEW, Public Health
    Service, 1970.

formula will express exposure in terms of milliroentgens per hour and is as follows:

$$mR/hr = \frac{5000\ CEf}{d^2}$$

where
    C = activity (in microcuries)
    E = energy in million electron volts (MeV)
    f = the fraction of disintegration emitting E
    d = the distance in cm

If the distance is to be calculated in feet, then the constant, 5000, must be replaced with the constant, 6. Further, if more than one level of photon energy is given off, each energy level (E) times its fraction of disintegration (f) must be calculated and a cumulative total of the exposure made.

This formula has two values. First, if a new source is being introduced, it is possible to calculate the exposure rate of that source at any distance. Second, in an emergency, it is possible to calculate the approximate safe distance that will not exceed the maximum permissible dose (MPD) limits. Table 6.5.7 presents data on typical radionuclides as found in the literature. This information will be used in subsequent examples and practice exercises.

Example
    A 50 microcurie source of Krypton-85 is to be used in a new industrial process being introduced in your facility. What is the exposure rate of an unshielded source at 25 cm?

Solution

$$mR/hr = \frac{5000\ CEf}{d^2}$$

where
        C = 50 microcuries
        E = 0.514 million electron volts
        f = 0.43%
        d = 25 centimeters

    Therefore

$$mR/hr = \frac{5000 \times (0.514 \times 0.0043) \times 50}{25^2}$$

$$= 0.885\ mR/hr\ at\ 25\ cm$$

It is also possible to perform the same calculation using the gamma ray constant (Γ) in the formula.

$$R/hr = \Gamma A/d^2$$

Table 6.5.7

Data on radionuclides referred to in problems.

Radionuclide	Symbol	Half-Life	Major radiations, energies (MeV) and percent of disintegrations	Specific gamma ray constant, R-cm^2/hr-mCi
Calcium-45	Ca-45	165 days	β⁻0.257 max; 0.077 avg	
Carbon-14	C-14	5730 yr	β⁻0.156 max; 0.049 avg	
Cesium-137	Cs-137	30 yr	β⁻1.174 max; (5.9%) 0.512 max; (94.1%) 0.188 avg/dis e⁻0.624 (7.8%); 0.656 (1.7%) γ 0.662 (85%) + low energy barium X-rays	3.3
Cobalt-60	Co-60	5.3 yr	β⁻1.49 max (0.12%) 0.318 max (100%) 0.087 avg/dis γ 1.332 (100%); 1.173 (100%)	13.2
Gold-198	Au-198	2.70 days	β⁻0.961 max (99%) 0.28 max (1%); 0.32 avg/dis e⁻0.33(2.9%); 0.40 (1.4%) γ 1.088 (0.2%) 0.676 (1%); 0.412 (95%)	2.35
Hydrogen-3	H-3	12.3 yr	β⁻0.0185 max; 0.0057 avg	
Iodine-131	I-131	8.05 days	β⁻0.807 max (0.7%) 0.606 max (90%) 0.33 max (7%); 0.18 avg/dis e⁻0.33 (1.7%); 0.046 (3%) γ 0.723 (1.6%); 0.637 (6.9%); 0.364 (82%) 0.284 (5.8%); 0.08 (2.5%)	2.18
Iron-59	Fe-59	45.6 days	β⁻1.57 max (0.3%); 0.47 max (53%) 0.27 max (46%) 0.188 avg/dis γ 1.292 (44%); 1.099 (56%); 0.192 (2.8%) 0.143 (0.8%)	6.13
Krypton-85	Kr-85	10.3 yr	β⁻0.67 max; 0.246 avg γ 0.514 (0.43%)	1.29

Table 6.5.7 (Continued)

Radionuclide	Symbol	Half-Life	Major radiations, energies (MeV) and percent of disintegrations	Specific gamma ray constant $R\text{-}cm^2/hr\text{-}mCi$
Molybdenum-99 + Technetium-99m	Mo-99	67 hr	β⁻1.23 max (80%); 0.454 max (19%) γ 0.392 avg/dis 0.78 (4.8%); 0.74 (14%) (4.8%); 0.74 (14%) 0.37 (1.5%); 0.18 (6.7%); 0.14 (90%) 0.04 (1.3%) 0.019 (12%); + low-energy Tc-99 X-rays	1.29
Phosphorus-32	P-32	14.3 days	β⁻1.71 max; 0.695 avg	
Potassium-42	K-42	12.4 hr	β⁻3.52 max (82%); 2.0 max (18%); 1.43 avg dis γ 0.31 (0.2%); 1.52 (18%)	1.50
Sodium-24 2.75	Na-24	15.0 hr	β⁻1.389 max; 0.55 avg γ 2.754 (100%); 1.369 (100%)	18.8 (11.7 from MeV and 7.1 from 1.37 MeV)
Sulfur-35	S-35	87.9 days	β⁻0.167 max; 0.049 avg	
Technetium-99m	Tc-99m	6.0 hr	e⁻0.138 (1.1%); 0.199 (8.8%); 0.0017 (98.6%); 0.017 avg/dis γ 0.140 (90%) + low- energy X-rays	0.70
Xenon-133	Xe-133	5.3 days	β⁻0.346 max (99.1%) 0.266 max (0.9%); 0.10 avg e⁻0.80 (2.4%); 0.075 (8.7%); 0.045 (52%) γ 0.081 (37%); Cs X-rays	

Sources: Martin and Blichert-Toft, 1970; Dillman, 1969; Hine and Brownell, 1956 (for values of specific gamma-ray constants)

where
Γ = gamma ray constant (R-cm²/hr-mCi)
A = activity (mCi)
d = distance (cm)

Using the tools of time, distance, and shielding, the exposure to employees can be minimized. By varying any of these factors, an increase or decrease in exposure can occur. In any instance, the exposure level can be minimized so that it is below established standards. The sample problems presented at the end of this chapter provide an opportunity to apply the concepts just presented on the shielding requirements of gamma radiation.

X-Radiation Shielding

When evaluating the potential radiation hazard produced by an X-ray machine, the following three components must be considered. The first component is the useful beam itself. This is the beam and its energy direct at a specified target. The second component is scattered radiation. This i the incident radiation that is reflecting off the target, the walls, etc. Finally, leakage radiation must be considered. This is the radiation that penetrates the tube housing and is not part of the useful beam. The degree shielding and protection required for an X-ray installation varies. X-ray shielding is based on the same principles as gamma shielding. However, dire calculation of half value layers for X-ray shielding are difficult. Factors such as the complexity of the X-ray spectrum, dependence upon the width of t beam and diffraction patterns, and factors contributing to the beam's scattering make HVL calculations difficult. Generally, when developing shielding patterns for the X-ray area, it is better to rely on the calculate values in the literature that are based on experiments that have a similar design. For example, Table 6.5.8 illustrates the half value layers for diagnostic X-rays for two shielding materials from 50 to 100,000 volts. The shielding is designed to limit the maximum exposure to 0.1 roentgens per wee at specified dose point.

Table 6.5.8

Half-value layers for diagnostic X-rays.

Tube Voltage	Lead (mm)	Concrete[a]
50,000	0.05	0.43
70,000	0.15	0.84
100,000	0.24	1.50
125,000	0.27	2.00

(a) The half-value layer will vary in different kinds of concrete and is given for illustrative purposes only.

Source: NCRP 1970, Report 34.

When evaluating the potential X-ray exposure that may be produced by a given installation, the following factors must be considered:

1. Work load (W)--The degree of use of the machine. This is usually expressed in terms of milliamp-minutes per week (mamp-min/wk).

2. Use factor (U)--Fraction of work load during which radiation under consideration is pointed in the direction of interest; e.g., toward personnel.

3. Occupancy factor (T)--Factor of occupancy of areas of interest.

4. Output (P)--The output of the direct beam.

5. The distance from the beam source to the employees of interest.

Figure 6.5.6 illustrates a typical X-ray installation.

Figure 6.5.6

Medical X-ray protection.

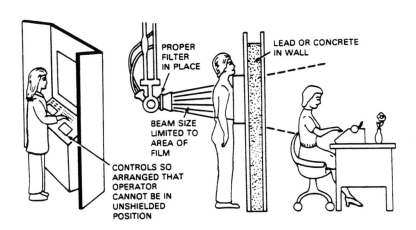

PROPER
FILTER
IN PLACE

LEAD OR CONCRETE
IN WALL

BEAM SIZE
LIMITED TO
AREA OF
FILM

CONTROLS SO
ARRANGED THAT
OPERATOR
CANNOT BE IN
UNSHIELDED
POSITION

If the output, work load, use factor, and occupancy factor are known, shielding requirements can be determined. First, it is necessary to calculate the output from the tube (TO). This can be done using tables found in the literature such as illustrated in Table 6.5.9. Then, it is necessary to calculate the product of W x U x T. Then, the attenuation can be calculated by determining the product of the output specified for the distance from the target to the point of interest and the three factors, W, U, T. This product is divided into the permissible weekly dose. The shield thickness is then calculated in the usual way from the number of half value layers required to produce the desired attenuation. For convenience, as previously mentioned, the protection handbooks contain tables for determining shielding thickness at installations operated at a given kilovolt peak.

Table 6.5.9

Average radiologic output*

Target Distance		Tube Potential (ρ)						
		50 Kvp	60 Kvp	70 Kvp	80 Kvp	90 Kvp	100 Kvp	125 Kv
inches	cm	R/100 mamp-sec						
12	30	1.8	2.8	4.0	5.8	8.0	9.8	15.2
18	46	0.8	1.3	1.8	2.5	3.4	4.2	6.7
24	61	0.4	0.7	1.1	1.4	1.9	2.3	3.8
36	91	0.2	0.3	0.5	0.6	0.9	2.1	1.7
54	137	0.1	0.1	0.2	0.3	0.4	0.5	0.7
72	183	0.1	0.1	0.1	0.2	0.2	0.3	0.4

* Measured in air with total filtration equivalent to 2.5 mm Al.
Source: NBS Handbook 76, 1961, Appendix A, Table 7.

Example

Determine the thickness of lead required on the wall of a radiographic installation with personnel working 12 feet from the source on the other side of the wall with the following conditions:
Kvp = 70
W = 200 milliamp minutes per week
U = 1
T = 0.25

Solution

A.   Calculate tube output (TO). (From Table 6.5.9)
     at 1 ft and 70 Kvp
         TO = 4.0 R/100 mamp-sec
     at 12 ft

$$TO = \frac{4.0 \text{ R/100 mamp-sec}}{(12)^2} = 0.028 \text{ R/100 mamp-sec}$$

B.   Calculate W x U x T
     W = 200 mamp-min/wk
     U = 1
     T = 0.25
W x U x T = 200 mamp-min/wk x 1 x 0.25
          = 50 mamp-min/wk

C.   Calculate attenuation

$$\text{attenuation} = 0.1 \text{ R/wk} \times \frac{1}{50 \text{ mamp-min/wk}} \times \frac{100 \text{ mamp-sec}}{0.028 \text{ R}} \times \frac{1}{60 \text{ sec/min}}$$

attenuation = 0.12

D.   Calculate HVL

$(0.5)^n = 0.12$

$$n = \frac{\log (0.12)}{\log (0.5)} = \frac{-0.9208}{-0.3010} = 3.06$$

From Table 6.5.8, it is found that 3.06 x 0.15 = 0.459 mm lead is required to shield this source.

The calculation for shielding requirements for incident radiation may also be calculated in the same manner. As previously mentioned, this procedure is somewhat simplified in the literature, but the same information is required to manipulate the data and calculate the shielding requirements.

The shielding requirements for beta radiation are somewhat less than for gamma and X-radiation because of the lesser penetrating capability of beta radiation. The range of the beta particle is a function of energy level of the beta particle and the composition of the absorbing material. The "range" of a beta particle refers to the thickness of material through which no beta particle emitted from a source can penetrate. Any shielding greater than the range specified for a given beta particle will prevent any emission of beta particles through the shield. In the literature, the range for the various energy levels of beta particles is given in terms of unit density material. Table 6.5.10 gives some properties of commonly used beta emitters including the unit density material. The range for the unit density material is based upon the assumption that the density of this absorbing material is one gram per cubic centimeter.

If an absorbing material with a density other than 1.0 gram per cubic centimeter is used, then the range can be calculated by dividing the unit density by the density of the shielding material. For example, if the minimal thickness of the wall of a glass test tube required to stop all beta particles from a Phosphorus-32 source is to be calculated, it is necessary to divide 0.8 cm (the unit density for P-32) by 2.3 grams/cm^3 (the density of glass) to get a value of 0.35 cm of glass as the range for Phosphorus-32 beta particles.

When considering the type of shielding material used for beta particle shielding, special consideration must be given to the atomic weight of the shielding material. Beta particles should be shielded by materials that are light or have small atomic weights; e.g., aluminum, water, glass. This is necessary because the beta particles convert to the more penetrating X-radiation in shielding materials like lead that have large atomic numbers. Because this production is more likely with heavier compounds, beta particle shielding should always be done with light atomic weight materials.

As with beta particles, alpha particles, because of their high atomic weight and charge, have a limited penetrating capability and range. This is true to the extent that alpha radiation cannot penetrate the outer layer of dead skin of the body. However, the danger with alpha radiation is the potential of the alpha emitter entering the body. Therefore, containment more than shielding is required when working with alpha emitters. Figure 6.5.7 illustrates a typical installation used for the containment of alpha particles; e.g., the glove box. The glove box will be discussed in greater detail in this chapter.

The final radiation form that has been discussed, neutrons, can be shielded following the same concepts of half value layer and attenuation coefficients as described with gamma photon shielding. The most efficient absorption materials used for neutron shielding are high (> 20%) in hydrogen content. Figure 6.5.8 illustrates the attenuation of hydrogen per energy level of neutrons.

To calculate the attenuation for other absorbing medium used as shielding it is first necessary to calculate the hydrogen density in that medium and then multiply that by the attenuation coefficient found on the table. To calculate the half value layer, it is then necessary to divide the attenuation coefficient calculated into the constant, 0.693, so that

$$HVL = \frac{0.693}{\text{attenuation coefficient}}$$

Table 6.5.10

Properties of some commonly used beta emitters.

Property	H-3	C-14	S-35	Ca-45	P-32	Sr-90
Half-Life	12.3 yr	5730 yr	88 d	165 d	14.3 d	28.1
Maximum beta energy (MeV)	0.018	0.154	0.167	0.254	1.71	2.24*
Average beta energy (MeV)	0.006	0.050	0.049	0.077	0.70	0.93
Range in air (ft)	0.02	1	1	2	20	29
Range in unit density material (cm)	0.00052	0.029	0.032	0.06	0.8	1.1
Half value layer, unit density absorber (cm)	--	0.0022	0.0025	0.0048	0.10	0.14
Dose from 100 beta particles/cm^2-sec (mrad/hr)	--	64	60	43	12	11
Fraction transmitted through dead layer of skin (0.007 cm)	--	0.11	0.16	0.37	0.95	0.97
Dose rate to basal cells of epidermis from 1 $\mu Ci/cm^2$ (mrad/hr)	--	2600	3600	5900	4300	3900

* From the Y-90 decay product.
Source: Shapiro, Jacob. Radiation Protection--A Guide for Scientists and Physicians, Harvard University Press, 1974.

Figure 6.5.7

Glove box.

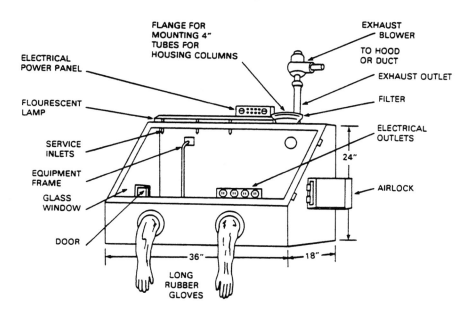

Figure 6.5.8

Hydrogen attenuation (cm^{-1}) vs. neutron energy.

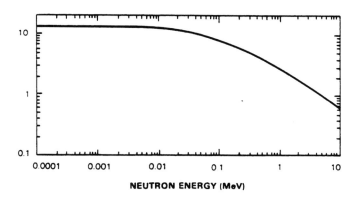

The following is an example of the calculation of the attenuation due to hydrogen in a water shield 150 cm thick for 8 MeV neutrons.

Water is 11% hydrogen by weight. Therefore, the density of hydrogen in the medium, water, is 0.11 grams/cc. From Figure 6.5.8, for neutrons with 8.0 MeV energy level, the attenuation coefficient equals 0.68 cm^{-1}. Therefore, for water the attenuation coefficient would be 0.68 x 0.11 or 0.075 cm^{-1}. The half-value layer would then be 0.693 divided by 0.075, or 9.24 centimeters. The number of half-value layers would be equal to 150 divided by 9.24, or 16.2. The attenuation caused by 16.2 half-value layers would be equal to $(0.5)^{16.2}$, or 1.3 x 10^{-5}.

Application of the previous formula can be used to calculate the effect of neutron shielding. However, neutron activity leads to the emission of gamma radiation. Therefore, neutron shielding also requires gamma shielding. Because of the sophistication of this problem, it is beyond the scope of this text. Any situations that require neutron shielding should be investigated further in the literature.

Survey and Monitoring Procedures for Radiation Hazards

The purpose of surveying and monitoring areas with potential radiation hazards is:

1.   To indicate the general level of radiation in the working environment.

2.   To monitor changes in the level of radiation.

An area surveyed would include an initial examination of the facility, laboratory operating procedures, personnel habits, types of radiation sources being used, methods used in handling the sources, and radiation levels that are observed. Special emphasis should be placed on identifying and quantifying those factors that determine the exposure rate for the personnel. These things include the average time of exposure during the operating procedure, average distance of the employee from the potential source, and areas of the body that may come in closer contact to the source than others, e.g., the hand. Area surveys are generally more interested in analyzing potential radiation hazards and identifying existing hazards without actually quantifying the hazard.

These surveys should be scheduled on a routine basis. Shields should be checked for cracks, excessive surface and airborne contamination should be evaluated, and factors such as improper disposal of waste should also be considered. Special emphasis should be placed on unlikely or remote areas that typically are not included in any type of daily monitoring procedure.

Routine measurements should be made at intervals during the performance of work. Measurements should be taken for all steps of the procedure and should include data such as the time of the procedure and exposure levels; distance from the source, including the mean body distance and specific areas of the body that are closer to the source, e.g., hands; the variations of exposure throughout the procedure to the employee, e.g., does the employee turn his back to the source during the procedure? From this information, a relative exposure rate for personnel can be determined and adjustments made accordingly. Care should be taken when taking these measurements to ensure that all potential exposed areas are analyzed.

Efforts should be made, if appropriate, to analyze the contamination that may occur during any given procedure. Specifically, three areas are of concern. First, any radioactive contamination that may settle on any surface in the laboratory in the form of dust or particulate matter. This may be evaluated by taking a smear or wipe test. Its purpose is to determine the amount of loose radioactive material that may potentially become airborne or be transferred to personnel and carried outside the radiation facility. If a specific surface area, for example 100 cm^2, is wiped off with a clean cloth or adhesive tape each time a smear test is performed, then the results may be quantified. Smear samples, once taken. should be removed to areas of low background radiation and a reading taken. If surface contamination is found beyond established limits, corrective action should be taken.

The second form of contamination that should be monitored is that of air contamination. Air samples may be collected by standard procedure, such as using filters, electrostatic precipitators, impingers, or impactors. Care must be taken to ensure that all particles of appropriate size are collected. Samples of 10 m^3 are usually adequate. Direct counting from the surfaces where air samples are collected is appropriate. Care must be taken when counting alpha particles because the alpha particles may be absorbed by the sample-collecting filter. In this instance, a correction factor must be determined. Assuming that the radionuclide is known, the concentration of radioactive contaminant in the air can be calculated in terms of microcuries per cubic centimeter ($\mu Ci/cc$). This value is then compared to the maximum permissible concentration (MPC) for unrestricted areas. These values may be found in Handbook 69. (See References.) Once the concentration has been calculated, the quantity of nuclide taken in by personnel can be roughly estimated by determining the exposure time and then determining the product of the exposure time, concentration, and the conversion factor of 10^7 cc per eight hours. This value can be compared to the maximum body burden, also found in Handbook 69. If the nuclide source is not known, arbitrary limits can be established such that gamma and beta sources should not exceed 10^{-9} $\mu Ci/cc$, and alpha sources should not exceed 10^{-12} $\mu Ci/cc$. In any instance where air contamination is a possibility, respirators should be used until radiation levels have been adequately determined. In some instances, naturally occurring radon and thoron may interfere with readings; specifically when counting alpha particles. In this instance, adjustments must be made for the interference.

Water sample analysis is similar to air analysis. The sample should be 100 to 500 ml. In analyzing the sample, the water is evaporated and a reading is taken. The concentration in microcuries per cubic centimeter is then calculated and the results compared to the maximum permissible concentration (MPC) values, also found in Handbook 69. If the nuclide is not known, qualitative tests can be performed to determine the source. In either the air or the water sample analysis, the minimum level for the critical organ should be used as a basis for comparison.

Personnel Monitoring

Personnel monitoring is the most direct method of calculating personnel exposure. As previously discussed, the common equipment used for personnel monitoring includes film badges, pocket ion chambers, and pocket dosimeters. Personnel monitoring should be used in any situation where it is possible that 25% of the MPD value for a 13-week period may be exceeded. Because of the potential liability of the instruments, the personnel devices should always be used in pairs.

The location of the personnel monitor is critical. If the whole-body radiation dose is of interest, the monitor should be worn between the waist and the neck, somewhere on the chest. It should be unshielded; that is, the monitor should not be covered by several layers of clothing. To maximize the value of the monitor, it should be at a point of maximum exposure. If, for example, the process requires the employee to handle the radioactive source with leaded gloves on, the monitor should be placed on the hands rather than somewhere on the body. Although the MPD value is greater for the hands and a body exposure may give a relative indication of exposure to the hands, the most accurate reading is necessary. The configuration of the employee's body to the radiation source must also be considered. If, for example, the person works 50 percent of the time with his left side facing the radiation source and 50 percent of the time facing the source directly, then the monitor should be placed such that readings are being taken at the points of maximum exposure and at no time does the worker's body shield the monitor from the radiation source.

Special effort must be made to ensure that the monitors selected match the type and energy level of the radiation being monitored. The use of monitors and dosimeters that are not correctly matched will give erroneous readings. Records on each employee should be maintained concerning cumulative doses received.

In some instances, it may be of value to receive a continuous recording of dose rate at a fixed location. In these instances, fixed monitors are used. These monitors may be equipped with visible or audible alarms that warn of increased radiation levels. If contamination is possible, a fixed monitor may be placed in the doorway of the radiation facility so that personnel are monitored for contamination of clothing before leaving the facility. Special monitors have been developed that survey the hands and shoes, including the soles. This type of monitoring capability is of value when large numbers of personnel are involved at the change of shifts. It limits the possibility of radioactive contamination outside the designated facility.

Controls can be designed into the system that minimize personnel exposure. These include warning systems, such as previously discussed, for high exposure levels. Also, it is possible to develop interlock systems so that radiation-producing equipment (X-rays) cannot be operated unless shielding is in place, or shielding cannot be moved until personnel are a designated distance from the source.

Facilities

When examining the design of the facility to be used for a radioactive procedure, steps must be taken to maximize containment of the radiation and to allow for the ease of cleanup in the event of contamination within the facility. Certain design factors can maximize this.

All surfaces involved in the radiation area should be smooth and nonporous; e.g., shelves, floors, sinks. It is unacceptable to have surfaces--such as uncoated wood, concrete, or soapstone--that would provide a porous surface for the collection of contaminants. Such surfaces as tile, polished stainless steel, and plate glass are acceptable. Although paints, varnishes, and lacquers do provide a somewhat nonporous surface, they are not recommended for use in radiation areas.

Any area that could be a dust collector should be eliminated. This includes things such as suspended lighting, suspended pipes, and roof trusses. Any shelving or storage areas should be enclosed by doors. Cove corners between the wall and floor will facilitate cleanup and reduce possible gathering of contaminated particles.

Any special piping or drainage systems that are necessary for the procedure and are involved in the radiation area should be plainly labeled, especially if used for radioactive waste.

The design of the facility and shielding should prevent any type of radiation leakage from the facility. For example, Figure 6.5.9 illustrates special precautions that must be taken in the construction of joints to prevent the leakage of incident radiation. Figure 6.5.10 illustrates a typical doorway maze that is used to minimize leakage.

Within the facility, special equipment is often required. For example, long-handled tools such as tongs and forceps are often used to increase the distance between personnel and the source and decrease the exposure rate (inverse-square law). In those instances when the radiation source is high-activity, it may be necessary to use remote control devices with protective lead glass windows such as displayed in Figure 6.5.5.

With respect to the facility design, there are two areas that should be given special consideration. First, when working with unsealed radioisotopes, hood and exhaust systems are needed to minimize airborne contamination. The airflow in the hood system should result in a minimum average face velocity of 100 feet per minute (fpm). If highly toxic radioisotopes are being used, then the flow rate should be adjusted to achieve a average face velocity of approximately 125 to 150 fpm. The hood should have its own exhaust system with appropriate filtering and decontamination systems. The air contamination should be monitored to ensure that it does not exceed established levels. (Note: The calculation of air contamination will be discussed later.) Airflow should also be monitored for cross drafts and leaks in the system. The development of the hood and exhaust system should follow the principles discussed in the Ventilation section.

Figure 6.5.9

Joint construction.

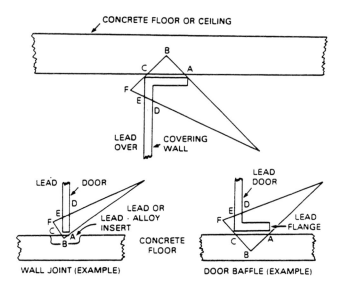

WALL JOINT (EXAMPLE)   DOOR BAFFLE (EXAMPLE)

Figure 6.5.10

Entrance maze.

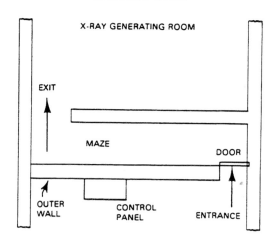

CONTROL ROOM
X-RAY ROOM LAYOUT USING A MAZE

When working with alpha and low-energy beta radiation, glove boxes, as shown in Figure 6.5.7, offer sufficient protection. This type of system prevents air contamination while allowing the employee to work closely with the radioisotope. As seen in the figure, hermetically sealed ports go into the box and allow for manipulation of the box contents using the glove. Air locks are also provided to allow for insertion and removal of samples without air contamination. For high-energy beta rays and gamma radiation, it is necessary to replace the gloves with some type of remote mechanical manipulator. Frequently, the glove boxes have exhaust ports and filters with exhaust volumes in the area of 20 to 30 cubic feet per minute. The personnel should be positioned so that any explosion would not be directed at them through exhaust and inlet ports.

Posting the Area

Warning signs are essential in radiation areas since individuals might otherwise be unaware of the presence of the radiation field. Areas need to be posted only if the radioactivity is to be present in that area for longer than eight hours. Each symbol or label should bear the three-blade radioactive caution symbol, either magenta or purple on a yellow background, as shown in Figure 6.5.11.

Figure 6.5.11

Radiation symbol.

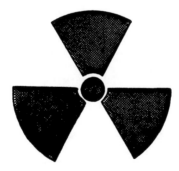

The labels and signs that accompany the radiation symbol are dependent upon the potential exposure in that given area. The following types of signs are required in areas where significant levels of radiation or radioactivity are present:

1.   "CAUTION RADIATION AREA"--This sign is used in areas accessible to personnel in which a major portion of the body could receive in any one hour a dose of 5 millirems, or in any 5 consecutive days, a dose in excess of 100 millirems.

2. "CAUTION RADIOACTIVE MATERIAL"--This sign is required in areas or rooms in which radioactive material is stored or used in an amount exceeding the quantities listed in Table 6.5.1.

3. "CAUTION RADIOACTIVE MATERIAL" (Label)--A durable, clearly visible label is required on any container that is transported, stored, or used for a quantity of any material greater than the quantity specified in Table 6.5.1. When containers are used for storage, the labels must state also the quantities and kinds of radioactive materials in the containers and the date of measurement of the quantities.

4. "AIRBORNE RADIOACTIVITY AREA"--This sign is required if airborne radioactive activity exceeds at any time concentrations in excess of the maximum permissible for 40 hours of occupational exposure, or if the average over a number of areas in any week during which individuals are in the area exceeds 25 percent of the maximum permissible concentration. (Table 6.5.1)

5. "HIGH RADIATION AREA"--This sign is required if the radiation dose to a major portion of the body to a person in the area could be in excess of 100 millirems in any one hour. These areas also require the audible or visible alarm signals that were discussed previously.

As stated, because radioactivity cannot be sensed by the human body, it is essential that signs be present in areas where radioactivity may exist. On the other hand, the signs should not be used when they are not needed.

In many instances, the handling procedures for radioisotopes or the operation of radiation-producing instruments have been specifically defined. In those instances, it may be of value to post the operating/handling procedures as illustrated in Figure 6.5.12.

Trays and Handling Tools. When working with radioisotopes, any procedure that may result in the contamination of a table top should be performed in a tray. This would negate the problem of having to replace counter tops rather than the contaminated trays. Also, even small amounts of radionuclides should not be handled directly, but tweezers and/or tongs should be used whenever possible to minimize exposure. This will reduce the potential of contamination on the hands and gloves and also decrease the exposure rate through the inverse-square law of distance.

Storage and Disposal of Radionuclides

Radionuclides should be stored in designated areas, protected against fire, explosion, or flooding. They should be stored in suitable containers that provide adequate shielding. In any type of storage situation, the radiation level should not exceed 5 millirems per hour at one foot in the storage area.

Figure 6.5.12

How to handle radioisotope shipments.

An Outline of Recommended Procedures to be
Followed When Receiving Radioactive Shipments

Open and inspect packages immediately upon receipt.
Radioactive solutions inadvertently stored upside down may
gradually leak and cause contamination problems; furthermore,
vendors often will not accept claims for shipments not inspected
within 15 days after delivery.

Monitor package for radiation field.
It is suggested that plastic gloves be worn while processing the
received package.

To Process Soft Beta, Hard Beta, and Gamma Emitters
1.   Wipe and test package for removable contamination.

2.   Note radiation units stated on package, verify and record in
     receipt log. (Hard beta and gamma only.)

3.   Place package in vented hood.

4.   Open outer package and remove packing slip. Open inner package
     and verify that the contents agree in name and quantity with the
     packing slip.

5.   Measure radiation field of unshielded container--if necessary,
     place container behind shielding to reduce field to allowable
     limits and proceed with remote handling devices. (Hard beta and
     gamma only.)

6.   Check for possible breakage of seals or containers, loss of
     liquid, or change in color of absorbing materials.

7.   Wipe test inner contents and document any pertinent findings on
     packing slip. Note: The liner, shield, and isotope container
     may have surface contamination; they should be discarded in hot
     waste disposal containers.

8.   Record type of activity, quantity present, and location of
     delivery in receiving log.

9.   Deliver processed package to proper laboratory. If delivery is
     delayed, notify recipient of its arrival and clearance.

10. If material has been packaged in dry ice, refrigerate or deliver
     immediately to ultimate user.

11. If contamination, leakage, or shortages are observed, notify the
     vendor's Customer Service Department immediately.

When concerned with disposal of radioactive wastes, there are four possible alternatives: release into the atmosphere, release into water, burial, or a contract arrangement with a commercially licensed radiation disposal firm. Each of these activities is controlled by the Nuclear Regulatory Commission.

The release of radioactivity in the air is limited by the Nuclear Regulatory Commission. The concentration released through exhaust system should not exceed the maximum permissible concentration (MPC) at the point of discharge. The exact concentration can be calculated, including the release of different nuclides at once.

Example

A radio chemist released 1 curie of tritium (tritiated water) through a hood while performing a synthesis. The hood face velocity was 100 feet per minute with a 1 foot by 4.5 foot hood opening. If the concentration is averaged over one week, was the MPC value exceeded?

Solution

Assuming 40 hours per week, the flow rate for the hood can be calculated to be 0.612×10^{10} cc/day or 3.06×10^{10} cc/week. From Table 6.5.11, the maximum permissible concentration for tritiated water (Hydrogen-3) is equal to 2.0×10^{-13} curies/cc. The radioactive release from the hood is equal to 1 Ci/week $\div$ 3.06×10^{10} cc/week = 3.26×10^{-11} Ci/cc. Therefore, the MPC has been exceeded.

Limited amounts of liquid radioactive waste can be deposited in unrestricted water or in sewage systems. Again. levels have been established by the NRC and must be met. Unlike the calculation of maximum level for air contamination, when calculating liquid disposal, both daily and monthly MPC values must be met. Further, disposal may not exceed 1.0 curies per year. An example of this is as follows:

Example

Determine how much Iodine-125 and Phosphorus-32 can be discharged into the sewerage system if the water flow (based on water bills) is 1.2×10^7 cubic feet per year.

Solution

From Table 6.5.11, the MPC value for Iodine-125 is 40×10^{-12} Ci/cc/wk, and the MPC value for Phosphorus-32 is 5.0×10^{-10} Ci/cc/day. The average daily water flow can be calculated based on the water bill to be equal to 9.31×10^8 cc/day (assume 365 day operation). Therefore, the daily limits for Iodine-125 and Phosphorus-32 would be equal to the product of the MPC value times the daily water flow, or 37.24 millicuries and 466 millicuries respectively. Therefore, these daily limits would be the maximum amount of radioactive waste that could be discharged into the sewerage system. However, this daily disposal rate could only continue until a maximum of 1 curie/yr limit for the disposal of gross activity has been reached.

When disposing of solid waste, the alternative of incineration, burial, or the commercial disposal firm are available. Incineration is a good bulk-reducing method. Again, this method is regulated by the NRC. The rule of thumb to follow is that the concentration released to the unrestricted areas should not exceed limits specified for continuous exposure. When calculating the release, the concentration may be averaged over a maximum of one year. The procedure for calculation is similar to that for air contamination, and to complete the calculation, the type of radionuclide, the quantity of radionuclide, and the airflow of the incinerator must be known. An important fact is that any ash left over after incineration must also be treated as radioactive waste.

Table 6.5.11

Maximum permissible concentrations of
radionuclides in air and water.

Radionuclide	Unrestricted Areas		Restricted Area (40 hr/wk)	
	Water (pCi/cc)	Air (pCi/cc)	Water (pCi/cc)	Air (pCi/cc)
C-14	80	0.1	20,000	4
H-3	3,000	.2	100,000	5
S-35	60	.009	2,000	0.3
I-131	0.3	.0001	60	0.009
I-125	0.2	.00008	40	0.005
P-32	20	.002	500	0.07
Ca-45	9	.001	300	0.03
Na-24	30	.005	800	0.1
K-42	20	.004	600	0.1
Cr-51	200	.08	50,000	2
Kr-85	--	.3	--	10
Xe-133	--	.3	--	10
Br-82	40	.006	1,000	0.2
Cl-36	60	.008	2,000	0.02

Note: The maximum permissible concentration depends upon several factors, including the degree of solubility of the contaminant. The lowest concentrations specified in the regulations have been listed.

Source: U.S. Code of Federal Regulations, Title 10, Part 20, as of December 10, 1969.

The NRC rules for burial are fairly simple. Each organization is permitted twelve burials per year. Burials must be at least six feet apart and a minimum of four feet deep. The total quantity of radionuclide buried at any location may not exceed 1000 times the level established in Table 6.5.1. If several nuclides are buried in a single burial, the sum of the radionuclide fractions cannot exceed one. For example, a user of radionuclides plans to dispose of 2 millicuries of Iron-59, 10 millicuries of Chromium-51, and 20 millicuries of Iodine-125 by burial. Is this possible?

Solution

He would be permitted to bury single (1000 times value in Table 6.5.1, third column):
Iron-59 = 10 millicuries
Chromium-51 = 1000 millicuries
Iodine-125 = 1 millicurie
Immediately it can be seen that the amount of Iodine-125 which is to be buried exceeds the limit. However, the Iron-59 requires only 20 percent of the allotted limit, and the Chromium-51 required only one percent of the allotted limit. Therefore, being sure that the sum of the nuclide fractions does not exceed 1, 0.79 of the Iodine limit, or 0.79 millicuries, could be buried in the same burial. However, the remaining 19.21 millicuries of Iodine would have to be buried in 19 separate burials. Because this exceeds the limit, it would seem more advisable to have the Iodine disposed of by a commercial firm.

In many instances, the guidelines for storage and disposal of wastes established by the NRC vary somewhat from state regulations. Therefore, state health departments must also be contacted when working with radioisotopes in production lines.

Personnel

Personnel have a responsibility to minimize their exposure to ionizing radiation. Although maximum exposure levels (MPD) have been established, every effort should be made to minimize exposure.

The Nuclear Regulatory Commission has established training requirements for those personnel directly involved with the use of radioisotopes or radiation-producing machinery. Each person potentially exposed to radioactivity should receive training in the potential dangers of radiation, operational procedures that minimize exposure, and procedures in case of accidents.

The protective clothing that is required of personnel is dependent on the level of radio toxicity of the nuclide. Specifically, the clothing should be such that it can be easily laundered or disposed of should contamination occur. The degree of protection that is required of the clothing is a function of the quantity and type of radioactivity, the nature of the operation, and the design of the laboratory. Sealed containers do not usually require protective clothing for use. In general, protective clothing of any kind is not required if the MPD value for the most critical organ (as defined by Handbook 69) is not and will not be exceeded. The amount of protective clothing, as previously mentioned, is dependent upon the radio toxicity. Figure 6.5.13 generally groups the radioisotopes according to toxicity.

Figure 6.5.13

Hazard from absorption into the body.

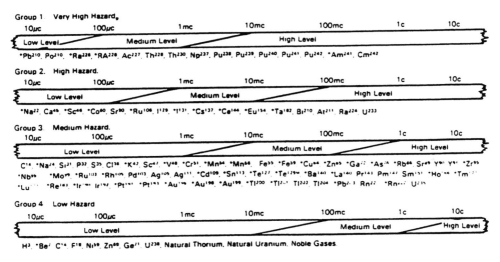

*Emits gamma radiation in significant amounts

For those personnel working with low level radioisotopes, laboratory coats or coveralls are recommended. Simple cloth or plastic bags on the shoes to reduce the potential contamination of the shoes is also recommended. Rubber or plastic gloves should be worn, and handling of the radioisotope without gloves should be avoided. Any isotope that is classified in the medium level requires the personnel to wear coveralls, caps, gloves, and shoe covers. Every effort should be made to minimize contamination of personal clothing. Should the individual be exposed to high level radioisotopes, a multi-layer of coveralls, shoes, etc., would be required. In most instances, high level radioisotopes should not be encountered during normal operation.

If the recommended MPC level is exceeded, it is required that some type of respiratory protection be used. The type of respirator employed may vary from a simple respirator, which merely filters out particles, to some type of self-contained breathing apparatus, which is a closed ventilation system for the employee. Typical respirators are illustrated in other chapters. One limitation of respiratory equipment must be mentioned; that is, in all instances the mask will leak approximately 1 to 2 percent. Growth of a beard or mustache may further affect the mask fit and leakage. Therefore, this potential leakage must be taken into consideration when the personnel are equipped with respiratory protection.

Shielding garments are somewhat different from protective clothing in that they not only serve to prevent and reduce contamination, but also they act as an absorbing or shielding material. They should be used for close contact work with radiation of low penetrating power. For example, leather or rubber gloves are often effective against most beta radiation. Fabrics loaded with high atomic material are used for shielding against X-radiation. Shielding garments should not be used solely for high-level beta or gamma radiation because the shielding cannot be designed to stop radiation of high penetrating power. Personal hygiene is also essential in minimizing exposure. Eating, smoking, food storage, pipetting by mouth should be prohibited in radioactive areas. Any work with unsealed sources requires a "wash up" before eating, smoking, or leaving the work area. Written procedures for personnel should include basic hygiene practices as mentioned.

Personnel monitoring has been discussed previously. As a review, any personnel who potentially may be in an area of radiation level that is 25 percent of the maximum permissible dose should carry personnel monitoring devices; e.g., film badges, dosimeters. As mentioned, these devices should be used in pairs at a minimum to ensure adequate coverage of the personnel.

Because of the physical hazards of ionizing radiation, medical supervision is essential. Each potential employee should have a pre-employment examination to identify his or her general physical condition. Efforts should be made at the pre-employment examination to quantify, if possible, previous radiation exposures including those involving medical examination; e.g., dental X-rays. Efforts should also be made to identify possible problems that may be magnified or potentially dangerous to the employee in a radioactive environment. Such problems might include dermatological diseases, impairment of pulmonary ventilation, or even cataracts. The decision of employment and placement should consider the above-mentioned factors. Once the employee has been hired and selected to work in a radioactive area, periodic medical examinations should be performed. They should occur at appropriate intervals based on the general health of the employee and the nature of work. These examinations should provide insight to any medical changes. However, the periodic examinations should not be used as a reliable method for monitoring radiation hazard. The examination should include a review of the occupational hazard records and the assessment of exposure doses. Medical advice should be followed with respect to continued radiation exposure for the employee.

In the event of a radiation accident, or even if the MPD value has been exceeded only slightly, it is important that followup examination continue. This is true even if the examinations must occur after the employee has resigned from the organization. This type of followup examination will provide extended coverage for the worker, along with adding information on the effect of radiation on the general population. Records should be established and maintained for each employee working in some type of radioactive environment. These records should include medical and radiation exposure history. Job assignments and hazards involved should also be recorded.

Radiation Accidents

Maximum efforts should be made to minimize accidents. For example, periodic review of operational procedures for potential hazards should be implemented. Further, equipment used in the handling and operation dealing with radioactive sources should also be checked periodically. For nonroutine or high level operations, a trial run of the operation should be performed. This trial run will evaluate the adequacy of the procedure and determine the exposure time to the personnel.

In the event of an accident, loose contamination should be minimized whenever possible. All spills should be cleaned up promptly. Cleaning tools should not be removed from the radiation area without being decontaminated. Any level of contamination is difficult to determine, and the impact of the contamination is also very complex.

When monitoring for contamination, a G–M counter is used for beta and gamma radiation, and a proportional counter is used when alpha contamination is suspected. The wipe or smear test is often performed when surface contamination is suspected.

When employees' hands, body surfaces, clothing, or shoes become contaminated, loose contamination should be removed as soon as possible. Care must be taken to minimize the spreading of the contamination. Initially, washing with mild soap or detergent is a good step. This may be followed up with a mild abrasive soap, complexing solution, or mild organic acid, whichever is appropriate. When the hands are involved in some type of contamination, clipping the fingernails may reduce contamination. In any instance, medical personnel should be notified and the employee examined. Because of potential medical treatment being based on the level of dose received and contamination involved, a relatively accurate determination of the level of exposure is necessary. With respect to specific procedures for decontamination, the following section provides a general overview for radiation accidents.

Emergency Instructions in the Event of Release of Radioactivity and Contamination of Personnel

Objectives of Remedial Action. In the event of an accident involving the release of significant quantities of radioactive material, the objectives of all remedial action are to:

a. Minimize the amount of radioactive material entering the body, by ingestion, inhalation, or through any wounds.

b. Prevent the spread of contamination from the area of the accident.

c. Remove radioactive contamination on personnel.

d. Start area decontamination procedures under qualified supervision. Inexperienced personnel should not attempt unsupervised decontamination.

Procedures for Dealing with Minor Spills and Contamination. Most accidents will involve only minor quantities or radioactivity (i.e., at the microcurie level).

a.   Put on gloves to prevent contamination of the hands. (Wash hands first if they are contaminated as a result of accident.)

b.   Drop absorbent paper or cloth on the spill to limit spread of contamination.

c.   Mark off contaminated area. Do not allow anyone to leave contaminated area without being monitored.

d.   Notify the radiation protection office of the accident.

e.   Start decontamination procedures as soon as possible. Normal cleaning agents should be adequate. Keep cleaning supplies to a minimum needed to do the job and place into sealed bags after use. Recommendations for difficult jobs may be found in the Radiological Health Handbook, listed in the References. Proceed from the outermost edges of the contaminated area inward, reducing systematically the area that is contaminated. (This principle may not apply in decontamination of highly radioactive areas, which would require supervision by a radiation protection specialist.)

f.   Put all contaminated objects into containers to prevent spread of contamination.

g.   Assign a person equipped with a survey meter to follow the work and watch for accidental spread of contamination.

Personnel Decontamination. If personnel contamination is suspected, first identify contaminated areas with a survey meter. Do not use decontamination methods that will spread localized material or increase penetration of the contaminant into the body; e.g., by abrasion of the skin. Decontamination of wounds should be accomplished under the supervision of a physician.

Irrigate any wounds profusely with tepid water and clean with a swab. Follow with soap or detergent and water (and gently scrubbing with a soft brush, if needed). Avoid the use of highly alkaline soaps (may result in fixation of the contaminant) or organic solvents (may increase skin penetration by contaminant).

Use the following procedures on intact skin:

a.   Wet hands and apply detergent.

b.   Work up good lather; keep lather wet.

c.   Work lather into contaminated area by rubbing gently for at least 3 minutes. Apply water frequently.

d.   Rinse thoroughly with lukewarm water (limiting water to contaminated areas).

e.   Repeat above procedures several times, gently scrubbing residual contaminated areas with a soft brush, if necessary.

f.   If the radiation level is still excessive, initiate more powerful decontamination procedures after consulting with the radiation protection office.

Reporting Radiation Accidents.   Those accidents involving radiation must be reported to the Nuclear Regulatory Commission. Reports must include information such as number of individuals exposed, names of individuals exposed, level of exposure, nuclides involved, and/or the concentration of nuclides released. The NRC has established notification requirements such that if an accident meets the following criteria, it must be reported immediately:

a.   Whole-body exposure of individual exceeds 25 rems.

b.   Skin exposure exceeds 150 rems.

c.   Exposure of hands, feet, ankles exceeds 375 rems.

d.   Release of radioactive materials exceeds 5000 times the specified limits over a 24-hour period.

e.   Loss of one or more working weeks due to radiation accident.

f.   Damage to property in excess of $100,000.

If the accident does not meet the above levels but meets the criteria below, the accident must be reported within 24 hours.

a.   Whole-body exposure in excess of 5 rems.

b.   Skin exposure exceeding 30 rems.

c.   Exposure of hands, feet, ankles exceeds 75 rems.

d.   Release of radioactive materials exceeding 500 times the specified concentration limits over a 24-hour period.

e.   Loss of one or more working days due to a radiation accident.

f.   Damage to property in excess of $1,000.

Responsibilities of the Industrial Hygiene Engineer

In some instances, the industrial hygiene engineer has direct responsibility for radioactive sources. In fulfilling this responsibility, the following activities should be performed:

1. Comply with all government regulations.

2. Ensure adequate supervision and training of personnel working with radioactivity.

3. Maintain inventory of radioactive sources being used, including type and amount.

4. Review operational procedures to evaluate potential:

    a. personnel exposure;
    b. accidents causing a radiation release.

5. Periodically survey radioactive areas for radiation levels.

6. Evaluate laboratory facility for proper design, construction, shielding, posting, labeling, etc.

7. Design alternative plans for containment and decontamination in the event of an accident.

8. Monitor the disposal of wastes.

9. Supervise the monitoring systems, including personnel monitoring procedures.

10. Maintain accurate records, including personnel cumulative exposure, radiation surveys, instrument calibration, waste disposal, and radiation incidents.

Summary

The last three chapters have presented an overview of the theory, use, monitoring, and control and management of ionizing radiation. Because of the potential health hazard of ionizing radiation, it is essential that the industrial hygiene engineer minimize the potential personnel exposure when working with radiation sources. These chapters were not intended to provide the reader with a complete and comprehensive understanding of ionizing radiation, but the material presented was designed to provide an initial understanding of the concepts of ionizing radiation.

6. References

American Conference of Governmental Industrial Hygienists. TLV's for Chemical Substances and Physical Agents in the Workroom Environment with Intended Changes for 1976. Cincinnati: American Conference of Governmental Industrial Hygienists, 1976.

Blaty, Hanson. Introduction to Radiological Health. New York: McGraw-Hill Book Company, 1976.

Department of the Air Force, AFM. Laser Health Hazards Control. Washington: 1971.

Departments of the Army and Navy TB Med 279/NAVMED P-5052-35. Control of Hazards from Laser Radiation. Washington.

International Commission on Radiation Units and Measurements. Radiation Protection Instrumentation and Its Application, ICRU Report 20. Washington: 1971.

___. Radiation Quantities and Units, ICRU Report 19. Washington: 1971.

Morgan, K. Z. and Turner, J. E. Principles of Radiation Protection. New York: John Wiley and Sons, Inc., March 1973.

National Bureau of Standards. Safe Handling of Radioactive Materials, Handbook 92. Washington: U. S. Government Printing Office, 1964.

National Committee on Radiation Protection. Maximum Permissible Body Burdens and Maximum Permissible Concentrations of Radionuclides in Air and Water for Occupational Exposure, National Bureau of Standards Handbook 69. Washington: U. S. Government Printing Office, 1959.

___. Medical X-ray and Gamma-ray Protection for Energies up to 10 MeV, Structural Shielding Design and Evaluation, NCRP Report No. 34. Washington: 1970.

___. Protection Against Neutron Radiation, NCRP Report No. 38. Washington: 1971.

___. Basic Radiation Protection Criteria, NCRP Report No. 39. Washington: 1971.

Olishifski, Julian B. and McElroy, Frank E., ed. Fundamentals of Industrial Hygiene. Chicago: National Safety Council, 1971.

Shapiro, Jacob. Radiation Protection--A Guide for Scientists and Physicians. Cambridge: Harvard University Press, 1974.

U. S. Department of Health, Education, and Welfare, Public Health Service, National Institute for Occupational Safety and Health. The Industrial Environment: Its Evaluation and Control. Washington: U. S. Government Printing Office, 1973.

U. S. Department of Health, Education, and Welfare, Public Health Service. Radiological Health Handbook. Washington: U. S. Government Printing Office, 1970.

Section 7

Ergonomics

1. Introduction to Ergonomics

<u>What is Ergonomics?</u>

In early times, man needed to use only simple tools to scratch out a living from the earth. With the coming of the industrial revolution, the complexity and number of tools that man must use in the workplace has increased astronomically. No longer is man subjected to only the natural environmental conditions. Workers must work in an industrial atmosphere where they are constantly subjected to conditions that may cause damage to their health and physical well being. Machinery in the workplace can cause noise and vibration as well as contamination of the atmosphere with toxic materials. In addition, the typical industrial environment is often not a serene atmosphere in which to work. The worker is bombarded by many auditory and visual stimuli and must react to these stimuli to perform tasks. Within this environment, the tasks that must be performed include both physical and mental activities. It is obvious that the stress placed on the worker is significant and that proper design is required to minimize the strain placed on the worker.

Ergonomics, though a recently identified discipline of study, has its basis in the study of Ramazzini who, in 1700, discussed the ill-effects of poor posture and poorly designed tools on the health of the worker. The term "ergonomics," is derived from the Greek words "ergos," meaning work, and "nomikos," meaning law. <u>Ergonomics</u> is, then, the study of work laws.

Some confusion exists concerning the field of ergonomics and the objectives toward which it is directed. Part of the confusion is a result of the fact that two general terms are used for essentially the same discipline. The term "ergonomics," which is used more widely in England, and the term "human factors," which is prevalent in use in the United States, essentially describe the same discipline or field of study. It might be argued that the field of human factors in the United States is broader in its applicability since it involves the design of products for the consumer market place as well as the design of work-related tasks and equipment. However, generally the major application of both fields is toward the use of bioengineering and biomechanics to improve the workplace environment for the worker.

Ergonomics draws from many fields or disciplines of study. Figure 7.1.1 illustrates the major disciplines from which ergonomics draws. In the physical sciences, both physics and chemistry provide basic information that is used in the field of ergonomics. Mathematics, through the use of statistics and biometrics (the measurement of body structure), is also widely applied in the study of work laws. The biological sciences give to the field

of ergonomics the studies of anatomy, physiology, and anthropometry.
Psychology provides a basis for learning theory as well as human reaction to
various stimuli. The field of engineering is important in the proper design
of equipment for use by humans in the workplace. Finally, the field of
systems analysis provides a basic structure whereby the analysis of the job
can be performed.

Figure 7.1.1

Major disciplines.

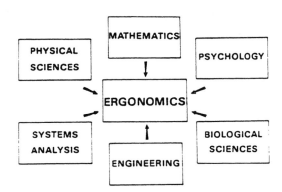

The <u>basic objective of ergonomics</u> is to obtain an optimum relationship
between the worker and the work environment. The worker, in performing a job,
must act to complete assigned tasks in a manner that will result in the
desired product being generated in the most efficient manner possible. At the
same time, the worker must be provided with protection against undue physical,
biological, and psychological strain that might occur as a result of the
performance of the required tasks.

In performing the tasks assigned, the worker is influenced by a number of
factors that must be considered in attempting to optimize the relationship
between the worker and the job. Among the important factors that must be
considered are the thermal conditions in the workplace, the amount of
illumination present, the physical and mental requirements of the job, the
noise level in the workplace, the worker's exposure to hazardous materials,
and the interaction between the worker and the equipment that is required for
the job.

Consider the worker who is working on an assembly line. This worker must
perform the assigned tasks in a manner so as to produce the desired quality
within a specified time period. If the worker does not perform the tasks
properly, then the product will be rejected, resulting in a loss to the
company of not only the materials in the product but also the cost of any
other workers' time invested in the product to the point of rejection. If the
worker does not perform the required tasks in the allowable time frame, the

assembly line will eventually slow to the pace of the worker, lowering the output and raising unit cost.

However, there are many factors that may act to affect the performance of the worker. For example, the assembly line may be located in an area of relatively high heat load, thus exposing the worker to thermal stress. At a minimum, this thermal stress can place a physiological strain on the worker, resulting in potential illness. The absence of adequate illumination can result in improper performance of the assigned tasks and a potential strain to the worker's vision. Inadequate illumination can also be a factor in accidents, resulting in potential injury to the worker.

Automation has had a major influence on the work that is performed in industry today. It has resulted in the elimination of many of the heavy physical tasks that must be performed. However, in spite of automation there are still many jobs that require physical tasks to be performed. The physical demands, though in many cases different in nature from those previously experienced in the workplace, can result in a stress being placed on the individual worker while performing a job. This stress can affect the worker's performance as well as his health and safety.

Perhaps one of the largest changes that has occurred in the industrial environment today when compared to the industrial environment of the past is the increased mental demands placed on the worker. Workers must be constantly monitoring and controlling equipment while making decisions related to the actions that are necessary. These mental demands can cause fatigue in the worker just as the more physical tasks of the past caused fatigue.

Another factor that is more important in today's industrial workplace than it was in the past is the necessity for workers to interact with mechanical and electrical equipment. During this interaction, the potential for accident and injury can exist. The worker must maintain vigilance and use appropriate procedures to assure his safety and health. Also, as a result of the use of mechanical and electrical equipment, noise and vibration are generated in the workplace. This noise and vibration can have a physiological as well as an injurious effect on the worker. Noise itself can make communication difficult while, at a high exposure level, both noise and vibration may be physically harmful to the human body.

With the many chemicals that are currently in use in industry today, workers are potentially exposed to hazardous materials during work. These hazardous materials can cause both acute and long-time injury or illness to the exposed worker.

As is evident from the above discussion, the worker in the industrial environment of today is subjected to many potentially harmful factors. It is the job of the industrial hygiene engineer to assure that these factors do not result in injury and illness to the worker. The field of ergonomics or human factors is involved with designing the workplace and job in such a manner that the potential harmful effects of these factors in terms of health, safety, and efficiency are minimized.

The Man/Machine System

Let's look at the workplace to determine those major characteristics that re present. First, the workplace will include various units of mechanical nd electrical equipment. The typical industrial workplace involves the use f such equipment as power presses, lathes, heat-treating equipment, and power aws. The nonindustrial work environment is not without the presence of echanical and electrical equipment. Included in the nonindustrial workplace e.g., office) is such equipment as typewriters, copy machines, and electronic ata processing equipment.   A second characteristic of most orkplaces is the fact that manual tools are often required to perform the ob. The manual tools can include hand power equipment, hammers, crewdrivers, and material handling equipment.

The third characteristic of the workplace is related to the jobs that are erformed. Often these jobs are described by standard sets of procedures that re to be used to produce a given output. These procedures may require strict dherence, or they may be subject to worker interpretation, depending upon the ype of job that is being performed.

The fourth characteristic of the workplace is that it is usually necessary or humans to act as operators or performers of tasks within the workplace nvironment. The workers interact with the equipment to perform many of the asks that are involved in producing the output.

Finally, the workplace must be serviced by various facilities. These acilities include such things as light, heat, water, and waste removal that re required for the work processes being carried out in the workplace.

Now let's look at the worker's functions within the workplace as the nterface with the various other characteristics or components. First, the worker acts to perform various physical tasks that are necessary to complete he job. These tasks might include such things as lifting and carrying aterials and finished products, positioning materials for work operations, nd using manual and power tools to perform the work functions.

A second function of the worker within the workplace is to act to control the processes that are performed by machines. The worker initiates the action that starts the machines to work and controls the processes so that the job is arried to completion properly. Finally, the worker acts to stop the process should something in the system fail, or at the completion of the process. In rder to control the equipment, it is necessary that the worker monitor the process being performed. This monitoring may be done on the work being erformed by others, such as is the case with an inspector; or the monitoring may be performed by the machine operator.

Finally, in addition to performing physical tasks and monitoring the work processes, the worker must also share the environment with the machines in the workplace. As a result, the worker is subjected to the potential hazards that exist as a result of the use of mechanical and electrical equipment to perform the job.

Ergonomics is concerned with this interface between the worker and the job. It is concerned with the physical and mental demands on the worker that are necessary to perform the job. Also, ergonomics is concerned with the manual tools that are used to perform the job and the mechanical equipment that must be monitored and controlled by the worker.

Finally ergonomics is concerned with the work space in which the worker must perform his tasks.

More specifically, then, ergonomics is concerned with the following:

1.   The design of tools that are used in order to match the physical characteristics of the worker with the functioning of the tools.

2.   The design of the workplace space itself to meet the physical characteristics of the worker.

3.   The analysis and design of controls and displays to allow the worker to operate and monitor processes efficiently with minimum error.

4.   The development of job procedures that meet the capabilities of the worker in the system.

5.   The minimization of external forces that can act to affect the worker in the workplace. These external forces include such things as noise, thermal conditions, illumination, and vibration.

The Systems Approach

Since we are concerned with the interface between the worker and the work environment, it is necessary that a logical procedure be developed to analyze this interface. The systems approach provides a method for investigating the worker/machine system in the work environment in such a logical manner. Using the systems approach, the total system is analyzed by dividing it into manageable subparts that can then be analyzed for the factors of concern.

The systems approach commonly uses a method that is called the "black box" method. In this approach, the major components of the system are considered to be the input, processes, and output of the system. In the workplace system, the input is in terms of the raw materials, data and information that are necessary to perform the job. The process involves the steps that are taken to convert the input to the desired output. The process may be many things such as the heat treating of metals, the multi-step fabrication of metal products, the manufacture of chemicals, or the processing of information that occurs in a data processing facility. Whatever the process, it results in a desired output, or product.

Using this black box approach, the first step is to define the desired output or purpose of the system. What output do we desire? What characteristics should the output have? What tolerances or error will be permitted? Questions such as these help to define what should be accomplished during the work process.

Figure 7.1.2

The black box.

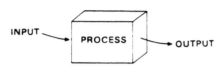

The second step of this approach is to define the inputs that are required to obtain the desired outputs. What materials are required to produce our product? What skills and knowledge are required of the worker to accomplish the desired result? What constraints are present within the system? These constraints may be environmental or mechanical factors, capital cost, or the need for adequately trained personnel.

Finally, after the outputs and inputs have been defined, the process itself can be described. How can the input be converted into the desired output, given the constraints that are present? What functions are required to convert the inputs into the outputs? What tasks are required to do the desired job?

Function and Task Analysis. One method for defining the process is through the use of function and task analysis. A job or group of jobs can be divided into functions and tasks or activities. These functions and tasks can then be analyzed. Job functions are themselves broad groups of activities that help to accomplish the objective or purpose of the organization. As an example of a function, consider driving an automobile. One function that is required is the observation of the road and surrounding conditions to determine what changes in operation are necessary. A second function is the steering of the automobile in order to assure the appropriate direction is being maintained. A third function includes acceleration and braking of the automobile to maintain the desired progress.

In some cases, higher order groupings of phases or stages is helpful. Such functional analysis is useful in the initial design of new processes and procedures. This approach has been commonly used in the space industry to define the various stages, phases, or functions within a mission.

A common set of functions that are useful in the initial analysis of a job is:

1.   Preparation--What steps are necessary to prepare the worker to perform the desired job?

2.   Observation--What information and data must the worker have in order to perform the job?

3.   Control--What steps must the worker take to control the processes
     involved? These steps include the mental processes or decisions tha
     must be made to activate given controls.

4.   Physical Demands--What physical tasks must the worker perform to
     accomplish the desired objective?

5.   Termination--What steps must be taken to terminate the job? This
     includes the cleanup after the job has been completed.

Functions 2 and 3 above are commonly considered in the feedback loop. I
the feedback loop, the worker is presented with certain information concernir
the status of the process. Using this information, the worker decides what
control must be exerted on the process to obtain the desired result and
institutes this control. Once the control is instituted, the process changes
and the information concerning th process change are fed back to the worker
enable evaluation of the outcome of the changes. This feedback loop exists
potentially in every job. It is not quite so obvious in some jobs as it isir
others; however, in all jobs, such a feedback mechanism must exist in order
for the worker to progress satisfactorily.

Figure 7.1.3

Feedback loop.

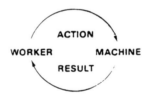

After the job has been divided into its major functions, each function c
then be subdivided into tasks or activities. These tasks define the smaller
steps that must be completed in order to obtain the desired output of the
job. For example, consider the operation of a small business. The function
that may be performed within such a business include marketing, production,
and accounting. Within the accounting function itself, further
functionalization exists. These functions may include such things as accoun
payable, accounts receivable, and payroll. Within the accounts receivable
function, various tasks can be identified such as mailing invoices and
maintaining a current status of unpaid invoices.

An even further breakdown of these tasks can be accomplished by breaking
down each task into elements. These elements are the smallest activities th
can be performed without considering simple psychomotor motions. For exampl

an element of the task of mailing invoices might be the stuffing of envelopes with the invoices. Finally, the elements themselves can be analyzed in terms of the micromotions that are necessary to perform the particular element involved. Such analysis of micromotions is typical of the work done by Gilbreth and Maynard in the study of industrial engineering.

Figure 7.1.4

Job analysis.

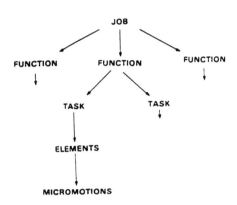

The purpose of the function and task analysis is to divide the job(s) into small, manageable segments that can be analyzed. How far the job must be divided is dependent upon the desired outcome. If a job is being analyzed to increase efficiency or to remove potential hazards, it may be necessary to go to the level of micromotions. On the other hand, if the objective is to outline the specific duties that must be performed, the task level may be sufficient.

In any case the tasks, elements, or micromotions can be analyzed. This analysis involves determining such things as:

1.   The man/machine interfaces.
2.   The initiating conditions.
3.   The required actions by the worker.
4.   The decision rules and required feedback.
5.   The potential errors.
6.   The time required to perform the task or element of interest.
7.   The potential harmful exposures.
8.   The work station requirements.
9.   The required skills and knowledge of the worker.

This approach can be used for the identification of many types of hazards that might exist within a given job. It can also be used to redesign existing jobs or to create designs for new jobs. Thus, it is both an identification and control technique that can be used by the industrial hygiene engineer.

Procedure for Conducting a Functional and Task Analysis. The first step
that must be performed is to subdivide the job into the major functions that
are necessary to accomplish the desired output. Remember the five general
functions or stages as the beginning point (i.e., the preparation stage, the
observation stage, the control stage, the physical requirement stage, and the
termination stage).

The second step is to divide the functions into the various tasks that
must be performed. Again, the five stages may be helpful in breaking each o
the major functions down into tasks.

For each task itself, it may be necessary to break it down further into
the elements and/or micromotions that are necessary, depending upon the
desired analysis. The five stages--preparation, observation, control,
physical requirements, and termination--may help to identify the groupings o
elements within the task itself, since it is likely that most of these stage
will be present in a given task. Once the desired lowest level has been
attained, the analysis can begin. This analysis involves asking a number of
questions about each of the individual tasks, elements, or micromotions that
are being analyzed. These questions include:

1. What are the initiating conditions? What is the cause or stimulus
    that results in the task being performed in the first place?

2. What actions must be carried out? What steps must be performed by
    the individual and/or machine to accomplish the desired result?

3. What feedback is required to assure that the results of the action
    are as desired?

4. What potential errors are possible? What is the cost of these erro
    occurring in terms of damage to equipment, materials, and/or the
    operator's physical well being?

5. What hazards are present that can cause illness or injury to the
    worker?

6. What is the required reaction time necessary to initiate the task?

7. What is the time frame in which the task must be completed?

8. What tools and equipment are required to complete the task or eleme

9. Where is the task or element being performed? What is the physical
    location and structure of the workplace in which the task or elemen
    is performed?

10. What physical demands are placed upon the worker to perform the tas
    or element?

11. What skills and knowledge are required of the worker to perform the
    task or element?

The objective of the analysis of the task or element is to define the task or element in such a way that an analysis can be made to determine the changes that can be introduced to that task or element to meet the desired result. This is done with the objective of also lowering the potential stress on the individual performing the task. If an existing job is being analyzed and the above questions have determined the current requirements of the job, it is desirable to answer some key questions that might help to obtain our objective.

First, we might want to consider if the physical demands of the task or element can be lowered. Is it necessary that the worker perform the job as it is currently outlined? Can equipment replace some of the physical demands on the worker? Can the worker be seated rather than standing to perform the task? Does the worker have to perform this task or element in close proximity to the mechanical process?

Second, can equipment be substituted to replace the operator totally? Can the entire process be automated to remove the worker from the workplace? Such action will eliminate the need for further consideration of potential strain on the worker.

Another question that might be asked is, "Does the equipment being used require redesign?" Are there potential hazards that are characteristic of the equipment? If so, can these potential hazards be designed out of the system by modifying or substituting for the equipment.

Can the workplace itself be changed? Can modifications be made to the work space, controls, displays, tools and equipment being used to allow for more efficient operation?

Finally, can the task or element procedures be changed to lower the potential for critical errors occurring? The removal of these critical errors will allow for a more efficient and less costly operation, while at the same time providing a safer environment for the worker.

Using functional and task analysis, certain benefits can be obtained. By analyzing the tasks and elements, the job, workplace, and tools can be designed to fit the worker's characteristics. The result is that there will be less possibility of injury or accident as well as lowering the fatigue occurring in the worker. Additional benefits are obtained by using this approach. These include improved production, lower costs, improved morale, and improved manpower utilization.

Summary

Ergonomics is the study of the worker's function within the workplace. The objective of ergonomics is to fit the worker and the job together in such a manner as to create a total system that is efficient and safe in producing the desired output. In order to begin an ergonomic study of a particular job, it is desirable that a functional and task analysis be conducted. This functional and task analysis provides a basis by which the job can be broken down into small segments that can then be analyzed for the critical components. After analyzing these components, the job can be designed in such a manner as to produce an efficient and safe worker/machine interface.

2. The Worker As the Physical Component

Introduction

In the preceding chapter, the discussion was centered on the fact that ergonomics is involved with the design of the job and the workplace in such a manner as to fit the worker into the system. There are essentially two ways in which the worker can be matched with the work environment. One way to accomplish this is to select only those workers who fit the work environment as it exists. However, this is generally not a satisfactory method for solving the problem. A much more satisfactory solution can be obtained by modifying the work environment to meet the characteristics of the great number of individuals who will be required to perform the job duties in this environment.

As was discussed in the last chapter, humans are required to perform physical and mental tasks while on the job. In addition, humans occupy physical space and must assume certain positions within the system. It is the objective of ergonomics to design jobs in terms of the physical and mental tasks required, the equipment that is used to perform these tasks, and the work space requirements in such a manner that the total job will meet the requirements of the human beings who must perform it.

The functioning of the muscles of the human body must be considered. The physical requirements must be within the limits of human capability in order for persons to be able to perform the work. The job must be designed to eliminate unnecessary stress on the physical functioning of the worker. In addition, the workplace must be designed to accommodate humans. It must be sized to allow for the performance of the tasks that are required on the job. It must be designed to eliminate unnecessary physical stress on the worker while performing these tasks.

Thus, it is the objective of ergonomics to design the work, the equipment and the workplace in such a manner that the job can be performed without unnecessary physical and mental stress being placed on the worker.

The Average Man

To design the job, the differences between individual workers must be considered. For example, the differences in workers' strength must be considered when designing a job. Differences in the size of workers require that the workplace be designed to accommodate different-sized individuals. The physical condition of the workers must also be considered when designing job.

Data has been gathered concerning the physical characteristics of human beings. These data can be used to determine the mean values and thus yield, as a result, the average man.

Figure 7.2.1

The average man.

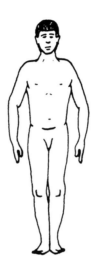

However, no single individual is average. Different ethnic groups and different generations tend to have different structural characteristics and measurements. Male and female workers have different structural measurements. Designing for the average results in problems for most individuals, since the average indicates that 50 percent of the population will be above its value, and 50 percent of the population will be below. Thus, only a few individuals will actually fit the average measurement for a given characteristic. In addition, no individual is average in all dimensions. An individual who is average in height and weight may possess arms that are above average length or legs that are below average length. Since it would be folly to design for only a few individuals, which would result in difficulty in obtaining the necessary personnel to perform the job, the design must accommodate most individuals for the important features required on the job.

This type of design requires that one look not at the average but at a range for the measurements of interest. Generally, a percentile distribution of the population is used, varying from 1 percent to 99 percent or from 5 percent to 95 percent, depending upon the particular job and the desire to utilize a maximum size labor pool. Where possible, adjustable equipment can be provided to allow for individual differences. An example is the adjustable office chair that allows for adjustments in height, tension, and angle of back support.

In designing the job, one must consider differences in strength and physical condition. These differences exist as a result of the sex of the

Figure 7.2.2

Design measurement range.

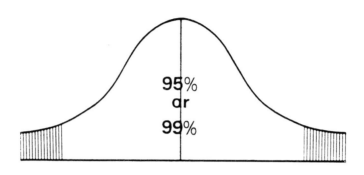

individuals as well as their age. Therefore, one objective of ergonomics is
to design the workplace in such a manner that the maximum number of
individuals can perform the job efficiently and safely. Jobs should not be
designed like positions on professional basketball and football teams where.
only those of large stature can perform adequately, thus limiting the
potential pool of employable individuals.

Using Anthropometrical Data

    The study of anthropometry involves the measurement of the physical
dimensions of the human body. Anthropometrical studies have been conducted on
various population groups. Measurements of various structural characteristics
have been taken, and the data gathered have been tabulated. These data have
been broken into percentile ranges for various physical characteristics.
Because of the differences that exist between generations, these data can
become outmoded after a period of time. As a result, it is necessary to be
sure that the population included in the studies is typical of the population
that will be required to perform in the workplace.

    To be useful, anthropometrical data must be collected in a standard
manner. Measuring techniques must be specified and consistent. The location
of the measurement must be clear; that is, from where to where is the
measurement being made. The conditions of the measurement must also be
indicated. Is clothing involved? What about body posture? The time of the
day may be important since it has been shown that, in terms of stature. the
individual height may vary up to one and one-half inches over a full day. The
chosen group must be representative of the population of interest. There is
no sense in taking measurements from existing studies concerning military age
groups when, in fact, the average age of the operator of the equipment is 50
years. Sex, age, race, etc., have been shown to exhibit differences in terms
of various body size measurements. Finally, the sample must be large enough
to yield statistical reliability.

    Structural Anthropometry. There are two types of anthropometrical
dimensions that are useful. The first of these types is structural

anthropometry, which is related to the body of the subjects in fixed standardized positions. On the other hand, functional anthropometry is involved with body dimensions taken during the performance of various physical movements that may be related to the particular types of work that the worker must perform.

Among the common structural anthropometrical measurements that are available are the following:

1. Stature--height
2. Weight
3. Sitting height
4. Body depth
5. Body breadth
6. Eye height
7. Shoulder breadth
8. Hip breadth
9. Elbow-to-elbow breadth
10. Elbow height sitting
11. Forearm-to-hand length
12. Arm reach
13. Popliteal height-sitting and standing

There are many other types of measurements and data that have been presented. The above is only a short list of types that are available. Some examples of the measurements are presented in the following Figures 7.2.3 - 7.2.5.

Functional Anthropometry

In the area of functional anthropometry, it is much more difficult to take the measurements that are required; thus, fewer studies are available and data are harder to obtain. Typical of functional anthropometrical data are:

1. Crawling height
2. Crawling length
3. Kneeling height
4. Prone length

5. Prone height
6. Bent torso height
7. Bent torso breadth
8. Overhead reach

Again, there are many measurements that can be taken. The above is only a sample that can be obtained when consulting anthropometric data. Figure 7.2.6 shows two measurements of the functional type.

Another type of anthropometrical data that is of the functional type and is useful is the measurement of the range of movement of various parts of the body. For example, the reach distance, which is important for work layout, depends upon the angle of reach horizontally away from the median plane of the body as well as the vertical angle of reach. It also depends upon the extent of the arms. The normal reach is generally related to that reach that can be obtained without moving the elbows away from the body. Maximum reach is that which can be obtained with the arms fully extended. Figure 7.2.7 illustrates these measurements.

Figure 7.2.3

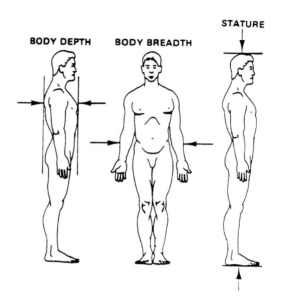

Figure 7.2.4

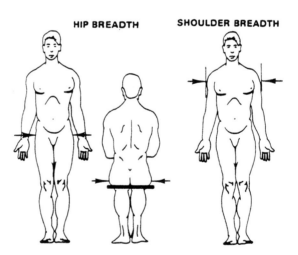

It is not the purpose of this discussion to present a complete tabulation and description of available anthropometrical data. There are many sources for such data. The most common source can be found in studies conducted by the military services. In addition, the National Health Survey of United States Adults, conducted by Stoudt, et. al., in 1965, presents twelve common

7.2.6

anthropometrical dimensions for a random sample selected on a nationwide
basis. Also, the revised edition of <u>Human Engineering Guide to Equipment</u>
<u>Design</u>, sponsored by the joint Army-Navy-Air Force Steering Committee, has a
large section on anthropometrical data as well as a discussion of principles
related to the gathering of such data.

Figure 7.2.5

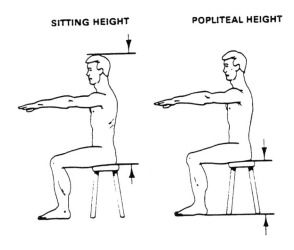

Figure 7.2.6

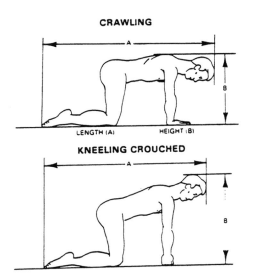

Figure 7.2.7

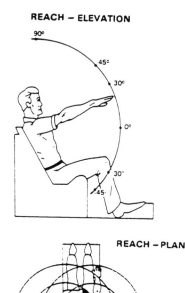

How can the industrial hygiene engineer use anthropometrical data in the design of the workplace? First, it is necessary to determine the body dimensions of interest. This determination is made after a functional and task analysis of the job has been accomplished to define what steps the job entails. Once this determination has been made, the next step is to determine who will use the equipment. Consider the age, sex, race, and any other important characteristics that may affect the measurements obtained.

The next step is to determine the basis of design. Will the workplace be designed to accommodate the extremes, or will it be designed to accommodate a percentile range? Though highly unlikely, it may be desirable to design the workplace to meet the average individual. In such a case, it will then be necessary to make much of the equipment adjustable to fit the percentile range who will likely be working within the workplace.

Existing anthropometric tables can be consulted to obtain the necessary data for the various measurements of interest. The designer should consider the clothing that will be required on the job and allow for this when using anthropometric data.

A sample of actual workers should be selected and measured to assure the validity of the tables. It may be that in the particular area in which the workplace is being designed the individuals who work on this job are different from those who are included in the study.

If appropriate data are not available, select and measure a representative sample from the population that will use the equipment. This sample should consider such variables as age, sex, race, and ethnic background. The size of the sample must be relatively large for some variables with a wide range of potential values such as height and weight.

Finally check out the prototype design on operators for finalizing. Make any necessary correction.

Biomechanics

Biomechanics is the study of the mechanical operation of the body. The functioning of the body members while performing various activities is of concern in the study of biometrics. The effects of internal and external stress on the body as a result of performing the various body motions are determined, and these data are used to modify the methods used on the job in order to reduce stress.

The musculoskeletal system of the human body is made up of a series of levers. The joints of the human body are the connection points of the levers. The bones themselves make up the levers while the muscles act as the moving force. There are three basic types of levers present in the human body that are of interest. These are discussed below.

The first-class lever, which is illustrated in Figure 7.2.8, is made up of a force and load located on opposite sides of a fulcrum. The force and load act in the same direction while the fulcrum acts in an opposing direction. As

Figure 7.2.8

First-class lever.

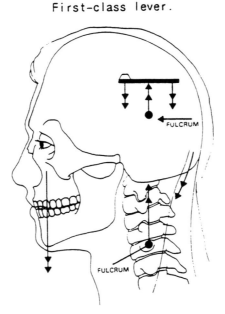

the figure illustrates, this type of lever can be found in the forward-backward motion of the head with the spine acting as the fulcrum and the neck muscles acting as the force downward counteracted by the force of gravity on the center of mass of the head.

The second-class lever, illustrated in Figure 7.2.9, has the fulcrum located at one end with the force acting upon the other end but in the same direction as the fulcrum. The figure illustrates an example of such a lever where the ball of the foot acts as the fulcrum and the weight of the body transmitted through the bone is counteracted by the upward force of the calf muscle.

Figure 7.2.9

Second-class lever.

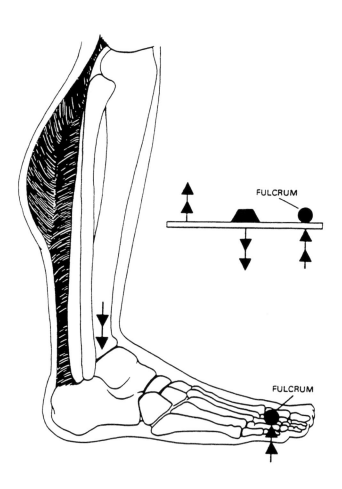

The third-class lever, illustrated in Figure 7.2.10, involves a fulcrum at one end of the lever and a force acting in the same direction at the other end of the lever. The upward force to balance the lever can be placed at any point between the fulcrum and weight force. As illustrated in the figure, such a lever can be found in the operation of the forearm where the elbow joint forms the fulcrum, and the weight is held in the hand with the counterbalancing force being a subgroup of muscles in the upper arm.

Figure 7.2.10

Third-class lever.

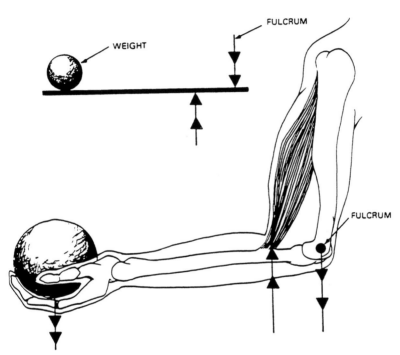

The importance of studying the body as a system of levers is the ability to describe the various motions and to match those motions to the tasks to assure that the motions and any postural adjustments to the body will occur efficiently. When such matching is not the case, the worker is subjected to excessive fatigue and the risk of accident or injury resulting from unnatural movements.

Classification of Body Movements. The classification of body movements has been previously discussed in Section 1, Chapter 3. However, it is worthwhile to review these classifications at this point. The classifications are as follows:

1.   Flexion-Extension. Flexion is the movement of a joint in which the angle between the bone is decreased, such as bending the arm at the

elbow. Extension is the opposite of flexion where the movement
increases the angle between the bone, such as straightening the arm.

Figure 7.2.11

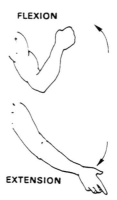

FLEXION

EXTENSION

2.   Abduction-Adduction. Abduction is the movement of a part away from
the center plane of the body or part of the body, such as lifting the
arm outward from the body. Adduction is the opposite of abduction; a
movement towards the center plane of the body or of a part of the
body.

Figure 7.2.12

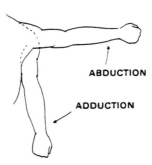

ABDUCTION

ADDUCTION

3.   Supination-Pronation. Supination is the turning of the hand so that
the palm faces upward; while pronation is the turning of the hand so
that the palm faces downward.

Figure 7.2.13

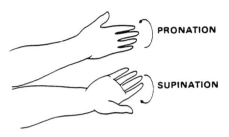

4.   Rotation. Rotation is a movement in which a part turns on its longitudinal axis, such as turning the head or turning the arm or leg outward.

Figure 7.2.14

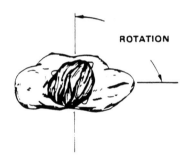

5.   Circumduction. Circumduction involves rotary movements which circumscribe an arc, such as swinging the arm in a circle.

6.   Inversion-Eversion. Inversion is the movement of the ankle joint in which the sole of the foot is turned inward. Eversion is the movement of the ankle in which the sole of the foot is turned outward.

7.   Elevation-Depression. Elevation is the movement in which the part is raised while depression is the movement in which the part is lowered. For example, the movement of the jaw upward and downward illustrates elevation-depression.

8.   Protraction-Retraction. Protraction is the movement of the part forward while retraction is the backward movement of the part; for example, jutting the jaw forward and pulling it backward.

Figure 7.2.15

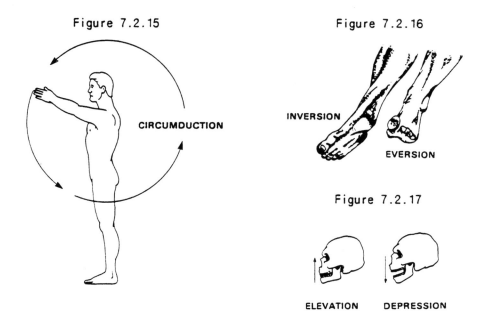

CIRCUMDUCTION

Figure 7.2.16

INVERSION

EVERSION

Figure 7.2.17

ELEVATION   DEPRESSION

Figure 7.2.18

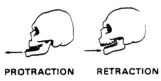

PROTRACTION   RETRACTION

9.   Hyperextension-Dorsiflexion. Hyperextension includes movements of
      the wrist and other joints in which the part is extended beyond a
      straight line and in the direction away from the normal movement of
      the joint. An example is to tilt the head backward to look up at the
      sky. Dorsiflexion is movement of the part to decrease the normal
      angle in the normal direction of movement.

Figure 7.2.19

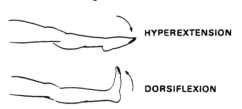

HYPEREXTENSION

DORSIFLEXION

For each of the various classifications of movements listed above, the range of movement will vary for different individuals. Data exist from functional anthropometrical studies that provide values for these ranges. However, these data are not nearly so extensive as data available for static anthropometrical studies because of the difficulty in collecting such data.

Another way in which movements can be viewed and classified is in terms of the operational definition. These operational definitions are discussed below.

1. Positioning. Positioning involves moving an extremity from one position to another. For example, the movement that is performed when an individual reaches for an object.

2. Continuous Movement. A continuous movement is any single movement involving muscle control to adjust or guide. An example of this is the movements that are necessary to steer an automobile on the desired course. Continuous adjustments in movements of the muscles are necessary to maintain the desired direction.

3. Manipulative Movements. Manipulative movements involve handling or assembling of parts, usually limited to hand or finger movement. Examples would include operating a typewriter, playing a piano, or assembling parts to build a machine.

4. Repetitive Movements. Repetitive movements are the same movements that are repeated over and over again. An example would be using a hammer or screwdriver where the pounding or twisting is a continuous repetition of the same movement.

5. Sequential Movements. Sequential movements are a series of separate movements that are joined together in a desired sequence to perform a given job. An example of sequential movements might be the reaching for an object with the left hand, reaching for a tool with the right hand, and bringing the two hands together to perform the desired adjustments using the tool.

6. Static Movements. These are not really movements but the maintenance of position of a body member to hold something in place. Though movement is not involved, the muscles are required to maintain the steady position of the object. An example would be holding a subassembly with one hand while attaching a part with the other hand.

Factors Affecting the Performance of Physical Tasks

A number of factors, some of which have been alluded to in the previous discussion, affect the performance of physical tasks by the worker. Among these are the range of movement of the body member, the strength of the muscles involved, the endurance of the individual performing the task, the speed of the performance that is required, and the accuracy of performance that is required. Not all tasks require equal emphasis on all factors. Some tasks, such as operating a typewriter, require very little strength or range of movement but do require speed and accuracy. On the other hand, lifting an object to feed a machine may require a particular range of movement as well as strength and endurance on the part of the worker. Speed and accuracy in such an operation may not be as important.

Range of Movement. As was previously discussed, individuals differ in size and build. As a result, the range of movement for these individuals will differ. For example, the height of reach of a large individual is likely to be greater than the height of reach of a smaller individual. The same would be expected in terms of length of reach.

However, even for individuals of the same approximate size, the range of movement will vary. Not all individuals have the same flexibility of the joints. Differences in range of movement for normal individuals vary widely. In general, as a person ages, the range lowers. This is a result of arthritic conditions that seem to be inherent with the aging of the human body.

In general, women exceed men in the range of joint movements at all joints except the knee. It should be pointed out that through physical training range of movement can be increased somewhat. An example familiar to all is the ability to bend at the waist and touch one's toes. When this is first attempted, many people have difficulty in coming within five or six inches of the toes. Through practice, the body becomes more supple and the gap between the fingers and toes decreases until, for most individuals, the toes can be reached. However, some individuals, no matter how hard they try, will never be able to touch their toes. There is a limit to how much physical training can accomplish in improving range of movement for a given individual.

Strength. The strength of an individual or the force that can be exerted is in many cases a result of the size and muscle structure of the individual. However, for a given sized individual, strength may still vary. For example, women in their mid-twenties and thirties will, in general, exert approximately two-thirds of the force of men in the same age category.

As a general rule, strength increases with age until it reaches a maximum in the mid-twenties. Strength remains approximately constant for a period of five to ten years after reaching its maximum. After this point as age increases, strength decreases. For men there is a slow decrease to approximately 80 percent of maximum strength in the fifty- to sixty-year age group. On the other hand, women decrease faster and exert about one-half the force of men in the fifty- to sixty-year age group. Age affects the strength of the legs and trunk much more than that of the hands and arms. Very little loss of strength in the hands and arms is experienced as a result of age, while the loss of leg and trunk strength is significant. Evidence of this is seen in the athlete who quit the sport because the legs gave way.

Of some concern is the difference in strength between the right and left arm, depending on the handedness of the person. Approximately 90 percent of the population is right handed. However, the difference in strength resulting from handedness is not nearly so critical as one might think since there is approximately only a 10 percent difference in strength between the right hand and the left hand.

A final factor that can affect strength is the conditioning of the individual. Through physical training or performance of tasks requiring the exertion of physical force, the muscle strength can be increased. The weight lifter who trains daily with barbells uses this principle to increase his total strength and ability to lift massive weights.

Endurance. As a muscle is maintained in a state of contraction or through repeated stimulation is caused to contract and expand, it loses its ability to contract and relaxation occurs. The muscle loses its irritability to the stimulus causing the contraction. Thus, the contractions are reduced or are absent during stimulation. This is the result of fatigue of the muscle.

Fatigue can be caused by a number of factors. Excessive activity that uses up energy-producing substances (glucose) stored in the muscle faster than this substance can be replenished will cause fatigue to occur. In such a situation, rest is the only answer to regenerate the muscles.

Malnutrition that is a result of a lack of food materials available as an energy source can also cause fatigue. In hot atmospheres, a lack of salt is a common factor resulting in muscle fatigue.

Circulatory problems that prevent distribution of an adequate supply of energy materials to the muscle (glucose and oxygen) and the removal of waste products generated during muscle functioning can also cause fatigue. Without adequate circulation, the worker will tire easily.

Another factor that can affect fatigue is the presence of a respiratory problem. Such a problem may be chronic or may just be the result of a cold or viral infection. Respiratory problems prevent the muscles from obtaining an adequate supply of oxygen and eliminating carbon dioxide as a waste product.

General infections of the body can also cause fatigue. This may be as a result of toxins built up by the organisms, or it may be a protective mechanism which the body uses to force the required rest needed for recuperation.

An endocrine imbalance can affect the metabolism rate. If the metabolism rate is slowed down, the result will be fatigue. Since many individuals differ in their metabolic rate, it is easy to see why some individuals tire more quickly than others, given an equivalent physical condition.

Psychogenic conditions resulting from emotional conflict, frustration, worry, and boredom can also be a cause of fatigue. Consider how tired you felt the last time you were performing a job which totally bored you. On the other hand, consider the exhilarating feeling that you were able to maintain during an exciting experience. You felt you had more energy than you knew what to do with.

The posture an individual assumes while performing a particular task can also contribute to fatigue. If the posture is such that the muscles have to work harder to overcome gravity, then this will result in a fatigue of these muscles.

The muscles can operate at 100 percent of their force for only a very short period of time, perhaps for only a few seconds. Generally, only about 20 percent of the maximum force can be exerted over a number of hours without excessive fatigue. These factors should be considered when designing a job that requires the worker to be physically active.

The amount of fatigue that is experienced by the worker can be reduced by lowering the application of force required of the worker. Allowing rest periods between heavy exertions will also allow the worker to recuperate and become less fatigued. Physical training can increase the worker's ability to perform tasks requiring physical exertion.

Speed. Another factor affecting the performance of physical tasks is the speed at which the tasks must be performed. How fast must the muscles react? This reaction involves both the reaction time of the worker and the actual movement time.

Reaction time involves observing a situation, deciding whether action is necessary, and transmitting that action to the muscles. The movement time involves the actual movement of the body part to accomplish the desired action. Reaction will vary with the number of stimuli received. In addition the expectancy of the individual for the stimuli can affect reaction time. Movement time varies with the mechanism of movement and the distance that the body part must move to engage the mechanism.

Accuracy. The final factor affecting the performance of physical tasks is the accuracy at which the task must be performed. How accurate must the performance be? This depends on a number of things. The type of movement involved can affect the accuracy. Where fingers and hands are used, accurate movements can be performed. On the other hand, where large forces must be exerted by the legs or other parts of the body, the accuracy will be less. Accuracy is also affected by the size of the objects that are to be manipulated. Small objects will require more accurate motions than large objects.

The work tolerances that are required in the performance of the task also affect the accuracy of motion needed. How much error is allowable before the resultant output is not useful? If the margin of error is small, the job requirements will differ significantly from the requirements where the margin for error is great.

The relative positioning of the task in relation to the body position also affects accuracy. It is much easier to be accurate in performing movements close to the body on, say, a worktable or a workbench than it is to reach over one's head and perform the same movements accurately.

The required speed of performance as well as the strength needed will also affect the accuracy of performance. It is difficult to perform a hard, physical task accurately. Also, it is very difficult to perform a task that must be done in a very short period of time with the same accuracy that a longer period of time might yield.

The effects of fatigue will also affect the accuracy of the performance of the task. As an individual becomes tired, it is much more difficult for that individual to perform small manipulative movements that may be required to yield the desired accuracy.

Summary

In this chapter, the worker as the physical component in the worker/machine system and the work environment has been discussed. Though changes have occurred that have lessened the need for the worker to perform physical tasks, the requirement for such performance is still present. When such tasks are being performed, it is necessary that the limitations and constraints resulting from the physical structure and physiology of the worker be considered. A knowledge of this structure and physiology is important to the engineer so that the design of the job is such that the assigned individual is capable of performing the desired operations.

3. The Worker As the Controlling Component

Introduction

In the previous chapter, the characteristics of the worker as part of the worker/machine system were discussed at some length. In this chapter, the role of the worker as the controlling component in the worker/machine system is discussed.

Within the worker/machine system, the worker can act as a controller. The worker senses where a modification in the operation is necessary. The worker determines the extent of the modification that is necessary and makes the adjustments that are required to modify the action. In this manner, the worker acts to control the operation of the mechanical or electrical system being utilized. The worker observes what is happening in the work environment, either by direct observation of the process or by observation of the displays that indicate the status of the process. The worker uses visual sense to identify the need for system adjustment. Also, the worker listens to hear what is going on while the process is under way. Various changes in system operation result in auditory stimuli indicating progress is as expected or that the system is not progressing satisfactorily. A common example of this is the driver of a car who hears a strange noise while driving down the road. This indicates to the driver that something mechanical is wrong with the automobile and that service may be necessary. In this manner, the driver uses his auditory sense to identify the need for system adjustment.

Finally, the worker can use other senses in particular situations to identify the need for system adjustment. These senses are termed the "somesthetic senses" and include the senses of touch, taste, smell, and temperature. Though these senses are seldom used as primary sensors in the work environment, they often come into play. For example, often the first indication of a problem is the fact that the sense of smell indicates an odor that is not normal in the environment.

After having used the senses to determine the fact that something is awry in the system, the worker must determine what adjustment, if any, should be made in the system. To accomplish this, the worker must use mental capacity. The worker decides on the action that is necessary based upon previous training and experience relating the observed sense stimulus to its potential cause.

Finally, to implement the adjustment, the worker communicates the change to the system. This communication may be accomplished by using language or signals to communicate to another worker who in turn makes the actual changes

in the system, or the communication may be made directly to the system by
adjusting the equipment controls.

The feedback loop is closed by providing information back to the worker's
senses regarding the results of the changes or adjustments made in the
system. From this information, the worker decides on the necessity for
further adjustment to the system.

The Worker as a Sensor--Visual

Humans employ two different types of vision to determine or sense changes
in the environment. The eye contains two types of sensing mechanisms. These
mechanisms are termed "cones" and "rods." The cones are sensitive to the wave
length of light; thus, cones are sensitive to color differences. On the other
hand, the rods are sensitive to the amount of light or brightness.

Colorblindness is a lack of the ability of the cones to function
properly. Colorblindness is seldom total. Most often, colorblindness is
related to the inability of the human to distinguish various hues of red,
green, and blue.

The ability to distinguish between colors is also affected by the
intensity of light in the environment. You may have noticed on a dark, dreary
morning how difficult it is to select the right color of socks from your
drawer. This problem is often identified only when you get into the light and
notice that one sock is brown and the other is black. The reason for this is
that in dark areas vision depends upon the rods that are not color sensitive,
and thus color discrimination is limited.

Visual Discrimination. There are two types of discrimination that can be
employed by the human. The first is relative discrimination where two objects
are viewed and their difference compared. The second is absolute
discrimination where comparative information is not available and only one
object is being viewed. Relative discrimination allows for a much greater
number of differences to be identified by the individual than absolute
discrimination does.

Some research has been conducted to identify the number of discriminations
that can be made in a relative mode and an absolute mode (Mobray and Gebhard,
1958). The results of this research indicated that for relative
discrimination, the following is found:

Relative Discrimination

1. Brightness--570 discriminable intensities were identified

2. Hues--128 discriminable hues at medium intensities were identified.

3. White light--375 discriminable interruption rates between 1 and 45
    seconds were identified.

Absolute Discrimination

1.   Brightness--3 to 5 discriminable intensities were identified.

2.   Hues--12 to 15 discriminable hues were identified.

3.   White light--5 to 6 discriminable rates were identified.

A similar situation was found for discrimination in the auditory senses. In a relative mode, 325 levels of loudness were discriminable. When an absolute discrimination was used, only 3 to 5 levels of loudness were discriminable by the subjects. In terms of pure tones, 1800 discriminable tones were identified in a relative mode while only 4 to 5 discriminable tones were identified in an absolute sense.

There are a number of factors that affect human visual sensitivity and ability to discriminate between various stimuli. Among the major factors are:

1.   Illumination--The amount of illumination that is present and measured in footcandles is a major factor in determining the ability to discriminate. The amount of illumination necessary depends upon the detail of the work required. Where fine motor skills are required. to assemble or produce the desired product, such as in mechanical drafting or inspection of finished product, the amount of illumination present must be high. On the other hand, if the worker is digging a ditch, illumination need not be nearly as intense.

2.   Glare--The amount of glare in the work area can affect the ability of the worker to discriminate. The eyes are adjusted to one level of light, while the glare is at a different level of light. This glare adversely affects the visual acuity of the worker and makes discrimination difficult if not impossible.

3.   Contrast--The ratio of difference between the reflectance of an object's background to the reflectance of the object is termed "contrast." Often the term used is "luminance contrast." This contrast can be calculated by the formula below.

$$\text{Contrast} = \frac{R_1 - R_2}{R_1 \ (100)}$$

where
   R_1 = the higher reflectance object
   R_2 = the lower reflectance object

4.   Changing light--As the light changes from bright to dark, the eye must adjust to allow for more light to enter. Time is required for the adjustment to occur. During this adjustment period, the ability to discriminate visually is greatly reduced.

5. Distance--The size of an object relative to the distance from which
    it is viewed is important in the ability of an individual to
    discriminate. Obviously the size must increase as the distance
    increases. However, this obvious fact is often overlooked in the
    preparation of materials for viewing by large audiences at a distance.

6. Angle of view--The angle of view can distort the visual stimulus
    being viewed. This is particularly the case when viewing through
    glass where a parallax distortion occurs when viewing at an angle. A
    90° angle is best for viewing accuracy.

7. Time to view--As the time increases, the discrimination increases to
    a point of diminishing returns. Time is also dependent upon other
    variables, such as the illumination, the distance of viewing, and the
    angle of view.

8. Movement--If the object being viewed is moving, the acuity of vision
    is not as great. The faster the movement of the object, the lower
    the visual acuity and the ability to discriminate.

9. Distractions--Distractions in the viewing area can cause a problem
    sometimes termed the "signal-to-noise ratio." The object being
    viewed is the signal, and any distractions are noise. If the
    signal-to-noise ratio is low, then the distraction stimuli will tend
    to mask the target stimuli that is being viewed. The viewer may then
    find it impossible to keep his attention directed to the signal
    object. This often happens when the viewer must split his attention
    between a number of displays. Errors are more likely, and
    identification of key situations is slower.

The Worker as a Sensor--Auditory

The reader will recall from previous discussions related to noise that the
sound intensity or sound-pressure level is measured in terms of the decibel.
The decibel is a logarithmic ratio of sound intensity or sound-pressure level
with a fixed standard base. Sound frequency, measured in hertz
(cycles/second) is related to the tones that are heard. The human ear is
sensitive in the range of 20 to 20,000 hertz.

Since human reaction to sound is a function of both pressure level and
frequency, some research has been done to determine equal loudness curves for
varying frequency and intensity as determined by human respondents. The phone
is basically a subjective equality of different sounds with varying frequency
and intensity. On the other hand, the sone is a measure of the relative
subjective loudness of sounds. If a sound is twice as loud, then the sones
are doubled.

Often in a work environment one sound will reduce the sensitivity of the
ears to another sound. This effect is termed "masking." Masking can cause
the threshold of audibility of the sound to be raised. The masking effect
depends on the frequency and intensity of the two sounds; that is, the masking
effect depends on the frequency of the signal versus the frequency of the
noise and the intensity of the signal versus the intensity of the noise.

Again, the signal-to-noise ratio is applicable. The noise acts in the environment to mask the signal. In the case where noise is a problem the signal can be increased in strength, or the noise level can be lowered. A general rule is that the signal should be increased in strength to a point one-half the way between the noise level and 100 decibels. At this point, the sound should be audible to most individuals. On the other hand, the noise can be decreased through the use of earmuffs that select out certain tones which act to mask the signal to be heard. Where electronic audio systems are present, electrical filters can be used to mask out noise or static that occurs, thus producing a clearer signal. Of course, there are also the many techniques that are available for noise reduction in the environment. These have been discussed previously in the section on the control of noise.

Auditory displays of a number of different types exist. First, there is voice communication where one individual communicates to another certain commands to be carried out. A second type of auditory display relates to the need for the operator to make adjustments to the system. A changing tone frequency can be used to indicate when adjustments are necessary and the results of these adjustments. The sound level itself can be varied to indicate the effect of adjustments to the system. Finally, an intermittent sound can be used as an auditory display. This type of auditory display is most commonly found where a warning signal is given to indicate that adjustments to the system are needed quickly.

The Worker as a Sensor--Tactual

The most common somesthetic sense that the worker is most likely to use in the work environment is the tactual or touch sense. In some cases it is necessary that the worker use his touch sense to determine system status and to exercise control. This may happen when it is necessary for an individual worker to reach and grasp a given object to be used while at the same time keeping his eyes fixed on another object.

Using the tactual sense, the worker can discriminate in a number of different ways. Using the tactual sense, man can discriminate between the sizes and shapes of objects. The texture of an object can also be determined by touch. In addition, the relative distance or location can often be determined by touch and positioning of the hands with the necessity of viewing the object.

Some of the other somesthetic senses that often come into play in the work environment are the sense of temperature, pain, vibration, and pressure. Although these senses are seldom used as a primary method for obtaining information concerning the state of the system, they can come into play when something goes wrong by providing the worker with an additional warning mechanism.

Displays

The purpose of a display in the workplace is to help the worker to sense changes in the state of the system where such changes might not be of a magnitude that normally would be sensed. There are basically three kinds of displays that are commonly used to assist the worker in sensing changes in the system. These types of displays are visual displays, auditory displays, and tactual displays.

Four basic types of visual displays are common. The type of visual display is based on the information obtained from the display. The types are:

1. Quantitative displays
2. Qualitative displays
3. Representational displays
4. Status displays

A quantitative display tells the operator or worker how much. It may measure a static variable, as a yardstick does; or it may measure a dynamic variable, as a gauge does. A common example of a quantitative display that measures a dynamic variable is the speedometer on an automobile. This instrument gives a readout to the operator concerning the actual velocity of the automobile as well as indicating the rate of change or acceleration of the automobile by the direction of movement of the pointer.

Figure 7.3.1

Quantitative display.

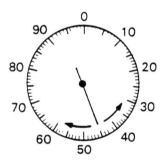

There are various types of display designs that are used for quantitative displays. The display may be presented as a circular scale or as a semi-circular scale. In some cases, vertical and horizontal scales might be used for the display. Finally, a digital display can be used. Research favors the use of a circular or semi-circular scale for display purposes. However, there are circumstances in which vertical and horizontal scales may have advantages and should be used. Digital scales have the advantage of both accuracy and time to read. However, the rate of change for a digital scale is not so easily determined as for scales of the other type.

Another concern is the type of display operation to be utilized. There are basically two types that can be used--the fixed-scale-moving-pointer display and the fixed-pointer-moving-scale display. In general, research has

Figure 7.3.2

Scales.

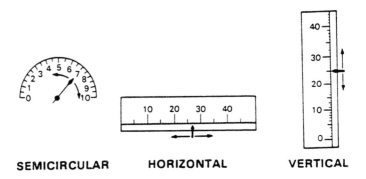

SEMICIRCULAR   HORIZONTAL   VERTICAL

shown that the fixed-scale-moving-pointer display is preferable in most cases. However, again there may be instances where the moving-scale-fixed-pointer provides the operator with information in a better form.

In terms of the general design of a quantitative scale, it is important that the scale displays the smallest and largest values possible. The interval between readings depends on the accuracy that is necessary. If, for example, a display is to be read to the nearest 10 feet, then 10 feet would the smallest unit of measurement. The scale would be constructed in such a manner that a given length of the scale would be equal to 10 feet. Research has indicated that the difference between scale units should be between .05 and .07 inches to assure acceptable accuracy in reading the scale. One mustconsider the conditions of use to determine the actual size of the numbe and the scale intervals to be used. Obviously if the visual acuity is lessened because of poor illumination or distance, the size of the numbers a the scale interval must be greater.

Scale markers can be used to indicate the units to be read. In general, the easiest progressions used are in terms of 1's, 10's, 100's, etc. With these types of scales, intermediate markers are generally shown at the 5, 15 25 levels. (See Figure 7.3.2.) In some cases, individual markers are shown between the intermediate marks. The preference for scales of this type is generally a matter of conditioning. Workers have become accustomed to readi scales of this type and need very little practice to read similar scales. I any case, the numbering should always progress from left to right, similar t the direction of reading.

The pointer should be close to the scale to avoid parallax distortion. The end of the pointer should just meet the smallest marker but should not overlap. It is generally recommended that the tip angle of the pointer be approximately 20°.

Qualitative Visual Displays

Qualitative visual displays are generally used for a relative determination of range or trend. One type of qualitative display can be obtained by color coding parts of a quantitative display. For example, the danger areas of a quantitative display may be color coded red while the normal operating areas are color coded green. Caution areas or areas immediately preceding the danger area can be color coded yellow.

An example of a qualitative type visual display is the temperature display found in most automobiles. Normally, temperature is no longer shown on such a display, and only hot and cold areas of the gauge are indicated. The pointer will move between the cold and hot areas. The driver need not be concerned about the particular temperature, only that the pointer is somewhere in the middle area of the gauge.

Qualitative displays have the advantage of providing the information that is necessary for the operator to take the required action quickly with very little chance of error. In the quantitative display, a great deal of information can be provided to the worker. However, it is not always necessary that the operator has such detailed information. In fact, research has shown that the addition of qualitative coding to a quantitative scale materially decreases the time required for recognition of certain key conditions. (Kurke, 1956.)

Figure 7.3.3

Qualitative displays.

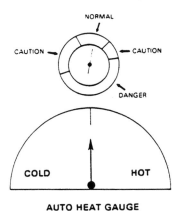

AUTO HEAT GAUGE

Status Indicators. Status indicators are generally used for discrete situations. Often a dichotomous output is obtained, such as on-off, hot-cool, charge-discharge, etc. Status indicators can be either labeled switches, such as are found in a circuit box, or signal lights that indicate the need for action.

Figure 7.3.4

Representational displays.

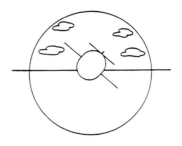

Figure 7.3.5

Status indicators.

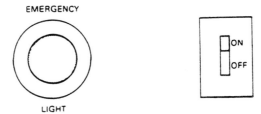

A special case of the status indicator is the auditory alarm. This alarm is the most common use of the auditory signal. Often an auditory alarm is used in conjunction with a visual signal. The auditory alarm is more likely to be noticed than the visual signal; however, the visual signal acts as a reinforcement of the auditory alarm to indicate the point where action is needed.

Auditory Range Displays. Auditory range displays are of two types. The intensity of the tone can be used to indicate the status of the system relative to the desired status by changes in the loudness or intensity of the tone. In another type of auditory display, different tones or patterns can be used to provide additional information, such as the status of the system being to the left or the right of the desired course. A constant signal can indicate that the system is on course. This type of system is commonly used for guidance in airplanes.

Tactual Display. Generally speaking, a tactual display is used as a display of information concerning the location of a control rather than system status. Control knobs are coded as to the function of the knob, either by shape or the location of the knob in question. Texture is another method of

coding control knobs in order that the operator can continue to maintain
visual contact with another target while determining if the proper knob is
being used.

Figure 7.3.6

Shape coding.

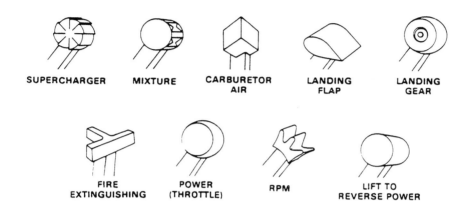

| SUPERCHARGER | MIXTURE | CARBURETOR AIR | LANDING FLAP | LANDING GEAR |

| FIRE EXTINGUISHING | POWER (THROTTLE) | RPM | LIFT TO REVERSE POWER |

Choosing the Type of Stimulus

In the design of a system for human control of a machine or a system of
machines, one of the major problems encountered is the type of stimulus that
should be provided to the operators. Should a visual signal be used or is an
auditory signal preferred? There are certain general rules that can be
applied to this determination.

In general, visual signals are preferred in the following cases:

1. Where relative values or quantitative values are desired.
2. Where the information is complex.
3. Where there is a need to refer to the information at a later point.
4. Where there are a number of displays that must be monitored.
5. Where the location of the object relative to another object is
    desired.
6. Where the display is representative of the actual situation.
7. Where noise limits the use of auditory signals.

On the other hand, an auditory signal is preferred in the following cases:

1. Where a warning is being given and action is desired.
2. Where too many visual stimuli are present.
3. Where information must be presented independent of head orientation.
4. Where visual acuity is limited.
5. By speech, where communication content may vary considerably.

Grouping of Visual Displays

Quite often it is necessary for the worker to monitor a number of displays. Multiple displays create the possibility of confusion to the work unless organized in some logical fashion. The general method is to organize the display such that the pointer is in the same direction for normal operation. Thus, it is easy to pick out abnormal situations when they occu The grouping tends to be viewed as a whole rather than individually, and variations in the pattern are easy to spot.

Figure 7.3.7

Pattern vs. non-pattern groups.

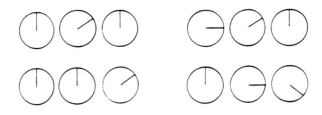

In terms of location of the display or groups of displays, the most significant displays--that is, those used most often--should be in the norma line of vision. Less important displays can be moved to an out-of-the-way position. Warning signals may allow some types of displays to be moved to a out-of-the-way position in which they need be read only if the warning signa goes off.

Summary

Within the worker/machine system, the worker often must act as a controller. In this position, it is necessary that information concerning t status of the system be presented to the worker. This information can be presented in such a way that the worker can use one of many senses to determine changes in the system. In general, the most common method for providing information to the worker is through visual displays. This type c display is normally either quantitative or qualitative in nature depending c the type of information required by the operator. Auditory displays are use in certain special conditions, particularly as warning devices where the worker's vision must be directed elsewhere. Generally, tactual displays are used to provide the worker with information concerning the appropriate contr to use in a given situation when it is necessary that the worker maintain visual contact with another area.

4. Design of the Job

The major question that should be asked is: "What does the worker do on the job?" If the job can be broken down into functions, the activities and tasks that are performed can be specified. These activities and tasks can then be analyzed. The analysis of the tasks provides information as to the optimum job design.

There are many purposes for the design or redesign of a job. The purpose of the design or redesign depends on the objectives that we wish to obtain. Among the possible objectives for job design are:

1. Increased efficiency
2. Increased productivity
3. Increased worker satisfaction
4. Decreased potential for hazard exposure

Though each of the first three reasons for job design is important in its own right, only the fourth reason for job design will be discussed here. Thus, the major objective of job design as related to this discussion is to decrease the potential hazard exposure of the worker on the job.

The Job Functions. Now let's look further to determine the answer to our original question; that is, "What does the worker do on the job?" Perhaps in determining the job functions that the worker performs, general rules for controlling the worker's exposure to potential hazards can be described.

The first step that the worker performs is to gather data and information on the situation as it currently exists. This data-gathering function may be limited, as is the case when a worker is performing basically a physical task and must only observe such things as obstacles in his path, the placement of hand tools, etc. On the other hand, the airline pilot is faced with a multitude of data and information that must be presented in a reasonable manner to allow for appropriate pilot action to control the airplane.

The second step that the worker must perform is the processing of the data and information that have been gathered. The purpose of this data processing is to make decisions concerning the future steps that will be taken. Again, in many cases this is a relatively simple process. Quite often, as is the case when driving an automobile, although basic data processing requirements may be somewhat complex, the actual processing itself goes on in the

741

background as an almost conditioned response to certain stimuli that the driver has learned to process through experience. On the other hand, in case such as nonstandard or emergency situations, data processing can become quite complex and the determination of the appropriate response to the system state can be critical to the health and safety of the individual as well as to others in the vicinity.

The next major step in performing a job is to implement the decision that has been reached in the data processing stage. This decision can be implemented in two separate ways. First, the decision can be communicated to another worker for final action. A second method is for the worker who makes the decision to take the action to control the situation.

The three functions discussed above are basically cognitive processes; that is, they involve the worker's mental process. In many jobs it is also necessary for the worker to perform physical tasks. These tasks may be required to implement the decision or they may be of a supportive nature. Typical of the types of physical tasks that might be performed are the physical operation of controls to maintain or adjust the system status, the physical movement and positioning of the materials used, and the application of various types of tools to the object in order to attain the desired result.

Finally, while performing the functions of the job, it may be necessary for the worker to assume different positions in the workplace. In some cases the worker may maintain a stationary position with only limited movement. Other types of jobs require the worker to be active with considerable movement throughout the work area.

A General Procedure for Determining Where Controls for Hazard Exposures Are Required

The first step in examining a job to determine where controls for hazard exposure are necessary is to review the functions and list the tasks that arerequired. As mentioned previously, it may be necessary to break the tasks further into elements and micromotions depending on the depth of the analysis needed.

Once the tasks have been listed and broken down into their components as necessary, the tasks or components should be analyzed to determine the requirements involved. What are the mental requirements that are present within the system? What information is required? What decisions must be made by the worker? What are the physical requirements of the jobs in terms of operating controls and other physical worker actions?

Now each of the individual tasks or components of the tasks should be analyzed to determine if potential hazard exposures exist. Are the requirements such that the worker cannot process the information that is presented? Is the worker provided with adequate information? Do the physical requirements of the job put an excess stress on the worker?

Next, alternate modes for performing the task, such as equipment, procedures, etc., should be identified where potential hazards exist. Can substitution of method be used to remove the potential hazard? Can the worker be removed from the job totally, thus eliminating any potential hazard? Can new equipment or materials be provided that are less likely to involve a hazard to the worker? Each individual task or component of a task in which a potential hazard is identified should be analyzed to determine the changes that might be made.

Finally, before selecting the appropriate alternatives to use, each of the alternatives presented should be compared in terms of the costs and benefits of the alternative. In addition, any potential hazards that may exist in the alternative proposed for substitution should also be considered. The substitution of one hazard for another is not good design. Finally, the efficiency of the job itself should be determined using the alternative methods. Even though a particular method may lead to a lower hazard potential, it will be difficult to sell if efficiency is adversely affected.

Now let us look at each of the major functions of the job in more detail to determine how the job might be redesigned to remove potential hazards.

The Data Gathering Function

One of the major objectives of the design of jobs is to provide the worker with the data that are required for efficient functioning on the job. In orderto do this, one must ask the question, "What data are required?" What does the worker need to know to perform the job? Without adequate data, it is virtually impossible to perform a job efficiently. One cannot drive an automobile without having a view of the road through the windshield. Consider what would happen if the hood latch broke and the hood flew up to obscure your view while you are driving an automobile. You no longer have sufficient data to make a decision concerning the course upon which you are steering the automobile. Unless quick action is taken to remove the automobile from the stream of traffic and stop, there is a high probability that an accident will occur. Likewise, without adequate data, the worker is operating blindly in performing the job. It is highly probable that something will go wrong as a result of this lack of data.

After determining what data are required, the next question that should be asked is, "In what form should the data be provided to the worker?" As previously discussed, the form of the data may be qualitative or quantitative. The data may be presented as a deviation from normal or as a warning when action is required. An analysis of the method of presentation of data is important. Qualitative data are useful in some situations. However, in some cases it is necessary that exact values and the indication of trends be presented to the worker so that action can be taken before it is too late. In these situations, quantitative data are necessary. Each of the various types of data that are to be presented to the worker should be analyzed to determine the form of the presentation. Care should be taken to provide only those data that are necessary for performance of the job and to assure that the data that are presented, are presented in the appropriate mode needed for operator decision.

The next step is to determine when the data are required. Is it necessary that the operator receive the data on a continuous basis, or can an intermittent supply of data be utilized? Again, using the example of driving an automobile, it is desirable that the operator have a clear view of the road ahead. However, intermittently the operator should view the rear of the automobile through the rear view mirror to assure that any traffic that is approaching from the rear is observed. In this case, some data are required continuously and some data are required intermittently.

The job designer should consider how much data are being presented to a given worker at a given point. Too much data can lead to a possible stressful situation in the worker. The visual and auditory channels can become overloaded, causing the worker to fail as a controller of the system. In such situations, it may be possible to modify the type of data presentation from a quantitative to a qualitative mode. Warning lights and auditory warning signals might be used to direct the worker's attention to a particular visual display, thus limiting the need for continuous monitoring of all displays. Finally, it may be necessary that additional workers be used to monitor the displays that are present.

Next, the job designer should consider how the data should be presented. Can the worker obtain the necessary data from the environment, or is a display necessary? If a display is required, should it be auditory or visual? What type of display should be used? Should a visual gauge be used? Consider the various kinds of displays available. Should the display be circular, semi-circular, vertical, horizontal, or digital? Consider the location of the display within the operator's viewing area. If a number of common displays are required, how can these be grouped in a manner to limit the necessity for continuous monitoring of each individual display?

Next, the need for an emergency warning system should be investigated. Should such a warning system be auditory or visual? At what point should such a warning system be provided in order to allow time for appropriate operator action to bring the system back into control?

In an emergency situation when a warning has been given to the operator, the designer must consider whether the operator can handle the abnormal conditions. What must the operator perform in an emergency situation? Can the operator perform this within the time allowed? If not, it may be necessary to provide a warning to the operator sooner, even though in some cases such a warning may prove to be a false alarm.

There are various ways in which the data-gathering phase can be modified to eliminate potential hazards or accidents. One way is to replace the human worker with automatic sensors. These sensors can provide for automatic shutdown when the situation so merits. Complete automation of the process, removing the need for worker interaction with the system, can be accomplished in such a manner. This is particularly useful in an emergency situation when it is impossible for the operator to react quickly enough to perform the many requirements to bring the system back under control.

The second method of modification can be to remove the monitoring of the process to a single location remote from the process itself. In this manner, an individual can monitor a number of systems at the same time. Again,

however, it is necessary to assure that this individual does not become
overloaded.

When one of the senses becomes overloaded, it may be necessary to provide
displays using one of the other senses. Most commonly, the visual sense will
become overloaded; and in such situations, the use of auditory signals,
vibration, or touch may be helpful to provide the worker with information
necessary to control the system.

Replacement of quantitative scales with qualitative displays or go-no-go
type displays may be advantageous. In this manner, the worker gathers
information in a simple form indicating when situations arise requiring
operator action.

The various types of data-display techniques should be analyzed to
determine the display facilities that are best for the particular situation.
Although in many cases the circular and semi-circular gauge are preferable for
a quantitative display, this is in no way a hard and fast rule. Vertical and
horizontal displays may provide the worker with the information more quickly.
The digital display, which has the advantage of accuracy of reading, can be
used in certain situations.

Finally, the designer must consider the need for redundancy. Should a
breakdown occur in one of the information gathering channels, what backup is
available to the worker to sense that something has gone wrong? What backup
can be implemented if the worker makes an error? What is the potential loss
that will be incurred if an error occurs and the system goes out of control?
Redundancy can be provided to take care of these situations. The redundancy
that is provided may be either parallel redundancy or series redundancy.

Processing Information

Once the data have been received by the worker, these data must be
processed. Of concern to the designer is the time that is necessary to
process the required data. Is sufficient time available to meet the time
requirements for data processing? How much of this time is reaction time. and
how much of this time is processing time? Can either the reaction time or the
processing time be reduced by changes in the system? Finally, are the
decisions that are required of the operator reasonable, considering the human
information processing capabilities of the operator?

In this modern era of electronic data processing, the job designer should
consider whether the data to be processed is best done by a human operator or
by a machine or computer. There are certain general principles that will help
the designer to make the appropriate determination.

In general, machines are best to perform the following functions.

1. Machines are best to sense low-level stimuli or small changes in the
   environment for certain types of stimuli.
2. Machines are best to handle standard situations without errors.
3. Machines are best to store and retrieve information quickly.

4. Machines are best to process large quantities of data.
5. Machines are best to make rapid and accurate calculations repetitively.
6. Machines are best to perform multiple functions simultaneously.
7. Machines are best to exert large physical forces. (Though not related to processing of data, this fact and should be considered.)
8. Machines are best to withstand stress without a decrement in service if an appropriate maintenance level is provided.
9. Machines are best to operate continuously without fatigue.
10. Machines are best to operate in a patterned manner, given known input and desired outputs.

On the other hand, humans provide certain advantages in the workplace, particularly in terms of data processing. In general--

1. Humans are best to sense changes related to visual, auditory, tactual, olfactory, and taste senses.
2. Humans are best to handle the unexpected.
3. Humans are best to store and recall principles and decision rules.
4. Humans are best to adapt procedures to meet the situation.
5. Humans are best to put contingency plans into effect.
6. Humans are best to perform various tasks which are required randomly.
7. Humans are best to apply new methods to create new solutions.
8. Humans are best to develop priorities for action.

In general, if the problem is a structured, repetitive one, a machine will be best in handling it. On the other hand, if the problem is unstructured and variable, the human operator is the best.

Controlling the System

The next major function of the worker in the workplace is to control the system. The first question the job designer must ask is, "What kind of controls are required?" This is dependent on the type of adjustment that must be made to the system by the operator. Some adjustments require intermittent control action by the operator; in other situations, it is necessary that a continuous adjustment to the system be made. Thus, the type of control that is required may be either in discrete settings or continuous settings, depending on the type of control action that is necessary.

The designer must decide where to place the control and identify it so that there is little chance for error on the part of the operator selecting the control that is used. Can the operator look for the control? If so, labeling of the controls or coding them may be sufficient to provide a key as to the type of control that the operator is using. If the operator must find the controls without looking, it will be necessary to code the controls in some manner. In such a situation, it is possible to code the controls by location. The controls should be spaced apart using standard location patterns where possible. Another method of coding the controls is to code by shape. The shape may be symbolic of the object being controlled as is often the case of airplane controls. In any case, the shapes should be significantly different from one another to assure that errors are not made. Where shape coding is used, it is advisable to conduct tests to determine those designs that are least likely to be confused.

Another method of coding controls is by size. Generally, a one-half difference in diameter and three-eighths difference in thickness will be sufficient to allow for discrimination between different controls. Finally, the coding of controls by texture has been used with some success. Research has indicated that three general types of texture coding can be discriminated by operators. These are a smooth surface, a fluted surface, and a knurled surface.

Figure 7.4.1

Texture coding.

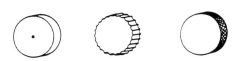

SMOOTH   FLUTED   KNURLED

If the mode of operation is discrete, there are two basic kinds of controls that might be used. First, if the situation is dichotomous, an on-off control can be used. Such a control can be a button that when in the down position is "on" and in the up position is "off." An additional visual cue might be provided by lighting behind the button when it is in the "on" position. A simple switch is another alternative for the on-off situation. In such a case, when the switch is in the up position it is on and may be labeled and lighted to provide an additional visual cue.

Where multiple discrete settings are required, a rotary selector switch with an arrow pointing to a marker for the appropriate setting can be implemented. Another example is the use of a lever that can be positioned to obtain various discrete settings. In either case, to provide for protection against inadvertent setting to the wrong position, the positioning may require two motions. Such a situation exists in the manual gear-shift lever of an automobile.

If the mode of operation is continuous, various types of control mechanisms can be used. The round knob can be used where it is desirable that the control be operated by the fingertips or hand. A hand wheel can be used where a larger force is required, and arm motion is necessary to provide the appropriate system response. In some cases, a crank may be necessary to control the system response. Where the hands are busy or wnere large forces are required, a foot pedal can be used to obtain the necessary control. Finally, a lever can be used as a method for control of the system.

Figure 7.4.2

Discrete controls--on-off.

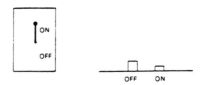

DISCRETE CONTROLS
MULTIPLE SETTINGS

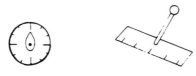

Figure 7.4.3

Continuous controls.

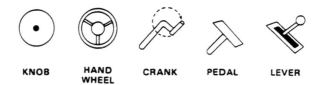

KNOB   HAND   CRANK   PEDAL   LEVER
        WHEEL

The Recommended Direction of Control Movements. There are recommended directions for control movements based upon previous conditioning that has occurred in humans. In general, humans expect controls to operate in certain manners. These recommendations should be implemented in the design of controls for the system.

In the case of on-off controls, the following directions as presented in Figure 7.4.4 are recommended.

General Control Design Principles

The following general control principles have been adapted from the book, Human Engineering Guide to Equipment Design, VanCott and Kinkade, 1972.

Figure 7.4.4

On-off control movement.

ON	OFF
Up	Down
In	Out
Right	Left
Pull	Push

For continuous or discrete controls, the direction of the knob or lever should be as shown in Figure 7.4.5.

Figure 7.4.5

Continuous control movement.

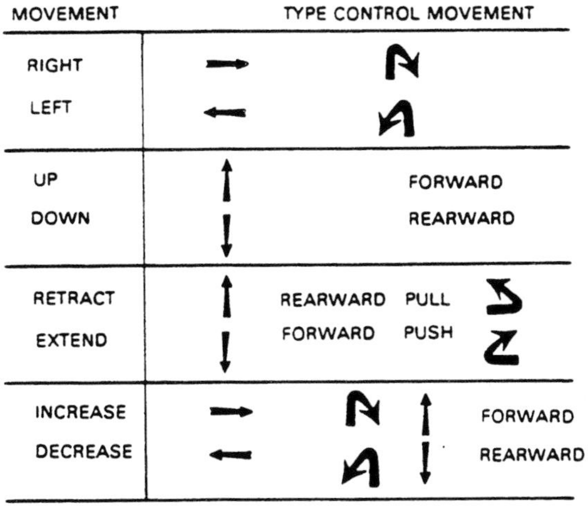

MOVEMENT	TYPE CONTROL MOVEMENT
RIGHT / LEFT	→ ←
UP / DOWN	↑↓ FORWARD REARWARD
RETRACT / EXTEND	↑↓ REARWARD PULL / FORWARD PUSH
INCREASE / DECREASE	→ ← ↑↓ FORWARD REARWARD

1. The maximum force, speed, accuracy, or range of the control should not exceed the limits of the least capable operator.
2. The normal control operation should be considerably less than the maximum capability of most operators.
3. The number of controls should be minimized.
4. Control movement should be simple and easy to perform.
5. Natural control movements are more efficient and less fatiguing.
6. Control movement should be as short as possible, consistent with the requirements of accuracy and feel.
7. Controls should have sufficient resistance to reduce the possibility of inadvertent activation.
8. Where a single application of force or short continuous force is required, the maximum resistance should be one-half the operator's maximum strength.

9. For continuously operated controls over long periods, the resistance should be low.
10. Where power assistance is required, artificial resistance cues shoul be provided.
11. Controls should be designed to withstand abuse.
12. Controls should provide a positive indication of activation so that malfunctions can be identified.
13. Controls should indicate a positive indication of system response.
14. The control surfaces should be designed to prevent slippage of the activating human appendage.
15. Hand controls are preferred in the following situations:

    - if the accuracy of the control is important
    - if the speed on control positioning is important
    - if continuous or prolonged force (greater than 20 pounds) is not necessary

16. The use of foot controls is recommended in the following cases:

    - when continuous, nonprecise control is required
    - where moderate to large forces are required (greater than 20 pound
    - when the hands are likely to become overburdened

Physical Requirements--Material Handling

One of the most common physical tasks performed by the worker on the job is the handling of material. Many injuries result from manual material handling by the worker. Improper handling of material often causes strains, sprains, fractures, and bruises.

There are many causes of improper lifting and carrying materials. Often the worker attempts to carry material that is too heavy. In some cases thoug the object may not be too heavy, it may be too bulky to maintain an adequate grip. The surface of the material may be slippery, thus causing the worker to lose grip during carrying. Rough or jagged surfaces of the material being handled can cause minor cuts and scratches which, when they occur, may cause the worker to drop the material, resulting in even a greater potential for serious injury. Finally, in some cases the worker must handle hazardous material, either manually or through the use of a system in which the worker must be in close proximity.

A major function of the industrial hygiene engineer who designs a job is controlling its material handling hazards. One of the questions that should be asked is, "Can the job be changed to eliminate the need to lift or carry the materials?" In some cases a gravity feed mechanism may be provided to move the materials into the machine from their locations. Mechanical or pneumatic conveyors can be used to move the material, either on a continuous or intermittent basis. One obvious method for material handling is the use of forklift trucks and/or hand trucks to move the material. The placement of the materials in a position for easy machine feeding is important. The materials should be placed at the same level as they are fed into the machine in order to remove the necessity for the operator to bend down and pick up the materials to be fed to the machine. Finally, bulk feeding of the materials in their packaged format may be possible.

The industrial hygiene engineer should consider if the objects being handled are hazardous to the worker. If these objects are hazardous and cannot be substituted for by other materials, then it is necessary to protect the worker from the hazardous materials. Automatic handling with the worker in a remote location is certainly a possibility. However, it may be necessary for the worker at times to come into physical contact with the materials. In such cases, personal protective equipment, such as gloves, aprons, respirators, etc., may be necessary to provide personal protection to the worker.

In some special types of material handling it may be necessary to design methods to provide assistance for handling the materials. Simple aids, such as tote boxes with handles, may be appropriate. Carts, pulleys, and hoists are also potential methods for assisting in the material handling process. If manual material handling is still necessary, it may be necessary that additional crew members be available to handle the material.

Finally, the employees involved in material handling should be trained to recognize potential material handling hazards. In this manner, the employeeswill become aware of the need to use proper techniques. The employee should be trained in the proper lifting and handling techniques to use for the various kinds of materials that are used on the job.

Summary

One of the major ways in which the field of ergonomics can be applied to the control of potential hazard exposures is in the design of the job itself. Such a job design should consider the various functions that the individual worker must perform while on the job. These functions will include data gathering, data processing, controlling of the system, and the various physical tasks required of the system. Each of these functions must be analyzed to determine how improvements can be made to protect the worker. Though not discussed in this chapter, a potential method for reducing ergonomic hazards is the proper design of hand tools used by the worker. However, this approach is beyond the scope of this discussion. Various texts on biomechanics and machine guarding have been written that cover this subject well. It is recommended that the industrial hygiene engineer consult these texts before completing a job design to eliminate potential hazards.

5. Design of the Workplace

After the industrial hygiene engineer has designed the job to meet the criteria of the desired output and provided the appropriate tools and procedures to protect the worker from potential hazards, it is necessary to design the work station in which the worker will perform the job. The general principle that should be followed on work station design is to provide an efficient and safe location in which the work can be performed. There are certain basic factors that must be considered when designing a workplace.

First, the designer must determine what the worker must see while on the job. What part of the work environment must be visible to the worker? While performing the job, what controls must the worker operate? Where should these controls be located, considering the type of operation that is necessary? Is it necessary for the worker to be able to view the action of the equipment being used on the job? What about the interaction of the job with other workers and their jobs? Is it necessary for the worker to be able to view other jobs and worker actions?

Third, the designer should consider what operations the worker must perform while on the job. Is it necessary for the worker to operate hand and/or foot controls? Will the worker be required to do lifting and carrying? While on the job, does the worker need to position materials in order to accomplish the task? What motions are required while performing the job? What special tools are used to perform the job? Are physical demands other than material handling placed upon the worker by the job?

The designer should consider the job procedure itself. What is the sequence of operation performed on the job? Is there any priority of operations that the worker must perform?

Important in the design of the workplace is the determination of clearances that are required to perform the job. Such clearances should consider the size of the workers who will perform in the workplace and include clearances for movement. Is there any chance for accidental injury by bumping objects in the workplace? The designer should consider the possibility of accidental activation of controls. What is the likelihood of such an event occurring and how can it be prevented?

Finally, the designer should consider what storage requirements are necessary for the job. Provision must be made for the storage of raw materials, in-process materials, and finished product. Also, the designer must consider what hand tools or other aids the worker will use that must be stored in the workplace.

Design for Visibility and Hearing

When designing the workplace for visibility and hearing, the first problem that the designer must face is where to locate the displays and controls that must be monitored and used by the operator. Displays and controls should be located in such a manner that the operator can perform the necessary monitoring and adjustment with a minimum disruption to other duties being performed on the job.

The first priority is the visual requirement of the job, and this requirement determines the general layout of the workplace. The operator should be positioned in order to face in the direction of the primary visual field. If it is necessary for the operator to view the operation of equipment, the operator should be faced in that direction with a clear and unobstructed field of vision between the operator and the equipment being viewed. If, as a part of the job, the operator must view certain displays or operate certain controls continuously, then these should be placed within the primary field of view.

The second priority is to locate the primary controls acting on the primary visual task. If, for example, the primary visual task is operating a crane to lift objects and it is necessary for the operator to view the crane operation while controlling the crane, the primary controls for operating the crane should be located in such a manner that the operator does not have to move positions from the primary viewing task.

Any emergency controls that are visual in nature should be located close to the primary field of vision. The operator should be able to observe any warning indications, such as blinking lights or pointers indicating danger, while viewing the primary task.

Displays that are related to the primary controls should be within or as close to the primary field of vision as possible. Where it is not possible to locate such displays in the direct field of vision, they should be located in such a manner that will require only the movement of the operator's eyes to observe them. Again using the automobile for an example, the speedometer and rear view mirror, though not located in the primary field of vision, are located where a quick glance of the eyes can ascertain the desired information.

Secondary controls or displays that are referred to infrequently can be placed in an out-of-the-way area. However, as much as possible, such controls should not require the operator to change body positions since this may interfere with the primary viewing task.

Auditory signals should be located in reference to the action causing the signal. If, for example, a warning is related to something happening to the right of the workplace, it is preferable to place the auditory signal on the right of the operator. This will automatically direct the worker's attention to that area of the workplace. The auditory signal itself should be pointed to the listener's ear and be close enough to overcome any noise masking that might occur in the workplace.

Finally, visual controls and displays should be grouped functionally. In this manner, it is possible for the worker to check a number of related controls and displays during one observation.

Once the controls and displays have been located, it may be necessary to label or code these controls and displays in some manner. One method of labeling is to color code the displays and controls. Generally, red is used for emergency situations, while yellow is often used for cautionary situations; and green is used for safe or normal operation.

The controls can be labeled if it is possible for the worker to observe the control panel while operating the equipment. If labels are used, they should be placed consistently relative to the controls. For example, all controls should be placed either above, below, to the right, or to the left of the control to which they refer.

It is useful to color the knobs of the controls differently than the background panel. This helps the operator to see quickly the actual location of the knob. Functional groups of controls can be offset in separate areas. and the background panel shaded or lined off to indicate the functional group Next, the designer should consider the amount of illumination that is present in the workplace. Is the illumination provided in the workplace adequate for the tasks required? If the tasks require fine adjustments and/or assembly, the illumination should be sufficient for the operator to discriminate between the fine differences in adjustment. The designer should take care to assure that glare will not be a problem while the worker is performing the job. Shiny surfaces are always subject to producing glare in the operator's eyes, particularly if the operator finds it necessary to move his position to perform certain tasks. In such cases, matte finished panels and glare resistant glass are useful.

Finally, the designer should consider the amount of illumination entering from outside the work area. In some cases, problems related to glare and visibility can result from the entrance of sunlight or floodlights from other areas. Where windows are located near the workplace, consider the angle of the sun during the work period throughout the year to determine if at any time the entry of sunlight will cause a visual problem.

Design for Worker Operations

While the worker is in the workplace, it may be necessary to perform certain physical or manual tasks. Certain types of equipment may also be required to perform the job. During the performance of the job, different motions will be required. The designer must design the workplace in such a manner as to provide for the motions that are required to operate the equipment. An additional consideration is the placement of the equipment itself. It should be placed in such a manner that it is easily accessible to the operator.

Of major consideration in the design of the workplace is the operator's position within it. Should the operator work from a sitting position, standing position, or a combined sitting and standing position? Certain general rules have been derived to determine which position is best, given the type of job to be performed. The following is adapted from the book, Human Engineering Guide to Equipment Design, VanCott and Kinkade, 1972.

The sitting position is best for:

1.   A high degree of operator stability.
2.   Precise controlling.
3.   Long work periods.
4.   Use of both feet for controlling.
5.   Large-force application or a range of movement for foot controls.
6.   Precise foot movements.

The standing position is best for:

1.   Mobility to reach and perform operations.
2.   Where large areas must be monitored.

A combined sit-stand position is often required by the job. In such cases it is generally best to provide a high stool since this enables the operator to move from one position to another quickly. When a high stool is provided in such a workplace, an adjustable footrest should be attached to the stool to enable the operator to maintain the proper position while sitting.

During the design of the workplace, it is necessary to determine the actual placement of manual controls to assure efficient and nonfatiguing operation. Primary controls should be located within the area of comfortable reach. In general, this area is determined by the arc of the arm with the elbow held near the body. In other words, it is an arc with the radius equal to the length of the worker's forearm and hand.

Secondary controls can be located beyond comfortable reach; that is, in an area circumscribed by an arc with a radius equal to the length of the individual's extended arm. Seldom used controls can be located in an out-of-the-way position that may require the operator to change positions to make adjustments.

Cranks should be placed at elbow level. Pull-up controls should be located below seat level or at near full extension of the arm when the operator is standing. Pull-out controls should be just short of full-arm extension for either the seated or standing operator.

Provision for Equipment in the Workplace. Where electrical power tools are going to be used by the operator, provision should be made for adequate electrical outlets. Each of the outlets should be of the three-prong grounded variety.

The designer should determine the adequate space that is necessary to operate the equipment in its most efficient manner. A clear work area should be available for the operation of the equipment. Consider each individual piece of equipment to be used as well as the particular operation performed b each piece of equipment. In order to develop a proper work space design, it may be necessary for the designer to observe a worker using the equipment to perform the required tasks.

The equipment used should be in logical order. Generally, such an order is according to the task performance sequence. The location in relation to the sequence should be either from left to right or top to bottom in the work station.

The designer should provide methods for stabilizing the work; such as jigs, vices, or built-in positioning frames. Such aids will enable the operator to free one hand to perform other tasks or to operate other controls

The designer should locate the most frequently used equipment nearest the worker. Less frequently used equipment can be located in an out-of-the-way position.

Standard Design. Where similar jobs are being performed by workers in different workplaces, the designer should consider standardizing the workplac layout and design for these operations. This provides the ability to shift workers back and forth between job duties with a minimum amount of training concerning the workplace layout. In addition, it reduces errors that will occur after a worker has been moved to a new job.

Provide Adequate Storage. An important consideration in design of the workplace is to provide adequate storage for both materials and equipment. A cluttered workplace causes errors and accidents as well as being detrimental to the worker's morale. Positions for tools and materials should be near their point of use. This will assist the worker in maintaining an uncluttere workplace since such a location will make it much more likely that the tool o material will be replaced when that particular part of the job is completed. Just as we often find in our own homes or apartments that there is never enough storage space, the worker often finds that the designer has not provided adequate space to store materials and tools.

Figure 7.5.1

Storage requirements.

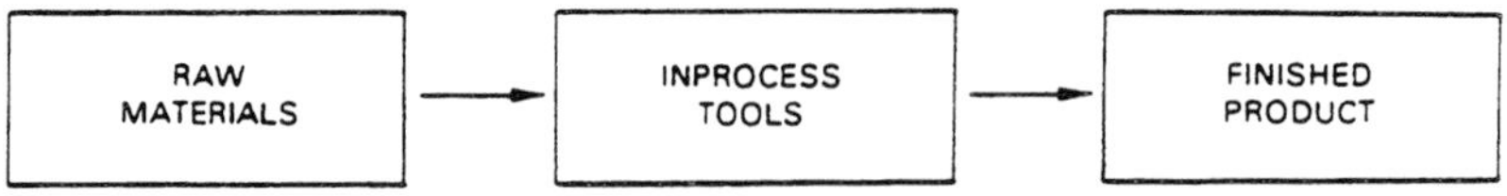

Workplace Space Considerations

Another consideration in the design of the workplace is how large it should be. In locating equipment within comfortable reach, what determines comfortable reach?

Generally, workplace space dimensions are based on anthropometric data that have been gathered. Normally, the workplace is designed to meet the requirements of those individuals between the fifth and ninety-fifth percentile range of the particular dimensions that are important to the job. Unless there is some known reason to vary, this approach should be used in the design of the workplace. A final checkout of data on a sample of workers may be helpful to determine the appropriateness of the anthropometric data that have been chosen.

Clearance requirements should be based on the largest dimensional data for the particular movements involved. For example, the overhead clearance should accommodate the largest person who might work in the work area. On the other hand, reach movements should be based on the smallest individual who will work in the workplace. In this manner, a maximum number of individuals will be able to perform the job efficiently.

The designer should allow for adjustability where possible. Most commonly, such adjustability can be obtained in the seating and height of the workbench. This will allow for the accommodation of both large and small workers.

When determining the space considerations, the designer should consider any clothing that will be worn by the worker that may increase the size dimensions or limit the motion of the worker. Also of importance are postural changes that may occur while the worker performs his job. As much as possible, the workplace should accommodate changes in posture, since these are necessary in order for the worker to prevent excessive fatigue.

In some cases, the work space may be in a vehicle or other moving systems; such as a crane, elevator, etc. In these situations, it is important for the designer to consider the clearance requirements in the case of a sudden stop or start. Swaying and turning are often problems in moving vehicles and should be considered for clearance requirements by the designer.

The workplace should be designed to provide a safe and healthful environment in which the worker can perform tasks. In order to do this, corners and angles that may be bumped by the worker should be round. Any projections should be removed as much as possible. Assurance should be made that the controls are protected from accidental bumping during the performance of other tasks, thus inadvertently activating equipment that could cause an accident or injury to the worker. Where the workplace is in motion, restraints--such as seat belts, guardrails, and other such devices--should be provided to prevent the worker from being moved from the normal work position.

A poorly designed work space can cause physical stress on the worker's body. Fatigue can set in if the worker is required to work in an awkward posture. The seat and workbench should be designed in such a manner as to encourage proper work posture. Certain types of seating can cause a dangerous limitation of blood flow to the lower extremities of the body. This can adversely affect the health of the worker after long periods of exposure.

In addition, where the work space itself is moving or where mechanical equipment is operating in close proximity to the workplace, there is the potential for vibration being transmitted to the worker. This vibration can be harmful to the worker if the exposure continues for an extended period of time. Methods should be provided to limit this vibration as much as possible.

The Design of the Plant Equipment Layout

The objective of plant layout is to locate the individual work stations within the plant such as to provide for efficient production, provide for efficient material flow, and provide a safe environment. Plant layout becomes important either when a new plant is being designed or when a renovation program of an existing plant is being considered. The industrial hygiene engineer should take an active part as a member of the task force charged with the plant layout. The involvement of the industrial hygiene engineer should be early in the design stage since the factors that are important for employee health and safety are most often related to major groupings of equipment. If the industrial hygiene engineer is involved in the design process, potential hazards to the health and safety of the workers can be prevented.

Generally the process layout is used to determine the general plant layout design. With such a layout, machines are arranged in functional groups. Material flow throughout the plant is then charted. The objective of such a layout is to reduce material handling costs and provide for efficient operation. Generally a layout that is efficient from a material handling viewpoint will provide for the safety of the worker since many of the accidents and injuries that occur on the job are as a result of material handling activities.

Where material handling activities cross paths going between functional areas of the plant, hazards exist. Also. inefficient material handling can make it difficult to meet production quotas, thus requiring that the workers within the plant operate at higher than safe speeds. Imagine a plant where fork trucks carrying materials are zipping to and fro randomly between operations. Such a plant layout is certainly highly likely to be unsafe.

In addition to material handling, other factors must be considered in the design and layout of the plant. In general, hot processes should be grouped together and isolated to limit the exposure to only a few workers. Noisy operations should be planned carefully and where possible isolated from the remainder of the plant. Noncompatible operations where there is a potential for hazardous materials to mingle should also be located in separate areas of the plant. In no case should operations requiring local exhaust ventilation be mixed in the same area with operations requiring general or dilution ventilation.

When looking at the location of each individual workplace within the plant, the designer should consider the protection of the worker and the equipment. Guardrails should be provided to eliminate the possibility of the operator entering the traffic area or vice versa. Adequate areas for maintenance of equipment should also be provided. Remember. it is the duty of the industrial hygiene engineer to protect the maintenance worker as well as the production worker. Space should be allowed around the work area for storage of raw materials, work in process, and finished materials: and these should be in such a location so as not to interfere with the normal operation of the equipment.

Use of Color Coding in the Plant. One method that is available to provide information concerning the potential hazards within the plant is to color code areas. equipment, and piping. Standard color codes are generally accepted for such coding. To code areas of the plant and equipment. the following codes are generally accepted:

1.   Red--Indicates a danger or fire protection equipment.
2.   Yellow--Indicates an area where caution should be exercised.
3.   Green--Indicates the location of first aid equipment.
4.   Black and White Stripes or Checks--Generally used for traffic markings. particularly where mobile traffic is present.
5.   Orange--Generally used to indicate hazardous parts of machinery where the operator must exert extreme care.
6.   Magenta--Used to indicate radiation areas.

In the same manner. piping may be color coded to indicate the contents of the pipe. This is particularly important since it is not always obvious which pipes contain which materials. The generally accepted color codes are as follows:

1.   Red--Indicates fire protection materials, most often water.
2.   Orange or Yellow--Indicates hazardous materials are contained within the pipe.
3.   Green--Indicates safe materials are transported in the pipe.
4.   Blue--Indicates protective materials are being transmitted.

Traffic Spaces

In addition to providing for appropriate location of equipment and work spaces within the plant, it is necessary to provide for the movement of traffic throughout the plant. Traffic movement involves the allowance for aisles and corridors. exits and entrances, as well as ladders. stairs. ramps. and elevators.

Aisles and Corridors. The designer should consider the purpose for which the aisle or corridor is to be used. Will one-way traffic likely exist in the area, or is it necessary to provide two-way traffic? Will the traffic be essentially pedestrian traffic. or will it be mechanical equipment: such as fork trucks and tractors pulling carts? In general, the dimensions shown in Figure 7.5.2 are recommended for aisles and corridors that will handle pedestrian traffic. The data presented in the figure are based on anthropometric data.

The designer should take into consideration other factors when designing aisles and corridors. As much as possible. blind corners should be avoided

Figure 7.5.2

Aisles and corridors.

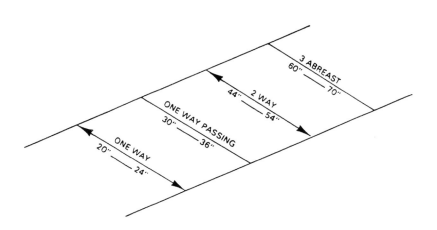

since there is the potential for accident or injury. This is particularly the
case when mechanical vehicles are using the aisles. The use of stop signs and
mirrors to indicate oncoming traffic around the corner can be helpful.

The designer should determine where dense traffic is likely to occur, both
in the normal working day and in times of emergency. The design should
provide for the maximum traffic expected in the area.

Aisles should be marked clearly to indicate the area in which traffic
should be constrained. The aisles should be kept clear of any obstructions.
This includes doors, which should not open into the corridor.

Corridors should be intersected at ninety degrees where possible. This
will conserve valuable space that can be used in the actual production
processes.

Exits and Entrances. It is important to provide adequate exits and
entrances to the facility or the various areas of the facility. Emergency
exits should be located to provide exit from the work area in case of
emergency. Multiple exit points are desirable to eliminate crowding at any
one exit and to provide alternate choices in case the emergency eliminates one
or more of the exits. A check should be made of the local building codes so
that sufficient exits are provided and properly located in order to be in
compliance.

In the case of emergency exits, the door should open outward. A panic bar
should be installed to assure that the push of the crowd will open the door
easily. In the case of an emergency, a jammed door can cause serious injury
and perhaps death to those trapped inside.

In general, ninety-degree corridors should be avoided for emergency exits. The straight line emergency exit is best. Where an intersection is necessary, the intersection should be from one aisle into two rather than from two aisles into one. This eliminates the possibility of congestion occurring, resulting in possible injury to the workers.

When designing the doors to be used as exits, the revolving door or spring-loaded swinging door should be avoided. These doors can cause unnecessary accidents or injury. If double doors are to be installed, each door should operate in only one direction. Where glass doors or panels are used, the glass should be frosted or marked with a pattern in order to prevent individuals from inadvertently assuming that the door is open and walking into the glass.

Figure 7.5.3 presents the dimensions for human traffic through entrances and exits for two-way flow.

Figure 7.5.3

Entrance and exit.

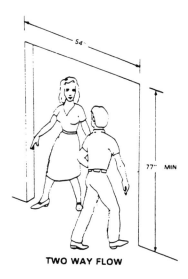

TWO WAY FLOW

Consideration should be given to the protection of individuals standing or walking near a hinged door. One method for accomplishing this is to place a glass window halfway up so that individuals on both sides of the door can view others approaching the door. Where possible, the door should open into a dead space or towards a wall. In any case, space should be allowed between the arc of the door and any equipment in order that a person can move out of the way of the swinging door and avoid injury.

Ladders, Stairs, and Ramps

The pitch of fixed ladders should be between 60 and 90 degrees. It is preferred that the pitch be in the area of 70 to 90 degrees. The rung diameter of the ladder should be between 1-1/4 and 1-3/8 inches with a distance between rungs of between 9 and 16 inches. The distance between side rails of a ladder should be between 12 and 21 inches, and the distance to the nearest object in front of the ladder should be 30 inches if the ladder is at a 90° angle and 36 inches if the ladder is at a 75° angle. Where ladders are located between floors, the ladder should be offset to prevent the possibility of the individual falling more than one floor.

Figure 7.5.4 shows the recommended dimensions for ladders.

Figure 7.5.4

Ladders.

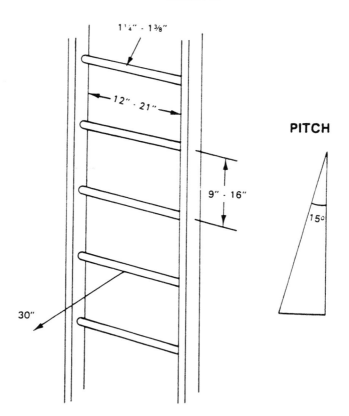

In the design of stairs, the rise between floors should be at a 20 to 35 degree angle. The riser height should be between 5 and 8 inches with the tread depth between 9-1/2 and 10-1/2 inches.

Where possible, landings should be provided every 10 to 12 steps. Stairs should be approximately 20 to 22 inches wide to allow for one-way traffic and 48 inches to 51 inches wide to allow for two-way traffic.

Figure 7.5.5

Stairways.

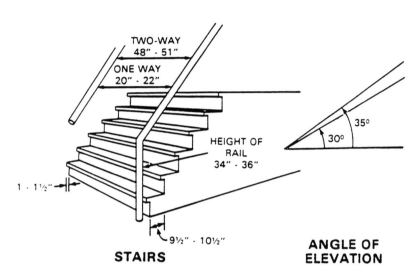

Handrails should be provided. These handrails should be at a height of 36 inches above the stair tread. Double rails and guard screens should be provided where 90 degree landings are present. This will prevent individuals from slipping and falling off the landings.

Where a ramp is used, the maximum slope should be 20 degrees. If the slope is to be greater than 15 degrees, cleats should be used to provide protection against slipping. Handrails should be provided along the side of the ramps to allow for pedestrian use. These rails also guard against the possibility of vehicles dropping off the side of the ramp.

Summary

It is important that the industrial hygiene engineer consider the design of the workplace. The workplace should be designed in such a manner that it provides a safe and healthful environment for the worker. Certain general principles concerning the workplace and station design have been presented that should assist in accomplishing this objective. In general, design of the workplace should be based on what the worker must see, what the worker must hear, what the worker must do, and what space requirements the worker must have to accomplish the required tasks. In addition, the overall plant layout is important to provide for a healthful work environment. The layout of equipment within the plant as well as traffic spaces must be considered. The industrial hygiene engineer must work closely as a member of the team that is charged with designing a new plant facility or the renovation of an existing facility. This involvement must begin early in the design process if it is to be effective in providing for the required safe and healthful environment.

6. References

Guyton, Arthur C., M.D. <u>Function of the Human Body</u>, 3d. ed. Philadelphia: W. B. Saunders Company, 1969.

International Labor Office. <u>Encyclopaedia of Occupational Safety and Health</u>, 2 vols. New York: McGraw-Hill Book Company, 1971.

Kurke, M. I. "Evaluation of a Display Incorporating Quantitative and Check Reading Characteristics." <u>Journal of Applied Psychology</u>, Vol. 40, pp. 233-236, 1956.

McCormick, Ernest J. <u>Human Factors Engineering and Design</u>, 4th. ed. New York: McGraw-Hill Book Company, 1976.

McElroy, Frank E., ed. <u>Accident Prevention Manual for Industrial Operations</u>, 7th. ed. Chicago: National Safety Council, 1975.

Mowbray, G. H. and J. W. Gebhard. "Man's Senses as Information Channels." Report CM-936. Silver Springs, MD: Johns Hopkins University, Applied Physics Laboratory, 1958.

Olishifski, Julian B. and Frank E. McElroy, eds. <u>Fundamentals of Industrial Hygiene</u>. Chicago: National Safety Council, 1971.

Patty, Frank A. <u>Industrial Hygiene and Toxicology</u>, 2d. ed. 2 vols. New York: Interscience Publishers, Inc., 1958.

Steen, Edwin B., Ph.D. and Ashley Montague, Ph.D. <u>Anatomy and Physiology</u>, 2 Vols. New York: Barnes and Noble Books, 1959.

Stoudt, H. W., A. Damon, R. A. McFarland and J. Roberts. <u>Weight, Height and Selected Body Dimensions of Adults, United States 1960-62</u>. Report 8, Series 11. Washington: U. S. Department of Health, Education, and Welfare, National Center for Health Statistics, 1965.

U. S. Department of Health, Education and Welfare, Public Health Service, National Institute for Occupational Safety and Health. <u>The Industrial Environment: Its Evaluation and Control</u>. Washington: U. S. Government Printing Office, 1973.

VanCott, Harold P. and Robert G. Kinkade, eds. <u>Human Engineering Guide to Equipment Design</u>, Rev. ed. Washington: U. S. Government Printing Office, 1972.

Section 8

Other Topics

1. Control of Industrial Water Quality

<u>Introduction</u>

Water, once thought to be an inexhaustible resource, is becoming more and more scarce. Each year we hear of areas of the world where drought has caused water to be at a premium. When one considers that approximately seventy-five percent of the earth's surface is covered with water, it is difficult to conceive of the possibility that water is in short supply. However, the problem is not with the quantity of available water but rather with its quality. Only a small percentage of the total supply of water covering the earth is directly usable by man either for intake into a municipal system or for industrial purposes.

The fact that a supply of relatively pure water is important to industry is obvious considering the number of industries that locate along rivers and lakes. In fact, the existence of an adequate water supply is perhaps the most important criterion considered when determining the location of a new industrial plant. Aside from the use of water as a transportation medium, large quantities of water are used in industrial processes.

Among the many uses of water in industry are:

1. As a product additive.
2. As a source of heat and cooling of the plant (boilers and evaporative cooling units).
3. As a source of heat exchange to remove unnecessary heat from the industrial process.
4. In the sanitary services of the industrial plant.
5. As a major component in product cleaning.
6. As the most commonly used method for providing fire protection within the plant.
7. As an additive for the preparation of food and as a source of fluid for the workers.
8. In the general housekeeping and cleanup around the plant.

When water is used within the industrial plant, it can become polluted with waste products. These waste products include disease-producing organisms, inorganic and organic solids. Chemicals may be added to the water, either in a liquid or gaseous form. In some special cases, radioactive material can become suspended within the waste water from the plant. Finally, in cases where the water has been used as a source of heat exchange, the heat that has been added to the water causes its temperature to be unnaturally high and acts as a pollutant.

The typical water cycle that occurs in an industrial operation includes an original source of water, a treatment of water to meet the requirements of the industry, the use of the treated water in the process, and a post-treatment of the water in order that it may flow back to the source in a relatively harmless condition. The source of water that the plant may use can include lakes, rivers, streams, wells which have been drilled in the locality of the plant, or municipal water systems. The source that is used depends upon the availability of one of the above types of water supply and the quality of water that is needed. Often more than one source may be utilized in the plant as in the case where a municipal system supplies potable water while a local lake supplies water used in the plant processes and fire protection system.

Figure 8.1.1.

The water cycle.

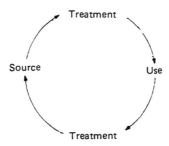

The treatment of water prior to use in an industrial plant varies depending on the ultimate use of the water and the source from which it was obtained. The source may be treated, or its water may be usable in its original form. Certain additives may be required before the water can be used, such as in the case of boiler feed water where additives are used to prevent calcium buildup within the boiler itself. Any industrial operation requires a potable water supply for the workers to drink. Some processes require that potable water be used, particularly those where water is added to a product intended for human consumption such as in food processing.

In some processes and in fire protection, the need for potable water does not exist. However, some pre-treatment may still be necessary to remove certain chemicals and solids which are present in the raw water supply.

During process use, water becomes contaminated. It can no longer be used in the process and must be removed from the plant, or treated for reuse.

Prior to disposal, the waste water must be post-treated to remove any environmentally hazardous pollutants. In the past such treatment was not common, and the water was returned to the source untreated. For obvious reasons, this approach was not satisfactory in terms of the environmental state of natural water sources. In more recent times, environmental laws have been enacted to control the pollutants that can be returned to the water source. Now, before the waste water can be returned to the source, it must be treated to remove potentially damaging pollutants. Such treatment may be accomplished by sending industrial waste water through a municipal sewerage system; or it may be necessary, depending upon the location of the plant and the type of pollutants in the water, that the water be treated in the plant before entry to either the source or a municipal sewerage system.

As water becomes more scarce, conservation of this precious resource is necessary. In some areas of the world, natural unpolluted water is at a premium today. Unless conservation methods are used, this situation will become more prevalent. The high cost of the treatment of source water can justify the need for conservation steps in the use of water in the plant. One method that is available to industry is the recycling of water within the plant. Using such an approach, water is recycled from one area to anotheruntil the contaminants that have been added make it no longer possible to recycle the water without treatment.

Water Treatment

The treatment of water depends to a great extent on the use to which the water will be put. It also depends upon whether the treatment is of a raw water supply or of waste water. Similar unit processes are used for treatment of raw water sources and waste water. However, some additional procedures and care are necessary when water is being treated to provide a potable water supply. In addition, some specific treatments may vary because of required additives or potential contaminants that are present within the waste water.

Certain general unit process steps are required when treating water, either from a source or to remove waste materials. These process steps are:

1. Sedimentation to remove large solids from the water.
2. Control of the acidity or alkalinity of the water.
3. Destabilization and conglomeration; coagulation and flocculation to remove smaller suspended solids.
4. Filtration to further remove solids.
5. Bacterial digestion to remove organic materials.
6. Disinfection using chemical additives to control disease-carrying organisms.
7. Aeration to remove odors and gases, as well as to control organisms.
8. Disposal of waste sludge that has been removed from the treated water.

Each of these steps will be discussed in more detail in the following material.

Sedimentation. The first step that must be taken in the treatment of water either from a source or as waste water from processes is to remove the large solids in suspension in the water. This step is accomplished through the use of sedimentation.

In the sedimentation process, large solids settle out of the water if an adequate time period is available for such settling to occur. Often this settling is accomplished by providing settling ponds, lakes, or tanks where the waste water or source water is pumped and held for a period of time.

As the water remains in these holding areas, the large solids tend to settle to the bottom of the storage area. Water is then removed from the surface of the tank for further treatment.

Settled sludge in the holding area must be removed occasionally or it will clog the holding tank or pond. In the case of a pond, periodic draining and removal of the sludge by bulldozers is necessary. Holding tanks often have sloping bottoms and are equipped with slowly rotating blades to push the sludge to the center where a small stream of water washes the sludge away.

In some cases, particularly in a municipal waste water plant, it is necessary to remove certain large solids such as waste paper, cans, etc., before further processing. In order to accomplish this, an initial screening removes the large solids, which, if allowed to continue through the system, might quickly clog the holding ponds or settling tanks.

Control of pH. The second step in the water treatment process is the control of the pH level of the water. This process step may be accomplished either before or after sedimentation. In general, pH control involves the treatment of highly acid water entering the treatment plant. This acid water must be neutralized in order to remove the potential for damage to piping and other equipment within the treatment plant. For this reason, pH control is often the first step in waste water treatment.

pH control for acid water is accomplished by adding alkali to the effluent. The most commonly used alkali additives are caustic soda, quicklime or sodium phosphate. These chemicals act to neutralize the acid in the water.

In many cases, pH control is required before waste water leaves an industrial plant to enter a municipal system. The municipal system will specify this control in order to protect the waste water collection piping system from potential damage.

Coagulation and Flocculation. The process of sedimentation removes large solids from the water being treated. However, many of the solids present within the water are so small that an extremely long period of time would be required for them to settle out. To remove these suspended solids, an approach is used to speed up the settling of the smaller solids.

The process of coagulation or destabilization which involves the addition of a chemical agent to cause the small solids to stick together to form larger solids, is used to accomplish this sedimentation. Small solids that have not precipitated during the original sedimentation process and which remain in suspension must be removed. The coagulant causes an electric or interionic force which makes the small particles of solids adhere when they come in contact with one another. Thus, larger solids are formed by the destabilization process.

Coagulation is a fast chemical process, and as a result rapid agitation is desirable during this phase of treatment to increase the potential contact of

the small particles with one another. A common coagulant that can be added to
the water being treated is alum, or aluminum salts.

Flocculation or conglomeration is the physical process in which the
particles become enmeshed with one another. In general, this process is a
slower process than coagulation. A gentle mixing or agitation over a longer
period of time is necessary to cause the solids to group together or
conglomerate. As the solids conglomerate, even larger particles are formed.
As the particles become larger, the probability of settling is increased.

Figure 8.1.2

Coagulation-flocculation.

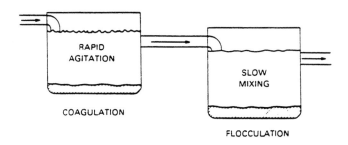

Generally, two tanks are used in the coagulation-flocculation process.
The first tank, or the coagulant tank, introduces a high agitation to the
water being treated as the destabilizer or coagulant is added. The water
being treated remains in this tank for only a short period of time. Thesecond
tank, the flocculation tank, involves a gentle mixing of the water over a
longer period of time to allow for conglomeration and settling to occur.

Filtration. After the conglomeration-flocculation process is completed,
it is often necessary to treat the water further to remove suspended solids.
In those cases where such further treatment is necessary, a filtration process
is used. The filters used consist of sand and gravel beds. Coarse gravel is
placed at the bottom of the filter, with finer mesh gravel and sand layers
used to build up the filter. The finest sand is used on the top layer. As
the water flows through this filter, the filter removes small suspended
solids. As the filter is used, it begins to load up with solids and the flow
of water through the filter slows. However, as the filter loads it becomes
more efficient and more solids are removed. Finally, the flow of water through
the filter slows to the point that the filter must be cleaned in order to
maintain the ability of the plant to treat a sufficient amount of water.

In order to remove the solids built up with the filter, it is necessary to
wash it. This washing is accomplished through the use of a backwash. Washing
must take place before the filter becomes clogged or before a break through
the fine layers can occur. Proper washing of a sand and gravel filter is

important to maintain the efficient flow and odor control function of the filtering process. Without proper washing, the probability of solids breaking through the upper layers of fine sand increases. When such a breakthrough occurs, the water being treated has direct access to the more coarse layers and fewer solids are removed.

Figure 8.1.3

Filtration.

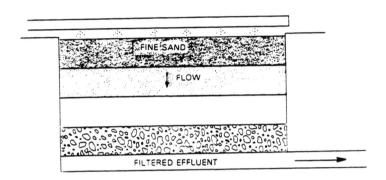

Bacterial Digestion. Even after processing to remove large suspended solids, it is often necessary to include a step to remove organic solids that still may exist in the water. This is accomplished by bacterial digestion. In this process step, bacteria feed on the organic solids in the water, yielding carbon dioxide and proteins. The bacteria themselves need oxygen, a controlled temperature, and food (sludge) to live.

Two types of bacterial digestion systems are used. The first is an anaerobic process in which the oxygen supply is obtained from the materials in the sludge. Anaerobic digestion often occurs at the bottom of a settling pond. The second type is an aerobic process which uses oxygen supplied by the air. The aerobic process is accomplished by aerating the settling tanks and is faster than an anaerobic process. The aerobic process is often used when the organic load within the waste water is low.

Often, the waste water treatment process involves either an aerobic system or an anaerobic system followed by an aerobic system.

In conjunction with bacterial digestion, settling tanks are often used. These tanks utilize skimmers to remove floating solids and to clarify the waste water. The settling tanks provide for control of the system by removal of excess bacteria in order that the digestion system does not become overpopulated.

Control of Disease-Causing Organisms. If the water is to be used for a potable supply, it is necessary to control any disease-causing organisms that may be present in the water supply. This is accomplished by the addition of chemicals that can kill the various organisms present. The most commonly used chemical in this case is chlorine. Chlorine is added to the water to provide both an immediate organism kill and a residual effect as the water is either stored for use in a potable water supply system or returned to the source.

Some other methods of disinfection have been tried and are used in particular cases. These include the use of ultraviolet light, heat, metal ions (silver), iodine, and ozone. In general, however, chlorine remains the most commonly used method for the control of disease-causing organisms.

Aeration. Aeration of the water being treated may be accomplished at various stages of the treatment. The purpose of aeration is to add oxygen and some other gases to the water. In addition, it can help to remove some of the gases that build-up during the treatment process, including carbon dioxide, hydrogen sulfide, and methane.

Various types of aerators are used. In some cases, a spray type aerator, in which the water is sprayed into the air in fine droplets, is used. Other methods include the waterfall and the multi-tray waterfall aerator. Finally, air may be introduced or bubbled into the treated water, as is often done during the bacterial digestion process.

If aeration is performed indoors, a potential hazard exists. The waste gases that are removed from the water during aeration (CO_2, H_2, and CH_4) can build up within a confined area. In order to remove these gases, it is necessary that adequate ventilation be provided to the enclosed area to prevent such a buildup from occurring.

Removal of Waste Sludge. The suspended solids removed from the water being treated result in a sludge that gathers at the bottom of the water treatment tanks of ponds. It is necessary to dispose of this sludge. Obviously this cannot be done by washing the sludge into the water source, since the treatment was performed to remove the sludge in the first place.

There are essentially two methods that can be used for removal of the waste sludge. The first method is incineration of the sludge. The second method is to remove the sludge to a landfill. In either case, it is necessary to remove excess water before the disposal of the sludge in order that a smaller volume is handled. Some potential does exist for reclamation of energy in a large industrial or municipal waste treatment plant by the incineration of the sludge. Incineration not only produces heat as well as various chemicals in the waste gases that may be potential energy, but also it has the advantage of reducing the volume of the sludge. Thus, a smaller quantity of sludge in the form of fly ash must be disposed of using the landfill process.

Other Water Treatment. In addition to the above general unit processes, it is necessary in some cases to provide special additives to water prior to its use. For example, in the case of general industrial process use of water it is often necessary to provide wetting agents and decalcifiers to the water before use in the process. In municipal water supply systems that treat water to obtain a potable supply, fluoridation is often performed. Salt is often added to industrial water supplies, especially in areas of thermal stress.

Thermal Pollution

Often during an industrial process heat is added to the water. This heat becomes a pollutant and can cause environmental damage if hot waste water is returned to a natural source. Among the effects of thermal pollution are:

1. An increased odor of organic materials in the waste water.
2. Potential failure of subsequent waste water treatment, particularly that of bacterial digestion.
3. An increased growth of algae in the natural source.
4. Potential harm to marine life in the natural water source.
5. A lack of dissolved oxygen in the heated water.

Two major methods of control can be used to remove the thermal pollution before entry to the natural source. These are the cooling tower and the spray pond.

The cooling tower is the most common method for removal of thermal pollution. In a cooling tower, water is pumped to the top of a tower and allowed to fall in a spray or a sheet of water through the tower. The tower contains baffles or decks that break the flow of water into smaller droplets. A source of upward motion of air through either natural draft or as a result of a fan drawing air through the tower at the top is available. The heat in the water is exchanged to the air through the evaporative cooling process.

The cooling tower is not without its problems. The evaporative cooling process produces a fog in the vicinity of the tower. If the water contains pollutants that are hazardous, these pollutants will be present in the fog. The effect of wind on the movement of the fog is termed "drift." This drift

Figure 8.1.4

Cooling tower.

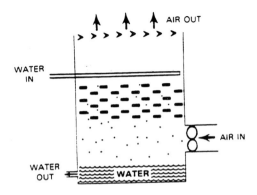

can cause fog to move away from the cooling tower to the surrounding area. If the fog contains hazardous pollutants, these pollutants can affect the health of those living in the vicinity of the cooling tower. Thus, pollutants that are hazardous should be removed from the water prior to cooling in a cooling tower.

Cross Connection of Water Sources

Within an industrial plant, various sources of water may be used. A potable water supply is necessary for drinking as well as for use in products that will be consumed by humans. Water must be supplied for cooling of hot industrial processes. Water is also used for fire protection within the industrial plant. If water conservation is practiced, water will be recycled from process to process. Finally, when the water becomes so contaminated it can no longer be used, the waste water must be disposed of by removing this waste water to a treatment facility. Each of these various uses of water requires a distribution system between the source and areas of the plant. As a result, large quantities of water distribution piping are required. Unless precautions are taken, inadvertent cross connection of water sources can occur. This may result in the misuse of water containing hazardous contaminants.

One method for controlling water distribution to prevent the cross connection of sources is to label each of the distribution pipes as to the type of water that it carries. In addition, piping layouts that are properly labeled should be prepared and consulted when any connections are to be made.

In some cases it is desirable to have cross connection of sources. In a case where it is necessary to add makeup water to recycled water, a cross connection must be provided. Where it is necessary to connect the public water supply to a plant to provide for additional water which may be needed, a cross connection will be present. In these cases certain precautions must be taken in order to assure that the cross connection does not result in contamination of the source of cleaner water.

Contamination from such a cross connection can occur when a back pressure is developed that causes the contaminated water to flow back into the public water supply system. This back pressure can be as a result of many different causes. For example, a reduced pressure in one of the public water supply lines can result in contaminated water flowing from a higher pressure area back through the public water system. This reduced pressure can be a result of an interrupted supply, an excessive demand, a break in the public water supply lines, freezing, or improper sizing of the piping.

In order to control cross connections, it is necessary that the industrial hygiene engineer take certain precautionary steps. All piping should be reviewed for existing cross connections. Where possible, these cross connections should be eliminated.

A method for control is to use a movable connection when the supply of clean water must not be directly connected at all times. Thus, when required, the movable connection can be attached to the source of potable water. Additionally, vacuum breakers and backflow preventers may be installed in the clean water supply line as an additional protection.

Control of Hazardous Materials in Water Treatment

The industrial hygiene engineer should be aware of the fact that some of the chemicals that are used in water treatment can be hazardous to the health of the workers exposed to them. For example, chlorine is well known as a hazardous chemical. The potential exposure to these hazardous chemicals of workers within the water treatment facility must be controlled.

The following table presents a selected list of chemicals used in the various water treatment processes. Special handling materials, threshold limit values, and flammable properties are indicated for these chemicals.

Table 8.1.1

Selected chemicals used in coagulation.

Name	Formula	Form	Handling	TLV	Flam.
Aluminum	$Al_2(SO_4)_3 \bullet 14H_2O$	Powder, lump, granular	dry—iron, steel; liquid—leadlined rubber, silicon asphalt, 316 stainless steel	Undetermined	—
Ammonium Aluminum Sulfate	$Al_2(SO_4)_3(NH_4)_2$ $SO_4 \bullet 24H_2O$	Powder, lump nut, pea	dureron, lead, rubber, silicon iron, stonewall	—	—
Bentonite	Colloidal Clay	Powder, pellet	iron, steel	Undetermined	—
Ferric Chloride	$FeCl_3$ $FeCl_3 \bullet 6H_2O$	Liquid, lump powder	glass, rubber, stoneware, synthetic resins	Undetermined	—
Ferric Sulfate	$Fe_2(SO_4)_3 \bullet 9H_2O$	Crystal, granule lump	ceramics, lead, plastic, rubber, 18—8 stainless steel	—	—

Table 8.1.1 (Continued)

Name	Formula	Form	Handling	TLV	Flam.
Potassium Aluminum Sulfate	$K_2SO_4AL(SO_4)_3\bullet$ 24 H_2O	Powder, lump, granule	lead, leadlined rubber, stone-ware	--	--
Anhydrous Ammonia	NH_3	Gas	glass, nickel, steel	25 ppm	yes
Chlorine	Cl_2	Liquified gas	glass, hard rubber, silver	1 ppm	yes
Ozone	O_3	Gas	aluminum, cera-mics, iron, steel, wood	.1 ppm	--
Chloride Dioxide	ClO_2	Gas	plastic, soft rubber	.1 ppm	--
Sulfur Dioxide	SO_2	Gas	aluminum, brass, 316 stainless steel	5 ppm	--

Selected chemicals for pH control.

Name	Formula	Form	Handling	TLV	Flam.
Disodium Phosphate	$Na_2HPO_4\bullet12H_2O$	Crystal	cast iron, steel	—	--
Sodium Hydroxide	NaOH	Liquid, flake, lump	cast iron, rubber, steel	$.2mg/m^3$	--
Sulfuric Acid	H_2SO_4	Liquid	iron, steel	$1mg/m^3$	--
Trisodium Phosphate	$Na_3PO_4\bullet12H_2O$	Crystal	cast iron, steel	--	--

Summary

The treatment of water both prior to use in an industrial plant and after use to remove waste before entry into a natural water source is important in the industrial process. Without proper treatment of the water supply or waste water effluent, potential hazards are introduced to the work and community environments. The industrial hygiene engineer must be aware of the appropriate steps that should be taken to control this potential hazard. Assurance that proper treatment of waste water is occurring is an important part of the industrial hygiene engineer's job. In addition, the industrial hygiene engineer must be aware of any potential hazards that are introduced to the workers within the plant as a result of poor water quality or the contamination of potable water with a contaminated water supply through cross connection of sources.

2. Control of Solid Waste

Introduction

In the "throw-away" age in which we live, the disposal of solid waste has become a major problem. It is a problem not only at the consumer level but also at the industrial level. The manufacturing process creates a significant amount of waste as a by-product of production. This waste must be removed from the process area and must be disposed of in some manner. The method of removal can create potential problems both in terms of the cost of removal and in terms of the potential health hazards present in waste materials of a hazardous nature. In addition, there is a further problem in terms of the environmental pollution that results from improper disposal of waste materials.

Solid waste has become a problem of such magnitude in industry that it can no longer be treated lightly. It is necessary that a complete program be developed to remove solid wastes from the production area and dispose of them in a nonpolluting and safe manner. The industrial hygiene engineer, because of his responsibilities for the health and safety of the worker and the community environment, must take an active part in such a solid waste disposal program.

The Objectives of a Solid Waste Disposal Program

The first objective of a solid waste disposal program is to dispose of the solid waste in such a manner that it does not cause a potential health hazard. In many cases the type of solid waste that is generated from the industrial process includes hazardous materials that are toxic to humans and animals. The method of disposal of the solid waste used must consider the effects of these toxic materials on the workers and the surrounding community. If the waste is allowed to build up in the production area or if appropriate measures are not taken to protect workers while removing the waste from the production area, the potential for exposure exists. Once the waste reaches its final destination, be that a landfill, incineration process, etc., the possibility exists for exposure to the surrounding community unless precautionary measures are taken.

The second objective of a solid waste disposal program is to dispose of the solid waste in such a manner that the effect on the environment is minimized. In today's society we must live with the fact that solid wastes are generated and that the environmental impact cannot be totally eliminated. The solid wastes must be disposed of in some manner, and the potential for harm to the environment does exist. However, all attempts should be made to minimize any harmful effects on the environment through the use of appropriate disposal methods.

The third objective of a solid waste disposal program is <u>to dispose of the solid waste in such a manner that the maximum utility and conservation of the waste is obtained before disposal</u>. Solid wastes from production processes often include valuable materials that are extracted during the production process. In a world of limited resources, the disposal of valuable materials as solid waste can be very costly. The decision to extract valuable materials from the waste before disposal is, in fact, an economic decision. In many cases the economics of extraction result in the disposal of valuable materials rather than performing a costly process to recover them.

The fourth objective of a solid waste disposal program is <u>to dispose of the solid waste in such a manner that the economic cost is minimized</u>. Handling and disposal costs of solid waste are high and must be incurred by industry to remove the waste from the production area. However, efficient methods can be utilized to dispose of solid wastes in such a manner as to minimize costs. In addition, reclamation costs for valuable materials contained in the waste being disposed of are important, as was mentioned previously.

The Sources of Industrial Waste

Now, let us look at the various industrial processes to identify the types of industrial waste that are generated by each process.

Raw Material Extraction. First, consider the raw material extraction process. Raw material extraction involves such industries as mining, lumber, agriculture, and fishing. In this type of industry the basic raw materials are obtained from the environment. As a by-product of the extraction process, massive amounts of waste products are generated since only a small part of the material extracted is usable. This waste or unwanted material must be properly disposed.

Consider deep mining, for example. In the mining process it is necessary to remove large amounts of rock and soil from the face of the mine through tunnels to the surface before the raw material—coal, salt, etc.,—can be reached. The removal of this rock and soil creates a significant amount of solid waste that must be disposed of so that it does not have a harmful effect on the environment. The cost of solid waste removal is significant in this case.

Another raw material extraction industry that has had great success in reclaiming waste products is the lumber industry. In the lumber industry today significant use is made of sawdust, chips, bark, and other wood products that are by-products of the lumber mill operations. Chip board, fiber board, and paper are manufactured from these waste materials.

Agriculture generates plant and animal waste, which, though organic, must be disposed of in some manner. A particular problem exists when animal wastes contain disease-causing bacteria which, unless properly controlled, can spread to the surrounding community.

Process Industries. A second type of industry in which solid waste products are generated is the process industry. In the process industry, basic raw materials are converted into usable products that may or may not require further processing. Included in the process industry grouping are chemical manufacture, basic iron and steel, plastics, oil refining, paper, paper, food processing, and power production. Process industries generate waste during the processing of materials into a usable form.

Figure 8.2.1

Extraction waste.

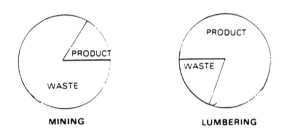

MINING   LUMBERING

An example of the waste that is generated from a process industry is the slag that results from iron and steel production. This slag is of significant quantity and has created significant disposal problems. Another example of solid waste generated is the particulate matter that are removed from air during an air cleaning operation. The collected particles must be disposed of properly. This problem can be particularly difficult if the particles are hazardous to the worker or the surrounding community.

One particular problem that is noteworthy is the need to dispose of spent fuel rods from nuclear power plants. This represents one of the most difficult solid waste disposal problems. Because of the long half-life of plutonium, the danger from such fuel rods is such that long-term protection must be provided.

Manufacturing and Assembly. Manufacturing and assembly involves the conversion of processed materials into usable products. Typical manufacturing and assembly industries include milling and machining, assembly operations, soft goods production, and construction.

In general, the waste products that are generated in the manufacturing and assembly process are a result of trimming and machining loss from materials and parts used in the assembly and manufacture of the usable end product. In addition, airborne particulates can occur as a result of milling and machining. Excess materials from the construction industry present a significant disposal problem for this industry. Observation of the waste material surrounding a newly constructed building provides an idea of the magnitude of this problem.

Packaging. Packaging can occur at any transfer point between the various stages of the production process, as well as at the final point of distribution to the consumer. As a result, packaging waste is a major problem. At each step in the production process materials that have been transferred from one industry to another and that are packaged must be opened and the packaging must be properly disposed. The packaging normally serves no useful function other protection of the product. When this protection is no longer needed the packaging is discarded, creating a major solid waste disposal problem.

Consumer Use. Finally, once the product has reached the consumer and has served its useful life, the product itself becomes waste material and is discarded. There has been a definite trend in society to move towards the disposable consumer product. Witness the development of the disposable razor, plastic cups, paper plates, throw-away pens, etc. In addition, the products seem to have a shorter lifetime in the hands of the consumer. This is perhaps a result of the desire of the consumer to upgrade to new and more modern products.

The cost of properly disposing of this waste material is significant. And the problems encountered are staggering. How do we remove and dispose of automobiles once their useful life has been reached? How can this be accomplished without adversely affecting the environment? The automobile graveyard or junkyard is probably one of the worst eyesores that modern technology has produced.

Society has only begun to face the problems involved with the disposal of solid wastes generated. The solutions are not easily found, and the costs are high.

Solid Waste Disposal Methods

There are essentially three methods that are available for the disposal of solid waste. These methods are:

1. Sanitary landfill
2. Incineration
3. Recycling

None of these methods is entirely satisfactory and without major problems. Let's look at each method in some detail to identify the problems that result from the use of that method.

Sanitary Landfill. Consider the sanitary landfill. Because of the need for large areas of available land and because of pressures exerted by the community, sanitary landfills are usually located at some distance from the plant facility. As a result, the transfer of solid waste to the sanitary landfill is time consuming and costly.

In many industrial areas, land is a scarce resource. It is difficult to find appropriate land areas that are satisfactory for the operation of a

sanitary landfill. Location is important. The landfill must be in such an
area that the drainage away from the fill can be controlled to prevent
contamination of nearby water resources or undue environmental damage to the
local ecology.

The sanitary landfill is built in layers. Generally, a large valley or
open pit mine area is filled with layers of solid waste and soil materials by
means of a bulldozer. In this way, the solid waste material is sandwiched
between the earth layers. Generally, the waste collected in a given day is
covered by about six inches of compacted soil.

Figure 8.2.2

Landfill design.

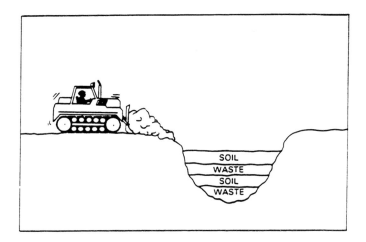

Toxic and radioactive solid waste presents a particular problem when using
a sanitary landfill. The potential for drain-off into surrounding water
sources can result in an exposure to the general population. In such cases
special care must be taken to provide protection to the general public. Toxic
materials and radioactive materials should be encased in containers to protect
against the potential for the materials to leak out into the surrounding
environment. In the special case of radioactive material, the selection of
the area must consider the geological structure and the potential for
earthquakes. Selection of such areas has been a major problem in determining
locations for the disposal of spent nuclear fuel rods. Potential locations
for the disposal of waste with toxic or hazardous properties are in abandoned
deep pit mines or caves.

Incineration. A second method for disposal of solid waste is through the
use of incineration. The objective of incineration is to reduce the volume of
the material that requires disposal. Incineration can also destroy some of
the potentially dangerous materials included in the solid waste.

However, a trade-off occurs during the incineration process. Potentially hazardous materials that are burned may contaminate the surrounding air. Thus, it is important that the emissions from an incineration system be controlled. Various types of air cleaners are required to remove particulates and gases resulting from the incineration process, significantly increasing the cost for this method of disposal. However, as sanitary landfills become more difficult to find and are located at greater distances from the plant, incineration becomes a more viable approach.

After the incineration process, the residual ash from incineration must be removed in some manner. Generally, the hazardous materials that may have been included in the original waste product have been destroyed at this point. The residual ash can then be transported to a landfill. Though the landfill is still required, the volume reduction that is obtained is such that the cost of transport is significantly lower.

Recycling. The third method available for the disposal of solid wastes is to recycle the solid waste in some manner to obtain any residual value from the materials. Waste products often contain valuable materials. If these materials can be extracted from the waste product at a low cost, the problem of solid waste removal is lessened. However, in many cases extraction can be difficult and costly. In such cases, the economics do not justify recycling, and solid waste disposal using alternate procedures results in the lowest cost.

As the cost of raw materials continues to increase, recycling becomes more attractive. Research is being conducted into the potential for recycling solid wastes that are being disposed of in a municipal system. Consideration is being given to the use of the combustion gases as well as the heat generated. Solid waste incineration may provide a potential energy source for the production of electric power in the future. As the price of oil and other natural resources increases, these alternatives may become economically feasible.

If waste recycling is to be successful, it is important to consider it in the initial product and process design. Perhaps the product can be designed in such a manner that recycling is simple to achieve. For example, consider the processing of a hazardous material. The hazardous material presents a potential danger to those required to handle it. The packaging of the hazardous material, which must be disposed of, will retain a residual quantity of the hazardous material.

One industry that continually faces the problem of solid waste disposal is the beverage container industry. Various attempts have been made to recycle containers. Glass containers, on which a redeemable deposit has been obtained, have always been used in the beverage industry. However, with the advent of the throw-away can, the waste problem has become more difficult. Some container manufacturers have offered a reward for the return of aluminum cans. This approach has met with mixed success.

Grinding-Compaction. When the landfill approach is used, a potential method for the reduction of the volume of material that must be transported to the landfill is to compact or grind the waste. Compaction reduces the volume but does not change the form of the waste material. Grinding reduces the volume and changes the form, generally to a slurry. Water is added to the waste being ground to form the slurry.

Certain advantages can be gained within the plant by using the grinding-slurry approach. The solid waste materials, after grinding and formation of the slurry, can be transported from one area of the plant to another in a sluice or in pipes, thus lowering the cost of the removal of waste materials from the original source. Water can be extracted at the destination point, and the sludge can be incinerated or carried to a landfill. Nongrindable materials must be removed in the normal fashion. This approach is applicable for certain types of waste, particularly those of an organic nature.

Meeting the Objectives of a Solid Waste Disposal Program

You will remember that the objectives stated at the beginning of this chapter for a solid waste disposal program were (1) the disposal of materials in such a manner as to eliminate potential health hazards; (2) the disposal of materials in such a manner as to minimize the effect on the environment; (3) the disposal of solid waste in such a manner as to obtain maximum utility and conservation of waste; and (4) the disposal of solid waste in such a manner as to minimize the economic cost of waste removal.

There is no easy answer by which attainment of the objectives stated above can be accomplished in a solid waste disposal program. The objectives in many cases compete with one another. To meet one objective completely may have a negative effect on another objective.

Since solid waste is a necessary by-product of most, if not all, of our modern production processes, we must face the problem of providing for its disposal in order to maximize the attainment of each of the objectives. A viable solid waste disposal program will attempt to meet each objective rather than maximizing one at the expense of the others. A system that minimizes the economic cost of waste removal by dumping the waste into an area, thus presenting a potential health hazard to the surrounding community, does not obtain the desired results. How can a viable solid waste management program be designed?

When designing a solid waste disposal system that will protect workers and the surrounding community from potential exposure to hazardous materials, the designer must consider not only the end destination of the solid waste, but also the method and route of transport. In removing the solid waste from the source through the plant and community to its final destination, the potential for exposure exists. Controls must be in force that prevent accidents or other occurrences from resulting in exposure to the hazardous waste material.

A second health hazard that must be considered is the potential air pollution that results from incineration. If the solid waste contains toxic material, the potential for this toxic material to be transferred to the air as a particulate or gas exists during incineration. Appropriate air cleaning equipment must be installed to remove these hazardous materials before the waste gases are dumped into the environment.

As has been discussed previously, the landfill method of disposal has the problem of protecting the general public from hazards as a result of drainage from the landfill. In addition, the potential development of disease organisms and rodent population at the site of the landfill may occur. This is particularly the case when it is necessary to dispose of nontoxic organic substances. Rodents and insects in the vicinity of the landfill can carry the disease-causing organisms to the general public unless proper controls are in place.

Public health agencies are charged with the control of waste disposal to promote this objective. These agencies are faced with a difficult job. It is impossible for agency workers to cover all potential problem areas. As a result, potential exposures can go unnoticed and uncorrected.

What is the responsibility of industry in this situation? Is it the responsibility of industry to protect the public health without governmental intervention? Will industry accept such a responsibility? Consider the recent incidences involving the disposal of waste products containing materials such as kepone and PCB's. Consider the problems that have resulted from acid mine drainage and the disposable beverage containers. These cases seem to indicate the need for some governmental intervention.

Although the cost of solid waste disposal to industry is great, the cost to the general public and the economy may be even greater. Since it is a difficult job to enforce regulations controlling the method of solid waste disposal, industry must assume responsibility in this matter. Although this objective is not easily met, industry must continue to develop and implement methods that are satisfactory in terms of protection of the health of workers and the general population, while at the same time minimizing the costs of solid waste disposal.

The second objective is to minimize the harmful effects on the environment. In this objective, the same dilemma exists in terms of the responsibility for the environment. Is it industry's job to police itself so as not to cause damage to the environment? Is it the job of governmentalagencies to enact and enforce environmental standards for industry? Again, ideally industry should police itself. The need for governmental control exists for those few individuals who would minimize the cost of handling solid waste at the expense of the environment and the health and safety of workers and the community.

The long-term effects of the environment should be considered as a part of the solid waste disposal system. Continual dumping of solid waste into the environment will, at some point, cause ecological damage. Though this may not occur in our lifetimes, we as citizens have a responsibility to future generations to provide a reasonably balanced ecological system.

This problem becomes even more acute when one considers the multitude of consumer products that are discarded after their useful life. Is industry responsible for the ultimate disposal of the product once it has reached the consumer? If so, how can the product be designed to provide for disposal that minimizes harmful effects on the environment?

The first problem that is encountered when one considers the attainment of the third objective--that is, utilizing and conserving valuable materials within waste products--is the fact that the cost to recycle or extract the products is high. However, this problem may be of lesser significance in the future as the natural resources that are available to our civilization become more scarce. As these natural resources become in short supply, it becomes more attractive to recycle or recover resources from solid waste. Perhaps in the future more efforts will be made to utilize and conserve valuable materials within solid waste products because of this situation.

The final objective is to minimize the cost of waste disposal. Waste disposal introduces a cost that must be borne by the industry. Industry wishes to maintain the lowest cost of disposal possible since this will impact on profits. In many cases, the lowest cost is to dump the materials into an uncontrolled landfill. However, this approach may result in the highest cost to the public.

Since industry management is responsible to its stockholders first in terms of maximizing profits and since the cost of waste removal lowers profits or increases production cost, it is unlikely that, unless economic incentives are available, industry on the whole will act responsibly to dispose of solid waste products. However, industry does have a responsibility to the community in which it lives. Poor practices may increase long-term costs involving land and wasted resources. The public relations of the industry within the local community may be harmed by irresponsible dumping. These poor public relations may in turn affect product sales which ultimately affects profits. Ideally, then, such a system would be self-policing. However, such is not always the case. The responsibility for enforcement, then, must lie with governmental agencies. Where costs do not justify responsible action on the part of industry, perhaps governmental incentives can be utilized to provide for such responsible action without affecting the profits of the industry.

Summary

The problems involving solid waste disposal are many and difficult to solve. Industry has a responsibility to protect the health of the worker and general public during and after disposal of waste products. Its responsibility also exists in terms of the effect of solid waste disposal on the environment. With natural resources becoming in short supply, industry must also assume some responsibility for conserving those valuable resources that can be extracted from materials which are currently being treated as waste materials. Finally, the cost of waste disposal can detrimentally affect profits and, as a result, management must select that method that results in the lowest cost while still attaining the objectives of protection of the health, environment, and conservation of natural resources.

3. Purchase, Handling, and Storage of Hazardous Materials

Introduction

What are hazardous materials? For the purposes of this discussion, hazardous materials will be considered to be any materials that can have an injurious effect on the health of the worker or that can result in a potential fire or explosion. The injurious effect of the materials may be either acute or chronic. A chronic effect is one in which a long period of exposure is necessary before injury to the functioning of the worker's physiological system results. For example, chlorine gas results in an acute effect to the worker while exposure to silica has a chronic effect.

The effects of the hazardous materials may range from relatively minor damage to the employee's health to extreme injury or death. For example, exposure to a particular hazardous chemical may result in a condition of dermatitis that is relatively minor. On the other hand, certain chemicals have been shown to be carcinogenic after prolonged exposure of the worker to them.

For purposes of this discussion, flammable or explosive materials have been included in the category of hazardous materials. In this case the hazard is not to the employee's health but to his safety as a result of the potential for fire and explosion.

Hazardous materials may take many forms. In some cases the hazardous material may be in the form of a liquid, such as carbon tetrachloride or other similar solvents. In other cases the hazardous material may be in the form of a solid, such as asbestos, silica, and radioactive material. The exposure to the solid may be as a result of the solid itself, in the case of a radioactive source; or it may be as a result of particulate matter that is generated during the processing of a solid, as in the case of asbestos and silica. Finally, the hazardous material may be gaseous in nature, such as methane, carbon monoxide, and chlorine.

The form in which the material is used will, to a great extent, dictate the handling and storage methods that are used. If the material is in the form of a solid, it is more likely that workers will come in direct contact with it during handling and transfer than if the material is in the form of a liquid or a gas. Liquids and gases are generally handled in closed systems which present a different type of exposure problem than that which is encountered when handling solid materials.

When considering the protection of workers from toxic and flammable material, it is necessary to determine the level of toxicity or flammability of the material. This level dictates the care that must be exercised in handling and storing particular materials. The more toxic or flammable the material, the more necessary it is to take precautions to protect the worker.

One of the major problems is the identification of potentially hazardous materials prior to exposure. This is not an easy task. A multitude of chemicals and chemical compounds are used in industry today. New chemicals and compounds are being introduced each day, either as a result of the process or as input into the process. Many of these compounds contain toxic or flammable materials that are not identified specifically. In addition, chemical manufacturers use a multitude of brand names that tend to obscure the fact that particular toxic substances are present.

Areas for Control of Hazardous Materials

Exposure to hazardous materials can occur at many points within an industrial operation. If the plant operation is divided into major functional areas, the significant operations involving potential exposure of workers to hazardous materials can be identified. The major functional areas are:

1. Entry to the plant.
2. Handling and movement within the plant.
3. Storage within the plant.
4. Use in plant processes.
5. Waste products generated from the process.

The first place to identify and control hazardous materials is at the entry to the plant. If hazardous materials are not identified at their entry point, control is difficult if not impossible. Therefore, the industrialhygiene engineer must determine at what point a hazardous material first enters the plant and, starting at that point, identify those areas and operations where potential exposure of the workers may be possible. Often hazardous materials are identified within the process and appropriate action for control is taken, while at the same time little concern is given for the initial handling and storage of these hazardous materials prior to their use in the process. If the material comes in by railroad tank car, care must be taken to assure that the transfer of the material from the tank car to internal storage or to the process is accomplished with a minimum of exposure to the worker.

Once the material has been transferred into the plant, the next potential exposure may occur during the handling and movement of the material within the plant itself. This is a most difficult area to control since during handling and movement in the plant a large number of workers are potentially exposed. As the material moves through the work area either in a solid, liquid or gaseous form, in tanks, carts, pipes, etc., the potential for accidental exposure exists. Particularly crucial are the transfer points where the material moves from storage to the material handling system and from the material handling system to storage or to the process itself. The probabilit of exposure at these points is significantly higher than at any other point within the material handling system in the plant.

The third major area of potential exposure to hazardous materials is in the storage areas for the materials. On the surface, storage of hazardous materials seems to be a relatively safe operation with little chance for exposure. However, even in storage, materials can present a potential hazard. Awareness of the potential danger is particularly important since a problem that develops in storage is likely to go unnoticed unless a positive action is taken to identify such potential exposures. Leaks in tanks, side-by-side storage of incompatible materials, overcrowded storage conditions, and other such factors can result in a potential exposure to workers in the plant.

Much of the emphasis of industrial hygiene is on the control of hazardous materials during process use. Obviously this is an important area for control since a number of workers may be exposed unless the proper precautions are taken. The major control of process exposures involving hazardous materials is accomplished through the use of local exhaust ventilation or general dilution ventilation. In terms of process control, the industrial hygiene engineer must be aware of the fact that it is possible that chemical changes will occur within the process. These chemical changes can result in in-process materials that may, in fact, not be known or identified and that may be potentially hazardous to the workers. It is important to be aware of this potential and take appropriate action to identify those materials that are generated in-process and that may be hazardous to the health of the worker.

Another area where potential exposure to hazardous materials can occur is in the removal of waste products resulting from the process. The process may convert harmless materials into hazardous waste. As has been previously discussed, these waste products cannot be dumped into the environment. Control is necessary to protect the environment and the workers from exposure to hazardous waste materials during handling and at the final point of disposition. The industrial hygiene engineer must be aware of the hazards that are a result of the removal and disposition of waste products and must take action to protect both the workers and the general public from exposure to such materials.

Finally, the product that is being produced must be considered. If there is a potential hazard involved with the product, this must be considered in terms of the shipment, handling, and ultimate use of the product. Care must be taken to assure protection of workers involved in transport and handling of potentially hazardous products. Also, the consumer of the product must be made aware of any dangers and precautions that should be taken concerning the use of the product. Product specification data should be supplied to the user.

The Purchase of Hazardous Materials

As was discussed above, the initial point at which exposure to hazardous materials must be controlled is upon entry to the plant. In order to identify hazardous materials upon entry to the plant and to provide for adequate

controls, it is necessary that these materials be known prior to their entry
The logical point to identify hazardous materials prior to entry is at the
point of purchase of the materials. If the industrial hygiene engineer is
aware that a hazardous material has been purchased and will be entering the
plant, then appropriate plans can be made and controls instituted to protect
plant personnel involved in handling and using the product from its first
entry to the plant. Obviously, the industrial hygiene engineer cannot provi
such protection if he or she is not aware that a problem exists.

As a result, it is necessary that the industrial hygiene engineer work
closely with the purchasing agent to develop procedures to handle the purcha
of hazardous materials. In order to accomplish this, it may be necessary to
educate the purchasing agent concerning the problems encountered when handli
and using hazardous materials and the need for control of exposures to these
materials. If a working relationship can be developed between the industria
hygiene engineer and the purchasing agent to identify hazardous materials at
the point of purchase, then the job of controlling exposures to the material
becomes much simpler.

Procedures should be developed to identify the responsibilities of both
the purchasing agent and the industrial hygiene engineer. These procedures
should identify the action that the purchasing agent should take when a
request for the purchase of a new material is made. It may be possible that
the purchasing agent can determine the potential hazards involved with the
material. Or it may be necessary that requests for the purchase of new
materials pass to the industrial hygiene engineer for identification of
potential hazards that may result from the handling, storage, and use of the
material. In any case, these procedures need to be clearly outlined and
followed.

The objective of such a system is to identify the hazardous materials
prior to purchase and entry to the plant. This allows the industrial hygien
engineer to exercise the maximum freedom in providing controls for the
protection of the worker. It may be possible that substitution of a less
hazardous material can be made that will accomplish the same result as the
hazardous material. The industrial hygiene engineer can take action to
develop procedures to be used to control the materials before they enter the
plant, during the transfer to plant storage, and in the production process.
Without such prior identification of hazardous materials, the probability of
exposure to the workers is greatly increased.

In many cases, potential hazards involved with the material are not
known. Because of particular brand names or the fact that the compound
composition is not always identified, the industrial hygiene engineer cannot
determine the extent of hazard present with the material. The manufacturer
supplier is a major source of information concerning such potentially
hazardous materials. The industrial hygiene engineer and the purchasing age
should arrange to discuss the potential problems with the supplier. A
material safety data sheet should be developed for chemicals and other
materials to be supplied. This data sheet can be requested along with any b
submitted for materials. The industrial hygiene engineer should attempt to
attain the establishment of a policy that requires the submission of such da

sheets on all materials being purchased before purchase can be approved. Since the ultimate responsibility for the use of the materials is with the purchaser, it is important that all information concerning a potentially hazardous material be known. The supplier has the responsibility to provide the purchaser with such information, and the purchaser has the responsibility to assure that such information is obtained before the material enters the plant.

Information Required for Potentially Hazardous Materials

Certain basic information should be obtained from the supplier. A product specification data sheet can be developed that includes this information. The components of such a specification sheet should include:

A. The material compound name.
B. The chemicals that are present in the compound.
C. Toxicity, including
   - level of toxicity
   - type of hazard
   - TLV, if applicable
D. Flammability
   - upper explosive limit (UEL)
   - lower explosive limit (LEL)
   - flash point
E. Any incompatible materials.
F. The form in which the material will be received.
G. The packaging of the material as delivered
   - type of packaging used
   - quantity per package
H. Any recommendations of the manufacturer or supplier concerning handling, storage, and use of the material.
I. An example of the label used on the product.
J. Other information, including
   - molecular weight
   - specific gravity
   - specific heat
   - solubility
   - vapor pressure

At the outset of the use of such a data sheet, similar information may not be available for many materials that are currently used in the plant. Many of these present materials may have hazards that are unknown. Because of this, an attempt should be made to obtain the same information for these materials from the current supplier.

A review of presently used materials should be conducted to determine the potential hazards involved in their use. As a result of this review, possible substitution materials can be identified and precautions can be established in the handling and use of these materials. The industrial hygiene engineer should also review the methods of control currently used for these materials to determine the adequacy of these methods to protect workers from potential exposure to the hazardous materials.

In a modern industrial plant, many compounds and materials are in use; and the data that is available or can become available through the use of such product specifications is voluminous. It will be necessary that a systematic approach be used to develop and organize the materials into a logical format that can be used on a day-to-day basis. Also, there is other information that is of use concerning a particular hazardous material that should be included in such a base of information. The resulting data base can be a tool that is a significant aid in the recognition, evaluation, and control of hazardous materials.

A Suggested Data Base for Hazardous Materials

In order for the data base to be useful, it is necessary that it be defined and the components to be included be identified.

The first major group of data that should be included within the data base is the data that have been obtained from the product specification data sheet submitted by the supplier. The information that should be included in the data base includes the chemical name and composition of the material, toxicity level of the material, the flammability of the material, the form of the material, any incompatibilities, packaging of the material, handling and use recommendations, labeling of the material, and other information concerning the chemical properties of the material. However, once this data base has been obtained from the manufacturer or supplier, the data base is not complete. Certain other information concerning the in-plant use of the product should also be included in the data base.

In order to complete the data base, the industrial hygiene engineer should ask certain key questions. Among these questions are:

1. Where is the material used?
2. When is the material used?
3. Why is the material used?
4. How is the material used?
5. Who is potentially exposed to the material?

In answering these questions, data will be obtained that completely define the material and its use within the plant. Each of these questions is briefly discussed below.

First, where is the material used? It is important to identify the locations in the plant where the material is used. What processes are involved in this use? Where is the material stored prior to use? Where is the material handled or moved, either from delivery to storage or from storage to process? Answers to these questions indicate the locations of possible problems involving exposure of the workers.

The second question to be asked is when is the material used? It is important to identify the time periods in which the material is used since it may not be used at all times. The material may be used on different shifts, or it may be used for different process schedules. As a result, the potential for exposure to the material will vary with its scheduled use.

The third question to ask is <u>why is the material used</u>? What is the planned use of the material? Is it used as a solvent, cleaner, product component, etc.? This information is useful in determining if potential, less hazardous substitute materials can be used to perform the same function.

The next question involves determining <u>how the material is used</u>. What procedures are followed in the use of the product? What are the loading and unloading procedures used when the material is transferred into and out of storage? What handling of the material is necessary? What procedures are used for this handling? Once the material enters the process, what process steps are involved in which workers may be potentially exposed? What equipment is used to process the material? The industrial hygiene engineer should describe the process and identify how it works. Is the process an open or closed process? Are any interim chemical reactions and materials generated that may be hazardous? What are the steps in the process?

The identification of potential exposures in the process used is not a simple job and will require significant research. The data base serves to provide a source of information that has been gathered as a result of the research preformed. Finally, it is necessary to identify the controls that are currently in use to protect the workers from exposure to the hazardous materials. The controls should not only be identified but also be described in such a manner as to indicate the proper operating criteria for the controls to provide a benchmark against which further measurements of system performance can be tested to determine the adequacy of the control operation.

Finally, the industrial hygiene engineer should determine <u>who is potentially exposed to the hazardous material</u>. Records should be kept on the employee's work history. As a minimum, these records should be kept from the point when the employee is employed by the plant until the employee ceases to work at the plant. Information concerning the individual's work area should be included in the data base. Procedures or process steps that the employee performs that may bring the employee into contact with the hazardous material should be noted. A record of the employee's health history should be kept, starting with the results of a pre-employment physical examination. This type of information is usable not only for identification of the exposure to hazardous materials but also for such things as noise, thermal stress, and other exposures.

The question must be asked, "What materials should be included in the data base?" Ideally, all materials used in the plant should be included in the data base. Practically, however, the number of materials that are used in the plant may be such that this ideal cannot be reached. Therefore, it is important that a priority be given to those materials to be included in the data base. Materials with a threshold limit value obviously should be included in such a data base. In addition, materials that are suspected carcinogens, materials that are flammable or explosive, and materials that have incompatible reactions with other materials used in the process should be included.

The data base might include other information that can be of assistance to the industrial hygiene engineer in performing duties. Items that might be included are the accepted methods for sampling a particular hazardous materia to determine the concentration of that material. A history of sampling data including when the sampling was done, where it was done, how it was done, and the results that were obtained is useful as a benchmark against which to compare future sampling results. A history of problems that have occurred as a result of the use of a particular material can be of value in identifying common problems and potential solutions to these problems. Finally, the type of problem that results from exposure to the hazardous material can be useful. Does a hazardous exposure result in dermatitis? What is the physiological reaction of the body when exposed to the hazardous material? I there any history of carcinogenic properties of the material?

Computerization of Data Base. The data base described above has potentia for implementation as part of a computer-based information system. Two major components of such a system would be developed; one involving the hazardous materials themselves and the other involving employee health and work history

Figure 8.3.1

Computerized data base.

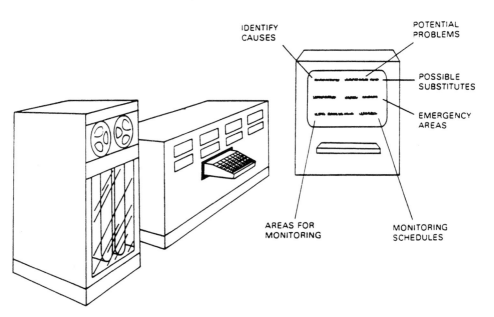

It would not be necessary to place all information on the computer since this would lead to inefficient use of the computer system. In such a compute data base, key information would be kept on the computer with background and descriptive information kept in cross-indexed files.

The industrial hygiene engineer could use such a system to identify possible causative agents when an illness appears. The system could be used

to identify potential problem areas where control may be necessary. Potential
areas where emergencies could occur can also be identified from the areas
where hazardous materials are being transferred from one point to another.
Such a system can be designed to indicate the need for monitoring on a regular
basis and, as such can provide reports on a regular basis indicating where
monitoring is needed and the type of monitoring that should occur. Schedules
for the monitoring of processes could be developed in such a manner. In
addition, an analysis of the data within the data base can indicate areas
where substitution of materials may be used as a potential method for control
of exposure to hazardous materials.

The possibilities for the use of such a system are far beyond those few
that have been mentioned above. The potential exists for the use of such a
computerized data base as a major tool in the recognition, evaluation, and
determination of appropriate control of hazardous material exposures.

Handling of Hazardous Materials

During the handling of hazardous materials, the potential for exposure to
workers is high. The worker who is involved in the actual handling of the
material will likely come into close contact with the material during its
handling. The danger of accidents or failure of equipment increases the
potential for exposure not only to the worker involved in the actual handling
of the material but also to those working in the vicinity of such an
accident. As material is transferred through the plant, many workers are
subjected to potential exposure in this manner.

One method for control that can be used to eliminate potential exposures
to the hazardous material is to eliminate the contact between the material and
the worker. This can be accomplished either by automating the process for
handling or by removing workers from the area where the material is being
handled. During normal day-to-day operations, the hazard exposure will then
be minimized.

However, even though contact between the worker and the hazardous material
has been minimized, the possibility still exists for accidents and resulting
injuries to workers. The use of Failure Mode and Effect Analysis can help to
identify those areas where potential exposure exists as a result of an
accident or failure within the system. In order to use Failure Mode and
Effect Analysis, it is necessary to determine where and how a failure in the
system can occur. What effect will such a failure have? What potential
controls can be instituted to reduce the possibility of failure and to protect
the workers in case of failure? As a result of identifying the possible
places where emergency situations can arise, it is possible to design controls
and emergency procedures to be instituted when a failure occurs.

In order to use Failure Mode and Effect Analysis, it is necessary to
determine at each point throughout a given system where a failure can occur.
What is the likelihood that such a failure will occur; and when it does occur,
what is likely to have caused it? The next step is to determine what controls
can be instituted to protect workers from any injurious effects as a result of

the failure. Obviously if controls can be instituted to eliminate the potential for the failure, this is the ultimate protection. However, such fail-safe operation is not easily accomplished. After all efforts have been made to protect against the occurrence of a failure, the potential effect of a failure must be considered. How can the workers be protected in the likely event of such an occurrence? What emergency procedures should be in place, and how can the workers be trained to use the emergency procedures?

Some Basic Rules for Handling of Hazardous Materials. There are some basic rules that can be implemented to protect workers when handling hazardous materials. These rules can help during the normal course of handling as well as in the case of an emergency resulting from a failure in the system.

1.   The workers should be provided with emergency protective equipment that can be used when a failure occurs.

2.   The workers should be provided with training as to the dangers in handling the material and any action that should be taken when an exposure is likely to occur.

3.   As much as possible, workers should be removed from contact with the material. If the system can be automated, thus removing the necessity for workers to be involved in the handling of the material, the potential exposure becomes significantly less.

4.   When handling material is being done in an open plant area, adequate ventilation should be provided to remove any contaminants that might escape into the workroom air.

5.   Maintenance and cleanup crews should be provided with training concerning the dangers involved with handling hazardous materials. Training should include the use of emergency procedures and equipment that are necessary in the case of an accidental exposure.

6.   Assurance should be made that outside factors do not affect the materials, resulting in a potentially dangerous situation. For example, sparking from equipment operating in a flammable area or the introduction of incompatible materials can result in a potentially harmful exposure to the workers.

7.   Proper maintenance of the handling equipment is important to assure that it is operating as designed and does not result in a potential exposure.

8.   The integrity of any packaging and/or transfer containers should be assured.

9.   The potential exposure to the work force during transfer and handling of the material can be minimized if this occurs during off hours or in relatively vacant areas of the plant.

Storage of Hazardous Materials

When determining where to store hazardous materials, it is important to identify the location in a plant area away from work areas as much as possible. Outside storage or underground storage often is the best for such materials. Incompatible materials should not be stored in the same area. In determining the area of storage, the industrial hygiene engineer must also be aware of the environmental conditions that exist in terms of both heat and humidity. These environmental conditions can act as a cause for failure within the storage system.

Within the storage area, proper storage containers and stacking procedures should be used. The containers should be well maintained and inspected regularly. Care should be taken in storing hazardous material in stacks to avoid the possibility that a container will become dislodged from the stack, fall to the floor and break open, thus causing a potential exposure.

Where hazardous materials are stored in tanks, proper cleaning is necessary when the tanks are emptied or when the material stored in the tank is changed. The process of cleaning tanks holding hazardous or volatile material can itself be a dangerous one. Proper precautions should be taken to protect workers involved in the cleaning process. Precautions include the use of appropriate personal protective equipment and work teams.

Where flammable materials are stored, it is necessary to provide adequate fire control. Emergency warning systems and sprinkling systems should be installed to identify the breakout of a fire and to control such a fire before it spreads to the rest of the plant. In some cases, chemical fire protection is necessary to control the fire. Bonded and grounded tanks should be used when storing flammable materials to prevent the buildup of static electricity with the accompanying potential for fire and explosion.

Finally, storage facilities should be inspected on a regular basis to identify potential problems. Just because the material is in a dormant state does not mean that it is harmless. It is still a hazardous material and must be treated as such. Undetected problems in a storage area can turn into large problems affecting the entire plant.

Summary

In this chapter, the purchase, handling, and storage of hazardous materials have been discussed. Emphasis was placed on the need to identify hazardous materials prior to their entry into the plant and to identify those areas where potential exposures might result either from handling of the materials or from failure of the handling system. A data base of information that should be gathered for hazardous materials has been discussed. This information can help to recognize, evaluate, and control hazardous materials from portal to portal within the plant.

4. Personal Protective Equipment

Introduction

The hazards that are encountered in the workplace take many forms. Workers may be exposed to toxic gases, hazardous vapors, mists and fogs, hazardous materials in the form of particulate matter, hazardous liquids, fumes and smoke, as well as other physical hazards such as noise and electromagnetic radiation. Throughout this text, various methods have been discussed to protect the workers from exposures related to these materials. In this chapter, the use of personal protective equipment as a potential method for controlling exposure to hazardous substances will be discussed.

One of the first important questions that must be asked before determining the type of personal protective equipment to use is the form in which the hazardous material exists. This is important in determining the route of entry of the material into the body and, as a result, the type of protection that is required.

Toxic gases are most likely to enter the body by being inhaled. These gases attack the respiratory system and through the respiratory system can enter the bloodstream. Carbon monoxide, for example, enters the body in this manner. A secondary exposure from gases can occur when the gases act on the skin and eyes of the worker.

Vapors, mists, and fogs act in essentially the same manner as gases in th respiratory system. There is an additional danger as a result of condensatio of the vapor, mist, or fog on the skin of the worker.

Particulate matter consists of solids suspended in the air. The very small particles may be inhaled and enter the respiratory system. These small particles can be passed into the bloodstream.

On the other hand, liquids, unless subject to vaporization, are more likely to attack the human body through the skin. Certain chemicals have a systemic action which, when entering the body through the skin, can cause har throughout the entire system. Additionally, liquids can be ingested either accidentally or as a result of failure to clean thoroughly before smoking or eating.

Fumes and smoke may be inhaled and enter the respiratory tract or they ma act on the skin. Fumes and smoke may also enter the eyes, causing damage.

Personal Protective Equipment as a Control

It should be noted that <u>personal protective equipment is a last resort control method</u>. Other controls should be attempted before using personal protective equipment. Can ventilation help solve the problem? Can a less hazardous material be substituted for a more hazardous one used in the process? Can engineering changes be made in the process and process equipment to eliminate the hazard? Can the worker be removed from contact with the source either by isolating the source or by isolating the worker? In those cases where the preferred methods of control do not provide adequate protection, then personal protective equipment should be prescribed until such time as permanent controls can be established.

Personal protective equipment provides a measure of control in the case of an emergency situation when a failure of the primary control method occurs. In such a case, personal protective equipment acts as emergency equipment. Personal protective equipment can also be used when no other control exists and the job is required to be performed by workers during the production process.

The basic categories of personal protective equipment that are available are:

1. Protection from inhalation of hazardous materials.
2. Protection from skin contact with hazardous materials.
3. Protection of the eyes from contact with hazardous materials.
4. Protection of the ears from hazardous exposure.
5. Protection from traumatic injury to a body part.
6. Protection from thermal stress.

Protection from Respirable Hazards

There are three basic types of personal protective equipment available for the protection of the worker from respirable hazards. These are:

1. Air purifying respirators
   - canister type
   - cartridge type
   - mechanical filter
2. Air supplied respirators
   - hose mask type
   - air-line respirator
   - abrasive blasting type respirator
3. Self-contained breathing type respirators
   - recirculating
   - open circulating

Before discussing each of these respirators in detail, let's look at the major criteria that should be considered when selecting the appropriate type of respirator.

The proper respirator must be used for a given situation. Otherwise, the respirator may provide a false sense of security and result in potential harm to the worker. The respirator used should be selected for the specific application involved.

There are many factors to consider in the selection of a respirator. The first question to consider is the hazardous material that is involved. What is its chemical makeup and its form? What are its characteristics? What are its chemical properties? What is the human physiological reaction to the material? What concentration of the material is present in the workplace?

Second, the conditions under which the worker will become exposed must be considered. Will the worker be required to perform normal work functions during exposure? This is likely to result when personal protective equipment is the final resort protection that is available. Or, is the respirator to be used only for emergency conditions; that is, when a failure of the existing controls or system occurs?

Closely related to the conditions in which the respirator will be used is the time or duration of the exposure. Will the respirator be required for quick escape as is the case in emergency use, or will the respirator be required for a longer period of time to perform work duties in the hazardous environment?

If the respirator is to be used during the performance of regular duties, it is important to determine the type of activity that must be performed while using the respirator. Will the work require much physical effort? If so, will the respirator inhibit the employee's ability to perform work in any way?

Another related question that must be asked but that does not directly involve the selection of the respirator is: "What is the need for additional protection?" While in the hazardous environment, will the employee be exposed in any way to the hazardous material? Is protection needed for the eyes or skin? Does the hazardous material act as a systemic agent through the exposed skin of the employee? If so, protection must be provided for those exposed parts of the body.

Finally, the selection of the respirator to be used must be based on approval standards. The National Institute for Occupational Safety and Health (NIOSH) and the Mine Safety and Health Administration (MSHA) test and certify respirators. Not all respirators being manufactured have been tested or approved by these bodies. In addition, the approval for the respirator may be limited to exposures occurring within a given environmental situation. The concentration of the substance as well as the duration of use must also be compared to that which is stated for an approved respirator.

The Air-Purifying Respirator. The first type of respirator that can be used is the air-purifying respirator. The purpose of this respirator is to remove contaminants from the air that is being respired. Sufficient oxygen must be present within the environment to support life. Air-purifying respirators come in three major types: the canister type, the cartridge type, and the mechanical filter type respirator.

The canister-type air-purifying respirator consists of a full facepiece with a hose connecting the mask to a canister. The canister is filled with the material that chemically reacts with the particular known contaminant to render it harmless. The type of materials that can be used to purify air containing contaminants varies with the type of contaminant in the air. Generally, the canister type respirator is limited to certain concentrations of a given substance. These concentrations are stated by the manufacturer in any data sheets involving the respirator and also on the canister itself.

The canisters involve various chemical sorbents for particular materials. For example, canisters exist for removal of acid gases, organic vapors, carbon monoxide, vinyl chloride, ammonia, hydrogen sulfide and chlorine.

Figure 8.4.1

Canister type.

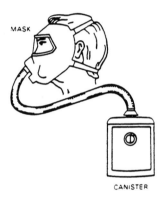

The canisters are color coded to indicate the type of toxic material for which the canister is effective. In general, the color coding is as follows:

- white--acid gases
- black--organic vapors
- green--ammonia
- blue--carbon monoxide
- various color stripes for specific compounds

The life of a canister varies and is generally specified based on a standard atmosphere and work rate. Factors that affect the life of a canister are the breathing rate of the individual using the canister, the temperature and humidity of the atmosphere in which the canister is being used, and the concentration of the contaminant in the atmosphere. Obviously each of these variables must be considered when determining how long a particular canister will provide protection for the worker. Standards for the life of canister type respirators have been specified by the Mine Safety and Health Administration. Generally, the typical canister life is approximately thirty minutes, but larger sizes can be purchased when a longer life is desired.

Some canisters come in a window design. The window indicates usage of the canister's capability for purifying the air. The window has a reference half circle of a given color. As the canister is used, the other half circle changes color. When the two colors match, the canister has lost its effectiveness.

Canisters that are used for carbon monoxide generate significant heat. This can provide an indication as to the proper functioning of the canister. If the air is hot when inhaled, the concentration of carbon monoxide in the atmosphere is too high for the canister to be effective, and the worker should immediately exit the area. An additional concern is the fact that the heat that is generated may be dangerous in a flammable atmosphere since it can act as an ignition source for flammable material.

Figure 8.4.2

Canister.

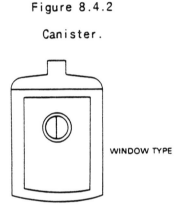

WINDOW TYPE

In general, the canister type respirator is for use in emergency situations only. The canister type respirator should not be used for regular work. When the canister is used in an emergency situation, sufficient warning should be given to the individuals so that the respirator can be put to use. The best warning is obtained when the gas has an odor or taste at or near the TLV. However, the odor threshold is most often above a hazardous level. In such cases, once the odor reaches the worker, it is too late to do anything about it. Thus, some type of system should be used to provide a warning when it is necessary for the worker to use a respirator.

After the canister has been used, no matter how long the use has been, it should be discarded. Canister sizes are selected for the appropriate needs of the individual, and a partially used canister can present a potential hazard to the worker unless discarded. The tendency is to assume that the canister is fully operational when in fact, if it has been partially used, it will operate for a shorter period of time to give the appropriate protection.

Cartridge Type Respirators. The cartridge type respirator is essentially a small canister that is attached directly to the facepiece or mask. A half mask with one or two cartridges is most common although a full mask may be used. Cartridge type respirators work in a manner similar to the canister type respirator. The major difference is the size of the smaller cartridge versus that of the canister.

Cartridges are generally approved for use in nonemergency situations only. Such situations involve an exposure to a material that is hazardous only after a prolonged period of time. Cartridge respirators are often used for protection against exposure to certain organic vapors and, in some cases, dust, fumes, and mist.

Mechanical Filter Type Respirator. The mechanical filter type respirator involves a half or full mask with filters attached to the mask in a manner similar to that of the cartridge type respirator. The filters, which are composed of fibrous materials, are connected directly to the mask.

Figure 8.4.3

Cartridge type.

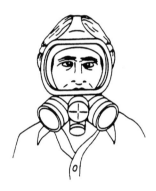

As with any filter, as it begins to clog or fill up, the efficiency is improved. However, as the filter loads, the resistance to breathing is increased and is a limiting factor for the use of the filter.

The filter medium that is used in a mechanical filter type respirator varies. The type of filter used is rated depending upon its efficiency in removing various particle sizes within the atmosphere. These ratings are available for each filter and should be consulted prior to selection.

Air-Supplied Respirators. This type of respirator involves a mask to which a supply of air is provided. The air-supplied respirator comes in three general types: the hose mask, the air-line respirator, and the abrasive blasting type respirator.

The hose mask involves a full facepiece with a one-inch collapsible hose attached. The hose is connected to a motor-driven or hand-operated pump outside the comtaminated atmosphere. The hose may also be connected to a

positive air pressure source. The blower intake is located in an
uncontaminated area and supplies air from that area to the worker through the
hose.

Figure 8.4.4

Hose mask.

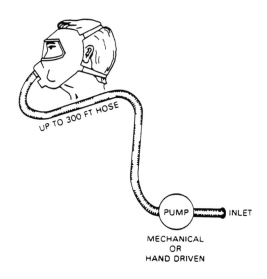

This type of system should be of a fail-safe nature to allow for breathing
in the event of a failure of the blower. Very little resistance to breathing
is encountered using the hose mask, and the worker can use it for a long
period of time without fatigue. In general, because of the dynamics of the
air within the hose itself, the hose cannot be too long. The maximum length
of hose is generally limited to 300 feet.

The air-line respirator is essentially the same as the hose mask except it
is connected to an air pressure line operating at a volume of between 2 and 20
cubic feet per minute. The connecting line is smaller in diameter and
supplies air under pressure. Filtering of compressed air is necessary to
assure that clean air is delivered to the worker.

Air-line respirators are often equipped with a demand type valve to
regulate the flow of air to the worker. This type of valve opens upon
inhalation and closes during exhalation. Exhaled air is discharged through a
separate valve.

The air-line respirator usually requires a pressure regulator and a relief
valve that is attached to the plant air supply. The pressure regulator lowers
the air pressure to that which should be supplied to the worker, and the
relief valve acts as a control should the air pressure regulator fail and the
pressure become so great as to cause harm to the user.

Figure 8.4.5

Demand valve.

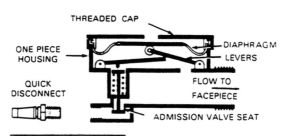

Courtesy of Mine Safety Appliances Co.

The air-line respirator offers low breathing resistance and is suitable for long wear in a contaminated atmosphere.

The abrasive blasting type respirator is composed of either a hose mask or an air-line respirator that is equipped with a helmet, hood, and inner collar that can be worn in an abrasive blasting operation. The hood and helmet protect the worker's face and head from the impact of the abrasive material in the atmosphere.

In an abrasive blasting type respirator, the air enters the hood from the hose and is exhausted at the neck collar or through an exhalation valve.

In certain situations where protection for the entire body is required, an air-supplied suit can be used. As an example, such suits can be used in high heat areas with conditioned air being supplied to the worker.

An additional advantage of the air-supplied respirator or air-supplied suit is that it can be utilized in an area where the oxygen level is such that it will not support life. For reasons of safety, such protection should be provided to the worker when the oxygen level is below 19.5% in the work area.

The Self-Contained Breathing Unit. As is the case with air-supplied respirators, the self-contained breathing unit can be used in areas where there is a deficiency of oxygen. The self-contained breathing unit has the additional advantage of being usable in an area where distance or movement prohibits the use of a hose mask or an air-line respirator.

The self-contained breathing unit is designed to allow the worker to carry a source of respirable air that is attached to the mask. The source of air may be supplied through oxygen-generating chemicals activated by moisture in the user's breath, liquid oxygen in a cylinder, or compressed air in a cylinder. Self-contained breathing units may be designed as either constant-flow type or demand valve operated.

There are two types of self-contained breathing units being manufactured. The first is a recirculating type unit in which a reservoir bag is attached. This bag collects air exhaled from the worker. Oxygen is added to the exhaled air by passing the exhaled air through a canister in which carbon dioxide is retained and oxygen is evolved. The oxygen may be added from compressed or liquid oxygen in a cylinder. This type of mask requires venting since an excess of oxygen is generally produced and must be vented.

The second type is the open circuit type. This type of respirator involves supplying air to the worker directly from a cylinder. The exhaled air is vented to the atmosphere from the mask.

Precautions That Should Be Taken When Using Respirators

There are certain precautions that should be taken when respirators are used by the workers. First, the industrial hygiene engineer should be sure that the appropriate equipment is being used. The mask should be selected to provide protection for those materials to which exposure can occur, and the appropriate type of canister or cartridge should be attached. For example, canister and cartridge type respirators are contaminant-specific. That is, if a canister is designed to remove a particular contaminant, it is not effective in removing another contaminant in the atmosphere. Consult "A Guide to Industrial Respiratory Protection," NIOSH Publ. 76-189, June 1976, and the latest edition of the "NIOSH Respirator Decision Logic" for further guidance on the elements of a respirator program and the selection of respirators.

The equipment should be maintained and cleaned on a regular basis. Equipment that is used regularly should be cleaned before and after each use. Equipment that is used in emergency situations only should be inspected and cleaned before and after each use and at least monthly to assure proper working condition in case an emergency arises. Maintenance should involve looking for defects and damage to the equipment. Any dirt that is present should be removed. The cartridge or canister should be checked to determine if it is the proper type. If an air-supplied respirator is being used, the operation of the pump, pressure-relief valve, pressure regulator, and other related equipment should be checked. After use, the mask should be placed in a plastic bag for storage in a clean, cool, dark, dry place.

When a worker is using a respirator inside a contaminated area, a second worker should be stationed outside the area. A lifeline should be attached to the worker in the contaminated area, and the worker outside the contaminated area should be supplied with respirator equipment.

Employees should be properly trained in the use of respirators. Such training should include why respirators are necessary and the necessity for proper handling of the equipment, proper fit, inspection, cleaning, and storage of the respirator. Where a respirator is used in an emergency condition, the workers should be familiar with emergency procedures and should drill using the procedures on a regular basis.

Workers who are required to use respirators should be in good physical condition. This is necessary since the use of a respirator presents an added burden on the worker in performing duties. In the case of a canister or filter type respirator, breathing is difficult and can result in problems for those individuals with cardiovascular disease.

Canisters that have been used should be discarded. When a respirator is needed, it is important that the worker be able to depend on the time of protection that a normal canister will give. A partially used canister will not provide adequate protection. In addition, once a canister has been used, it is subject to loss of effectiveness more quickly than a closed and sealed canister.

Warning should be provided to the worker when exhaustion of the supply of air or canister service life is nearing. This warning should provide the worker with adequate time to exit the contaminated area without harm to health.

New canisters that are purchased should be checked and stored in a dry place. Before storing, the canisters should be weighed and this weight compared to the weight of the canister immediately prior to use. Such weighing provides data on the moisture absorbed, which is an indication of the loss of effectiveness of the canister. If the seal on the canister has been broken, it should not be kept over one year.

Other Personal Protective Equipment

In addition to respirators, other personal protective equipment can be used to protect the worker from health and safety hazards. For protection of the face and eyes, safety glasses, goggles, face shields, and hoods can be provided to the workers.

Safety glasses are used in situations where the impact of particulate matter may result in damage to the eyes. The objective of safety glasses is to act as a barrier to protect the eyes from particulates. Safety glasses should be equipped with side shields to protect the eye from entry of particulates at the sides of the glasses. Plastic or metal frames can be used. The lenses should be constructed of impact and shock resistant glass. If a significant number of particles are impacting the worker in the facial area, more protection is required.

Goggles protect a larger area of the worker's eyes and can be worn over glasses. The tighter fit offers more protection in the case where more particles are present in the atmosphere.

Where a high incidence of particles are impacting on the face or where there is a potential for minor explosion, the face shield can be used. Face shields offer protection to the entire face, including the eyes. Face shields should cover the side of the head as well as the forehead, face and chin. Safety glasses should be worn underneath the shield for added protection.

In those cases where an extreme hazard exists, the worker can be equipped
with a hood covering the face and head as well as the shoulders and upper
body. Such a hood is often utilized in welding operations.

In order to protect the worker's head from blows, a hard hat or helmet can
be used. These helmets should be constructed in such a manner as to protect
the workers not only from the impact of the blow but also should be designed
to absorb any shock that might be transferred to the cervical spine. The type
of helmet varies and should be chosen for the particular hazards of the job.

As was mentioned earlier, one route of entry for hazardous materials is
through the skin. Thus, it is necessary that protective clothing be provided
to the worker where the skin is exposed to the systemic action of a toxic
material. Where a less toxic material is used in which the physiological
result is dermatitis, skin protection is also necessary. Skin protection can
also be necessary to protect the worker from radiant heat loads. In this
case, reflective type clothing is utilized.

The various types of protective clothing involve gloves, aprons, and full
suits. The types of material and design of this clothing are important. The
clothing should be chosen in such a way that the fabric does not react to the
contaminants. The fabric should also be impervious to the contaminants in
order to provide protection from absorption and contact with the skin. The
fabric that is involved in such clothing should be flame resistant and of
anti-static type. The fabric must also be of sufficient flexibility and
design of the clothing such that the worker is able to function with a minimum
of retardation to work processes.

Other types of protective equipment can be provided for various types of
hazards. Included among these are protection from noise exposure which
involves the use of earplugs or earmuffs. The feet can be protected from
traumatic injury by using hard-toed shoes, steel sole shoes, instep guards,
and in those cases where static electricity is important, conductive soles.
In addition, safety showers and eye baths can be provided to flush away any
toxic or hazardous substances to which the worker is exposed.

Summary

Personal protective equipment is used as a last resort mechanism for
protection of the worker. Other types of controls such as substitution,
engineering, and isolation should be instituted before resorting to personal
protective equipment. However, there are situations where personal
protectiveequipment can and should be used. Where other methods of control
are not adequate or in those special cases where an emergency condition
arises, the use of personal protective equipment is justified.

Personal protective equipment in the form of respirators can be used to
protect the employee from respirable hazards. Three major types of
respirators available are: The air-purifying respirator, the air-supplied
respirator, and the self-contained breathing unit. Each of these is usable in
a particular situation, and certain selection criteria must be utilized when
determining which respirator should be used.

Other types of personal protective equipment can be utilized to protect the worker from various potential causes of illness and injury. Among these are protective clothing to protect the skin, eyeglasses and face shields to protect the eyes and face, and earplugs to protect the ears from excessive noise.

5. Costs of Industrial Hygiene Control

Introduction

Because of an involvement and commitment to protecting the worker's health and safety, the industrial hygiene engineer often takes for granted that particular controls are needed to protect the worker. The fact that a worker may be exposed to a particular hazard is sufficient reason to justify the need for control. However, management may not have the same viewpoint. The objective of management is to maximize profits. Industrial hygiene controls cost money and do not necessarily result in added profit to the firm. Management is more likely to be desirous of considering the risks of not controlling a particular hazard versus the costs and effects on profit to obtain these controls.

One of the jobs of the industrial hygiene engineer is to convince management of the need for control. The industrial hygiene engineer must become a salesman of a product, the control of exposure to occupational health hazards. In order to do this, a logical decision process and approach to problems must be used in the same manner as management approaches other decisions. Since the economics of decisions are important to management in other areas, they must also be important to the when related to the implementation of a given control method.

In order to sell industrial hygiene controls to management, the industrial hygiene engineer must approach management on its own ground. A case must be made for why a particular control is required. The benefits must be clearly outlined as well as the costs that are involved. It may not always be possible to sell industrial hygiene control as a method for improving the firm's profitability. However, it may be possible to minimize the costs of the controls required and to outline those costs associated with the risks that are taken by not instituting the controls even though, on a purely economic basis, they do not pay for themselves. In other cases. the decision can be made on pure economics. Thus, it is important to have an understanding of the costs of industrial hygiene control and be able to utilize basic economic analysis tools to present the case.

A number of factors are important when selling an industrial hygiene control program to management. From the economic standpoint, the costs of control versus the costs of no control must be considered and compared. Other factors that enter the picture are the legal requirements as stipulated by the Occupational Safety and Health Act as well as any state or local provisions. Also, the moral responsibility of the employer to the worker must be considered. The industrial hygiene engineer must consider the risk factor of

Figure 8.5.1

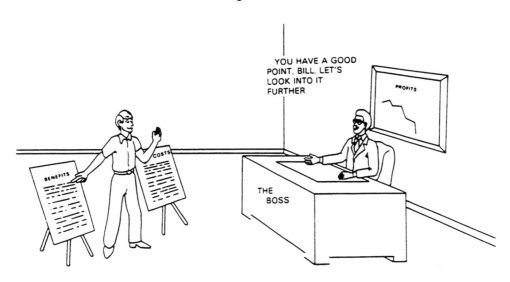

exposure in order to determine the costs involved. Finally, the industrial
hygiene engineer must be aware of the level of danger to the worker that
results from a particular exposure. Is the level of danger extreme, resulting
in death, disability, or physical impairment; is the danger moderate,
resulting in illness with lost time; or is the danger low, resulting only in
discomfort to the worker but not lost time or accompanying harm to the
worker's health?

Economic Cost of Not Providing Controls

First, consider the costs of not providing controls for hazards. That is,
what costs accrue to the organization when appropriate controls are not
present, and an exposure occurs?

Workers' Compensation. The purpose of workers' compensation is to remove
the risk of the loss of employment, as a result of injury, from the employee.
Workers' compensation insurance provides a fund base from which to compensate
a worker when a job-related accident or illness occurs. Prior to the
institution of workers' compensation, such protection was provided only as a
result of a common law suit filed by the employee with the employer as the
defendant. This dependence upon common law provided little protection to the
worker. Workers' compensation insurance was developed and exists throughout
this country to provide such protection to the worker.

Workers' compensation laws are governed by the individual state in which
the business resides. In general, most industries are required to have
coverage of their employees. There is some variance among states as to the

number of employees and the type of industry that require coverage. The type of coverage and the payment schedule also vary among states. In most states, the law covers both occupational illness and injury.

The premium costs that must be paid by a particular industry for workers' compensation depend upon the risks of the industry group in which the company operates, the experience of the company in terms of illness and injury, and an adjusted annual gross payroll based upon a maximum amount of compensation per week for each employee. The basic rate is established for a particular industry group as a result of the experience of that industry group. The experience of a particular company is evaluated and compared to the industry group, and a rating is determined. This rating is called the experience modification factor. If the experienced loss has been less than the average for the industry over a historical period (generally three years), then the experience modification factor is less than 1. If the experienced loss has been the same as the average for the industry over the historical period, the experience modification factor equals 1. If the experienced loss is greater than the industry over the historical period, the experience modification factor is greater than 1. The premium cost is determined by multiplying the base rate times the annual payroll (calculated for determination of rate) and the experience modification factor.

For example, consider a firm in which the base industry rate is $1.65 per $100 payroll and which has a $360,000 adjusted annual payroll after deductions for wages in excess of the maximum annual rate. If the experience modification factor for this firm is 1.8, then the premium would be determined as follows:

Premium = $1.65/100 x 360,000 x 1.8
Premium = $10,692

The premium that results from a high experience modification factor is a cost of not providing controls. In terms of actual dollars, it is the difference between the industry average with an experience modification factor of 1 and the rate being paid. In the above example, the cost to the particular plant involved is $4,752. An additional cost involving workers' compensation is the cost of processing claims against the workers' compensation benefits.

Disability Insurance. Many companies pay for disability insurance in addition to premiums for workers' compensation. This fringe benefit continues to become more prevalent in industry. The cost of higher premiums for such insurance may be a cost of not providing industrial hygiene controls. In addition, any sick leave that is incurred but not insured and that results from occupational illness or injury is also a cost of not providing controls.

Legal Costs. Specific laws may be in existence to specify the requirement for controls. The absence of proper control may result in potential losses, either from law suits or from penalties assessed by enforcement agencies. The absence of controls can result in such costs being incurred by the organization.

Replacing Lost Employees. As a result of occupational illness or injury, employees may be lost to the organization either for short periods of time or, in the case of disability or death, forever. Assuming that such employees are productive and have been properly trained, the cost of replacing these employees is significant. Included in this cost factor are the costs for recruiting, interviewing, and hiring new employees and the cost of training these new employees to become productive. A hidden cost is the loss of production which results from the replacement of an older, well-trained employee with a new employee. In the case of short-term absence, the cost of overstaffing which is needed to provide for such short-term absence is also a part of this factor.

Medical Insurance. Medical insurance coverage is almost universally provided by employers today. In many cases, medical insurance premiums are a result of group experience. Increased medical costs as a result of occupational injury or illness can raise the cost of such premiums.

Availability of Labor Pool. The risk of illness and injury which is assumed by a worker on a particular job can affect the size of the labor pool available. If the job appears to be a high-risk job, few applicants will be willing to consider such a job. As the labor pool becomes smaller, it is necessary to raise the pay in order to attract applicants to the job. Thus, though difficult to assess, this situation can lead to a cost of not providing controls for occupational hazards.

Production Losses. Production losses can result from the absence of controls which cause occupational illness and injury. High turnover rate and employee absence can detrimentally affect production, resulting in a loss of profits to the organization. In addition, because of legal action or a feeling that the company is indifferent to the needs of the worker, employee morale and general attitude can become a problem which in turn may affect production.

Public Relations. The lack of necessary controls to protect the worker from occupational hazards can detrimentally affect the public image of the organization. This detrimental effect on the organization can result in a loss of sales, which affects the profitability of the firm.

Social Costs. Though not directly related to the profitability of the firm, there are certain social costs that result from a lack of control of occupational hazards. The first loss is to the family in terms of the loss of a wage earner. This results in a cost to the government to support families whose source of earning power has been removed. Though not directly a cost to an individual organization, industry in total helps to support such costs through taxes.

The Assessment of Risk

In order to determine the necessity for controls, the industrial hygiene engineer must assess the risks involved and the extent of illness or injury which will result from an absence of control. This assessment is necessary because it is impossible to control all possible exposures to the worker. To do so would result in an astronomical cost. In general, the principle that should be used is to control the highest risk exposures first. The control of those exposures with the greatest loss potential will minimize the costs incurred as a result of not controlling the exposures.

For example, consider an organization employing 3500 employees with the following exposures:

Exposure A
>   Loss per occurrence is estimated at $1,000 with a probability of exposure of 1 in 100 for a given year.

Exposure B
>   Loss per occurrence is estimated at $10,500 with a probability of exposure of 1 in 500 for a year.

Exposure C
>   Loss per occurrence is estimated at $250,000 with a probability of exposure of 1 in 2500 for a year.

The question is, "Which exposure should be controlled first?" For the purpose of this illustration, it is assumed that the same cost is necessary to institute the controls for each of the three situations. In this example, the following calculations can be made:

Expected Loss (A) = $1,000 x .01 x 3500
Expected Loss (A) = $35,000 per year

Expected Loss (B) = $10,500 x .002 x 3500
Expected Loss (B) = $73,500 per year

Expected Loss (C) = $250,000 x .0004 x 3500
Expected Loss (C) = $350,000 per year

In the above example, it can be seen that the control of Exposure C should be undertaken first. If sufficient dollars are available to control another exposure, then Exposure B should be controlled. Finally, when dollars are available to control Exposure A, this can be done. Although the above analysis was based upon pure economics and did not consider the potential exposure level directly, an indirect consideration of the exposure level was made in terms of the cost per occurrence. It is likely that a higher cost per occurrence is a result of the more serious loss, thus indirectly the seriousness of the exposure is considered.

The Economic Cost of Providing Industrial Hygiene Controls

On the other side of the coin, certain costs are incurred as the result of providing industrial hygiene control. The following discussion centers around these costs.

Equipment Costs. The installation of industrial hygiene controls may require equipment. The cost of equipment includes not only the capital expenditure for the equipment itself but also any delivery and installation costs as well as the space that is used by the equipment. Purchasing and engineering costs must be considered. Any modifications that must be made to the plant and other production equipment to accommodate the control equipment must also be considered to be a cost of control.

Effects on Production. The installation of industrial hygiene controls can have a detrimental effect on the production of the plant. First, there is a potential for lost production during the installation of the controls themselves. In addition, any downtime necessary for the maintenance of the controls may result in the necessity to shut down production. Finally, in some cases, the controls themselves may limit the productive capacity of the facility. Such a situation might be the case where special handling of toxic materials is required and where such handling is accomplished at a rate slower than the process equipment using the materials.

Costs of Control Operation. Many of the controls which are used to protect workers from occupational hazards involve mechanical and electrical equipment. This equipment does not operate without a cost. The cost of the power to operate the equipment as well as the cost of maintenance in terms of both hours and replacement parts must be considered. Any personal protective equipment for maintenance and production personnel, which is necessary should the controls fail, must also be considered.

Cost of Training. When an industrial hygiene control has been installed, it is necessary to provide training to the workers in precautions concerning the use of the control equipment. Training in the operation of the equipment as well as training of the maintenance crew is also necessary. This training involves the man hours of both a trainer and the crews and, as a result, is a cost of installing the control.

Equipment Life. Once the control has been put in place, it in effect becomes a necessary part of the production facility. At some time, this equipment must be replaced. Replacement of this equipment is a cost of providing control in the first case.

Other Related Costs. Other costs that are related to the provision of industrial hygiene controls involve special packaging which may be required to protect workers from toxic substances, warning or monitoring equipment which may be necessary to indicate when the control is no longer working, and waste removal costs for toxic substances which have been removed from the work area.

Not all costs will be incurred for all methods of control. The costs for various controls will differ. For example, the operating cost may be high while the cost of obtaining and installing the equipment is low. Such would be the case in terms of a dilution ventilation system where the installation and purchase of such a system is relatively low while the operating cost is high. On the other hand, in the case of a local exhaust system, the opposite may be the case. The purchase and installation of a local exhaust system usually involves a high capital expenditure while the operating costs are low relative to a dilution ventilation system.

Selecting a Control Method

Various general methods are available for use in the control of occupational hazards. These methods include:

1. Elimination
2. Substitution
3. Process or procedure change
4. Isolation or enclosure of the source or worker
5. Ventilation
6. Administrative control
7. Personal protective equipment

Within each of these general methods of control, various alternative approaches are available for use to control a particular occupational hazard. It is important to consider the various alternatives in some logical manner to assure that the best choice is made for control of hazards. In order to do this, it is important that a logical and systematic approach be used. Such a systematic procedure involves a number of steps, which are discussed below.

Identify the Exposure. The first step in selecting a control method to be implemented for a particular occupational hazard is to identify the hazard exposure. To identify the hazard exposure, a number of questions should be answered. What is the exposure? Who is exposed, when are they exposed, where does the exposure occur, and how does the exposure occur? What is the extent of the hazard involved? Is the loss severe, moderate, or low? What is the estimated cost of the loss? What risks are involved with the exposure? Is the likelihood of exposure high or low? What personnel are subjected to the exposure when it occurs? What specifically is the objective of the control method?

By answering these questions, the industrial hygiene engineer has clearly defined the problem that is faced and identified the result which he wishes to obtain. The importance of specifying the result that is desired cannot be overemphasized. It is difficult to compare various methods of control when the desired result is unknown.

Choosing Alternatives. After the problem has been clearly identified and the objectives for control stated, the industrial hygiene engineer should identify those alternatives that can be implemented to obtain the stated objective. It cannot be emphasized too much that the first choice alternative should not be selected without comparing this choice to other alternatives. Often the first choice is not the best method for control, either in terms of the desired result or in terms of the cost involved. For this reason, it is necessary that alternative methods for control be considered.

As a starting point for identifying various alternatives, consider the seven general methods of control previously listed. Each of these general methods of control can act as an organizer from which alternative control procedures may be identified. Within each general method of control, specific alternatives can be identified.

Once the initial list of alternatives has been developed, the search process should not stop. It may be possible to improve upon the list of alternatives by identifying modifications to the selected alternatives. By modifying the alternatives, new and better alternatives may result.

When an alternative has been identified, the possibility of modifying it to obtain another alternative can be accomplished by the following:

1. Consider if any part of the alternatives can be eliminated.
2. Can two or more alternatives be combined?
3. Can the procedures for use be changed?
4. Can changes be made in some parts of the alternative to make it more attractive?

By answering these and other questions, it may be possible to improve upon the alternative list used for comparison.

One technique that can be utilized to generate alternatives involves a group process. Based upon the old adage that two heads are better than one and that there is a synergistic effect within a group, the technique of brainstorming may be used to identify alternative methods of control. Brainstorming operates on the principle that, initially, the quantity of ideas is more important than quality. Ideas are not evaluated until an exhaustive list has been developed. Then, by either combining or modifying the various approaches suggested during the brainstorming session, perhaps a new and more creative alternative, resulting in better control for a lower cost, can be developed.

Predicting Results. After the list of alternative controls has been developed, it will be obvious that not all alternatives are equal in terms of either their effects or their costs of implementation. To determine which alternative is best, it is important to be able to predict the results of selecting and implementing a particular alternative control. The prediction can be made as a result of experience. If experience with a particular control has not been obtained, the experience of others or experimental results may provide the data necessary for the prediction. The objective of such prediction is to determine as much as possible the result that will be obtained by instituting the particular alternative control; that is, how much will the risk factor be lowered? Also, what will be the cost of implementing the alternative?

Evaluation of Alternatives. After predictions have been made for the results of each of the alternatives, it is necessary to evaluate the alternatives to determine the best or most acceptable alternative. The most important question to ask is, "What alternatives will result in reaching the objective stated for the control of the hazard?" By asking this question, the list of alternatives can be pared down through the elimination of those alternatives that do not meet the desired criteria stated in the objective.

The next step is to determine, from those alternatives which attain the objective, the one that provides the best economic advantage. Some basic techniques of economic analysis can be used to carry out this step.   These techniques are discussed in the next chapter.

Finally, once the alternatives have been compared in terms of the desired result and the economics of implementation, the decision can be made concerning which alternative provides the best approach to controlling the occupational hazard. In most cases, the decision will be obvious, based on the use of the appropriate analysis techniques.

Summary

In this chapter, the cost of industrial hygiene control has been discussed from two points of view. From the first point of view, the cost of not providing controls for occupational hazards has been considered. Among the costs that are important are the increased costs of workers' compensation, production losses, training and recruitment costs, and medical and disability premium increases. When it is determined that an industrial control is desired, certain costs necessary to implement the control are incurred. Among the costs involved are the cost of the equipment, its operation and maintenance, as well as any production losses that may result from the installation of the equipment in the production process.

The industrial hygiene engineer is often tempted to recommend the installation of controls whenever a worker is exposed to an occupational hazard. Though such a recommendation certainly is to be applauded in terms of the desired outcome, that of a safe and healthful workplace, the facts do not always indicate that management will take the same viewpoint. The industrial hygiene engineer must be aware of the manager's view that to operate an industrial concern involves certain risks that must be taken. As a result, it becomes incumbent to sell the need for such controls to management. In order to perform this job in a credible fashion, the industrial hygiene engineer must approach the institution of a particular control from the viewpoint that management is likely to take. This includes the need to consider the economic costs involved in providing the control versus those involved with not providing the control. Though this situation is not ideal from the standpoint of the occupational safety and health professional, realization of the need to sell industrial hygiene control may, in the long run, maximize the desired objective--that of providing a safe and healthful environment for the worker.

6. Basic Economic Analysis

<u>Introduction</u>

From the discussion presented in the previous chapter, it is clear that it is necessary to determine a method for comparing alternatives in a standard manner. The alternatives being compared may have different costs of implementation. Given the same result in meeting the objective stated for control, it is desired that the best alternative be chosen. In the simplest case, this is done by selecting the lowest cost alternative.

However, the lowest cost alternative is not always easy to determine at first glance. The initial investment may differ between alternatives, and the operational costs may vary. The life of the equipment between two alternatives being considered or compared may also vary. Labor costs to operate and maintain the equipment as well as space requirements for each of the alternatives may be different. A method is needed to put these costs on an equal basis for comparison.

The first step in comparing alternatives is to determine those alternatives that meet the objective. If two alternatives meet a given objective, then these alternatives are comparable. If, on the other hand, one of the alternatives does not meet the objective, then it is not comparable to another alternative that does meet the objective. This fact emphasizes the need to state clearly the objectives of control. The objectives of control should be stated so that:

a. the desired result is specified,
b. the desired result can be measured,
c. the required conditions of performance are specified,
d. the method for determining whether the desired result has been reached is specified, and
e. the acceptable tolerances are identified.

Once the objective has been stated and clearly defined, the various alternatives can be compared to this objective to determine if the objective will be attained. If an alternative results in meeting the objective, it can be considered further. If the objective is not reached by implementation of an alternative, then this alternative can be eliminated from any further comparison.

Finally, after eliminating those alternatives that do not meet the objective, the remaining alternatives must be compared in some manner. An economic analysis provides the best method for making such a comparison. This economic analysis considers the initial investment cost, the yearly operating cost, and the savings generated over existing methods. That alternative which results in the best economic advantage to the organization is the alternative that should be implemented.

In this chapter, two methods of economic analysis will be discussed; the N-year payback method and the present-worth approach. Variations of these methods, as well as other methods, have been developed and will provide equally useful analysis techniques. However, it is felt that, for the most part, these two methods are sufficient for conducting an economic analysis of capital investments.

The N-Year Payback

The N-Year payback approach for comparing capital investments is perhaps the simplest technique to use. This approach is particularly useful when it is necessary to compare a new method of control to an existing method of control. Using the N-Year payback, the costs that are incurred for the present method of control are compared to the projected costs for the new method being considered. The difference in cost between the methods, i.e., the savings, is then compared to the required investment to implement the new method of control. This comparison results in a payback for the new method being considered. When using this approach, the assumption is made that the savings are equal for each year of life of the new investment. The payback formula can be stated as

$$(8.6.1) \quad \text{Payback (P)} = \frac{I}{S}$$

where

I = the capital investment cost to obtain the savings
S = the savings generated by the new method as compared to the existing method
P = the number of years required to pay back the investment

In using the N-year payback method, it is necessary to choose a cutoff payback period. This varies to some degree upon the type of investment. Generally, three to five years is used for equipment; whereas, plant investments may use a ten-year or greater payback period. Most organizations have specific desired payback periods for different types of investments. To illustrate the N-year payback, the following example is presented.

Example Problem

A plant operates with an intermittently cleaned bag house to remove particulates from the exhausted air. The bag house requires cleaning daily, involving production shutdown for one hour and an operator at $12 per hour including fringe benefits. The bag house was purchased one (1) year ago at an installed cost of $50,000. A newly-designed bag house can be obtained for $160,000 installed. The new design will not require shutdown for cleaning since it is cleaned continuously. The new design will operate at the same efficiency in removing particulates but will cost $50 per day more to operate. One hour's production has an estimated value of $300 profit to the firm. Assuming a three (3) year payback is required for investments of this type, answer the following questions.

a. If the plant is now operating to capacity (3 shifts), 365 days per year, and if additional capacity can be sold, should the investment be made?

b. If the plant is operating two shifts per day on a 365 day basis, should the investment be made?

c. Is any other alternative available, and if so, is this alternative a better investment than the new equipment?

Using the N-year payback method, the first step is to determine the investment involved. In this case, the investment is $160,000. The reader should be cautioned not to consider the $50,000 spent on the existing equipment since this represents a "sunk" cost. The concept of "sunk" costs involves costs or investments that have been made in the past. These costs do not in any way effect the determination as to whether to implement a given new alternative.

The savings to be generated in the first case where the plant is operating at full capacity and where additional capacity provided by removing the need for production downtime can be sold is as follows:

Savings

a. Labor Cost = $12 per hour x 365 days = $4,380
Production Revenue = $300 per hour x 365 days = $109,500
The costs of operating the new equipment must be determined since these costs will result in a lower net savings to the firm. These costs are:

Operating Cost = $50 per day x 365 days = $18,250

The savings are then:

Net savings = savings - cost
Net savings = ($4,380 + 109,500) - $18,250
Net savings = $95,630

The payback can be calculated by the formula:

Payback = I/S
Payback = $160,000/95,630
Payback = 1.67 years

b. In the second case, the additional capacity is not needed. The invest- ment remains the same at $160,000. However, the savings now involve only the labor cost since no production revenue will be obtained by eliminating the need for downtime. The cost of operating the new

equipment is still $18,250. In this case, the net savings is--$13,87
Obviously, the investment under this situation is a losing propositio

c. One alternative that was not specifically stated in the problem but
which can be considered is to install a second intermittent-type bag
house in parallel with the first. The second bag house can be operat
to clean the air while the first bag house is shut down for cleaning.
This will not require a shutdown of the production facility.

To compare this alternative with the existing situation and assuming that
the installed cost has not changed over the last year, the following is
developed:

Investment = $50,000

Savings:

Labor Cost = Same as present method (alternate day cleaning)
Production Revenue = $300 per hour x 365 days
Production Revenue = $109,500

$$\text{Payback} = \frac{\$50,000}{\$109,500}$$

Payback = 0.46 years

This is clearly the best economic alternative. This situation points out
the necessity to consider other alternatives to make sure that the best
alternative will be chosen. If only the obvious alternative had been
considered and chosen, then a significant opportunity cost would have been
incurred by the company.

Economic Analysis Using the Present Worth Approach

The simple method of the N-year payback does not always provide the best
approach for conducting an economic analysis. The cost and savings flow may
vary from year to year between the alternatives being compared. In addition,
unequal life cycles may be present. In order to consider these factors, it i
necessary to look at the investment in another way.

One method is to consider the average savings that are generated.
However, using this approach does not consider the fact that a dollar earned
today is worth more than a dollar earned tomorrow. Let's look at this concep
a little further.

If a firm earns a dollar today, that dollar can be invested in such a
manner that additional money can be made. For example, consider the simple
case of putting a dollar in a savings bank. If the rate of interest earned. i
a savings bank is 6%, then the dollar will be worth $1.06 at the end of the
year. A dollar earned next year cannot be invested until it has been earned
and, therefore, is still only worth a dollar. Thus, the dollar earned this
year is worth six cents more than the dollar earned next year. It is on this
concept that the present worth approach is based.

The objective of the present worth approach is to put all costs and savings in terms of current dollars. This is done by using a compound interest rate to discount the money back to its equivalent worth in dollars today. Inflation is not considered since it is assumed that it will equally affect costs and profit. The rate that is used to discount the money to its present worth is determined by either looking at the cost to borrow capital or determining an acceptable rate of return on investment from the profit return rate the organization earns.

Let's look at a simple example to see how the present worth approach works. Consider $10 invested today. How much more is this $10 worth than $10 earned in one year or $10 earned in two years, if it is assumed that a return of 5% can be obtained on any investments made?

Ten dollars will yield $10.50 in one year at 5% interest. This is shown by the following:

Value = $10 + 10(.05) = $10.50

This can be generalized for any interest rate and investment by:

(8.6.2) Value = $(1 + i)I$

Ten Dollars in two years can earn:

Value = 10(1 + .05) + 10(1 + .05)(.05)

Generalizing from this, we obtain the following:

Value = $I(1 + i) + I(1 + i)(i)$
Value = $I[1 + i + i + i^2]$
     = $I[1 + 2i + i^2]$
     = $I(1 + i)^2$

This can be generalized for N years in the following way:

(8.6.3) Value = $I(1 + i)^n$

Now, the question must be asked, "How much money would have to be earned in the future to be worth the same as money earned today?" This can be stated as:

(8.6.4) Future Earnings = $I(1 + i)^n$

Future earnings are then worth what value today? Transposing the formula above, the following is obtained:

$$(8.6.5) \quad I = \frac{\text{Future Earnings}}{(1 + i)^n}$$

This is the basis for the present-worth approach. The formula for determining
the present worth of a dollar earned or saved in the future is as follows:

$$(8.6.6) \quad PW_i = S \times \frac{1}{(1 + i)^n}$$

where

PW_i = the present worth of a future savings at a rate of interest
S = the savings earned at some future point in time
i = interest rate
n = years until savings are earned

Consider the following example which illustrates the use of the present
worth approach. A series of savings are earned at a rate of return of 8
percent.

At the End of Year	Savings($)
I	400
2	200
3	500
4	300

Using the present worth approach, the following calculation can be made:

Year	Savings($)	x	Factor	=	Present Worth(
1	400		$1/(1 + 0.08)$		370.37
2	200		$1/(1 + 0.08)^2$		171.47
3	500		$1/(1 + 0.08)^3$		396.42
4	300		$1/(1 + 0.08)^4$		220.51
					$1,159.27

To determine the rate of return on an investment, the present worth of the
investment at a given rate of return minus the present worth of the savings
earned at this same return must be equal to 0. In the above case, to earn a
rate of return of 8 percent, the investment today must be equal to $1,159.27
for the investment and present worth of savings to be equal. Perhaps this
method can be better shown by considering another problem involving present
worth.

Example

A manufacturer has been using a dilution ventilation system for control of
nuisance dusts in a work area. However, with the cost of fuel rising, a
local exhaust system is being considered as a replacement for the existing

system. It is estimated that the cost of tempering makeup air will be reduced to one-fourth of the present cost of $50,000 annually using the local exhaust system. Also it is expected that the present dilution system will require a major overhaul at the end of 5 years at a cost of $50,000. The investment cost for the new system is $300,000. If the desired rate of return for the firm is 6%, should the investment be recommended? Assume a 10-year life for the project.

Solution

In each year, the savings obtained by making the investment will be as follows :

Heating + power = Total savings
$50,000 x 3/4 + $8,000 = $45,500

In year 5, the additional overhaul costs of $50,000 will also be saved. The resulting savings and present worth at 6% are shown in the following table.

Year	Savings($)	Present Worth Factor $[1/(1 + i)^n]$	Present Worth($) (Savings)
1	45,500	.94339	42,925
2	45,500	.88999	40,495
3	45,500	.83961	38,203
4	45,500	.79209	36,040
5	45,500	.74725	34,000
6	95,500	.70496	67,324
7	45,500	.66505	30,260
8	45,500	.62741	28,547
9	45,500	.59189	26,931
10	45,500	.55839	25,407
			$370,132

Since the following is the case:

$PW_{.06}$ (Savings) > $PW_{.06}$ (Investment)
That is, $370,132 > $300,000, then the rate of return criterion is exceeded and the investment should be recommended.

If it were desired to determine the actual rate of return that is obtained from this investment, it would be necessary to make a trial and error calculation using different rates of return until the present worth of the savings is equal to the present worth of the investment. The rate at which the two values are equal is the rate of return for the investment.

Effects of Taxes on Economic Analysis

Taxes play an important part in the economic decisions that are made in industry. Since taxes affect profits and are paid after expenses and depreciation are deducted, they can have an appreciable effect on an economic analysis, given that certain conditions exist involving the investments. The major factor that can affect the tax structure is the use of depreciation. Depreciation is the method for charging the cost of equipment purchased over the useful life of the equipment. Expenses are charged as they are incurred since they have no life beyond the present year.

The amount which can be depreciated for a capital investment is calculate as the difference between the capital investment minus any salvage value that the equipment has at the end of its useful life. The depreciation can then b obtained in a number of ways. Two methods that are commonly used are the straight line depreciation method and the declining balance method. In the straight line depreciation method, the difference between the capital investment and the salvage value is distributed equally over each year in the life of the equipment. Thus, if an investment has a capital cost of $10,000 with a $2,000 salvage value and an expected life of 10 years, the depreciatio chargeable each year would be $800.

In the declining balance method, an attempt is made to depreciate the larger amount of money during the early life of the equipment. This is done based upon the principle that a dollar today is worth more than a dollar tomorrow and any charges made will reduce the tax liability of the corporation, thus, in effect earning dollars for the corporation. The formul for calculating depreciation based upon the declining balance method is

$$(8.6.7) \quad D = \frac{2}{n} + (1-2/n)^{j-1} \quad \text{for } j = 1, \ldots, n$$

where

D = the depreciation for year j

$\dfrac{2}{n}$ = the maximum allowable percentage depreciation, n = number of years life of the investment

I = investment
j = year depreciation

This formula includes the salvage value as a part of the original investment since this money will not be returned until year n. That is, the salvage value is $I(1 - s/n)^n$ in terms of present dollars.

Using this depreciation method for a $5,000 investment with an expected life of 5 years and a salvage value of $500, the depreciation and tax write-off at a 50% tax are as follows:

Year	Depreciation($)	Tax Write-Off($)
1	2,000	1,000
2	1,200	600
3	720	360
4	432	216
5	148*	74

*Since you cannot depreciate more than (I - SV), you must use straight line depreciation over the last two years.

Other depreciation methods have been approved for use by the Internal Revenue Service. One of the major of these is the sum-of-the-years-digit-method. However for the purposes of this discussion, other methods will not be discussed. The reader may refer to a basic accounting book for a further explanation of depreciation methods.

In order to stimulate the economy, over the past few years the Federal government laws have given an investment credit for capital expenditures. This investment credit can be charged against the current year's taxes and is an incentive for purchasing equipment.

Taxes can affect the decision to make an investment. The effect of taxes depends upon the flow of capital versus expense dollars. The investment credit can have an effect on the decision. The tax laws are constantly changing; and, as a result, it is advisable for the industrial hygiene engineer to consult an expert in the area of tax laws to interpret the current law and its effects on an investment.

Problem

What will be the effect of taxes on the problem presented in the previous example if the desired after-tax rate of return is 6% and if the $50,000 overhaul cannot be expensed? Use a straight line depreciation for the 10-year life of the local exhaust system, a 7.5% investment credit, and a tax rate of 50%. Assume no salvage value for the local exhaust system after its life and 5-year life on the $50,000 overhaul.

Year	After Tax Savings Depreciation ($)	x	Present Worth $_{.06}$	= Present Worth $_{.06}$ (S)($)
1	(22,750 + 15,000)		.94339	35,613
2	(22,750 + 15,000)		.88999	33,597
3	(22,750 + 15,000)		.83961	31,695
4	(22,750 + 15,000)		.79209	29,901
5	(22,750 + 15,000)		.74725	28,209
*6	(22,750 + 6,250)		.70496	20,444
7	(22,750 + 10,000)		.66505	21,780
8	(22,750 + 10,000)		.62741	20,548
9	(22,750 + 10,000)		.59189	19,384
10	(22,750 + 10,000)		.55839	18,287

$$\$259,458$$

*Includes 7.5% investment credit on overhaul in year 6 and the difference in depreciation between the overhaul and the new equipment for the remaining years.

Since
$PW_{.06}$ (Savings) < $PW_{.06}$ (Investment − .075 Investment), the investment is not recommended.

In the above example, it is obvious that a different present worth would be obtained if a declining balance depreciation were used since this would load the savings in the early life of the equipment. The student is encouraged to work out the problem in this manner to observe the effect.

Summary

In this chapter, the need for economic analysis of various alternative investments has been presented. Two methods for analyzing investments have been discussed: the N-year payback method and the present worth approach. The N-year payback method is applicable where the savings are equal over the life of the equipment, while the present worth approach takes into consideration varying rates of savings and expense. In addition, the effect of taxes on an investment may be of concern. Of particular importance is the distribution of costs in terms of capital investment which must be depreciated and expenses which can be charged in the year when they are incurred. Depending upon the flow of investments versus expenses, taxes can have a major effect on an investment decision.

7. References

ANSI, American National Standard Practices for Respiratory Protection. ANSI
Z88.2-1969, New York: American National Standards Institute, Inc., 1969.

Anthony, Robert N. Management Accounting--Text and Cases, Ref. ed. Homewood,
Illinois: Richard D. Irwin, Inc., 1960.

Baumeister, Theodore, ed. Marks Standard Handbook for Mechanical Engineers,
7th ed. New York: McGraw-Hill Book Company, 1967.

Committee on Respirators. Respiratory Protection Devices Manual. Lansing:
Committee on Respirators.

Mine Safety Appliances Company. Basic Elements of Respiratory Protection.
Pittsburgh: Mine Safety Appliances Company. 1976.

____. Safety Equipment Catalog. Pittsburgh: Mine Safety Appliances Company.

Morris, William T. The Analysis of Management Decisions. Homewood, Illinois:
Richard D. Irwin, Inc., 1964.

NIOSH, MESA. "Code of Federal Regulations, Title 30, Part II," Washington:
U.S. Government Printing Office.

U.S. Department of Health, Education, and Welfare, Public Health Service,
National Institute for Occupational Safety and Health. The Industrial
Environment. Its Evaluation and Control. Washington: U.S. Government
Printing Office, 1973.